Myeloma Therapy

CONTEMPORARY HEMATOLOGY

Judith E. Karp, SERIES EDITOR

For other titles published in the series, go to
www.springer.com/humana
select the subdiscipline
search for the series title

Myeloma Therapy
Pursuing the Plasma Cell

First Edition

Edited by

Sagar Lonial, MD
Winship Cancer Institute
Atlanta, GA

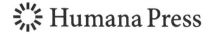 Humana Press

Editor
Sagar Lonial
Emory University
Winship Cancer Institute
B3307 Clifton Road
Atlanta, GA 30322
USA
sloni01@emory.edu

Series Editor
Judith E. Karp
The Sidney Kimmel Comprehensive Cancer
   Center at Johns Hopkins
Division of Hematologic Malignancies
Baltimore, Maryland 21231

ISBN: 978-1-934115-82-4   e-ISBN: 978-1-59745-564-0
DOI: 10.1007/978-1-59745-564-0

Library of Congress Control Number: 2008933590

Dedication

To my Parents and Teachers who provided the tools,
To the Patients who provided the motivation,
To Jennifer, Hallie, and Ben who provided the inspiration.
This book would not have been possible without you.

Sagar Lonial

Preface

Therapeutic options for patients with myeloma have dramatically changed over the past 10 years. Beginning with the advances in therapy resulting from the use of high-dose therapy and autologous bone marrow or stem cell transplant, we have more than doubled the median survival for patients as a whole, and have now have a wealth of different biology -based treatment approaches for our patients in all disease stages.

This book represents state-of-the-art information from many of the leaders in the plasma cell disorders world. Sections focusing on disease pathogenesis and biology, chemotherapy-based approaches, immune -based therapies, currently approved novel agents, developing targets, supportive care, and other plasma cell disorders provides a comprehensive collection and an excellent resource in this time of rapid change in clinical and preclinical disease knowledge.

It is important to realize that these changes did not occur in a vacuum. Partnerships between academic institutions, the pharmaceutical industry, patient advocacy groups, the National Cancer Institute, community oncologists, and ultimately our patients worked closely together to realize these advances, and to effect the radical changes in therapy we have witnessed over the past few years. This book would not have been possible without contributions from each of the gifted scientists and clinicians who worked tirelessly to prepare their individual chapters all the while maintaining commitment to the scientific and clinical mission of advancing care. Finally, all of us in clinical practice owe a great debt of gratitude to our patients, without whose efforts all of this would be pure basic science without real-world clinical relevance.

Sagar Lonial

Contents

Section 6   Supportive Care

Section 7   Other Plasma Cell Disorders

Contributors

Sikander Ailawadhi
Department of Medicine, Roswell Park Cancer Institute, Buffalo, NY, USA

Kenneth Anderson,
Department of Medical Oncology, Dana-Farber Cancer Institute, Harvard
Medical School, Boston, MA, USA

Ashraf Badros
University of Maryland, Greenebaum Cancer Center, Baltimore, MD, USA

Peter Leif Bergsagel
Mayo Clinic Comprehensive Cancer Center, Scottsdale, AZ, USA

Esteban Braggio
Mayo Clinic, Scottsdale, AZ, USA

Sara Bringhen
Divisione di Ematologia dell'Universita di Torino, Italy

Francis K. Buadi
Mayo Clinic College of Medicine, Rochester, MN, USA

Dharminder Chauhan
Department of Medical Oncology, The LeBow Institute for Myeloma
Therapeutics and Jerome Lipper Center for Myeloma Research,
Dana-Farber Cancer Institute, Boston, MA, USA

Wee Joo Chng
Mayo Clinic Comprehensive Cancer Center, Scottsdale, AZ, USA

Yun Dai
Department of Medicine, Virginia Commonwealth University and Massey
Cancer Center, Richmond, VA, USA

Madhav V. Dhodapkar
Laboratory of Tumor Immunology and Immunotherapy, The Rockefeller
University, New York, NY, USA

Angela Dispenzeri
Division of Hematology, Mayo Clinic, Rochester, MN, USA

Brian G.M. Durie
Department of Medicine, Division of Hematology/Oncology, Cedars-Sinai
Comprehensive Cancer Center, Los Angeles, CA, USA

Rafael Fonseca
Mayo Clinic, Scottsdale, AZ, USA

Dixil Francis
Winship Cancer Institute, Emory University School of Medicine, Atlanta,
GA, USA

Patrick Frost
Department of Medicine, UCLA, The Jonsson Comprehensive Cancer Center
and Department of Hematology-Oncology, VA Medical Center, Los Angeles,
CA, USA

Morie A. Gertz
Mayo Clinic, Rochester, MN, USA

Irene Ghobrial
Dana-Farber Cancer Institute, Boston, MA, USA

Steven Grant
Department of Medicine, Biochemistry and Pharmacology, Virginia
Commonwealth University and Massey Cancer Center, Richmond,
VA, USA

Jean-Luc Harousseau
Centre Hospitalier Universitaire Hotel-Dieu, Place Alexis Ricordeau, France

Donald Harvey
Winship Cancer Institute, Emory University School of Medicine, Atlanta,
GA, USA

Leonard T. Heffner
Winship Cancer Institute, Emory University School of Medicine, Atlanta,
GA, USA

Teru Hideshima
Department of Medical Oncology, Jerome Lipper Multiple Myeloma Center,
Dana-Farber Cancer Institute and Harvard Medical School, Boston, MA, USA

Jonathan L. Kaufman
Winship Cancer Institute, Emory University School of Medicine, Atlanta,
GA, USA

Asher Chanan-Khan
Department of Medicine, Roswell Park Cancer Institute, Buffalo, NY, USA

Shaji Kumar
Mayo Clinic, Rochester, MN, USA

Robert A. Kyle
Mayo Clinic, Rochester, MN, USA

Amelia A. Langston
Winship Cancer Institute, Emory University School of Medicine, Atlanta,
GA, USA

Alan Lichtenstein
UCLA, The Jonsson Comprehensive Cancer Center and Department of
Hematology-Oncology, West Los Angeles, VA Medical Center, Los Angeles,
CA, USA

Sagar Lonial
Winship Cancer Institute, Emory University School of Medicine, Atlanta,
GA, USA

M. V. Mateos
Cancer Research Center, University Hospital of Salemanca, Spain

Tomer M. Mark
Weil Medical College of Cornell University, New York, NY, USA

J. San Miguel
Cancer Research Center, University Hospital of Salemanca, Spain

Constantine S. Mitsiades
Dana-Farber Cancer Institute, Boston, MA, USA

Faustino Mollinedo
Centro de Investigacion del Cancer Instituto de Biologia Molecular y Celular
del Cancer, Consejo Superior de Investigaciones Cientificas-Universidad de
Salamanca, Spain

Nikhil C. Munshi
Dana-Farber Cancer Institute, Boston, MA, USA

Sandra Narayanan
Emory University Hospital, Atlanta, GA, USA

Antonio Palumbo
Divisione di Ematologia dell'Universita di Torino, Italy
Azienda Ospedaliera S. Giovanni Battista, Ospedale Molinette, Turin, Italy

Roger N. Pearse
Weil Medical College of Cornell Univeristy, New York, NY, USA

Marc Raab
Department of Medical Oncology, Dana-Farber Cancer Institute, Harvard
Medical School, Boston, MA, USA

S. Vincent Rajkumar
Mayo Clinic College of Medicine, Rochester, MN, USA

Noopur Raje
Dana-Farber Cancer Institute, Boston, MA, USA

Tiffany A. Richards
Anderson Cancer Center, Houston, TX, USA

Paul G. Richardson
Dana-Farber Cancer Institute, Boston, MA, USA

Vaishali Sanchorawala
Boston University Medical Center, Boston, MA, USA

Robert Schlossman
Dana-Farber Cancer Institute, Boston, MA, USA

Michael Sebag
Mayo Clinic, Scottsdale, AZ, USA

Jeannine Silberman
Winship Cancer Institute, Emory University School of Medicine,
Atlanta, GA, USA

Lijo Simpson
Mayo Clinic, Rochester, MN, USA

Ajita Singh
Dana-Farber Cancer Institute, Boston, MA, USA

A. Keith Stewart
Mayo Clinic College of Medicine, Scottsdale, AZ, USA

Sheeba K. Thomas
Anderson Cancer Center, Houston, TX, USA

Frank Tong
Emory University Hospital, Atlanta, GA, USA

Edmund K. Waller
Winship Cancer Institute, Emory University School of Medicine,
Atlanta, GA, USA

Fengrong Wang
Bone Marrow and Stem Cell Transplant Center, Winship Cancer Institute,
Emory University School of Medicine, Atlanta, GA, USA

Donna Weber
Department of Lymphoma and Myeloma, The University of Texas M.D.
Anderson Cancer Center, Houston, TX, USA

Victor Hugo Jimenez-Zepeda
Department of Hematological Malignancies, Mayo Clinic College
of Medicine, Scottsdale, AZ, USA

Section 1

Biologic Consideration and Myeloma

Chapter 1

Staging in Multiple Myeloma

Leonard T. Heffner

A useful staging system should define a specific point in the course of a disease that can be characterized by a certain group of clinical or laboratory findings. Among the values of a uniformly accepted staging system are the ability to predict responses to treatment and survival, as well as having a system that allows for retrospective analyses of therapies and prospective planning of clinical trials. As useful treatments became available for myeloma, the search for parameters that might predict outcomes among these patients became more important. Initially, individuals presenting clinical features were considered for prognostic importance, including mainly renal function, hemoglobin, calcium, presence of Bence-Jones proteinuria, and immunoglobulin subtype.[1–5] However, Carbone was among the first to group a series of such features that represented good or poor prognosis and found that performance status, level of anemia, calcium level, and renal function correlated with survival.[1] This was corroborated by Alexanian in a large series from the Southwest Oncology Study Group.[6] Soon it became apparent that combinations of these individual prognostic factors might be used as a myeloma staging classification. However, the first useful staging system for myeloma was proposed by Durie and Salmon in 1975.[7]

The Durie–Salmon (DS) staging system was created by direct measurement of myeloma cell burden calculated from measurements of M-component synthesis and metabolism. This measured myeloma cell mass was then correlated with presenting clinical features, response to treatment, and survival to create a clinical staging system (Table 1). The DS three-stage system became widely accepted and has endured over 30 years primarily because of the ease of obtaining the four components of the system, that is, level of serum and/or urine M-component, hemoglobin, serum calcium, and extent of bone lesions. Serum creatinine correlated very well with survival, but not with measured cell mass. Therefore, subcategories of A and B were included for each of the three stages to indicate near normal (<2.0 mg/dL) or abnormal (≥2.0 mg/dL) renal function, in effect, creating a five-stage system (no patients in stage IB).

Over the ensuing years, other prognostic factors have emerged including C-reactive protein, albumin, plasma cell labeling index, and cytogenetics. But the single most powerful prognostic factor has turned out to be beta-2

From: *Contemporary Hematology Myeloma Therapy*
Edited by: S. Lonial © Humana Press, Totowa, NJ

Table 1 Durie–Salmon staging system.

	Stage I All of the following	Stage II Not meeting criteria	Stage III At least 1 below
Hgb	>10 gm/dL	for I or III	<8.5 g/dL
Calcium	12 mg/dL		>12 mg/dL
Skeletal survey	Normal or single plasmacytoma		Advanced lytic bone lesions
M-spike	IgG < 5 g/dL IgA < 3 g/dL Urine < 4 g/24 h		IgG > 7 g/dL IgA > 5 g/dL Urine > 12 g/24hrs
A = serum creatinine < 2.0 mg/dL			
B = serum creatinine > 2.0 mg/dL			

Modified from Durie and Salmon [7]

Table 2 Southwest Oncology Group (SWOG) multiple myeloma staging system.

Stage	No. (%)	β2M (mg/L)	Albumin (g/L)	Survival (months)
1	197 (14)	<2.5		55
2	614 (43)	2.5 < 5.5		40
3	447 (32)	5.5	≥30	24
4	152 (11)	5.5	<30	16

microglobulin (β2M).[8–10] Combinations of these factors, generally including the β2M, have been proposed. Most of these proposals have been limited to some extent by small numbers of subjects in the analyses, including the DS system. As early as 1986, Bataille recognized the predictive power of the combination of β2M and albumin, but the proposed staging system using these two elements failed to gain widespread acceptance.[11] However, in 2003, the Southwest Oncology Group (SWOG) presented a new staging system for myeloma using β2M and albumin alone.[12] This study utilized data on 1,555 previously untreated myeloma patients who had been enrolled in four phase III SWOG trials. Four stages were defined, as outlined in Table 2. While this system used the same variables as Bataille did much earlier, the SWOG system had a larger database and utilized different statistical methods to select cutoff points for β2M and albumin. The four stages corresponded reasonably well with the DS system in complete remission and overall survival when stage III of DS was divided into IIIA and IIIB categories corresponding to stage 3 and 4, respectively, of SWOG. Using this approach, both systems identified a group (IIIB and stage 4) with high 1-year mortality of 35% and 40%, and low ≥5-year event-free survival of 8% and 4%, respectively. However, in this population, the SWOG stage 1 identified a group with a low 1-year mortality of 8%, while the DS system failed to distinguish a difference in this parameter among stage I–IIIA (16–18%). Still, both systems did identify a superior long-term event-free survival of 29% and 24%, respectively, in the earliest stage.

Table 3 International staging system.

Stage	Beta 2-microglobulin	Albumin	% of patients	Median survival (months)
I	<3.5 mg/L	≥3.5 mg/dL	28	62
II	β2M < 3.5 mg/L or 3.5 to < 5.5 irrespective of albumin	<3.5 mg/dL	33	44
III	β2M ≥ 5.5		39	29

Modified from Greipp et al.[13]

This large data set from the SWOG study has now been incorporated into an even larger database of 10,750 patients from Asia, Europe, and North America to create the International Staging System (ISS) published in 2005.[13] Using a rigorous statistical analysis of multiple patient characteristics in this large data set, again β2M and albumin emerged as a simple, yet powerful and reproducible means of creating a three-stage classification system that could be used worldwide Table 3. Importantly, the three stages have very comparable size with clearly different median survival times. A notable difference is seen in the ISS that the inclusion of serum albumin in each stage defined 12.5% of the population as stage II rather than as stage I by using β2M alone in early stage disease by the SWOG system. Also the ISS stage III clearly defined a poor risk group (median survival 29 months) compared to the DS stage III that had widely differing median survival depending on renal function (median survival 49 months IIIA vs 24 months IIIB). The ISS has been validated independently by a multicenter European group as well.[14]

As research produces new insights into the pathogenesis of myeloma, undoubtedly new variables will become part of more accurate staging systems that will help to predict outcomes and individualize therapy. Most notably, cytogenetic changes are now able to be found in almost all myeloma patients with currently available sophisticated techniques. While specific chromosomal changes have been associated with better or worse outcomes (see Chapter 5), these findings have not yet been widely enough available to incorporate into a useful staging system. Similarly, emerging other genomic and proteomic data may in the future be applied to staging systems. Recently, Bergsagel has proposed a molecular classification of myeloma based on the almost universal activation of one or the three cyclin D genes, a possible early, initiating event in the pathogenesis of the disease.[15,16] Using RNA expression levels of eight genes, tumors were assigned to one of eight different translocation/cyclin D (TC) groups that appear to be associated with differences in prevalence of bone disease, relapse, and progression to extramedullary disease. Whether this approach will ultimately result in a reproducible staging system or actually identify several different, but related, diseases remains to be seen.

One of the major criticisms of the DS staging system has been the difficulty in reproducibly defining the extent of bone disease, an observer-dependent exercise. With the advent of more sensitive imaging techniques, the DS PLUS myeloma staging system has recently been proposed to answer that criticism.[17] Magnetic resonance imaging (MRI) has proven to be a much more sensitive technique for identifying focal bone lesions compared to conventional metastatic bone survey with the number of bone lesions identified by this technique having independent prognostic significance.[18],[19] PET/CT scanning is a relatively new imaging technique but appears superior to conventional bone radiographs in identifying both medullary and extramedullary myelomatous lesions.[20] By enumerating the number of bone lesions through either MRI or PET/CT, the DS PLUS system again defines a three-stage classification with A and B divisions based on renal function. Although this approach addresses one of the limitations of the original DS staging system, the technical and financial constraints involved currently limit its widespread application.

Although a number of staging systems for myeloma have been proposed in recent years, the ISS appears to be the current standard and should be utilized in current and future studies of the disease. However, it is clear that further refinements of the ISS will be needed for the ever-expanding knowledge base of myeloma, especially the inclusion of better imaging techniques for detection of bone disease and the use of emerging genomic and proteomic data.

References

1. Carbone, P.P., L.E. Kellerhouse, and E.A. Gehan, *Plasmacytic myeloma. A study of the relationship of survival to various clinical manifestations and anomalous protein type in 112 patients.* Am J Med, 1967. **42**(6): pp. 937–48.
2. Dawson, A.A and D. Ogston, *Factors influencing the prognosis in myelomatosis.* Postgrad Med J, 1971. **47**(552): pp. 635–8.
3. *Report on the first myelomatosis trial.* I. Analysis of presenting features of prognostic importance. Br J Haematol, 1973. **24**(1): pp. 123–39.
4. Bergsagel, D.E., P.J. Migliore, and K.M. Griffith, *Myeloma proteins and the clinical response to melphalan therapy.* Science, 1965. 148: pp. 376–7.
5. *Correlation of abnormal immunoglobulin with clinical features of myeloma.* Arch Intern Med, 1975. **135**(1): pp. 46–52.
6. Alexanian, R., et al., *Prognostic factors in multiple myeloma.* Cancer, 1975. **36**(4): pp. 1192–201.
7. Durie, B.G. and S.E. Salmon, *A clinical staging system for multiple myeloma. Correlation of measured myeloma cell mass with presenting clinical features,* response to treatment, and survival. Cancer, 1975. **36**(3): pp. 842–54.
8. Bataille, R., B.G. Durie, and J. Grenier, Serum beta2 *microglobulin and survival duration in multiple myeloma: a simple reliable marker for staging.* Br J Haematol, 1983. 55(3): pp. 439–47.
9. Gobbi, P.G., et al., *A plea to overcome the concept of staging and related inadequacy in multiple myeloma.* Eur J Haematol, 1991. **46**(3): pp. 177–81.
10. Merlini, G., P.G. Gobbi, and E. Ascari, *The Merlini, Waldenstrom, Jayakar staging system revisited.* Eur J Haematol Suppl, 1989. 51: pp. 105–10.
11. Bataille, R., et al., *Prognostic factors and staging in multiple myeloma: A reappraisal.* J Clin Oncol, 1986. **4**(1): pp. 80–7.
12. Jacobson, J.L., et al., *A new staging system for multiple myeloma patients based on the Southwest Oncology Group (SWOG) experience.* Br J Haematol, 2003. **122**(3): pp. 441–50.
13. Greipp, P.R., et al., *International Staging System for multiple myeloma.* J Clin Oncol, 2005. **23**(15): pp 3412–20
14. Krejci, M., et al., *Prognostic factors for survival after autologous transplantation: A single centre experience in 133 multiple myeloma patients.* Bone Marrow Transplant, 2005. **35**(2): pp. 159–64.

15. Bergsagel, P.L., et al., *Cyclin D dysregulation: An early and unifying pathogenic event in multiple myeloma*. Blood, 2005. **106**(1): pp. 296–303.

16. Bergsagel, P.L. and W.M. Kuehl, *Molecular pathogenesis and a consequent classification of multiple myeloma*. J Clin Oncol, 2005. **23**(26): pp. 6333–8.

17. Durie, B.G., *The role of anatomic and functional staging in myeloma: Description of Durie/Salmon plus staging system*. Eur J Cancer, 2006. **42**(11): pp. 1539–43.

18. Walker, R., et al., *Magnetic resonance imaging in multiple myeloma: Diagnostic and clinical implications*. J Clin Oncol, 2007. **25**(9): pp. 1121–8.

19. Ghanem, N., et al., *Whole–body MRI in the detection of bone marrow infitteration in patients with plasma cell neoplasms in comparison to the radiological skeletal survey*. Eur Radiol, 2006. **16**(5): pp. 1005–14.

20. Zamagni, E., et al., *A prospective comparison of 18F-fluorodeoxyglucose positron emission tomography-computed tomography, magnetic resonance imaging and whole-body planar radiographs in the assessment of bone disease in newly diagnosed multiple myeloma*. Haematologica, 2007. **92**(1): pp. 50–5.

Chapter 2

Epidemiology of Multiple Myeloma

Amelia A. Langston and Dixil Francis

Introduction

Multiple myeloma represents about 0.8% of all cancer cases worldwide, with incidence rates ranging from 0.4 to 5 per 100,000 persons in different parts of the world.[1] The highest rates of myeloma are observed in Australia, New Zealand, North America, northern and western Europe, while the lowest rates are seen in Asia. Modest increases in both incidence and mortality for myeloma have been observed over the last few decades, without an apparent explanation.[1]

As with other forms of cancer, there is great interest in the role of environmental, immunologic, and genetic risk factors for myeloma. Unlike some subtypes of leukemia and lymphoma for which environmental and/or infectious risk factors have been clearly defined, there are few generally accepted predisposing insults leading to the development of mycloma. There are anecdotal cases of myeloma occurring in spouses,[2–6] as well as rare reports of community clusters of myeloma cases.[7,8] These observations imply the existence of environmental exposures capable of dramatically influencing the risk of myeloma, although the insult(s) remain to be defined. Nevertheless, a number of epidemiologic observations offer clues regarding the etiology and pathogenesis of myeloma. We will review the epidemiology of myeloma and monoclonal gammopathy of unknown significance (MGUS), with particular attention to known associations with race, environmental exposures, genetics, immunologic function, and infection.

General Epidemiology

In 2006, there were an estimated 16,500 new myeloma cases, and 11,310 deaths with myeloma in the United States, translating to an overall age standardized incidence rate of 7 per 100,000 persons.[9] The median age at diagnosis of myeloma is ~70 years, and the risk increases exponentially with age, with over 75% of cases occurring in individuals over the age of 50, as shown in Fig. 1.[9] In the United States, the incidence of myeloma varies substantially by

From: *Contemporary Hematology Myeloma Therapy*
Edited by: S. Lonial © Humana Press, Totowa, NJ

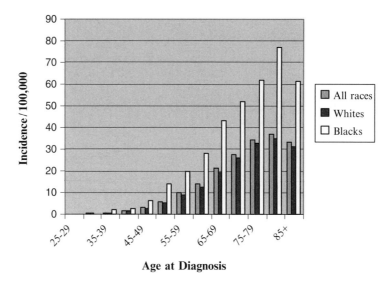

Fig. 1 Incidence of multiple myeloma according to age (SEER Data, 2000–2004). (*see* Plate 1).

race, where it is greatest among blacks, intermediate for whites, and least in Asians.[10,11] Incidence rates in the Caribbean and Central America are similar to those of US residents of African decent,[1] lending support to the idea that some of the disparity in incidence by race may be genetic in origin.

Much has been written about the relationship between myeloma and MGUS, and a separate chapter in this volume is devoted to a detailed discussion of MGUS. Risk factors for MGUS parallel those identified for myeloma, with age being the dominant predisposing factor. In a large population-based study of 21,463 older adults in Olmstead County, MN, the prevalence of MGUS was 3.2% among persons age 50 and older, 5.3% for age 70 and older, and 7.5% for age 85 and older.[12] The risk of progression from MGUS to myeloma appears to be constant over time, occurring at a rate of ~1% per year. [13–15] It is difficult to determine the proportion of myeloma cases that are preceded by MGUS, given that MGUS is typically asymptomatic and is not usually detected on routine blood analyses.

Racial Differences in the Incidence of Multiple Myeloma

The incidence of myeloma among blacks is approximately twice that of their white counterparts, as shown in Table 1. Differences in both genetic suscepti-bility and environmental factors have been postulated to explain the disparity in incidence according to race.[16] In addition, age-adjusted incidence rates have increased for both blacks and whites over the past three decades, and the explanation for this observation remains unclear.

In a detailed examination of Surveillance Epidemiology and End Results (SEER) data, Francis has shown that both incidence rates and racial disparities vary by geographic location.[17] Over the time period of 1975–2002, Detroit had

Table 1 Incidence, mortality, and survival rates for multiple myeloma over various time periods by race and gender.

	Incidence (1975–2002)			Mortality (1975–2002)			Five-year survival (1974–2001)		
	Total	Males	Females	Total	Males	Females	Total	Males	Females
All races	5.5	6.8	4.5	3.6	4.5	3.0	30.0	31.0	29.0
Whites	5.1	6.4	4.1	3.3	4.1	2.7	29.5	30.6	28.2
Blacks	11.2	13.6	9.7	6.8	8.3	5.8	32.4	33.2	31.7

the highest incidence of myeloma regardless of race, followed by Atlanta, in comparison with seven other geographic regions: San Francisco, Connecticut, Hawaii, Iowa, New Mexico, Seattle, and Utah. In eight of the nine geographic locations, the incidence rate for blacks was approximately twofold that of their white counterparts. In contrast, the corresponding difference was approximately threefold among Iowans. These differences imply the existence of environmental or lifestyle factors that influence the incidence of myeloma; however, there are not yet firm data identifying specific factors that can account for the observed differences.

Several studies also suggest an increased risk of MGUS among blacks. [18–21] In the largest study to date, Landgren et al.[21] examined the prevalence of MGUS and subsequent risk of myeloma among 4 million men who were admitted to Veterans Affairs (VA) hospitals. The age-adjusted prevalence ratio of MGUS for African Americans versus whites was 3.0 (2.7–3.3; 95% CI). In that study, the cumulative risk of progression to myeloma during the first 10 years of follow-up was similar between the two groups (17% for African Americans and 15% for whites, $p = 0.37$). These results suggest similar degrees of increased risk for both MGUS and myeloma in blacks, without evidence of racial differences in the risk of progression from MGUS to myeloma.

Socioeconomic Status, Diet, and Tobacco

Baris et al.[22] examined the effect of socioeconomic status (SES) on the incidence of myeloma in a population-based case-control study. They observed an inverse correlation between occupation-based SES and myeloma risk for both black and white persons. Risk was significantly increased for individuals in the lowest category of SES (OR = 1.71, 95% CI = 1.16, 2.53). Among blacks, 37% of myeloma occurred in low-SES persons versus 17% of myeloma in whites, largely due to a higher representation of blacks in the lowest SES category. The authors concluded that occupation-based SES may account for about half of the excess occurrence of myeloma in blacks.[22] The explanation for an association with SES remains unclear, but differences in diet, occupational or environmental insults, or infectious exposures have been proposed as possibilities.

Nutritional status and diet have also been associated with the risk of myeloma in a number of studies and are undoubtedly linked to differences in SES. Obesity, defined in terms of body mass index, has been associated with an increased risk of myeloma in a number of studies.[23,24] In a case-control study, Brown et al.[23] observed an association of obesity with increased risk of myeloma among both blacks and whites of both genders. Friedman et al.[24] also observed an association with obesity, but only for white men. There are modest racial differences in the prevalence of obesity, particularly among women; however, this cannot explain the magnitude of difference in the incidence of myeloma among blacks versus whites.

Data on dietary factors and risk of myeloma are mixed, but some studies suggest a protective effect of green vegetable and fish intake. A large Italian study showed an inverse correlation between intake of green vegetables and risk of myeloma.[25] More specifically, the study of Brown et al.[23] suggested a protective effect associated with intake of cruciferous (mustard, broccoli, cauliflower, and cabbage family) vegetables, fish, and vitamin C. Several case-control studies suggest an inverse correlation between fish consumption and myeloma.[23,25–27] In contrast, Svensson et al.[28] reported an increased risk of mortality from myeloma among eastcoast Swedish fishermen, who have a high intake of fatty fish.[29] The significance of this observation is obscured by the demonstration of high levels of organochlorine compounds in the plasma of fishermen from this region.[29]

Several large studies have examined the effect of tobacco use on the risk of hematologic malignancies, and there is little evidence of an increased risk of myeloma among current or past smokers. Three large prospective surveillance studies followed a total of over 500,000 persons over periods spanning several decades, and each failed to demonstrate an association between smoking and myeloma, although there was some evidence of a weak association between tobacco use and lymphoma.[30–32] In a case-control study, Brown et al. also failed to demonstrate an association between smoking and myeloma, although this study again suggested an association with non-Hodgkin's lymphoma.[33] The only large study suggesting an association between tobacco use and myeloma is a German case-control study of smoking and hemato-lymphoid malignancies, which showed an odds ratio for myeloma of 2.4 (95% CI = 0.98–5.74) for current male smokers and an odds ratio of 2.9 (95% CI = 1.1–7.4) for women smokers.[34] It should be pointed out, however, that this analysis included only 76 myeloma cases; thus, the confidence intervals are wide.

Ionizing Radiation

Ionizing radiation is a well-established risk factor for acute myelogenous leukemia; however, its role in the pathogenesis of other hemato-lymphoid malignancies is less clear, and the effects less dramatic. The largest body of data regarding acute radiation exposure and the risk of myeloma comes from studies of survivors of the Hiroshima and Nagasaki atomic bomb exposures. Early studies from the Atomic Bomb Casualty Commission observed an increased risk of myeloma, and this was most evident in individuals exposed to an estimated marrow dose of at least 50–100 rad.[35,36] The magnitude of increased risk correlated with the estimated radiation dose to the marrow, was demonstrable in survivors between ages 20 and 59 years at the time of exposure, and had a latent period between exposure and diagnosis of at least 20 years.[35,36] Preston et al.[37] extended the analysis of cancer incidence through

1987, and, in contrast to earlier studies, did not observe an excess risk of myeloma among bomb survivors. The analysis was limited to first cancers, but beyond this the study was similar in methods and population to the previous studies. Pierce et al.[38] examined cancer mortality through 1990 and did observe an increased risk of myeloma-related mortality among exposed individuals. Another recent study suggested a marginally increased incidence of MGUS among bomb survivors, without clear evidence of an accelerated rate of progression of MGUS to multiple myeloma.[39]

Studies of cancer mortality among individuals receiving radiation therapy for ankylosing spondylitis[40] and metropathia hemorrhagia[41] indicate an increased incidence of myeloma among exposed individuals. In another case-control study, an increased risk of plasmacytoma was observed among persons exposed to the old contrast agent thorotrast.[42] Taken together, these studies coupled with those from the Atomic Bomb Casualty Commission suggest a dose-dependent effect of acute radiation exposure on the subsequent risk of both myeloma and MGUS.

The effects of chronic low-level radiation exposure are less clearly defined, both for myeloma and for other cancer types. Several studies examining cancer-related mortality following chronic low-level occupational radiation exposure have identified myeloma as one of the malignancies that occurs in excess in radiation exposed individuals.[43–47] In one of the early studies, a threefold excess of myeloma-related death was observed among female radium dial workers.[43] More recently, a 15-country collaborative study examined cancer risk among over 400,000 nuclear industry workers with individual exposure data and long-term medical follow-up. There was a dose-dependent increase in cancer mortality, and a trend toward a dose-dependent increase in the risk of myeloma-related death among chronically exposed workers.[47] On the contrary, other large studies of radiation workers have failed to identify an increased risk of myeloma among exposed persons.[48–51] Overall, the data suggest that if there is an effect of chronic low-level exposure, it is modest compared with the risks associated with more intensive acute radiation exposure. Furthermore, with modern industrial protections and regulations, it is unlikely that occupational radiation exposure remains a major risk factor for myeloma.

Other Occupational and Environmental Risk Factors

Although organic solvents, pesticides, and other chemicals have all been investigated as potential risk factors for myeloma, studies have generally failed to show consistent and compelling associations with the risk of myeloma. Lack of accuracy in defining the types of exposures for a given workforce, challenges in quantifying an individual's exposure, and the relatively low-baseline incidence of myeloma all contribute to difficulties in designing appropriately powered studies and interpreting results.

Farmers and other agricultural workers have been extensively studied because of their exposure to chemicals and pesticides, as well as peculiarities in diet and lifestyle associated with rural living. Three meta-analyses have compiled data from available epidemiologic studies of farmers,[52–54] and taken together their results suggest that the age-adjusted risk of myeloma among farmers is similar to that of the general population.

Pesticide exposure has also been specifically studied, and results have been inconsistent, with some studies suggesting positive and others negative associations with myeloma. These data have been reviewed in detail by Alexander et al.[55] In the large US Agricultural Health Study, exposures to atrazine, alachlor, chlorpyrifos, and glyphosate, a total of over 160,000 persons were evaluated, and no association with myeloma could be identified for any cohort of applicators.[56–59] Herbicides such as dioxin and TCDD have received public attention as possible carcinogens, and a few studies suggest modest increases in the risk of myeloma associated with occupational or accidental exposure.[60–62]

Exposure to organic solvents does not appear to be a major risk factor for myeloma. In a recent meta-analysis of multiple myeloma mortality among solvent-exposed workers, the summary relative risk estimate was 1.14 (95% CI, 0.83–1.15).[63] An early study of California petroleum workers suggested an excess of myeloma-related mortality,[64] but the excess was limited to workers enrolled before 1949. Studies of more recent cohorts of workers do not suggest significant increases in myeloma among exposed individuals in the petroleum industry.[65–70]

Immunology, Infection, and Myeloma Risk

Although myeloma is not considered an AIDS-defining malignancy, several large surveys have shown a significantly increased risk of myeloma among persons living with AIDS.[71–75] In a case-control study of elderly persons with AIDS, the increased risk became apparent at about 2 years after the onset of AIDS.[75] Similarly, in a cohort study of AIDS patients in New South Wales, the risk of myeloma and other malignancies increased over time after the original AIDS-defining illness.[73]

Following the discovery of human herpesvirus-8 (HHV-8) DNA sequences in Kaposi's sarcoma tissue from patients with AIDS,[76–78] several studies suggested a possible relationship between HHV-8 and several hemato-lymphoid malignancies including primary effusion lymphoma, plasmacytic lymphoma, multicentric Castleman's disease, and myeloma. More rigorous epidemiologic studies suggest a role for the virus in a subset of cases of primary effusion lymphoma, plasmacytic lymphoma, and multicentric Castleman's disease, but do not support a relationship between HHV-8 and myeloma.[79–83] Thus, it is difficult to invoke HHV-8 as the explanation for an increased risk of myeloma among AIDS patients. It is more likely that failure of immune surveillance mechanisms plays a role in enabling the emergence of overt myeloma in some patients.

Historically, there has been great interest in the hypothesis that chronic or recurrent antigenic stimulation might serve as a possible predisposing factor for development of multiple myeloma. Results of epidemiologic studies offer only weak support for this hypothesis. Most case-control studies examining medical history in relation to myeloma have failed to identify strong and consistent associations with prior infections, autoimmunity, or inflammatory conditions.[11,84–87] On the contrary, in one case-control study from four geographic areas of the United States, risk of myeloma was inversely related to the number of diseases for which the person reported having been immunized.[86] It is unclear whether this observation relates to an immunologic effect, or to differences in SES. One of the largest studies examining infection as a risk factor included all myeloma patients diagnosed in Denmark over a 20-year period (more than 4,000 cases and 16,000 matched controls). A history of pneumonia was associated with a 1.6-fold (95% CI 1.3–2.0) increased risk of myeloma, with the increased risk limited to pneumonia episodes occurring within 5 years of the diagnosis of myeloma.[88] Although the observed association in this study is statistically robust, it may simply be a reflection of the humoral immune compromise associated with myeloma, rather than a causative factor in its development.

Inherited Predisposition to Myeloma

Available data from both case-control and cohort studies suggest a two- to fourfold increased risk of myeloma among persons with affected family members.[89–93] Some studies also suggest a more modest increased risk of myeloma in association with a family history that includes other hemato-lymphoid malignancies.[90,91,94,95] Reports of the occurrence of myeloma in monozygotic twins add additional evidence of a genetic contribution in some cases.[96–98]

The possibility of an association between HLA antigens or haplotypes and myeloma has been widely studied, based on the general hypothesis that immune recognition mechanisms might somehow be involved in the pathogenesis of the disease. Early studies were hampered by limited understanding of the HLA genes and by primitive testing reagents.[99–103] In a case-control study from Lousiana, Leech et al.[104] observed an increased frequency of HLA-CW5 among black men with myeloma. More recently, a larger study from the NCI observed an increased risk of myeloma among both blacks and whites associated with the HLA-CW2 antigen.[105] The relative risk associated with the CW2 antigen was 5.7 (95% CI, 1.5–26.6) for blacks and 2.6 (95% CI, 1.0–7.2) for whites. The antigen frequencies among black and white controls were similar, but the data raise the possibility of a stronger risk modifying effect associated with CW2 in blacks. Taken together, studies of HLA associations with myeloma support the hypothesis that the incidence of myeloma may be affected by "genetic background," leaving open the question of whether the effect is immunologic or a result of linkage disequilibrium with particular alleles of other genes in the same region.

The most compelling evidence for the existence of inherited predisposition to myeloma comes from reports of rare families with numerous members affected with myeloma and/or MGUS. Some of these families display patterns of occurrence consistent with autosomal dominant inheritance of a weakly penetrant phenotype.[95,106–108] Several reports suggest the possibility of genetic anticipation, which refers to the earlier onset of disease with successive generations.[95,108–110] The latter possibility is particularly interesting in light of the association of inherited disorders showing anticipation with mutations involving instability of trinucleotide repeats.

In the largest series of 39 multiple myeloma families, Lynch et al.[108] described 10 families in which myeloma occurred in the context of clustering of other tumor types. The most common other cancer types were lymphoma, leukemia, breast, colon, and pancreatic carcinomas. A significant increase in the incidence of myeloma has been described in a survey of cancers among

Ashkenazi Jewish BRCA1 and BRCA2 mutation carriers.[111] In addition, Sobol et al.[110] identified a likely mutation in BRCA2 in the proband of a family with multiple cases of both breast cancer and myeloma. Finally, Dilworth et al.[112] described a germline mutation in CDKN2A with loss of the normal allele in the bone marrow of a myeloma patient from an otherwise typical family with multiple cases of melanoma. Thus, it is likely that a modest increase in the risk of myeloma may be part of the spectrum of several familial cancer syndromes, the specifics of which will require much larger genetic epidemiological studies.

Conclusions

The most undisputed risk factor for myeloma is increasing age, which is undoubtedly a surrogate marker for genetic insults that contribute directly to the pathogenesis of the disease. Acute high-level radiation exposure (>50–100 cGy) is a predisposing factor, but accounts for few cases of myeloma today. The role of other environmental pathogens in the pathogenesis of the disease is unclear, although there is a suggestion that herbicides may play a role.

The observation of a twofold difference in incidence between blacks and whites is intriguing, and available data suggest that both genetic and environmental or lifestyle factors likely play a role in the higher incidence of both myeloma and MGUS among blacks. Obesity, diet, and occupational risk factors have all been identified as potential contributors to the observed differences in incidence, but these are likely surrogate markers for as yet unidentified specific factors.

An increased risk of myeloma among AIDS patients has been a consistent observation in cohorts from around the world. It remains to be shown whether this observation reflects immunologic or infectious mechanisms, or a failure in immune surveillance mechanisms. In any event, with the aging of the AIDS population as a result of better antiviral and supportive therapies, we will undoubtedly see more multiple myeloma in the context of AIDS.

Inherited predisposition to myeloma remains poorly understood, although several distinct mechanisms are likely in play. It appears that there may be a rare gene (or genes) predisposing to a relatively "pure" myeloma phenotype; inheritance is autosomal dominant, penetrance is incomplete, and there is some suggestion of genetic anticipation in successive generations. In addition, myeloma may be part of the spectrum of several of the cancer family syndromes such as BRCA1, BRCA2, and familial melanoma. Finally, there may be additional more common, but less penetrant genes that predispose to a variety of hemato-lymphoid malignancies including myeloma, non-Hodgkin's and Hodgkin's lymphomas, and leukemias.

With the aging of the population upon us, we can expect that the prevalence of myeloma will continue to increase over the next few decades. Enormous progress has been made over the last decade in the development of novel strategies for treatment of myeloma, as discussed elsewhere in this volume. As we move forward, the challenge will be to continue to translate knowledge gained from the Human Genome Project and other basic science research into a greater understanding of the pathogenesis of myeloma, with development of effective strategies for prevention, prognostication, and more effective management of the disease and its complications.

References

1. Bray F, Ferlay J, Parkin M, Pisani P. Global Cancer Statistics, 2002. CA A Cancer Journal for Clinicians 2005;55(2).
2. Kyle RA, Greipp PR. Multiple myeloma. Houses and spouses. Cancer 1983;51(4):735–9.
3. Kyle RA, Heath CW, Jr., Carbone P. Multiple myeloma in spouses. Archives of Internal Medicine 1971;127(5):944–6.
4. Brugiatelli M, Comis M, Iacopino P, et al. Multiple myeloma in husband and wife. Acta Haematologica 1980;64(4):227–9.
5. Kanoh T. Multiple myeloma in spouses. European Journal of Haematology 1988;41(4):397.
6. Kanoh T, Ohno T, Usui T, Inamoto Y. Multiple myeloma in husband and wife. Nippon Ketsueki Gakkai Zasshi 1989;52(4):763–6.
7. Kyle RA, Finkelstein S, Elveback LR, Kurland LT. Incidence of monoclonal proteins in a Minnesota community with a cluster of multiple myeloma. Blood 1972;40(5):719–24.
8. Ende M. Multiple myeloma: A cluster in Virginia? Virginia Medical 1979; 106(2):115–6.
9. Howe HL, Wu X, Ries LA, et al. Annual report to the nation on the status of cancer, 1975–2003, featuring cancer among U.S. Hispanic/Latino populations. Cancer 2006;107(8):1711–42.
10. Schwartz J. Multinational trends in multiple myeloma. Annals of the New York Academy of Sciences 1990;609:215–24.
11. Lewis DR, Pottern LM, Brown LM, et al. Multiple myeloma among blacks and whites in the United States: The role of chronic antigenic stimulation. Cancer Causes Control 1994;5(6):529–39.
12. Kyle RA, Therneau TM, Rajkumar SV, et al. Prevalence of monoclonal gammopathy of undetermined significance. The New England Journal of Medicine 2006;354(13):1362–9.
13. Cesana C, Klersy C, Barbarano L, et al. Prognostic factors for malignant transformation in monoclonal gammopathy of undetermined significance and smoldering multiple myeloma. Journal of Clinical Oncology 2002;20(6):1625–34.
14. Kyle RA, Therneau TM, Rajkumar SV, et al. A long-term study of prognosis in monoclonal gammopathy of undetermined significance. The New England Journal of Medicine 2002;346(8):564–9.
15. Kyle RA, Therneau TM, Rajkumar SV, et al. Long-term follow-up of IgM monoclonal gammopathy of undetermined significance. Blood 2003;102(10):3759–64.
16. Benjamin M, Reddy S, Brawley OW. Myeloma and race: A review of the literature. Cancer Metastasis Reviews 2003;22(1):87–93.
17. Francis D. Racial variation in the incidence, mortality, and survival rates of multiple myeloma patients through the eyes of the fundamental theory. 2006.
18. Cohen HJ, Crawford J, Rao MK, Pieper CF, Currie MS. Racial differences in the prevalence of monoclonal gammopathy in a community-based sample of the elderly. Erratum in: The American Journal of Medicine 1998;105(5):362.
19. Singh J, Dudley AW, Jr., Kulig KA. Increased incidence of monoclonal gammopathy of undetermined significance in blacks and its age-related differences with whites on the basis of a study of 397 men and one woman in a hospital setting. The Journal of Laboratory and Clinical Medicine 1990;116(6):785–9.
20. Schechter GP, Shoff N, Chan C, McManus CD, Hawley HP. The frequency of monoclonalgammopathy of unknown significance in Black and Caucasian veterans in a hospital population. In: Obrams GI, Potter M, eds. Epidemiology and Biology of Multiple Myeloma. New York, N.Y.: Springer; 1991:83–5.
21. Landgren O, Gridley G, Turesson I, et al. Risk of monoclonal gammopathy of undetermined significance (MGUS) and subsequent multiple myeloma among African American and white veterans in the United States. Blood 2006;107(3):904–6.

22. Baris D, Brown LM, Silverman DT, et al. Socioeconomic status and multiple myeloma among US blacks and whites. American Journal of Public Health 2000;90(8):1277–81.

23. Brown LM, Gridley G, Pottern LM, et al. Diet and nutrition as risk factors for multiple myeloma among blacks and whites in the United States. Cancer Causes Control 2001;12(2):117–25.

24. Friedman GD, Herrinton LJ. Obesity and multiple myeloma. Cancer Causes Control 1994;5(5):479–83.

25. Tavani A, Pregnolato A, Negri E, et al. Diet and risk of lymphoid neoplasms and soft tissue sarcomas. Nutrition and Cancer 1997;27(3):256–60.

26. Fernandez E, Chatenoud L, La Vecchia C, Negri E, Franceschi S. Fish consumption and cancer risk. The American Journal of Clinical Nutrition 1999;70(1):85–90.

27. Fritschi L, Ambrosini GL, Kliewer EV, Johnson KC. Dietary fish intake and risk of leukaemia, multiple myeloma, and non-Hodgkin lymphoma. Cancer Epidemiology Biomarkers Prevention 2004;13(4):532–7.

28. Svensson BG, Mikoczy Z, Stromberg U, Hagmar L. Mortality and cancer incidence among Swedish fishermen with a high dietary intake of persistent organochlorine compounds. Scandinavian Journal of Work, Environment & Health 1995;21(2):106–15.

29. Svensson BG, Nilsson A, Jonsson E, Schutz A, Akesson B, Hagmar L. Fish consumption and exposure to persistent organochlorine compounds, mercury, selenium and methylamines among Swedish fishermen. Scandinavian Journal of Work, Environment & Health 1995;21(2):96–105.

30. Heineman EF, Zahm SH, McLaughlin JK, Vaught JB, Hrubec Z. A prospective study of tobacco use and multiple myeloma: Evidence against an association. Cancer Causes Control 1992;3(1):31–6.

31. Fernberg P, Odenbro A, Bellocco R, et al. Tobacco use, body mass index, and the risk of leukemia and multiple myeloma: A nationwide cohort study in Sweden. Cancer Research 2007;67(12):5983–6.

32. Adami J, Nyren O, Bergstrom R, et al. Smoking and the risk of leukemia, lymphoma, and multiple myeloma (Sweden). Cancer Causes Control 1998;9(1):49–56.

33. Brown LM, Everett GD, Gibson R, Burmeister LF, Schuman LM, Blair A. Smoking and risk of non-Hodgkin's lymphoma and multiple myeloma. Cancer Causes Control 1992;3(1):49–55.

34. Nieters A, Deeg E, Becker N. Tobacco and alcohol consumption and risk of lymphoma: Results of a population-based case-control study in Germany. International Journal of Cancer 2006;118(2):422–30.

35. Nishiyama H, Anderson RE, Ishimaru T, Ishida K, Ii Y, Okabe N. The incidence of malignant lymphoma and multiple myeloma in Hiroshima and Nagasaki atomic bomb survivors, 1945–1965. Cancer 1973;32(6):1301–9.

36. Ichimaru M, Ishimaru T, Mikami M, Matsunaga M. Multiple myeloma among atomic bomb survivors in Hiroshima and Nagasaki, 1950–76: relationship to radiation dose absorbed by marrow. Journal of the National Cancer Institute 1982;69(2):323–8.

37. Preston DL, Kusumi S, Tomonaga M, et al. Cancer incidence in atomic bomb survivors. Part III. Leukemia, lymphoma and multiple myeloma, 1950–1987. Radiation Research 1994;137(2 Suppl):S68–97.

38. Pierce DA, Shimizu Y, Preston DL, Vaeth M, Mabuchi k. Studies of the mortality of atomic bomb survivours. Report 12, part I. Cancer: 1950–1990. Radiation Research 1996;146(1):1–27.

39. Neriishi K, Nakashima E, Suzuki G. Monoclonal gammapathy of undetermined significance in atomic bomb survivors: Incidence and transformation to multiple myeloma. British Journal of Haematology 2003;121(3):405–10.

40. Weiss HA, Darby SC, Doll R. Cancer mortality following X-ray treatment for ankylosing spondylitis. International Journal of Cancer 1994;59(3):327–38.

41. Darby SC, Reeves G, Key T, Doll R, Stovall M. Mortality in a cohort of women given X-ray therapy for metropathia haemorrhagica. International Journal of Cancer 1994;56(6):793–801.

42. van Kaick G, Dalheimer A, Hornik S, et al. The German Thorotrast study: Recent results and assessment of risks. Radiation Research 1999;152(6 Suppl):S64–71.

43. Stebbings JH, Lucas HF, Stehney AF. Mortality from cancers of major sites in female radium dial workers. American Journal of Industrial Medicine 1984;5(6):435–59.

44. Smith PG, Douglas AJ. Mortality of workers at the Sellafield plant of British Nuclear Fuels. British Medical Journal (Clinical research ed) 1986;293(6551):845–54.

45. Gilbert ES, Petersen GR, Buchanan JA. Mortality of workers at the Hanford site: 1945–1981. Health Physics 1989;56(1):11–25.

46. Cardis E, Gilbert ES, Carpenter L, et al. Effects of low doses and low dose rates of external ionizing radiation: Cancer mortality among nuclear industry workers in three countries. Radiation Research 1995;142(2):117–32.

47. Cardis E, Vrijheid M, Blettner M, et al. The 15-Country Collaborative Study of Cancer Risk among Radiation Workers in the Nuclear Industry: Estimates of radiation-related cancer risks. Radiation Research 2007;167(4):396–416.

48. Douglas AJ, Omar RZ, Smith PG. Cancer mortality and morbidity among workers at the Sellafield plant of British Nuclear Fuels. British Journal of Cancer 1994;70(6):1232–43.

49. Muirhead CR, Goodill AA, Haylock RG, et al. Occupational radiation exposure and mortality: Second analysis of the national registry for radiation workers. Journal of Radiological Protection 1999;19(1):3–26.

50. Omar RZ, Barber JA, Smith PG. Cancer mortality and morbidity among plutonium workers at the Sellafield plant of British Nuclear Fuels. British Journal of Cancer 1999;79(7–8):1288–301.

51. Iwasaki T, Murata M, Ohshima S, et al. Second analysis of mortality of nuclear industry workers in Japan, 1986–1997. Radiation Research 2003;159(2):228–38.

52. Acquavella J, Olsen G, Cole P, et al. Cancer among farmers: A meta-analysis. Annals of Epidemiology 1998;8(1):64–74.

53. Blair A, Zahm SH, Pearce NE, Heineman EF, Fraumeni JF, Jr. Clues to cancer etiology from studies of farmers. Scandinavian Journal of Work, Environment & Health 1992;18(4):209–15.

54. Khuder SA, Mutgi AB. Meta-analyses of multiple myeloma and farming. American Journal of Industrial Medicine 1997;32(5):510–6.

55. Alexander DD, Mink PJ, Adami HO, et al. Multiple myeloma: A review of the epidemiologic literature. International Journal of Cancer 2007;120(Suppl 12):40–61.

56. Rusiecki JA, De Roos A, Lee WJ, et al. Cancer incidence among pesticide applicators exposed to atrazine in the agricultural health study. Journal of the National Cancer Institute 2004;96(18):1375–82.

57. Lee WJ, Hoppin JA, Blair A, et al. Cancer incidence among pesticide applicators exposed to alachlor in the agricultural health study. American Journal of Epidemiology 2004;159(4):373–80.

58. De Roos AJ, Blair A, Rusiecki JA, et al. Cancer incidence among glyphosate-exposed pesticide applicators in the agricultural health study. Environmental Health Perspectives 2005;113(1):49–54.

59. Blair A, Sandler DP, Tarone R, et al. Mortality among participants in the agricultural health study. Annals of Epidemiology 2005;15(4):279–85.

60. Steenland K, Piacitelli L, Deddens J, Fingerhut M, Chang LI. Cancer, heart disease, and diabetes in workers exposed to 2,3,7,8-tetrachlorodibenzo-p-dioxin. Journal of the National Cancer Institute 1999;91(9):779–86.

61. Bertazzi PA, Consonni D, Bachetti S, et al. Health effects of dioxin exposure: A 20-year mortality study. American Journal of Epidemiology 2001;153(11):1031–44.

62. t Mannetje A, McLean D, Cheng S, Boffetta P, Colin D, Pearce N. Mortality in New Zealand workers exposed to phenoxy herbicides and dioxins. Occupational and Environmental Medicine 2005;62(1):34–40.

63. Chen R, Seaton A. A meta-analysis of mortality among workers exposed to organic solvents. Occupational Medicine (Oxford, England) 1996;46(5):337–44.

64. Satin KP, Bailey WJ, Newton KL, Ross AY, Wong O. Updated epidemiological study of workers at two California petroleum refineries, 1950–95. Occupational and Environmental Medicine 2002;59(4):248–56.

65. Collingwood KW, Raabe GK, Wong O. An updated cohort mortality study of workers at a northeastern United States petroleum refinery. International Archives of Occupational and Environmental Health 1996;68(5):277–88.

66. Raabe GK, Collingwood KW, Wong O. An updated mortality study of workers at a petroleum refinery in Beaumont, Texas. American Journal of Industrial Medicine 1998;33(1):61–81.

67. Huebner WW, Chen VW, Friedlander BR, et al. Incidence of lymphohaematopoietic malignancies in a petrochemical industry cohort: 1983–94 follow up. Occupational and Environmental Medicine 2000;57(9):605–14.

68. Huebner WW, Wojcik NC, Rosamilia K, Jorgensen G, Milano CA. Mortality updates (1970–1997) of two refinery/petrochemical plant cohorts at Baton Rouge, Louisiana, and Baytown, Texas. Journal of Occupational and Environmental Medicine/American College of Occupational and Environmental Medicine 2004;46(12):1229–45.

69. Gun RT, Pratt NL, Griffith EC, Adams GG, Bisby JA, Robinson KL. Update of a prospective study of mortality and cancer incidence in the Australian petroleum industry. Occupational and Environmental Medicine 2004;61(2):150–6.

70. Tsai SP, Chen VW, Fox EE, et al. Cancer incidence among refinery and petrochemical employees in Louisiana, 1983–1999. Annals of Epidemiology 2004;14(9):722–30.

71. Fordyce EJ, Wang Z, Kahn AR, et al. Risk of cancer among women with AIDS in New York City. AIDS & Public Policy Journal 2000;15(3–4):95–104.

72. Goedert JJ, Cote TR, Virgo P, et al. Spectrum of AIDS-associated malignant disorders. Lancet 1998;351(9119):1833–9.

73. Grulich AE, Li Y, McDonald A, Correll PK, Law MG, Kaldor JM. Rates of non-AIDS-defining cancers in people with HIV infection before and after AIDS diagnosis. AIDS (London, England) 2002;16(8):1155–61.

74. Grulich AE, Wan X, Law MG, Coates M, Kaldor JM. Risk of cancer in people with AIDS. AIDS (London, England) 1999;13(7):839–43.

75. Biggar RJ, Kirby KA, Atkinson J, McNeel TS, Engels E. Cancer risk in elderly persons with HIV/AIDS. Journal of Acquired Immune Deficiency Syndromes 2004;36(3):861–8.

76. Chang Y, Cesarman E, Pessin MS, et al. Identification of herpesvirus-like DNA sequences in AIDS-associated Kaposi's sarcoma. Science (New York, NY) 1994;266(5192):1865–9.

77. Cesarman E, Chang Y, Moore PS, Said JW, Knowles DM. Kaposi's sarcoma-associated herpesvirus-like DNA sequences in AIDS-related body-cavity-based lymphomas. The New England Journal of Medicine 1995;332(18):1186–91.

78. Memar OM, Rady PL, Tyring SK. Human herpesvirus-8: Detection of novel herpesvirus-like DNA sequences in Kaposi's sarcoma and other lesions. Journal of Molecular Medicine (Berlin, Germany) 1995;73(12):603–9.

79. Patel M, Mahlangu J, Patel J, et al. Kaposi sarcoma-associated herpesvirus/human herpesvirus 8 and multiple myeloma in South Africa. Diagnostic Molecular Pathology 2001;10(2):95–9.

80. Brander C, Raje N, O'Connor PG, et al. Absence of biologically important Kaposi sarcoma-associated herpesvirus gene products and virus-specific cellular immune responses in multiple myeloma. Blood 2002;100(2):698–700.

81. Drabick JJ, Davis BJ, Lichy JH, Flynn J, Byrd JC. Human herpesvirus 8 genome is not found in whole bone marrow core biopsy specimens of patients with plasma cell dyscrasias. Annals of Hematology 2002;81(6):304–7.

82. Zhu YX, Li ZH, Voralia M, Stewart AK. Antigenic open reading frames from HHV-8 are present in multiple myeloma patients and normal individuals at similar frequency. Leukemia & Lymphoma 2002;43(2):369–75.

83. Tedeschi R, Luostarinen T, De Paoli P, et al. Joint Nordic prospective study on human herpesvirus 8 and multiple myeloma risk. British Journal of Cancer 2005;93(7):834–7.

84. Cohen HJ, Bernstein RJ, Grufferman S. Role of immune stimulation in the etiology of multiple myeloma: A case control study. American Journal of Hematology 1987;24(2):119–26.

85. Linet MS, Harlow SD, McLaughlin JK. A case-control study of multiple myeloma in whites: Chronic antigenic stimulation, occupation, and drug use. Cancer Research 1987;47(11):2978–81.

86. Koepsell TD, Daling JR, Weiss NS, et al. Antigenic stimulation and the occurrence of multiple myeloma. American Journal of Epidemiology 1987;126(6):1051–62.

87. Gramenzi A, Buttino I, D'Avanzo B, Negri E, Franceschi S, La Vecchia C. Medical history and the risk of multiple myeloma. British Journal of Cancer 1991;63(5):769–72.

88. Landgren O, Rapkin JS, Mellemkjaer L, Gridley G, Goldin LR, Engels EA. Respiratory tract infections in the pathway to multiple myeloma: A population-based study in Scandinavia. Haematologica 2006;91(12):1697–700.

89. Brown LM, Linet MS, Greenberg RS, et al. Multiple myeloma and family history of cancer among blacks and whites in the U.S. Cancer 1999;85(11):2385–90.

90. Bourguet CC, Grufferman S, Delzell E, DeLong ER, Cohen HJ. Multiple myeloma and family history of cancer. A case-control study. Cancer 1985;56(8):2133–9.

91. Eriksson M, Hallberg B. Familial occurrence of hematologic malignancies and other diseases in multiple myeloma: A case-control study. Cancer Causes Control 1992;3(1):63–7.

92. Dong C, Hemminki K. Second primary neoplasms among 53 159 haematolymphoproliferative malignancy patients in Sweden, 1958–1996: A search for common mechanisms. British Journal of Cancer 2001;85(7):997–1005.

93. Landgren O, Linet MS, McMaster ML, Gridley G, Hemminki K, Goldin LR. Familial characteristics of autoimmune and hematologic disorders in 8,406 multiple myeloma patients: A population-based case-control study. International Journal of Cancer 2006;118(12):3095–8.

94. Paltiel O, Schmit T, Adler B, et al. The incidence of lymphoma in first-degree relatives of patients with Hodgkin disease and non-Hodgkin lymphoma: Results and limitations of a registry-linked study. Cancer 2000;88(10):2357–66.

95. Grosbois B, Jego P, Attal M, et al. Familial multiple myeloma: Report of fifteen families. British Journal of Haematology 1999;105(3):768–70.

96. Cutting RJ, Snowden JA. Myeloma in monozygotic twin. British Journal of Haematology 2006;134(6):646.

97. Judson IR, Wiltshaw E, Newland AC. Multiple myeloma in a pair of monozygotic twins: The first reported case. British Journal of Haematology 1985;60(3):551–4.

98. Ogawa M, Wurster DH, McIntyre OR. Multiple myeloma in one of a pair of monozygotic twins. Acta Haematologica 1970;44(5):295–304.

99. Jeannet M, Magnin C. HL-A antigens in haematological malignant diseases. European Journal of Clinical Investigation 1971;2(1):39–42.

100. Bertrams J, Kuwert E, Bohme U, et al. HL-A antigens in Hodgkin's disease and multiple myeloma. Increased frequency of W18 in both diseases. Tissue Antigens 1972;2(1):41–6.

101. Smith G, Walford RL, Fishkin B, Carter PK, Tanaka K. HL-A phenotypes, immunoglobulins and K and L chains in multiple myeloma. Tissue Antigens 1974;4(4):374–7.

102. Mason DY, Cullen P. HL-A antigen frequencies in myeloma. Tissue Antigens 1975;5(4):238–45.
103. Saleun JP, Youinou P, Le Goff P, Le Menn G, Morin JF. HLA antigens and monoclonal gammopathy. Tissue Antigens 1979;13(3):233–5.
104. Leech SH, Bryan CF, Elston RC, Rainey J, Bickers JN, Pelias MZ. Genetic studies in multiple myeloma. 1. Association with HLA-Cw5. Cancer 1983;51(8):1408–11.
105. Pottern LM, Gart JJ, Nam JM, et al. HLA and multiple myeloma among black and white men: Evidence of a genetic association. Cancer Epidemiology Biomarkers Prevention 1992;1(3):177–82.
106. Lynch HT, Sanger WG, Pirruccello S, Quinn-Laquer B, Weisenburger DD. Familial multiple myeloma: A family study and review of the literature. Journal of the National Cancer Institute 2001;93(19):1479–83.
107. Shoenfeld Y, Berliner S, Shaklai M, Gallant LA, Pinkhas J. Familial multiple myeloma. A review of thirty-seven families. Postgraduate Medical Journal 1982;58(675):12–6.
108. Lynch HT, Watson P, Tarantolo S, et al. Phenotypic heterogeneity in multiple myeloma families. Journal of Clinical Oncology 2005;23(4):685–93.
109. Deshpande HA, Hu XP, Marino P, Jan NA, Wiernik PH. Anticipation in familial plasma cell dyscrasias. British Journal of Haematology 1998;103(3):696–703.
110. Sobol H, Vey N, Sauvan R, Philip N, Noguchi T, Eisinger F. Re: Familial multiple myeloma: A family study and review of the literature. Journal of the National Cancer Institute 2002;94(6):461–2; author reply 3.
111. Struewing JP, Hartge P, Wacholder S, et al. The risk of cancer associated with specific mutations of BRCA1 and BRCA2 among Ashkenazi Jews. The New England Journal of Medicine 1997;336(20):1401–8.
112. Dilworth D, Liu L, Stewart AK, Berenson JR, Lassam N, Hogg D. Germline CDKN2A mutation implicated in predisposition to multiple myeloma. Blood 2000;95(5):1869–71.

Chapter 3

Basic Biology of Plasma Cell Dyscrasias: Focus on the Role of the Tumor Microenviroment

Marc S. Raab and Kenneth C. Anderson

Introduction

B-cell development involves several mechanisms of remodeling Ig genes: VDJ recombination, somatic hypermutation, and Ig heavy chain (IgH) switch recombination. Once matured, B-cells reside in secondary lymphoid tissues. Antigen interaction induces proliferation and differentiation to lymphoblasts, leading to the generation of short-lived pregerminal center plasma cells. An antigen-activated lymphoblast entering a germinal center undergoes a unique modification of Ig genes through sequential rounds of somatic hypermutation and antigen selection, as well as by IgH switch recombination. Postgerminal center B-cells may become plasmablasts that have successfully completed somatic hypermutation and IgH switching before migrating to the bone marrow (BM), where stromal cells enable terminal differentiation into nonproliferating long-lived plasma cells.[1,2]

Multiple myeloma (MM) is a malignant disease of terminally differentiated B-cells that may be preceded by a premalignant condition called monoclonal gammopathy of undetermined significance (MGUS). This is present in 1% of adults over the age of 25 years, the prevalence increasing with age. MGUS cells, like MM cells, secrete a monoclonal immunoglobulin and progress to malignant MM at a rate of 1% per year. Compared to MM, MGUS is characterized by a lower tumor burden (intramedullary tumor cell content less than 10%) and the absence of osteolytic lesions. Another disease related to aberrant plasma cells is amyloidosis, which shares most of the pathologic features of MGUS except that the secreted monoclonal immunoglobulin forms pathological deposits in various tissues.

Myeloma Genetics: A Brief Overview

Both MGUS and MM are characterized by the accumulation of transformed plasma cells at multiple sites in the BM. These cells show a marked karyotypic complexity with gains and losses of whole chromosomes, nonrandom chromosomal translocations causing dysregulation of genes at the breakpoints, and point mutations of genes, all contributing to disease pathogenesis.[6,7] In addition, small focal lesions of the MM genome as well as epigenetic changes have recently been identified[8–11] Briefly, MM patients can be subdivided into two groups based on the pattern of chromosomal gains and losses.[12] Approximately 55% of patients have a hyperdiploid karyotype (number of chromosomes 48–74) with trisomies of odd-numbered chromosomes including 3, 5, 7, 9, 11, 15, 19, and 21. The remaining cases (summarized as the nonhyperdiploid group) consist of patients with hypodiploid, near-diploid, pseudodiploid, or near-tetraploid chromosome numbers with less than 48 or more than 74 chromosomes.[12,13]

In addition to whole chromosome gains and losses, nonrandom, early-onset reciprocal chromosomal translocations are a hallmark of myeloma genetics, involving the IgH locus (at 14q32.3), or occasionally the IgL light chain locus (at kappa 2p12 or lambda 22q11).[14,15] In these primary translocations, various genes are juxtaposed to and dysregulated by a strong Ig enhancer.[16] In 15–20% of MM patients, this leads to cyclin D1 overexpression by a translocation t(11;14), in 12% an overexpressed MMSET and/or FGFR3 gene can be detected due to t(4;14), 5–10% show the dysregulated oncogene MAF with t(14;16), and 5% of the patients display elevated cyclin D3 or MAFB because of t(6;14) or t(14;20), respectively.[6,17–22] These chromosomal rearrangements appear to be mutually exclusive in the majority of patients, although two independent translocations could be found in the same patient in 5% of MGUS and 25% of advanced MM tumors.[23] In general, chromosomal translocations are associated with a nonhyperdiploid karyotype. The translocations t(6;14) as well as t(4;14) have been shown to confer a poor prognosis, whereas patients presenting with t(11;14) have a longer survival.[24,25]

The fact that at least one of the D-type cyclins is overexpressed in virtually all MM tumors, caused either directly or indirectly by translocation, or by a yet-to-be-defined mechanism within the hyperdiploid group, suggests a major role for D-type cyclins in the early pathogenesis of MM.[18]

Additional genetic changes have been shown to affect prognosis, such as chromosome 13 monosomy, loss of the short arm of chromosome 17 (locus of TP53, usually occurring later in the disease course) as well as gains and losses of the short arm of chromosome 1.[1,18,26–29]

Although the underlying mechanism leading to these genetic alterations remains to be elucidated, it is worth noting that the gross pattern of ploidy status rarely changes during disease progression.[30] In addition, genetic lesions in MM may not only confer enhanced proliferative capacity and increased resistance to apoptosis but also modulate the ability of MM cells to interact with their BM milieu. For example, MM cells with a t(14;16) translocation overexpress the transcription factor MAF, which both transactivates the cyclin D2 promoter, thereby increasing MM cell proliferation, and upregulates β1-integrin expression, thereby enhancing tumor cell adhesion to bone marrow stroma cells (BMSCs).[31] Furthermore, hyperdiploidy with cyclin D1 overexpression in the absence of Ig translocations renders MM cells uniquely dependent on the BM microenvironment.[18] These examples highlight the biological significance of the interplay between specific genetic lesions and those signaling pathways which mediate the effects of MM cell– microenvironment interactions.

There is now increased understanding of how the adhesion of MM cells to BM further impacts gene expression in MM cells and in BMSCs, thereby increasing tumor growth, drug resistance, and migration in the microenvironment.

Here, we aim to review the recent progress of these studies with emphasis on how the various constituents of the bone marrow modulate MM cell growth, survival, resistance to therapy, as well as bone resorption.

The Role of the Bone Marrow and Its Components in MM Pathogenesis

The interplay between neoplastic cells and their local microenvironment is not exclusively restricted to MM, but is shared by a wide spectrum of other hematologic neoplasias and solid tumors.[32–35] Nonetheless, the concept of tumor–microenvironment interaction is closely linked to MM, a prototypical disease model and ongoing research has already provided several new molecular targets and corresponding therapeutic strategies.

The BM microenvironment is composed of a variety of extracellular matrix (ECM) proteins, such as fibronectin, collagen, laminin, and osteopontin, as well as cell components including hematopoetic stem cells, progenitor and precursor cells, immune cells, erythrocytes, BMSCs, BM endothelial cells, as well as osteoclasts and osteoblasts. The close interaction between MM cells and both ECM proteins and accessory cells in the BM milieu plays a crucial role in MM pathogenesis, both by tumor cell adhesion to the ECM and accessory cells, and by secretion of cytokines, growth factors, and chemokines by tumor cells (autocrine loop) or BM cells (paracrine loop). Cytokines include interleukin-6 (IL-6), insulin-like growth factor-1 (IGF-1), vascular endothelial growth factor (VEGF), B-cell activating factor (BAFF), fibroblast growth factor (FGF), stromal cell-derived factor (SDF-1α), and tumor necrosis factor-a (TNF-α).[36–51] Interactions between MM cells and their microenvironment activate signaling pathways mediating growth, survival, drug resistance, and migration of MM cells,[52,53] as well as osteoblastogenesis and angiogenesis[56,57] in the BM (Fig. 1).

Homing and Adhesion of MM Cells to the BM

Homing to the bone marrow and adhesion to the microenvironment is a critical event for MM cells which leads to the activation of pathways mediating proliferation and survival. In MM, this process is mediated by SDF-1α, a chemokine which interacts with its receptor CXCR4 on MM cells. SDF-1α induces motility, internalization of CXCR4, and cytoskeletal rearrangement in MM cells. Conversely, specific inhibition by CXCR4 inhibitors abrogates MM cell migration in vitro, confirming the critical role of this receptor–ligand interaction for MM homing.[36,58] Adhesion to ECM proteins or BMSCs is then mediated by several adhesion molecules. CD44, VLA-4 (very late antigen-4, CD49d), VLA-5 (CD49e), LFA-1 (leukocyte function-associated antigen-1, CD1 1α), NCAM (neuronal adhesion molecule, CD56), ICAM-1 (intracellular adhesion molecule, CD54), syndecan-1 (CD 138), or MPC-1 mediate the adhesion of MM cells to the BM, thereby triggering MM cell proliferation and enhanced viability through distinct, but mutually complementary mechanisms.

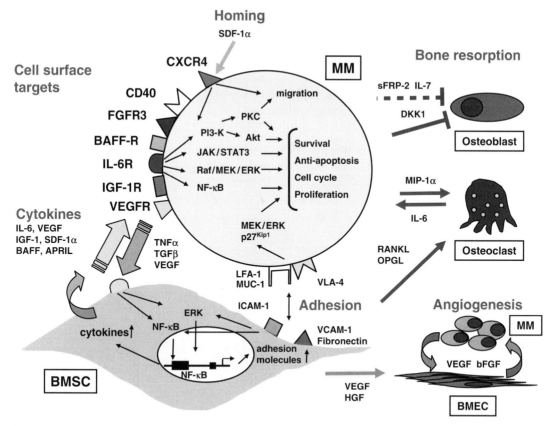

Fig. 1 Interaction of multiple myeloma (MM) cells with their bone marrow microenvironment. The adhesion of MM cells to bone marrow stromal cells (BMSCs) triggers cytokine-mediated tumor cell growth, survival, drug resistance, and migration. In both MM cells and BMSCs, adhesion mediates activation of NF-KB, thereby further upregulating adhesion molecules including intercellular adhesion molecule (ICAM-1) and vascular cell adhesion molecule-1 (VCAM-1). Binding of MM cells to BMSCs upregulates cytokine secretion from both BMSCs and tumor cells. These cytokines activate via their cell surface receptors major signaling pathways, such as extracellular signal-regulated kinase (ERK), Janus kinase (JAK) 2/signal tranducers and activators of transcription (STAT)-3, phosphatidylinositol-3 kinase (P13-K)/Akt, and nuclear factor-id3 (NF-κB). Their downstream targets include cytokines, such as interleukin-6 (IL-6), insulin-like growth factor-1 (IGF-1), and vascular endothelial growth factor (VEGF), antiapoptotic proteins, and cell cycle modulators. Homing of MM cells to their BM milieu is mediated by stromal-derived factor-la (SDF-la) and its receptor CXCR4 on MM cells. Osteoclastogenesis is stimulated by receptor activator of NF-κB ligand (RANKL) and osteoprotegerin ligand (OPGL) from BMSCs, as well as macrophage inflammatory protein 1α (MIP-1α) from MM cells. In addition, MM cells inhibit osteoblastogenesis via the secretion of IL-7 and Dickkopf 1 (DKK1), thereby further enhancing osteolysis. Secretion of factors like VEGF and basic fibroblast growth factor (bFGF) stimulates angiogenesis (*see* Plate 2).

For example, VLA-4 expressed on MM cells mediates binding both to ECM and to BMSCs through fibronectin and VCAM-1 (CD 106), respectively. Binding to fibronectin upregulates p27Kipl and induces nuclear factor (NF)-κB activation in MM cells, which confers cell adhesion-mediated drug resistance (CAM-DR) to conventional therapy.[40,60–63] Furthermore, adhesion of MM cells to ECM via type I collagen through syndecan-1, a heparin-sulfate proteoglycan, induces the expression of matrix metalloproteinase-1, thereby promoting bone resorption and tumor invasion, as well as concentrates heparin-binding growth factors on the surface of MM cells, thereby ensuring proliferation and survival. Elevated serum soluble syndecan-1 correlates with increased tumor cell mass, decreased metalloproteinase-9 activity, and poor prognosis.[64–66] Delineating the mechanisms of MM cell homing and adhesion may lead to new potential therapeutic strategies to overcome CAM-DR by targeting SDF-1α/CXCR4 and adhesion molecules, respectively (Fig. 1).

Interactions of MM Cells with BMSCs

Adhesion of MM cells to BMSCs has important functional sequelae. The secretion of IL-6 by stroma cells is triggered upon MM cell adhesion in an NF-κB-dependent manner, further promoting MM cell growth, survival, drug resistance, and migration.[51,67] Moreover, MM cells localized in the BM milieu secrete cytokines, such as TNF-α, transforming growth factor-13 (TGF-13), and VEGF, which further upregulate IL-6 secretion. Specifically, IL-6 binds to its receptor, which is present on normal plasmablasts, MGUS, and MM cells, and mediates growth survival and drug resistance via activation of MEK/MAPK signaling, Janus kinase/signal transducer and activator of transcription 3 (JAK/STAT3), as well as phosphoinositol 3-kinase(PI3K)/AKT-1 pathways.[68,69] IL-6 triggered activation of JAK/STAT upregulates the antiapoptotic proteins Mcl-1, Bcl-xl, Piml, and c-Myc. In addition, IL-6 downregulates three major isoforms of the pro-apoptotic BH3-only protein Bim, which, in turn, is neutralized by the formation of a complex with Mcl-1. Conversely, triggering the MEK/MAPK cascade via IL-6 activates nuclear proteins, such as c-Myc, c-Jun, and c-Fos, ultimately influencing MM cell cycle progression.

IGF-1 is another important paracrine growth factor that induces proliferation, survival, migration, and drug resistance in MM cells. Compared to IL-6, IGF-1 plays an equally important role in proliferation and is an even more powerful pro-survival factor for MM cells. Specifically, IGF-l exerts its effects on MM cells via activation of MAPK and PI3K/Akt-l signaling cascades and sustained NF-κB activation. Importantly, there is a close interplay between IL-6 and IGF-1 receptors, which are in close proximity at lipid rafts on the plasma membrane, facilitating cross-activation of IGF-1 receptors by IL-6.[76] Consequently, inhibition of IGF-1 receptor has also been shown to block IL-6- triggered response in MM cells. IGF-l also induces MM cell migration and invasion via a P13K-dependent, though Akt-1-independent, pathway, via protein kinase D, RhoA, and β1-integrin.

VEGF is produced by MM cells as well as by BMSCs and contributes to the increased angiogenesis in MM patient's BM.[78,79] The adhesion of MM cells to both BMSCs and exogenous IL-6 upregulates VEGF secretion.[80,81] VEGF triggers Flt-1 phosphorylation, resulting in activation of a P13K/protein kinase Ca-dependent cascade mediating MM cell migration on fibronectin, activation of the MEK/ERK pathway leading to MM cell proliferation, and survival signaling via upregulating Mcl-1 and survivin.[82,83]

TNF-α is expressed by both MM cells and BMSCs. While it seems to have only modest direct impact on MM cells, it significantly upregulates IL-6 secretion by BMSCs via binding to a TNF-α response element in the IL-6 promoter. Moreover, TNF-α secreted by MM cells induces NF-κB-dependent upregulation of adhesion molecules on both MM cells and BMSCs, like LFA-1, CD54, VCAM-1, VLA-4, thereby increasing the specific binding of MM cells to BMSCs and associated CAM-DR.[67]

The list of paracrine/autocrine factors in the BM enhancing MM cell growth and survival is continuously expanding. In addition to those already mentioned, this list includes the growth factors IGF-1, hepatocyte growth factor (HGF), basic fibroblast growth factor (bFGF), granulocyte colony-stimulating factor (G-CSF), SCF, and heparin-binding EGF-like growth factor (HB-EGF); the cytokines IL-1, IL-10, IL-1l, IL-15, IL-21, ciliary neutropic factor, LIF, oncostatin M, TGF-, macrophage inflammatory protein-lcx (MIP-lcx), and interferon-α (IFN-α).

Despite the different starting points of the signaling cascades of these various cytokines, chemokines, and adhesion molecules, their functional sequelae are not dissimilar, since they eventually converge to the same downstream PI3K/Akt-1, NF-κB, Ras/Raf/MAPK, and JAKISTAT3 pathways. These pathways, in turn, result in cytoplasmic sequestration of many transcription factors (i.e., FKHRL-1), upregulation of cell cycle proteins (i.e., Bcl-1, Bcl-xL, Mcl-1 or FLIP, cIAP-2, survivin), and increased activity of telomerase.[52]

Novel agents (like bortezomib, thalidomide, and lenalidomide) targeting not only MM cells directly but also tumor–host interaction as well as the BM milieu can overcome CAM-DR and the growth advantage conferred by the BM and hold great promise to overcome conventional drug resistance to improve patient outcome.

Furthermore, the bidirectional MM cell–BM interactions have important clinical sequelae, including enhanced osteoclastogenesis and suppressed osteoblast activity as well as increased blood vessel formation, resulting in osteolytic lesions and angiogenesis, respectively.

Interactions of MM Cells with Endothelial Cells

Angiogenesis in the BM is associated with disease activity. Angiogenesis levels, assessed by grading and microvessel density, are low in primary amyloidosis and MGUS, increased in smoldering myeloma, and markedly high in active MM. The extent of angiogenesis is directly correlated with the degree of plasma cell proliferation and infiltration, and is therefore an adverse prognostic factor. Angiogenesis promotes MM cell growth by enhancing the delivery of oxygen and nutrients, and by removing catabolites. Furthermore, bone marrow endothelial cells secrete growth factors, such as VEGF and bFGF, that promote tumor cell growth, and SDF-1α, which mediates the initial homing of MM cells to the BM stromal compartment through CXCR4. Conversely, bone marrow angiogenesis is sustained by VEGF, bFGF, and matrix metalloproteinases (MMPs) secreted by MM cells, allowing recruitment of new blood vessels to the BM.[81,84,85] Thus, these autocrine/paracrine loops in the BM milieu facilitate progression of MM. Other pro-angiogenic factors expressed by bone marrow endothelial cells include angiopontin-1, TGFβ, platelet-derived growth factor (PDGF), HGF, and IL-1 (Fig. 1). Importantly, BM angiogenesis can be targeted by novel agents. Thalidomide is the prototypic novel agent that came into use empirically because of its antiangiogenic properties. It has been shown to inhibit the secretion of VEGF, bFGF, and HGF, as well as abrogate endothelial cell proliferation and capillarogenesis in MM patients.[86]

Interactions of MM Cells with Osteoclasts

Osteolytic lesions, a hallmark feature of active disease in MM, occur predominantly at the interface of MM cell accumulations within the bone. At these sites, increased osteoclast activity, triggered by tumor cells, has been reported.[87–89] In this context, two major factors regulate bone resorption: osteoprotegerin (OPG) and its ligand (OPGL). OPG binds to the receptor activator of NF-κB ligand (RANKL) secreted by BMSCs and inhibits bone resorption while mediating MM cell survival, whereas OPGL stimulates osteoclast differentiation and activity.[90–92] MM cells affect the OPG/RANKL ratio in the BM microenvironment, thereby promoting bone disease. Specifically, BMSCs secrete OPG, serving as a decoy receptor which competes with RANK for RANKL binding, thereby inhibiting osteoclast maturation and bone destruction. However, the binding of VCAM-1 on BMSCs to α4 β1- integrin on MM cells decreases the secretion of OPG and, in turn, increases expression of pro-osteolytic RANKL.[96,97]

In addition to the OPG/RANKL ratio, macrophage inflammatory protein-1α (MIP-1α) secreted by MM cells mediates bone destruction in MM. MIP-1α levels are elevated in the BM plasma of MM patients and correlate with osteolytic lesions. A potent inducer of osteoclast formation independently of RANKL, MIP-1α also enhances both RANKL-stimulated and IL6-stimulated osteoclast formation.[98] MIP-1α binds to CCR1 on OCL and CCR5 on MM cells, thereby contributing to OCL formation and MM cell adhesion to BMSCs, respectively. Conversely and importantly, osteoclasts produce a variety of factors that stimulate growth of MM cells, including IL-6. In turn, IL-6 secretion triggered by MM cell adhesion to BMSCs also stimulates osteoclastogenesis and contributes, together with IL-1β, IL-11, VEGF, and HGF, to the increased bone resorption observed in MM.[100,101] These findings suggest that paracrine loops between osteoclasts and MM cells confer MM cell growth and bone destruction in the BM milieu (Fig. 1).

Interactions of MM Cells with Osteoblasts

Despite the multi-factorial induction of bone resorption by osteoclasts in the MM BM, decreased osteoblasts activity also contributes to MM bone disease and the formation of osteolytic lesions. Soluble factors secreted by MM cells, such as Dickkopf 1 (DKK1) and IL-7, contribute to the inhibitory effects of MM cells on osteoblast differentiation, in part via inhibition of the transcription factor Runx2/Cbfal, which is required for the formation and differentiation of mesenchymal stem cells into osteoblastic cells. In addition, this pathway is abrogated in osteoprogenitor cells via cell-to-cell contact mediated by VLA-4 on MM cells and VCAM-1 on osteoblast progenitors.[102–105] Furthermore, DKK1 inhibits canonical WNT signaling, which is also required for the differentiation of osteoblast progenitors. This may contribute to MM bone disease, since it could be shown that BM plasma containing elevated DKK1 levels as well as recombinant human DKK1 are able to inhibit the differentiation of osteoblast precursor cells in vitro, and elevated DKK1 levels in BM plasma and peripheral blood of MM patients are associated with the occurrence of focal bone lesions.[106]Another WNT inhibitor produced by MM cells is Frizzled-related protein 2 (sFRP-2), which is also capable of suppressing osteoblast differentiation.[107]

Multiple other cytokines mediate the imbalance of osteoblast/osteoclast activity in MM.[108] For example, HGF directly inhibits osteoblastogenesis in vitro and is elevated and inversely correlated to markers of osteoblast activity in patient sera with MM; TGFβ produced by MM cells augments IL-6 secretion from BMSCs and osteoblasts, thereby further stimulating OCL activity[55,109,110]; and IL-3 has recently been shown to counteract the stimulatory effect of bone morphogenic protein-2 (BMP-2) on basal osteoblast formation (Fig. 1).[111]

Proteasome inhibitors, a novel class of highly effective anti-MM agents, activate osteoblasts, thereby enabling new bone formation while achieving responses in advanced MM.[112–114]

Targeting MM Cells in Their BM Microenvironment: A Brief Overview

Despite the relative success of conventional and high-dose therapy in MM, disease inevitably relapses due to the acquisition of drug resistance. Even in cases where MM cells do not harbor detectable genetic lesions conferring drug resistance early in the disease, the BM microenvironment may provide epigenetic protection and allow some MM cells to finally develop those additional genetic alterations, ultimately conferring clinical resistance. While salvage therapy may then achieve transient responses, few, if any, patients are cured. In vitro and in vivo (animal) model systems of MM cells in the BM milieu have been developed to identify promising novel, biologically based therapies, targeting both homing to the BM and the interactions with BMSCs, endothelial cells, osteoclasts, and osteoblasts, as well as the tumor cell directly. Table 1 summarizes targets currently addressed by novel agents in clinical trials.

However, given the enormous complexity of constitutive and microenvironmentally induced genetic events and interactions in and between the MM cells and the BM milieu, combination therapies will be required to finally overcome drug resistance and improve patient outcome.

One of the first agents used as a platform for combination therapies was the proteasome inhibitor bortezomib. Genetic and proteomic profiling has provided the rationale for the evaluation of specific combinations. For example, bortezomib induces cleavage of DNA repair enzymes. Clinical trials have, therefore, successfully validated the clinical relevance of combining bortezomib with alkylating agents or anthracyclines.[115–118] Furthermore, bortezomib induces expression of hsp90, and its combination with the hsp90 inhibitor 17AAG enhances cytotoxicity by abrogating this stress response.[119,120] This was also found to be a promising clinical strategy to overcome bortezomib resistance. Moreover, combined bortezomib and lenalidomide treatment has achieved clinical responses even in MM patients resistant to either agent alone. This regimen was based on the in vitro finding that bortezomib induces apoptosis primarily via caspase-9, whereas lenalidomide exerts its cytotoxicity via caspase-8.[121] While simultaneously inhibiting several pathways involved in MM cell growth and survival, bortezomib activates Akt-1 and its downstream signaling molecules in vitro. This rescue mechanism can be abrogated by the addition of the Akt inhibitor perifosine, thereby inducing synergistic MM cell cytotoxicity. Similarly, proteasome inhibition leads to increased degradation

Table 1 New therapeutic agents in MM, currently in clinical trial targeting cell surface molecules and cytokines.

Target	Agent
CD40	SGN4O
CD56	huN9Ol-DM1
CD52	Alemtuzumab
FGF, PDGF	CH1R258
IL-6, IL-6R	CNT0328
	Altizumab
IGF-1R	CP-571
	EM164
MHC class II	1D09C3
MUC 1	AR2O.5 (BrevaRex)
RTK	SU6668
RANKL	Denosumab (AMG 162)
Serotonin	Fluphenazin
TRAIL	PR01672
	Mapatumunab (HGS-ETR1)
TACI	TACI-Ig
VEGF, VEGFR	Bevacizumab
	Semaxanib (SU54 16)
	Vatalanib (PTK-787)
	Zactima (ZD6474)
Akt	Perifosine (KRX-0401)
Bcl-2	Genasense (G3139)
CDK1	Alvocidib (NSC649890)
DNA	VPN4O11O1M
	Brostallicin (PNU-166196)
	PNU-108 112
	Temozolomide
	O-6-benzylguanine
	Bendamustine (SDX-105)
Farnesyltransferase	Tipifamib (Ri 1577)
HDAC	Vorinostat
	SAHA
	Romidepsin
	Panobinostat (LBH-589)
	Belinostat (PDX 101)
Heparanase	P1-88
Hsp90	Tanespimycin (K0S953)
	1P1504
IKK	RTA4O2 (CDDO-Me)
Inosine monophosphate dehydrogenase	AVN944
Mitochondria	Plimexon (Imexon)
	GCS-100
mTOR	Defibrotide
	AP23 573
	Temsirolimus (CCI-779)
	Everolimus (RADOO1)
	Rapamycin
Multi-kinases	Atiprimod
	VQD-001
	zIo-lOi

(continued)

Table 1 (continued)

Target	Agent
	Arsenic trioxide
	2ME2
Oxidative stress-related proteins	Motexafihin gadolinium
Proteasome	NPI-0052
	PR-171
Purine nucleoside phosphorylase	Fludosine (BCX-1777)
Src, Rae 1, JNK	Plitidepsin (Aplidin)
Superoxide dismutase 1	ATN-224
Thioredoxin	PX-12

Source: www.clinicaltrials.gov; www.multiplemyeloma.org; www.myeloma.org
FGF Fibroblast growth factor, *PDGF* platelet-derived growth factor, *IL* interleukin, *IGF* insulin-like growth factor, *RANKL* receptor activator of NF-KB ligand, *VEGF* vascular endothelial growth factor

of proteins via the aggresome /autophagy pathway, which can be synergistically blocked by the histone deacetylase inhibitors tubacin or LBH-589.[122]

Lenalidomide, like bortezomib, has been used as a platform for several combination strategies. For example, dexamethasone, with its caspase-9-dependent apoptotic pathway, has been shown to synergize with lenalidomide, which induces cell death via caspase-8 activation. This concept has already been clinically proven and resulted in significantly higher response rates in plasma cell diseases.[123,124] The immunomodulatory effect of lenalidomide markedly enhances antibody-dependent cell-mediated cytotoxicity (ADCC) induced by humanized monoclonal antibodies in vitro.[125] This led to the ongoing clinical evaluation of lenalidomide in combination with the humanized anti-CD40 monoclonal antibody in MM patients. Other agents combined with lenalidomide in preclinical studies include mTOR inhibitors,[126] VEGF inhibitors,[127,128] the PKC inhibitor enzastaurin,[129] and the Akt inhibitor perifosine. The results of these studies will inform the design of rational combination clinical trials to improve patient outcome.

References

1. Kuehi WM, Bergsagel PL. Multiple myeloma: Evolving genetic events and host interactions. Nat Rev Cancer 2002; 2(3):175–187.
2. Rajkumar SV, Fonseca R, Dewald GW et al. Cytogenetic abnormalities correlate with the plasma cell labeling index and extent of bone marrow involvement in myeloma. Cancer Genet Cytogenet 1999; 113(1):73–77.
3. Cohen HJ, Crawford J, Rao MK, Pieper CF, Currie MS. Racial differences in the prevalence of monoclonal gammopathy in a community-based sample of the elderly. Am J Med 1998; 104(5):439–444.
4. Kyle RA, Beard CM, O'Fallon WM, Kurland LT. Incidence of multiple myeloma in Olmsted County, Minnesota: 1978 through 1990, with a review of the trend since 1945. J Clin Oncol 1994; 12(8):1577–1583.
5. Kyle RA, Rajkumar SV. Monoclonal gammopathies of undetermined significance. Hematol Oncol Clin North Am 1999; 13(6):1181–1202.
6. Chesi M, Nardini E, Brents LA et al. Frequent translocation t(4;14)Q,16.3;q32.3) in multiple myeloma is associated with increased expression and activating mutations of fibroblast growth factor receptor 3. Nat Genet 1997; 16(3):260–264.

7. Trudel S, Ely S, Farooqi YC et al. Inhibition of fibroblast growth factor receptor 3 induces differentiation and apoptosis in t(4;14) myeloma. Blood 2004; 103(9):3521–3528.

8. Gonzalez-Paz N, Chng WJ, McClure RF et al. Tumor suppressor p16 methylation in multiple myeloma: Biological and clinical implications. Blood 2007; 109(3): 1228–1232.

9. Pompeia C, Hodge DR, Plass C et al. Microarray analysis of epigenetic silencing of gene expression in the KAS-6/1 multiple myeloma cell line. Cancer Res 2004; 64(10):3465–3473.

10. Carrasco DR, Tonon G, Huang Y et al. High-resolution genomic profiles define distinct clinico-pathogenetic subgroups of multiple myeloma patients. Cancer Cell 2006; 9(4):313–325.

11. Takahashi T, Shivapurkar N, Reddy J et al. DNA methylation profiles of lymphoid and hematopoietic malignancies. Clin Cancer Res 2004; 10(9):2928–2935.

12. Smadja NV, Fruchart C, Isnard F et al. Chromosomal analysis in multiple myeloma: Cyto genetic evidence of two different diseases. Leukemia 1998; 12(6):960–969.

13. Debes-Marun CS, Dewald GW, Bryant S et al. Chromosome abnormalities clustering and its implications for pathogenesis and prognosis in myeloma. Leukemia 2003; 17(2):427–436.

14. Bergsagel PL, Chesi M, Nardini E, Brents LA, Kirby SL, Kuehi WM. Promiscuous translocations into immunoglobulin heavy chain switch regions in multiple myeloma. Proc Natl Acad Sci USA 1996; 93(24):13931–13936.

15. Smadja NV, Bastard C, Brigaudeau C, Leroux D, Fruchart C. Hypodiploidy is a major prognostic factor in multiple myeloma. Blood 2001; 98(7):2229–2238.

16. Bergsagel PL, Kuehi WM. Chromosome translocations in multiple myeloma. Oncogene 2001; 20(40):5611–5622.

17. Bergsagel PL, Kuehi WM. Critical roles for immunoglobulin translocations and cyclin D dysregulation in multiple myeloma. Immunol Rev 2003; 194:96–104.

18. Bergsagei PL, Kuehl WM, Zhan F, Sawyer J, Barlogie B, Shaughnessy J. Cyclin D dysregulation: An early and unifying pathogenic event in multiple myeloma. Blood 2005; 106(1):296–303.

19. Chesi M, Bergsagel PL, Brents LA, Smith CM, Gerhard DS, Kuehi WM. Dysregulation of cyclin Dl by translocation into an IgH gamma switch region in two multiple myeloma cell lines. Blood 1996; 88(2):674–681.

20. Chesi M, Nardini E, Lim RS, Smith KID, Kuehl WM, Bergsagel PL. The t(4;14) translocation in myeloma dysregulates both FGFR3 and a novel gene, MMSET, resulting in IgH/MMSET hybrid transcripts. Blood 1998; 92(9):3025–3034.

21. Gabrea A, Bergsagel PL, Chesi M, Shou Y, Kuehi WM. Insertion of excised IgH switch sequences causes overexpression of cyclin Dl in a myeloma tumor cell. Mol Cell 1999; 3(1):119–123.

22. Shaughnessy J, Jr., Gabrea A, Qi Y et al. Cyclin D3 at 6p2l is dysregulated by recurrent chromosomal translocations to immunoglobulin loci in multiple myeloma. Blood 2001; 98(1):217–223.

23. Bergsagel PL, Kuehl WM. Molecular pathogenesis and a consequent classification of multiple myeloma. J Clin Oncol 2005; 23(26):6333–6338.

24. Avet-Loiseau H, Daviet A, Brigaudeau C et al. Cytogenetic, interphase, and multicolor fluorescence in situ hybridization analyses in primary plasma cell leukemia: A study of 40 patients at diagnosis, on behalf of the Intergroupe Francophone du Myelome and the Groupe Francais de Cytogenetique Hematologique. Blood 2001; 97(3):822–825.

25. Fonseca R, Blood E, Rue M et al. Clinical and biologic implications of recurrent genomic aberrations in myeloma. Blood 2003; 101(11):4569–4575.

26. Zhan F, Huang Y, Colla S et al. The molecular classification of multiple myeloma. Blood 2006; 108(6):2020–2028.

27. Hanamura I, Stewart JP, Huang Y et al. Frequent gain of chromosome band 1q21 in plasma-cell dyscrasias detected by fluorescence in situ hybridization: incidence

increases from MGUS to relapsed myeloma and is related to prognosis and disease progression following tandem stem-cell transplantation. Blood 2006; 108(5):1724–1732.

28. Shou Y, Martelli ML, Gabrea A et al. Diverse karyotypic abnormalities of the c-myc locus associated with c-myc dysregulation and tumor progression in multiple myeloma. Proc Natl Acad Sci USA 2000; 97(1):228–233.

29. Stewart AK, Fonseca R. Prognostic and therapeutic significance of myeloma genetics and gene expression profiling. J Clin Oncol 2005; 23(26):6339–6344.

30. Chng WJ, Winkler JM, Greipp PR et al. Ploidy status rarely changes in myeloma patients at disease progression. Leuk Res 2006; 30(3):266–271.

31. Hurt EM, Wiestner A, Rosenwald A et al. Overexpression of c-maf is a frequent oncogenic event in multiple myeloma that promotes proliferation and pathological interactions with bone marrow stroma. Cancer Cell 2004; 5(2):191–199.

32. Mitsiades CS, Koutsilieris M. Molecular biology and cellular physiology of refractoriness to androgen ablation therapy in advanced prostate cancer. Expert Opin Investig Drugs 2001; 10(6):1099–1115.

33. van Kempen LC, Ruiter DJ, van Muijen GN, Coussens LM. The tumor microenvironment: a critical determinant of neoplastic evolution. Eur J Cell Biol 2003; 82(11):539–548.

34. Munk Pedersen I, Reed J. Microenvironmental interactions and survival of CLL B-cells. Leuk Lymphoma 2004; 45(12):2365–2372.

35. Zhou J, Mauerer K, Farina L, Gribben JG. The role of the tumor microenvironment in hematological malignancies and implication for therapy. Front Biosci 2005; 10:1581–1596.

36. Hideshima T, Chauhan D, Hayashi T et al. The biological sequelae of stromal cell-derived factor-1{alpha} in multiple myeloma. Mol Cancer Ther 2002; 1(7):539–544.

37. Mitsiades CS, Mitsiades NS, McMullan CJ et al. Inhibition of the insulin-like growth factor receptor-1 tyrosine kinase activity as a therapeutic strategy for multiple myeloma, other hematologic malignancies, and solid tumors. Cancer Cell 2004; 5(3):221–230.

38. Moreaux J, Cremer FW, Reme T, Raab M, Mahtouk K, Kaukel P, Pantesco V, De Vos J, Jourdan E, Jauch A, Legouffe E, Moos M, Fiol G, Goldschmidt H, Rossi JF, Hose D, Klein B. The level of TAC1 gene expression in myeloma cells is associated with a signature of microenvironment dependence versus a plasmablastic signature. Blood. 2005; 106(3):1021–1030. Epub 2005 Apr 12.

39. Chauhan D, Catley L, Li G et al. A novel orally active proteasome inhibitor induces apoptosis in multiple myeloma cells with mechanisms distinct from Bortezomib [In Process Citation]. Cancer Cell 2005; 8(5):407–419.

40. Damiano JS, Cress AE, Hazlehurst LA, Shtil AA, Dalton WS. Cell adhesion mediated drug resistance (CAM-DR): Role of integrins and resistance to apoptosis in human myeloma cell lines. Blood 1999; 93(5):1658–1667.

41. Akiyama M, Hideshima T, Hayashi T et al. Cytokines modulate telomerase activity in a human multiple myeloma cell line. Cancer Res 2002; 62(13):3876–3882.

42. Chauhan D, Li G, Hideshima T et al. Blockade of ubiquitin-conjugating enzyme CDC34 enhances anti-myeloma activity of Bortezomib/Proteasome inhibitor PS341. Oncogene 2004; 23(20):3597–3602.

43. Hideshima T, Catley L, Yasui H et al. Perifosine, an oral bio active novel alkyl-phospholipid, inhibits Akt and induces in vitro and in vivo cytotoxicity in human multiple myeloma cells. Blood 2006; 107(10):4053–4062.

44. Mitsiades CS, Mitsiades NS, Munshi NC, Richardson PG, Anderson KC. The role of the bone microenvironment in the pathophysiology and therapeutic management of multiple myeloma: Interplay of growth factors, their receptors and stromal interactions. Eur J Cancer 2006; 42(11):1564–1573.

45. Freund GG, Kulas DT, Mooney RA et al. Insulin and TGF-1 increase mitogenesis and glucose metabolism in the multiple myeloma cell line, RPMI 8226. J Immunol 1993; 151(4):1811–1820.

46. Vanderkerken K, Asosingh K, Braet F, Van Riet I, Van CB. Insulin-like growth factor-1 acts as a chemoattractant factor for 5T2 multiple myeloma cells. Blood 1999; 93(1):235–241.

47. Podar K, Tai YT, Davies FE et al. Vascular endothelial growth factor triggers signaling cascades mediating multiple myeloma cell growth and migration. Blood 2001; 98(2):428–435.

48. Podar K, Tai YT, Lin BK et al. Vascular endothelial growth factor-induced migration of multiple myeloma cells is associated with beta 1 integrin- and phosphatidylinositol 3-kinase-dependent PKC alpha activation. J Biol Chem 2002; 277(10): 7875–7881.

49. L'Hote CG, Knowles MA. Cell responses to FGFR3 signalling: Growth, differentiation and apoptosis. Exp Cell Res 2005; 304(2):417–431.

50. Otsuki T, Yamada O, Yata K et al. Expression of fibroblast growth factor and FGF-receptor family genes in human myeloma cells, including lines possessing t(4; 14)(q16.3; q32. 3) and FGFR3 translocation. Tnt J Oncol 1999; 15(6): 1205–1212.

51. Chauhan D, Uchiyama H, Akbarali Y et al. Multiple myeloma cell adhesion-induced interleukin-6 expression in bone marrow stromal cells involves activation of NF-kappa B. Blood 1996; 87(3):1104–1112.

52. Hideshima T, Bergsagel PL, Kuehi WM, Anderson KC. Advances in biology of multiple myeloma: Clinical applications. Blood 2004; 104(3):607–618.

53. Hideshima T, Anderson KC. Molecular mechanisms of novel therapeutic approaches for multiple myeloma. Nat Rev Cancer 2002; 2(12):927–937.

54. Roodman GD. New potential targets for treating myeloma bone disease. Clin Cancer Res 2006; 12(20 Pt 2):6270s–6273s.

55. Roodman GD. Pathogenesis of myeloma bone disease. Blood Cells Mol Dis 2004; 32(2):290–292.

56. Ribatti D, Nico B, Vacca A. Importance of the bone marrow microenvironment in inducing the angiogenic response in multiple myeloma. Oncogene 2006; 25(31):4257–4266.

57. Jakob C, Sterz J, Zavrski I et al. Angiogenesis in multiple myeloma. Eur J Cancer 2006; 42(11):1581–1590.

58. De CE. Potential clinical applications of the CXCR4 antagonist bicyclam AMD3 100. Mini Rev Med Chem 2005; 5(9):805–824.

59. Alsayed Y, Ngo H, Runnels J . Mechanisms of regulation of CXCR4/SDF-l (CXCL 12)-dependent migration and homing in multiple myeloma. Blood 2007; 109(7):2708–217.

60. Landowski TH, Olashaw NE, Agrawal D, Dalton WS. Cell adhesion-mediated drug resistance (CAM-DR) is associated with activation of NF-kappa B (RelB/p50) in myeloma cells. Oncogene 2003; 22(16):2417–2421.

61. Hazlehurst LA, Damiano JS, Buyuksal I, Pledger WJ, Dalton WS. Adhesion to fibronectin via betal integrins regulates p27kipl levels and contributes to cell adhesion mediated drug resistance (CAM-DR). Oncogene 2000; 19(38): 4319–4327.

62. Damiano JS, Dalton WS. Integrin-mediated drug resistance in multiple myeloma. Leuk Lymphoma 2000; 38(1-2):71–81.

63. Hazlehurst LA, Enkemann SA, Beam CA et al. Genotypic and phenotypic comparisons of de novo and acquired melphalan resistance in an isogenic multiple myeloma cell line model. Cancer Res 2003; 63(22):7900–7906.

64. Yang Y, Yaccoby S, Liu W et al. Soluble syndecan-1 promotes growth of myeloma tumors in vivo. Blood 2002; 100(2):610–617.

65. Mahtouk K, Hose D, Raynaud P et al. Heparanase influences expression and shedding of syndecan-1, and its expression by the bone marrow environment is a bad prognostic factor in multiple myeloma. Blood 2007; 109(11):4914–4923.

66. Mahtouk K, Cremer FW, Reme T et al. Heparan sulphate proteoglycans are essential for the myeloma cell growth activity of EGF-family ligands in multiple myeloma. Oncogene 2006; 25(54):7180–7791.

67. Flideshima T, Chauhan D, Schlossman R, Richardson P, Anderson KC. The role of tumor necrosis factor alpha in the pathophysiology of human multiple myeloma: therapeutic applications. Oncogene 2001; 20(33):4519–4527.

68. Hideshima T, Nakamura N, Chauhan D, Anderson KC. Biologic sequelae of interleukin-6 induced P13-K/Akt signaling in multiple myeloma. Oncogene 2001; 20(42):5991–6000.

69. Pene F, Claessens YE, Muller O et al. Role of the phosphatidylinositol 3-kinase/Akt and mTORIP70S6-kinase pathways in the proliferation and apoptosis in multiple myeloma. Oncogene 2002; 21(43):6587–6597.

70. Puthier D, Bataille R, Amiot M. IL-6 up-regulates mcl-1 in human myeloma cells through JAK/STAT rather than Ras/MAP kinase pathway. Eur J Immunol 1999; 29(12):3945–3950.

71. Puthier D, Derenne S, Barille S et al. Mcl-1 and Bcl-xL are co-regulated by IL-6 in human myeloma cells. Br J Haematol 1999; 107(2):392–395.

72. Catlett-Falcone R, Landowski TH, Oshiro MM et al. Constitutive activation of Stat3 signaling confers resistance to apoptosis in human U266 myeloma cells. Immunity 1999; 10(1):105–115.

73. Kiuchi N, Nakajima K, Ichiba M et al. STAT3 is required for the gpl3O-mediated full activation of the c-myc gene. J Exp Med 1999; 189(1):63–73.

74. Shirogane T, Fukada T, Muller JM, Shima DT, Hibi M, Hirano T. Synergistic roles for Pim-1 and c-Myc in STAT3-mediated cell cycle progression and antiapoptosis. Immunity 1999; 11(6):709–719.

75. Ge NL, Rudikoff S. Insulin-like growth factor I is a dual effector of multiple myeloma cell growth. Blood 2000; 96(8):2856–2861.

76. Abroun S, Ishikawa H, Tsuyama N et al. Receptor synergy of interleukin-6 (IL-6) and insulin-like growth factor-I in myeloma cells that highly express IL-6 receptor alpha. Blood 2004; 103(6):2291–2298.

77. Tu Y, Gardner A, Lichtenstein A. The phosphatidylinositol 3-kinase/AKT kinase pathway in multiple myeloma plasma cells: Roles in cytokine-dependent survival and proliferative responses. Cancer Res 2000; 60(23):6763–6770.

78. Rajkumar SV, Kyle RA. Angiogenesis in multiple myeloma. Semin Oncol 2001; 28(6):560–564.

79. Xu JL, Lai R, Kinoshita T, Nakashima N, Nagasaka T. Proliferation, apoptosis, and intratumoral vascularity in multiple myeloma: Correlation with the clinical stage and cytological grade. J Clin Pathol 2002; 55(7):530–534.

80. Dankbar B, Padro T, Leo R et al. Vascular endothelial growth factor and interleukin-6 in paracrine tumor-stromal cell interactions in multiple myeloma. Blood 2000; 95(8):2630–2636.

81. Gupta D, Treon SP, Shima Y et al. Adherence of multiple myeloma cells to bone marrow stromal cells upregulates vascular endothelial growth factor secretion: Therapeutic applications. Leukemia 2001; 15(12):1950–1961.

82. Le Gouill S, Podar K, Amiot M et al. VEGF induces Mcl-1 up-regulation and protects multiple myeloma cells against apoptosis. Blood 2004; 104(9):2886–2892.

83. Podar K, Anderson KC. The pathophysiologic role of VEGF in hematologic malignancies: Therapeutic implications. Blood 2005; 105(4):1383–1395.

84. Vacca A, Ribatti D, Presta M et al. Bone marrow neovascularization, plasma cell angiogenic potential, and matrix metalloproteinase-2 secretion parallel progression of human multiple myeloma. Blood 1999; 93(9):3064–3073.

85. Kline M, Donovan K, Wellik L et al. Cytokine and chemokine profiles in multiple myeloma; significance of stromal interaction and correlation of IL-8 production with disease progression. Leuk Res 2007; 31(5):591–598.

86. Singhal S, Mehta J, Desikan R et al. Antitumor activity of thalidomide in refractory multiple myeloma. N Engl J Med 1999; 341(21):1565–1571.

87. Dallas SL, Garrett IR, Oyajobi BO et al. Ibandronate reduces osteolytic lesions but not tumor burden in a murine model of myeloma bone disease. Blood 1999; 93(5):1697–1706.

88. Callander NS, Roodman GD. Myeloma bone disease. Semin Hematol 2001; 38(3):276–285.

89. Roodman GD. Biology of osteoclast activation in cancer. J Clin Oncol 2001; 19(15):3562–3571.

90. Sezer O, Heider U, Zavrski I, Kuhne CA, Hofbauer LC. RANK ligand and osteoprotegerin in myeloma bone disease. Blood 2003; 101(6):2094–2098.

91. Hofbauer LC, Schoppet M. Clinical implications of the osteoprotegerin/RANKL/RANK system for bone and vascular diseases. JAMA 2004; 292(4):490–495.

92. Shipman CM, Croucher PI. Osteoprotegerin is a soluble decoy receptor for tumor necrosis factor-related apoptosis-inducing ligand/Apo2 ligand and can function as a paracrine survival factor for human myeloma cells. Cancer Res 2003; 63(5): 912–916.

93. Giuliani N, Bataille R, Mancini C, Lazzaretti M, Barille S. Myeloma cells induce imbalance in the osteoprotegerin/osteoprotegerin ligand system in the human bone marrow environment. Blood 2001; 98(13):3527–3533.

94. Giuliani N, Colla S, Rizzoli V. New insight in the mechanism of osteoclast activation and formation in multiple myeloma: Focus on the receptor activator of NF-kappaB ligand (RANKL). Exp Hematol 2004; 32(8):685–691.

95. Croucher PI, Shipman CM, Lippitt J et al. Osteoprotegerin inhibits the development of osteolytic bone disease in multiple myeloma. Blood 2001; 98(13):3534–3540.

96. Michigami T, Shimizu N, Williams PJ et al. Cell-cell contact between marrow stromal cells and myeloma cells via VCAM-1 and alpha(4)beta(1)-integrin enhances production of osteoclast-stimulating activity. Blood 2000; 96(5):1953–1960.

97. Pearse RN, Sordillo EM, Yaccoby S et al. Multiple myeloma disrupts the TRANCEL osteoprotegerin cytokine axis to trigger bone destruction and promote tumor progression. Proc Natl Acad Sci USA 2001; 98(20):11581–11586.

98. Choi SJ, Oba Y, Gazitt Y et al. Antisense inhibition of macrophage inflammatory protein 1-alpha blocks bone destruction in a model of myeloma bone disease. J Clin Invest 2001; 108(12):1833–1841.

99. Oba Y, Lee JW, Ehrlich LA et al. MIP-l alpha utilizes both CCR1 and CCR5 to induce osteoclast formation and increase adhesion of myeloma cells to marrow stromal cells. Exp Hematol 2005; 33(3):272–278.

100. Roodman GD, Kurihara N, Ohsaki Y et al. Interleukin 6. A potential autocrine/paracrine factor in Paget's disease of bone. J Clin Invest 1992; 89(1):46–52.

101. Nguyen AN, Stebbins EG, Henson M et al. Normalizing the bone marrow microenvironment with p38 inhibitor reduces multiple myeloma cell proliferation and adhesion and suppresses osteoclast formation. Exp Cell Res 2006; 312(10): 1909–1923.

102. Giuliani N, Colla S, Morandi F et al. Myeloma cells block RUNX2/CBFA1 activity in human bone marrow osteoblast progenitors and inhibit osteoblast formation and differentiation. Blood 2005; 106(7):2472–2483.

103. Giuliani N, Rizzoli V, Roodman GD. Multiple myeloma bone disease: Pathophysiology of osteoblast inhibition. Blood 2006; 108(13):3992–3996.

104. Karsenty G, Ducy P, Starbuck M . Cbfal as a regulator of osteoblast differentiation and function. Bone 1999; 25(1):107–108.

105. Ducy P, Karsenty G. Transcriptional control of osteoblast differentiation [Record Supplied By Aries Systems]. Endocrinologist 1999; 9(1):32–35.

106. Tian E, Zhan F, Walker R et al. The role of the Wnt-signaling antagonist DKK1 in the development of osteolytic lesions in multiple myeloma. N Engl J Med 2003; 349(26):2483–2494.

107. Oshima T, Abe M, Asano J et al. Myeloma cells suppress bone formation by secreting a soluble Wnt inhibitor, sFRP-2. Blood 2005; 106(9):3160–3165.

108. Standal T, Abildgaard N, Fagerli UM . HGF inhibits BMP-induced osteoblastogenesis: Possible implications for the bone disease of multiple myeloma [In Process Citation]. Blood 2007; 109(7):3024–3330.

109. Franchimont N, Rydziel S, Canalis E. Transforming growth factor-beta increases interleukin-6 transcripts in osteoblasts. Bone 2000; 26(3):249–253.

110. Urashima M, Ogata A, Chauhan D et al. Transforming growth factor-betal: differential effects on multiple myeloma versus normal B cells. Blood 1996; 87(5):1928–1938.

111. Ehrlich LA, Chung HY, Ghobrial I et al. IL-3 is a potential inhibitor of osteoblast differentiation in multiple myeloma. Blood 2005; 106(4):1407–1414.

112. Garrett IR, Chen D, Gutierrez G et al. Selective inhibitors of the osteoblast proteasome stimulate bone formation in vivo and in vitro. J Clin Invest 2003; 111(11):1771—1782. 26

113. Heider U, Kaiser M, Muller C et al. Bortezomib increases osteoblast activity in myeloma patients irrespective of response to treatment. Eur J Haematol 2006; 77(3):233–238.

114. Murray EJ, Bentley GV, Grisanti MS, Murray SS. The ubiquitin-proteasome system and cellular proliferation and regulation in osteoblastic cells. Exp Cell Res 1998; 242(2):460–469.

115. Berenson JR, Yang HH, Sadler K et al. Phase 1/11 trial assessing bortezomib and meiphalan combination therapy for the treatment of patients with relapsed or refractory multiple myeloma. J Clin Oncol 2006; 24(6):937–944.

116. Orlowski RZ, Voorhees PM, Garcia RA et al. Phase 1 trial of the proteasome inhibitor bortezomib and pegylated liposomal doxorubicin in patients with advanced hematologic malignancies. Blood 2005; 105(8):3058–3065.

117. Hideshima T, Mitsiades C, Akiyama M et al. Molecular mechanisms mediating antimyeloma activity of proteasome inhibitor PS-34 1. Blood 2003; 101(4):1530–1534.

118. Mitsiades N, Mitsiades CS, Richardson PG et al. The proteasome inhibitor PS-341 potentiates sensitivity of multiple myeloma cells to conventional chemotherapeutic agents: Therapeutic applications. Blood 2003; 101(6):2377–2380.

119. Mitsiades CS, Mitsiades NS, McMullan CJ et al. Antimyeloma activity of heat shock protein-90 inhibition. Blood 2006; 107(3):1092–1100.

120. Mitsiades N, Mitsiades CS, Poulaki V et al. Molecular sequelae of proteasome inhibition in human multiple myeloma cells. Proc Nati Acad Sci U S A 2002; 99(22):14374–14379.

121. Mitsiades N, Mitsiades CS, Poulaki V et al. Apoptotic signaling induced by immunomodulatory thalidomide analogs in human multiple myeloma cells: Therapeutic implications. Blood 2002; 99(12):4525–4530.

122. Hideshima T, Bradner JE, Wong J . Small-molecule inhibition of proteasome and aggresome function induces synergistic antitumor activity in multiple myeloma. Proc Natl Acad Sci U S A 2005; 102(24):8567–8572.

123. Rajkumar SV, Hayman SR, Lacy MQ . Combination therapy with lenalidomide plus dexamethasone (Rev/Dex) for newly diagnosed myeloma. Blood 2005; 106(13):4050–4053.

124. Dispenzieri A, Lacy MQ, Zeldenrust SR et al. The activity of lenalidomide with or without dexamethasone in patients with primary systemic amyloidosis. Blood 2007; 109(2):465–470.

125. Tai YT, Li XF, Catley L . Immunomodulatory drug lenalidomide (CC-5013, IMiD3) augments anti-CD4O SGN-40-induced cytotoxicity in human multiple myeloma: Clinical implications. Cancer Res 2005; 65(24):11712–11720.

126. Raje N, Kumar S, Hideshima T et al. Combination of the mTOR inhibitor rapamycin and CC-5013 has synergistic activity in multiple myeloma. Blood 2004; 104(13):4188–4193.

127. Podar K, Tonon G, Sattler M et al. The small-molecule VEGF receptor inhibitor pazopanib (GW786034B) targets both tumor and endothelial cells in multiple myeloma. Proc Natl Acad Sci U S A 2006; 103(51):19478–19483.

128. Podar K, Catley LP, Tai YT et al. GW654652, the pan-inhibitor of VEGF receptors, blocks the growth and migration of multiple myeloma cells in the bone marrow microenvironment. Blood 2004; 103(9):3474–3479.

129. Podar K, Raab MS, Zhang J et al. Targeting PKC in multiple myeloma: in vitro and in vivo effects of the novel, orally available small-molecule inhibitor enzastaurin (LY3 17615.HC1). Blood 2007; 109(4):1669–1677.

Chapter 4

Biology-Based Classification and Staging of Multiple Myeloma

Wee Joo Chng and Peter Leif Bergsagel

Introduction

While staging in solid tumor describes the anatomical spread of the tumor, for example, to the lymph nodes or distant sites, this concept is not applicable to hematological malignancies as the malignant cells by default are already distributed throughout the body. In hematological malignancies such as multiple myeloma (MM), an incurable late B-cell malignancy characterized by bone marrow infiltration with malignant plasma cells (PCs), and lytic bone lesions, staging provides a measure of how advance the tumor is and often reflects tumor burden.

There is a close link between disease stage and prognosis, and in hematological malignancies, prognostic systems are often built around factors that reflect disease stage. As such staging system and prognostic system are synonymous. Ultimately, the importance of staging and classification is in the ability to define clinically relevant heterogeneity within a tumor type and their clinical utility as guide to treatment decision and prognosis. In this regard, examples abound in other hematological malignancies such as non-Hodgkin lymphoma, myelodysplastic syndrome, and acute leukemias where the International Prognostic Index, the International Prognostic Scoring System, and cytogenetic classification, respectively, are established clinical tools.

Conventional Prognostic Factors

To establish risk categories, one must define a set of reliable and practical prognostic factors. Conventional prognostic factors are predominantly surrogates for tumor burden. They reflect various aspects of disease phenotype such as PC characteristics and end organ involvement.

Tumor Burden

β_2-microglobulin (B_2M), which simultaneously measures cell proliferation, cell mass, and renal function, is one of the most consistent and powerful prognostic factor.[1,2] Patients with high-serum B_2M levels have

From: *Contemporary Hematology Myeloma Therapy*
Edited by: S. Lonial © Humana Press, Totowa, NJ

shorter survival whether treated by chemotherapy, high-dose therapy (HDT) and autologous stem cell transplantation,[3–7] or allogeneic stem cell transplantation.[8,9] Different studies used different cutoff values, with 2.5, 3.5, and 4 mg/dl being the most common.

An elevated serum lactate dehydrogenase (LDH) has been associated with an aggressive phenotype,[10] poorer response to chemotherapy,[11] and shorter survival following chemotherapy[10,11] and HDT.[7] Although LDH is a powerful prognostic factor, its clinical utility is limited by being elevated in only a very small subset of patients (<5–10%).

Albumin was introduced as a prognostic factor in the 1980s.[12] It is a simple and routine clinical test which indirectly reflects serum interleukin-6 (IL-6) levels (inverse relationship), liver function, and nutritional status.[13] Therefore, a low-serum albumin probably correlate with rapid MM growth due to higher IL-6 levels[14] and a reduction in patient's performance status.

PC Characteristics

PC Proliferation

Proliferation of bone marrow PC in myeloma can be measured by a slide-based immunofluorescent assay (PC labeling index, PCLI)[15] or enumeration of S-phase PC by flow cytometry.[16] The PCLI has been validated as a powerful prognostic factor for survival in chemotherapy-treated patients by various groups.[17] Although it is a robust prognostic factor, its use has been limited to specialized centers due to the technical complexity of the assay. Cell cycle analysis and enumeration of S-phase PCs using flow cytometry as a surrogate for proliferation has also been shown to be an independent prognostic factor,[16] although overall there is less literature of its validation and technical limitations have prevented the widespread application of the technique. An Eastern Cooperative Oncology Group (ECOG) study showed that the PCLI is a more powerful prognostic factor than S-phase cell enumeration by flow cytometry. A recent study of elderly MM patients showed that the number of S-phase PCs was the most powerful prognostic factor and can further refine the prognosis of patients classified as stage III according to the new International Staging System (ISS).[18]

Circulating PCs

Circulating PCs can be detected in the peripheral blood by slide-based fluorescent immunocytochemistry[19] or flow cytometry.[20,21] Detection of PCs in peripheral blood above certain threshold is associated with short survival.[19,22] In a recent study, detection of more than 10 circulating PCs per 50,000 mononuclear cells using flow cytometry is also prognostic independent of the ISS.[22]

PC Morphology

Plasmablastic morphology is an independent poor prognostic factor in patients undergoing both chemotherapy[23] and HDT.[24] Because of the precise morphologic examination required for classification of plasmablastic PCs, this marker has not been widely adopted in clinical use. A simpler morphological classification system based on identification and enumeration of mature PCs with prognostic relevance has been proposed. [25]

Imaging

The radiographic skeletal survey has been the mainstay in diagnosing features of myeloma-related bone disease such as osteopenia, focal lytic lesion, and fractures. New imaging technologies, such as magnetic resonance imaging (MRI), have made anatomic and functional staging much more precise.

In a large prospective study, including 611 newly diagnosed patients uniformly treated with total therapy II, a treatment regimen including tandem HDT with a median follow-up of 55 months, MRI was found to be much more sensitive at picking up focal lesion compared to skeletal survey. It identifies more lesions per patients and more patients with focal bone lesions. The number of MRI-defined focal lesions (MRI-FL) correlated with serum levels of c-reactive protein, albumin, and LDH, suggesting that extent of bone disease is a surrogate for tumor burden. On multivariate analysis, MRI-FL number was an independent adverse prognostic factor for overall survival (OS). [26]

Staging/Prognostic Systems Based on Conventional Prognostic Factors

Many prognostic systems using a combination of the aforementioned prognostic factors have been proposed by various groups. While effective in identifying high-risk groups, these prognostic systems do not provide insights into biology.

Durie—Salmon and Durie—Salmon Plus Staging System

The Durie—Salmon staging system[27] incorporates commonly available clinical parameters, such as level and type of monoclonal protein, hemoglobin, calcium level, and number of bone lesions, and is widely used (Table 1). The uneven distribution of patients across the stages (majority of newly diagnosed MM falling into stage III), complexity of the system, and subjectivity of radiological evidence of lytic lesions are major shortcomings.

In a German study including 77 patients, integration of MRI findings and the Durie—Salmon staging system (Table 1) show stronger correlation with survival than do MRI or the Durie—Salmon staging alone. None of the Durie—Salmon plus MRI stage I patients have died while the median survival was 59 months and 15 months for stage II and III patients, respectively. [28]

Mayo Clinic

A prognostic system incorporating PCLI and B_2M was proposed by the Mayo Clinic in 1993 based on a study of 107 patients treated with combination chemotherapy who had a minimum follow-up of 4.5 months. The low-risk patients (PCLI < 1 and B_2M < 2.7) had a median survival of 71 months, the intermediate-risk patients (PCLI ≥ 1 or B_2M ≥ 2.7) had a median survival of 40 months, whereas high-risk patients (PCLI ≥ 1 and B_2M ≥ 2.7) had a median survival of 17 months.[15]

Table 1 Durie—Salmon and Durie—Salmon plus MRI staging.

Durie—Salmon staging criteria	Durie—Salmon plus MRI staging criteria
Stage I (low cell mass)	Stage I (low cell mass)
All of the following:	All of the following:
Hemoglobin > 10 g/dl	Hemoglobin < 10 g/dl
Serum calcium normal or < 10.5 mg/dl	Serum calcium normal or < 10.5 mg/dl
Normal skeletal survey or solitary bone plasmacytoma only	Normal skeletal survey or solitary bone plasmacytoma only
IgG < 5.0 g/dl	IgG < 5.0 g/dl
IgA < 3.0 g/dl	IgA < 3.0 g/dl
Urine light-chain M component < 4 g/day	Urine light-chain M component < 4 g/day
	MRI show no focal lesion in spine or diffuse infiltration
Stage II (intermediate cell mass)	Stage II (intermediate cell mass)
Fitting neither Stage I nor Stage III	Fitting neither Stage I nor Stage III
Stage III (high cell mass)	Stage III (high cell mass)
One or more of the following:	One or more of the following:
Hemoglobin < 8.5 g/dl	Hemoglobin < 8.5 g/dl
Serum calcium > 12 mg/dl	Serum calcium > 12 mg/dl
Advance bone lesion	Advance bone lesion
IgG > 7.0 g/dl	IgG > 7.0 g/dl
IgA > 5.0 g/dl	IgA > 5.0 g/dl
Urine light-chain M component > 12 g/day	Urine light-chain M component > 12 g/day
	MRI show more than 10 focal lesions in spine or marked diffuse infiltration[a]
Subclassification (either A or B)	Subclassification (either A or B)
A: Creatinine < 2.0 mg/dl	A: Creatinine < 2.0 mg/dl
B: Creatinine ≥ 2.0 mg/dl	B: Creatinine ≥ 2.0 mg/dl

MRI magnetic resonance imaging
[a]Signal intensity of the bone marrow is markedly decreased and reaches the signal intensity of intervertebral discs.

Southwest Oncology Group

The Southwest Oncology Group (SWOG) derived a staging system based on serum B_2M and albumin levels from 1,555 newly diagnosed patients entered into four different chemotherapy induction and maintenance trials.[13] Four stages are defined. Stage I patients had median OS of 55 months compared to 16 months for stage IV patients.

International Staging System

A major international collaborative effort resulted in the ISS (Table 2).[29] This staging system is derived from and validated on 5,383 and 5,367 newly diagnosed MM patients, respectively. Different statistical modeling was applied and patients included were treated with various modalities (conventional and HDT), from different geographical regions (including Asia, Europe, and North America), age groups (greater or less than 65 years of age) and clinical settings

Table 2 The ISS staging.

Stage I
$B_2M < 3.5$ mg/dl and serum albumin < 3.5 g/dl
Stage II
$B_2M < 3.5$ mg/dl and serum albumin > 3.5 g/dl Or B_2M 3.5–5.5 mg/dl
Stage III
$B_2M < 5.5$ mg/dl

(single institutions or cooperative groups). The prognostic power of the ISS is maintained in all these situations, highlighting its reliability and wide application. The ISS is now being widely adopted and forms the basis for risk-stratification in future clinical trials. A major drawback of the ISS is the noninclusion of genetic factors as cytogenetic or the fluorescent in situ hybridization (FISH) data is available only for 390 patients (3.6% of total cohort) in the study. Integration of genetic factors into prognostic systems would be an important area for future collaborative studies.

Biology-Based Prognostic Factors

As opposed to prognostic factor relating to tumor burden and PC phenotype, biology-based prognostic factors provide direct information relevant to disease pathogenesis and biology. With the availability of molecular techniques and global genomic techniques, we are increasingly able to dissect myeloma into molecularly and biologically distinct subgroups. But more important, by identifying the specific genes or pathways deregulated and understanding the biological basis of these clinically relevant subgroups, novel therapeutic targets can be unearthed and individualized targeted risk-adopted therapy can be implemented.

Genetics

Metaphase Versus Interphase Cytogenetics

In any karyotyping study, abnormal karyotypes can be detected in about 10% of MM.[30,31] The presence of abnormal metaphase is correlated with PCLI and extent of bone marrow involvement,[32] and confers a poor prognosis.[33,34] Interphase FISH may be preferred in the study of MM genetics due to its ability to detect abnormalities in nonproliferating cells (no metaphase) and hence information on recurrent genetic abnormalities in a large number of patients. Furthermore, some of the recurrent abnormalities with important prognostic implication such as t(4;14)(p16.3;q32) are karyotypically silent. However, it is important to note that cytogenetics remain a commonly requested clinical test due to its widespread availability. If abnormal metaphases are obtained, the prognosis conferred is very poor when abnormalities such as monosomy 13[34–36] or hypodiploidy[37–39] are observed. The net effect on prognosis is greater if chromosome 13 abnormalities are detected than when detected by FISH,[40,41] but the test is limited in that only a very small minority of patients will have informative metaphases.

Recurrent Cytogenetic Abnormalities

Among the recurrent genetic abnormalities in MM, hypodiploid,[37–39] t(4;14)(p16.3;q32), [39–45] t(14;16)(q32;q23),[43] Δ13,[46] and chromosome 17p13 (*p53* locus) deletion[43,45,47,48] have been shown by many studies to confer poor prognosis across all treatment modalities. In addition to the aforementioned abnormalities, other monosomies have been associated with an adverse outcome, particularly that of chromosomes 2, 3, 14, and 19.[37] A large study from the Intergroup Francophone du Myelome (IFM) group comprising more than 900 patients entered into clinical trials showed that high-risk genetic abnormalities such as t(4;14) and 17p13 deletion significantly dichotomize survival in each of the ISS stages, showing conclusively that genetic factors are powerful prognostic factors that should be incorporated into routine clinical practice.[49].

In addition, there are still some controversies surrounding which is the most relevant genetic prognostic marker. Several of these poor prognostic genetic markers are closely associated. t(4;14)(p16.3;q32) and t(14;16)(q32;q23) are highly associated with Δ13,[50,51] and nonhyperdiploidy[52], although their relationship with hypodiploidy per se is less studied. We recently investigated the prognostic impact of Δ13 in hyperdiploid (HRD) MM and found that Δ13 status does not alter survival in these patients.[53] Therefore, the overall prognostic significance of Δ13 is likely linked to the presence of t(4;14)(p16.3;q32) and t(14;16)(q32;q23).

Recently, elevated CKS1B expression has been identified by gene expression studies as a significant adverse prognostic factor. Furthermore, the same authors showed that elevated gene expression is mechanistically linked to amplification of chromosome 1q21 where the gene is located.[54] CKS1B is a cell cycle-associated gene and its product favors cell cycle progression by promoting degradation of *p27* with release of the cyclin-dependent kinases and entry into mitosis.[55] In a study using FISH probes bracketing CKS1B on 1q21 conducted at the Mayo Clinic, CKS1B gene amplification (in majority of cases gene duplication rather than true amplification) was observed in a third of patients studied. Although significant on univariate analysis, CKS1B amplification did not emerge as an independent prognostic factor on multivariate analysis.[56] Further study is required to ascertain the prognostic importance of elevated CKS1B expression in MM.

Molecular Profiling

Gene Expression-Defined High-Risk Molecular Signature

Recently, a molecular signature that defines high-risk disease was identified using gene expression profiling (GEP). Using log-rank tests of expression quartiles, 70 genes were linked to early disease-related death. The ratio of mean expression levels of the 51 upregulated to 19 downregulated genes defined a high-risk score present in 13% of patients with shorter durations of event-free and overall survival, with a hazard ratio exceeding 4.5. The high-risk score was also an independent predictor of outcome endpoints in a multivariate analysis that included the ISS and high-risk translocations. Interestingly, 30% of these genes mapped to chromosome 1, with the majority of upregulated genes mapped to chromosome 1q and downregulated genes mapped to chromosome 1p. Multivariate discriminant analysis revealed that a 17-gene subset (12 upregulated) could predict outcome as well as the 70-gene model.[57] We have validated this 17-gene signature in two additional datasets of newly diagnosed (Mayo Clinic cohort) and relapse (patients entered into an international phase III bortezomib trial) patients. In both settings, it was significantly associated with poorer survival.[79]

The biological significance of this high-risk signature is not yet fully understood. As mentioned above, it is enriched for chromosome 1 genes. In addition, the upregulated genes are markedly enriched for proliferation-related genes and the signature is correlated with that of the proliferation index ($r^2 = 0.63$). Yet it is a stronger prognostic factor than both 1q amplification and a gene expression-based proliferation index that is closely correlated with the slide-based PCLI. Understanding the biological basis of this high-risk signature will aid in the selection of novel therapy for these patients with abysmal survival with currently available therapies.

MGUS-Like MM

Recently, Zhan and colleagues identified a monoclonal gammopathy of undetermined significance (MGUS) signature and when applied to a large dataset of MM patients could identify about 30% of MM cases that also express this MGUS signature, which they termed MGUS-L (MGUS-like) MM. They found that MGUS-L MM has more benign clinical features and despite lower complete response to treatment have better survival.[58] The study is hampered by the technical difficulty of extricating molecular signature related to contaminating nonmalignant PCs. Although the results were interpreted in the context of these technical limitations, it is unclear how the effects of contamination are defined and excluded. Therefore, while compelling, the existence of MGUS-L MM as a biological entity is unclear.

Centrosome Index

MM is characterized by genomic instability. Possible mechanisms underlying this have been investigated and centrosome amplification leading to asymmetric spindle poles and mitosis has been demonstrated in PC neoplasm starting from the premalignant MGUS stage.[59,60] A gene expression-based index that correlated strongly with centrosome amplification was derived. A high index was an independent prognostic factor in multiple datasets comprising of patients treated with either conventional or novel therapy.[59]

Biology-Based Staging

Several classification/prognostic/staging systems based on genetics that directly relate to critical alterations in gene and pathways underlying different tumors have been developed. The ability to pinpoint genetic abnormalities relating to pathogenesis and therapeutic resistance based on these models offer the potential of selecting the optimum treatment for individual patient.

Cytogenetic Based

ECOG Genetics

In an ECOG study including 351 patients treated with combination chemotherapy with a median follow-up of 40.5 months, t(4;14), t(14;160), and 17p13 deletion were significant prognostic factors on univariate analysis. Using hierarchic modeling of the prognostic impact of recurrent genetic abnormalities, including these three factors, a prognostic system was constructed. The poor prognostic group consists of patients with t(4;14) and/or t(14;16) and/or 17p13 deletion; the intermediate-prognostic group consists of patients with chromosome 13 deletion but not t(4;14), t(14;16), or 17p13 deletion; and the good prognosis group consists of all other patients. Their median survival times were 24.7 months, 42.3 months, and 50.5 months, respectively.

Intergroup Francophone du Myelome Genetics

The IFM group derived a prognostic system based on serum B_2M and $\Delta 13$ by interphase FISH from 110 newly diagnosed patients treated with HDT upfront.[3] The median OSs of the high-, intermediate-, and low-risk groups are 25 months, 47 months, and more than 111 months, respectively.

In a more recent study comprising more than 900 patients, the IFM refined this prognostic system. The group found that patients with t(4;14) and/or 17p13 deletion and $B_2M > 4$ mg/l had poor prognosis with median survival of only 19 months; patients with t(4;14) and/or 17p13 deletion or $B_2M > 4$ mg/l had intermediate prognosis; and patients without any of these factors had the best prognosis with an expected survival of 83% at 4 years.

A Model with Hypoploidy and B_2M

In a French study that identified hypodiploidy as a significant poor prognostic factor, a prognostic model including hypodiploidy and B_2M was proposed. The low-risk group without hypodiploidy and with low B_2M had median OS of 44.4 months; the intermediate-risk group with either hypodiploidy or a high B_2M had a median OS of 23.3 months; and the high-risk patients, who had both hypodiploidy and high B_2M, had a median OS of only 10.9 months.

A Model Using MRI-FL and Presence of Abnormal Cytogenetics

In the study that identified MRI-FL as an independent prognostic factor, a prognostic model incorporating MRI-FL and presence of abnormal cytogenetics by karyotyping (CA, chromosome analysis) was also proposed. Five-year survival estimates are 76% in the absence of CA and seven or fewer MRI-FL, about 61% in the presence of one of these adverse features, and 37% among patients with higher MRI-FL number and CA ($p > 0.001$).

Classification by Array Comparative Genomic Hybridization

When the abnormalities detected by array comparative genomic hybridization (aCGH) were used to cluster MM, two groups of patients corresponding to HRD and nonhyperdiploid (NHRD) MM could be identified. In addition, HRD MM could be further divided into two groups with significantly different event-free survival but not OS (when treated with total therapy II). The main differences between these groups are the enrichment of 1q gain, and chromosome 13 loss in the group with poorer prognosis and the enrichment of chromosome 11 gain in the group with better prognosis. The NHRD MM can also be split into two groups based on chromosome 1, 8, and 16q abnormalities. However, the subgroups of NHRD MM have similar survival.[61].

These observations require further validation as the sample size is small and follow-up relatively short. The importance of chromosome 13 deletion in survival of HRD patients is inconsistent with the results of two large series.[49,53] The poor prognostic impact of chromosome 1q gain is well established and is probably mediating most of the differences in survival. The classification of MM by aCGH therefore recapitulates previous FISH findings and does not provide additional prognostic information.

Gene Expression Profiling-Based Staging/Classifications

Translocation and Cyclin D Classification[62]

Translocation and cyclin D (TC) classification is based on spiked expression of genes deregulated by primary immunoglobulin heavy-chain translocations and the universal overexpression of cyclin D genes either by these translocations or by other mechanism. The resultant classification identifies eight groups of tumors: those with primary translocations (designated 4p16, 11q13, 6p21, and maf), those that overexpressed *CCND1* and *CCND2* either alone or in combination (D1, D1 & D2, D2), and the rare cases that do not overexpress any cyclin D genes ("none"). Most of the patients with HRD MM fall within the D1 and D1 & D2 groups.

The advantage of this classification system is that it focuses on different kinds of mechanisms that dysregulate a cyclin D gene as an early and unifying event in pathogenesis. The underlying cyclin D deregulation potentially has an important therapeutic implication as differential targeting of cyclin D may be very useful and may add specificity to treatment. Indeed, some potential agents targeting cyclin D2 have been identified in a drug library screen (Stewart AK, personal communications).

This classification has great potential for translation into the clinic as it involves the measurement of relatively few markers, and most of the translocations can be detected by FISH.

On the downside, the TC classification does not identify patients with HRD myeloma clearly, with the majority of these patients falling into the D1 and D1 & D2 group. D1 & D2 HRD MM appears to have more proliferative disease, but the survival of these patients is not different from the survival of those who fall into the D1 group. In addition, the clinical and biological significance of the D2 group is unclear.

UAMS Molecular Classification of Myeloma

Recently, the group from the University of Arkansas for Medical Sciences (UAMS) derived another MM classification using an unsupervised approach and identified seven tumor groups characterized by the co-expression of unique gene clusters.[63] Interestingly, these clusters also identify tumors with t(4;14), maf translocations, t(11;14), and t(6;14) corresponding to the MS, MF, and CD-1 and/or CD-2 groups, respectively. In this analysis, t(11;14) and t(6;14) can belong either to the CD-1 or to the CD-2 group, depending on expression of CD20 and other B-cell-related genes. This is consistent with the finding that t(11;14) and t(6;14) have very similar expression profiles, clinical profiles, and outcome. In contrast to the TC classification, the UAMS classification identifies HRD MM as a distinct HY group. However, this may be somewhat misleading since the HY group, which is about 28% of MM tumors, includes only about 60% of HRD tumors. The distribution of the remaining HRD tumors among the other six groups has not been clarified, although most are probably in the LB and proliferation (PR) groups. Besides these groups which correspond to the major genetic subtypes of MM, there are two further groups: PR, defined by increased expression of proliferation related genes, and LB, defined by low-bone disease and lower expression of genes associated with bone disease in MM such as FRZB and DKK1.[64] The PR, MS, and MF groups identify patients with poor prognosis. The PR group, containing patients with t(4;14), t(11;14), and HRD patients, identifies the patients within these categories with more proliferative disease associated with poorer outcome.

The advantage of the UAMS molecular classification is that it is clinically relevant. It identifies the main genetic subtypes and other clinically relevant subtypes such as the high-risk PR subgroup and the CD20-expressing CD-2 group. It is also interesting that an unsupervised analysis of GEP data essentially identifies the main genetic subtypes of MM, suggesting that the predominant transcriptional heterogeneity seen within MM is driven by these pivotal primary genetic events and/or by progression events such as proliferation in the PR group. One of the deficiencies of this classification is that samples with white cell and normal PCs contamination were excluded from the classification, as the expression signatures from these contaminating cells may affect assignment to the different groups. Furthermore, classification is based on composite expression of large sets of genes. It is therefore uncertain how this can be applied clinically.

Genetic Subtype Specific Heterogeneity: HRD MM as a Model

In a recent analysis of GEP data of HRD MM, four reproducible molecular signatures could be identified: first, overexpressing cancer testis antigen and proliferation genes; second, overexpressing HGF, IL6, SOCS3, and PTP4A3; third, overexpressing NF-KB genes; while the last signature includes underexpressing genes associated with the first three signatures. Importantly, patients expressing the different signature have different survival, with the group expressing cancer testis antigen having a median survival of 27 months after diagnosis compared to not yet reached for the group expressing the NF-KB signature after a median follow-up of 3 years.[65] A separate study, using aCGH, identifies a group of HRD MM patients with chromosome 1q amplification, 13 deletion, and 11 trisomies who have significantly shorter progression-free survival than do other HRD MM patients.[61] Interestingly, 1q amplification is a common feature of high-risk HRD MM groups identified by both the GEP and aCGH studies. These studies highlight the presence of molecular and genetic heterogeneity within HRD MM and the importance of defining genetic subtype-specific prognostic factors. Similar heterogeneity probably exists in other genetic subgroups. For example, in the UAMS classification, the t(11;14) can belong to the CD-1, CD-2, or PR group.

Integration of Genetic and Gene Expression Prognostic Models

When analyzing the same dataset from which the previously mentioned high-risk molecular signature was derived (see section "Gene Expression-Defined High-Risk Molecular Signature" above), we found that the presence of t(4;14) could further dissect the survival of the high-risk but not the low-risk patients defined by this molecular signature. Combining the use of t(4;14) and the high-risk 17-gene signature, three groups of patients with significantly different survival could be identified. The high-risk group defined by presence of high-risk molecular signature and t(4;14) has a median OS of 16.7 months, the intermediate-risk group ($n = 45$) defined by the presence of the high-risk molecular signature but without t(4;14) has a median OS of 39.8 months, and the low-risk group ($n = 289$) defined by the absence of high-risk molecular signature has yet to achieve the median survival.[79]

Implication on Therapy

The ability to stage myeloma biologically has two main clinical implications: the implementation of risk-stratified therapy and identification of novel-targeted therapy for high-risk patients who do not seem to benefit from any of the currently available therapy.

Risk-Stratified Therapy

A number of robust and biologically relevant prognostic factors have been identified in recent years. Emerging is a number of factors which consistently define patients with very poor prognosis when treated by the current standard of care, HDT (Table 3).[66] With the expansion in therapeutic armamentarium in recent years, it is now possible to consider different therapeutic approaches for patients in different risk categories. Recently, several studies have shown that treatment with bortezomib overcomes the poor prognosis associated with t(4;14) in both newly diagnosed and relapse patients.[63,67,68] For these reasons, t(4;14) should be assessed routinely for all patients as it provides important prognostic information and offers opportunities to tailor therapy, for example, using a bortezomib-containing regimen rather than HDT upfront. Risk-stratified therapy is therefore currently a distinct possibility for MM. One such risk-adopted treatment strategy, based on underlying tumor genetics, has already been proposed by the Mayo Clinic.[69]

Table 3 Factors used to define high-risk patients by Mayo Clinic.

Any of the following:
t(4;14) by FISH
t(14;16) or t(14;20) by FISH
Deletion 17p13 by FISH
Deletion 13 or aneuploidy by metaphase cytogenetics
Plasma cell-labeling index < 3.0

FISH fluorescent in situ hybridization

Novel-Targeted Therapy

Patients most in need of new therapeutic approaches are those who do not benefit from currently available therapy. The understanding of the biological basis of poor-risk patients provide an avenue for specifically targeting deregulated gene/pathways to benefit these patients. The prime examples are specific inhibitors of FGFR3, one of the genes deregulated by the high risk t(4;14), which have shown efficacy in vitro and in vivo and are currently in clinical testing.[70–73].

Similarly, targeting p53 in patients with 17p13 deletion or TP53 mutation is attractive. Onyx-015,[74] a permitting viral replication exclusively in cells with defective p53 and induction of tumor-specific cell lysis, or a gene therapy approach using ad5CMV-p53 (INGN 201; ADVEXIN; Introgen Therapeutics Inc., Houston, TX),[75] a replication-defective adenoviral construct containing the wild-type *TP53* gene that delivers a normal *TP53* gene into p53-defective tumor cells, thereby restoring p53 function, has already shown promise in early clinical studies.[76,77].

By analyzing global gene expression profiles, we found that patients with a high-centrosome index overexpresse aurora kinases, which are novel anti-cancer targets.[80] Initial study of aurora kinase inhibitors in MM has already shown promising results,[78] suggesting that these novel treatments may benefit the high-risk patients with very poor survival following currently available therapy.

Conclusion

Recent years have seen the marked expansion of our understanding of the molecular basis of MM as well as therapeutic options. In many ways, progress in both areas has been complementary. Using biologically relevant factors to stage and classify patients, personalized therapy is a distinct possibility for MM patients within the next few years.

References

1. Bataille R, Durie BG, Grenier J. Serum beta2 microglobulin and survival duration in multiple myeloma: a simple reliable marker for staging. Br J Haematol. 1983;55:439–447.
2. Durie BG, Stock-Novack D, Salmon SE, et al. Prognostic value of pretreatment serum beta 2 microglobulin in myeloma: A Southwest Oncology Group Study. Blood. 1990;75:823–830.
3. Facon T, Avet-Loiseau H, Guillerm G, et al. Chromosome 13 abnormalities identified by FISH analysis and serum beta2-microglobulin produce a powerful myeloma staging system for patients receiving high-dose therapy. Blood. 2001;97:1566–1571.
4. Attal M, Harousseau JL, Facon T, et al. Single versus double autologous stem-cell transplantation for multiple myeloma. N Engl J Med. 2003;349:2495–2502.
5. Desikan R, Barlogie B, Sawyer J, et al. Results of high-dose therapy for 1000 patients with multiple myeloma: Durable complete remissions and superior survival in the absence of chromosome 13 abnormalities. Blood. 2000;95:4008–4010.
6. Tricot G, Spencer T, Sawyer J, et al. Predicting long-term (> or = 5 years) event-free survival in multiple myeloma patients following planned tandem autotransplants. Br J Haematol. 2002;116:211–217.

7. Shaughnessy J, Jr., Tian E, Sawyer J, et al. Prognostic impact of cytogenetic and interphase fluorescence in situ hybridization-defined chromosome 13 deletion in multiple myeloma: Early results of total therapy II. Br J Haematol. 2003;120:44–52.

8. Bensinger WI, Buckner CD, Anasetti C, et al. Allogeneic marrow transplantation for multiple myeloma: An analysis of risk factors on outcome. Blood. 1996;88:2787–2793.

9. Gahrton G, Tura S, Ljungman P, et al. Prognostic factors in allogeneic bone marrow transplantation for multiple myeloma. J Clin Oncol. 1995;13:1312–1322.

10. Barlogie B, Smallwood L, Smith T, Alexanian R. High serum levels of lactic dehydrogenase identify a high-grade lymphoma-like myeloma. Ann Intern Med. 1989;110:521–525.

11. Dimopoulos MA, Barlogie B, Smith TL, Alexanian R. High serum lactate dehydrogenase level as a marker for drug resistance and short survival in multiple myeloma. Ann Intern Med. 1991;115:931–935.

12. Bataille R, Durie BG, Grenier J, Sany J. Prognostic factors and staging in multiple myeloma: A reappraisal. J Clin Oncol. 1986;4:80–87.

13. Jacobson JL, Hussein MA, Barlogie B, Durie BG, Crowley JJ. A new staging system for multiple myeloma patients based on the Southwest Oncology Group (SWOG) experience. Br J Haematol. 2003;122:441–450.

14. Bataille R, Jourdan M, Zhang XG, Klein B. Serum levels of interleukin 6, a potent myeloma cell growth factor, as a reflect of disease severity in plasma cell dyscrasias. J Clin Invest. 1989;84:2008–2011.

15. Greipp PR, Lust JA, O'Fallon WM, Katzmann JA, Witzig TE, Kyle RA. Plasma cell labeling index and beta 2-microglobulin predict survival independent of thymidine kinase and C-reactive protein in multiple myeloma. Blood. 1993;81:3382–3387.

16. San Miguel JF, Garcia-Sanz R, Gonzalez M, et al. A new staging system for multiple myeloma based on the number of S-phase plasma cells. Blood. 1995;85:448–455.

17. Fonseca R, Conte G, Greipp PR. Laboratory correlates in multiple myeloma: How useful for prognosis? Blood Rev. 2001;15:97–102.

18. Garcia-Sanz R, Gonzalez-Fraile MI, Mateo G, et al. Proliferative activity of plasma cells is the most relevant prognostic factor in elderly multiple myeloma patients. Int J Cancer. 2004;112:884–889.

19. Witzig TE, Gertz MA, Lust JA, Kyle RA, O'Fallon WM, Greipp PR. Peripheral blood monoclonal plasma cells as a predictor of survival in patients with multiple myeloma. Blood. 1996;88:1780–1787.

20. Rawstron AC, Owen RG, Davies FE, et al. Circulating plasma cells in multiple myeloma: Characterization and correlation with disease stage. Br J Haematol. 1997;97:46–55.

21. Witzig TE, Kimlinger TK, Ahmann GJ, Katzmann JA, Greipp PR. Detection of myeloma cells in the peripheral blood by flow cytometry. Cytometry. 1996;26:113–120.

22. Nowakowski GS, Witzig TE, Dingli D, et al. Circulating plasma cells detected by flow cytometry as a predictor of survival in 302 patients with newly diagnosed multiple myeloma. Blood. 2005;106(7):2276–2279.

23. Greipp PR, Leong T, Bennett JM, et al. Plasmablastic morphology — an independent prognostic factor with clinical and laboratory correlates: Eastern Cooperative Oncology Group (ECOG) myeloma trial E9486 report by the ECOG Myeloma Laboratory Group. Blood. 1998;91:2501–2507.

24. Rajkumar SV, Fonseca R, Lacy MQ, et al. Plasmablastic morphology is an independent predictor of poor survival after autologous stem-cell transplantation for multiple myeloma. J Clin Oncol. 1999;17:1551–1557.

25. Goasguen JE, Zandecki M, Mathiot C, et al. Mature plasma cells as indicator of better prognosis in multiple myeloma. New methodology for the assessment of plasma cell morphology. Leuk Res. 1999;23:1133–1140.

26. Walker R, Barlogie B, Haessler J, et al. Magnetic resonance imaging in multiple myeloma: Diagnostic and clinical implications. J Clin Oncol. 2007;25:1121–1128.

27. Durie BG, Salmon SE. A clinical staging system for multiple myeloma. Correlation of measured myeloma cell mass with presenting clinical features, response to treatment, and survival. Cancer. 1975;36:842–854.

28. Baur A, Stabler A, Nagel D, et al. Magnetic resonance imaging as a supplement for the clinical staging system of Durie and Salmon? Cancer. 2002;95:1334–1345.

29. Greipp PR, San Miguel J, Durie BG, et al. International staging system for multiple myeloma. J Clin Oncol. 2005;23:3412–3420.

30. Dewald GW, Kyle RA, Hicks GA, Greipp PR. The clinical significance of cytogenetic studies in 100 patients with multiple myeloma, plasma cell leukemia, or amyloidosis. Blood. 1985;66:380–390.

31. Sawyer JR, Waldron JA, Jagannath S, Barlogie B. Cytogenetic findings in 200 patients with multiple myeloma. Cancer Genet Cytogenet. 1995;82:41–49.

32. Rajkumar SV, Fonseca R, Dewald GW, et al. Cytogenetic abnormalities correlate with the plasma cell labeling index and extent of bone marrow involvement in myeloma. Cancer Genet Cytogenet. 1999;113:73–77.

33. Rajkumar S, Fonseca R, Lacy M, et al. Abnormal cytogenetics predict poor survival after high-dose therapy and autologous blood cell transplantation in multiple myeloma. Bone Marrow Transplant. 1999;24:497–503.

34. Tricot G, Sawyer JR, Jagannath S, et al. Unique role of cytogenetics in the prognosis of patients with myeloma receiving high-dose therapy and autotransplants. J Clin Oncol. 1997;15:2659–2666.

35. Tricot G, Barlogie B, Jagannath S, et al. Poor prognosis in multiple myeloma is associated only with partial or complete deletions of chromosome 13 or abnormalities involving 11q and not with other karyotype abnormalities. Blood. 1995;86:4250–4256.

36. Seong C, Delasalle K, Hayes K, et al. Prognostic value of cytogenetics in multiple myeloma. Br J Haematol. 1998;101:189–194.

37. Debes-Marun CS, Dewald GW, Bryant S, et al. Chromosome abnormalities clustering and its implications for pathogenesis and prognosis in myeloma. Leukemia. 2003;17:427–436.

38. Smadja NV, Bastard C, Brigaudeau C, Leroux D, Fruchart C. Hypodiploidy is a major prognostic factor in multiple myeloma. Blood. 2001;98:2229–2238.

39. Fassas AB, Spencer T, Sawyer J, et al. Both hypodiploidy and deletion of chromosome 13 independently confer poor prognosis in multiple myeloma. Br J Haematol. 2002;118:1041–1047.

40. Shaughnessy J, Jacobson J, Sawyer J, et al. Continuous absence of metaphase-defined cytogenetic abnormalities, especially of chromosome 13 and hypodiploidy, ensures long-term survival in multiple myeloma treated with Total Therapy I: Interpretation in the context of global gene expression. Blood. 2003;101:3849–3856.

41. Dewald G, Therneau T, Larson D, et al. Relationship of patient survival and chromosome anomalies detected in metaphase and/or interphase cells at diagnosis of myeloma. Blood. 2005;106(10):3553–3558.

42. Chang H, Sloan S, Li D, et al. The t(4;14) is associated with poor prognosis in myeloma patients undergoing autologous stem cell transplant. Br J Haematol. 2004;125:64–68.

43. Fonseca R, Blood E, Rue M, et al. Clinical and biologic implications of recurrent genomic aberrations in myeloma. Blood. 2003;101:4569–4575.

44. Keats JJ, Reiman T, Maxwell CA, et al. In multiple myeloma, t(4;14)(p16;q32) is an adverse prognostic factor irrespective of FGFR3 expression. Blood. 2003;101:1520–1529.

45. Gertz MA, Lacy MQ, Dispenzieri A, et al. Clinical implications of t(11;14)(q13;q32), t(4;14)(p16.3;q32), and -17p13 in myeloma patients treated with high-dose therapy. Blood. 2005;106(8):2837–2840.

46. Fonseca R, Barlogie B, Bataille R, et al. Genetics and cytogenetics of multiple myeloma: A workshop report. Cancer Res. 2004;64:1546–1558.

47. Chang H, Qi C, Yi QL, Reece D, Stewart AK. p53 gene deletion detected by fluorescence in situ hybridization is an adverse prognostic factor for patients with multiple myeloma following autologous stem cell transplantation. Blood. 2005;105:358–360.

48. Drach J, Ackermann J, Fritz E, et al. Presence of a p53 gene deletion in patients with multiple myeloma predicts for short survival after conventional-dose chemotherapy. Blood. 1998;92:802–809.

49. Avet-Loiseau H, Attal M, Moreau P, et al. Genetic abnormalities and survival in multiple myeloma: The experience of the Intergroupe Francophone du Myelome. Blood. 2007;109(8):3489–3495.

50. Fonseca R, Oken MM, Greipp PR. The t(4;14)(p16.3;q32) is strongly associated with chromosome 13 abnormalities in both multiple myeloma and monoclonal gammopathy of undetermined significance. Blood. 2001;98:1271–1272.

51. Avet-Loiseau H, Facon T, Grosbois B, et al. Oncogenesis of multiple myeloma: 14q32 and 13q chromosomal abnormalities are not randomly distributed, but correlate with natural history, immunological features, and clinical presentation. Blood. 2002;99:2185–2191.

52. Fonseca R, Debes-Marun CS, Picken EB, et al. The recurrent IgH translocations are highly associated with nonhyperdiploid variant multiple myeloma. Blood. 2003;102:2562–2567.

53. Chng WJ, Santana-Davila R, Van Wier SA, et al. Prognostic factors for hyperdiploid-myeloma: Effects of chromosome 13 deletions and IgH translocations. Leukemia. 2006;20:807–813.

54. Zhan F, Sawyer J, Gupta S, et al. Elevated expression of CKS1B at 1q21 is highly correlated with short survival in myeloma. Blood. 2004;104:77a.

55. Zhan F, Colla S, Wu X, et al. CKS1B, over expressed in aggressive disease, regulates multiple myeloma growth and survival through SKP2- and p27Kip1-dependent and independent mechanisms. Blood. 2007;109(11):4995–5001.

56. Fonseca R, Van Wier SA, Chng WJ, et al. Prognostic value of chromosome 1q21 gain by fluorescent in situ hybridization and increase CKS1B expression in myeloma. Leukemia. 2006;20:2034–2040.

57. Shaughnessy JD Jr., Zhan F, Burington BE, et al. A validated gene expression model of high-risk multiple myeloma is defined by deregulated expression of genes mapping to chromosome 1. Blood. 2006;109:2276–2284.

58. Zhan F, Barlogie B, Arzoumanian V, et al. Gene-expression signature of benign monoclonal gammopathy evident in multiple myeloma is linked to good prognosis. Blood. 2007;109:1692–1700.

59. Chng WJ, Ahmann GJ, Henderson K, et al. Clinical implication of centrosome amplification in plasma cell neoplasm. Blood. 2006;107:3669–3675.

60. Maxwell CA, Keats JJ, Belch AR, Pilarski LM, Reiman T. Receptor for hyaluronan-mediated motility correlates with centrosome abnormalities in multiple myeloma and maintains mitotic integrity. Cancer Res. 2005;65:850–860.

61. Carrasco DR, Tonon G, Huang Y, et al. High-resolution genomic profiles define distinct clinico-pathogenetic subgroups of multiple myeloma patients. Cancer Cell. 2006;9:313–325.

62. Bergsagel PL, Kuehl WM, Zhan F, Sawyer J, Barlogie B, Shaughnessy J Jr. Cyclin D dysregulation: An early and unifying pathogenic event in multiple myeloma. Blood. 2005;106:296–303.

63. Zhan F, Huang Y, Colla S, et al. The molecular classification of multiple myeloma. Blood. 2006;108:2020–2028.

64. Tian E, Zhan F, Walker R, et al. The role of the Wnt-signaling antagonist DKK1 in the development of osteolytic lesions in multiple myeloma. N Engl J Med. 2003;349:2483–2494.

65. Chng WJ, Kumar S, Vanwier S, et al. Molecular dissection of hyperdiploid multiple myeloma by gene expression profiling. Cancer Res. 2007;67:2982–2989.

66. Stewart AK, Bergsagel PL, Greipp PR, et al. A practical guide to defining high-risk myeloma for clinical trials, patient counseling and choice of therapy. Leukemia. 2007;21:529–534.

67. Chang H, Trieu Y, Qi X, Xu W, Stewart KA, Reece D. Bortezomib therapy response is independent of cytogenetic abnormalities in relapsed/refractory multiple myeloma. Leuk Res. 2007;31(6):779–782.

68. Mateos MV, Hernandez JM, Hernandez MT, et al. Bortezomib plus melphalan and prednisone in elderly untreated patients with multiple myeloma: Results of a multicenter phase 1/2 study. Blood. 2006;108:2165–2172.

69. Dispenzieri A, Rajkumar SV, Gertz MA, et al. Treatment of newly diagnosed multiple myeloma based on mayo stratification of myeloma and risk-adapted therapy (mSMART): Consensus statement. Mayo Clin Proc. 2007;82:323–341.

70. Paterson JL, Li Z, Wen XY, et al. Preclinical studies of fibroblast growth factor receptor 3 as a therapeutic target in multiple myeloma. Br J Haematol. 2004;124:595–603.

71. Trudel S, Ely S, Farooqi Y, et al. Inhibition of fibroblast growth factor receptor 3 induces differentiation and apoptosis in t(4;14) myeloma. Blood. 2004;103:3521–3528.

72. Trudel S, Li ZH, Wei E, et al. CHIR-258, a novel, multitargeted tyrosine kinase inhibitor for the potential treatment of t(4;14) multiple myeloma. Blood. 2005;105:2941–2948.

73. Trudel S, Stewart AK, Rom E, et al. The inhibitory anti-FGFR3 antibody, PRO-001, is cytotoxic to t(4;14) multiple myeloma cells. Blood. 2006;107:4039–4046.

74. Bischoff JR, Kirn DH, Williams A, et al. An adenovirus mutant that replicates selectively in p53-deficient human tumor cells. Science. 1996;274:373–376.

75. Zhang WW, Fang X, Mazur W, French BA, Georges RN, Roth JA. High-efficiency gene transfer and high-level expression of wild-type p53 in human lung cancer cells mediated by recombinant adenovirus. Cancer Gene Ther. 1994;1:5–13.

76. Kirn D, Hermiston T, McCormick F. ONYX-015: Clinical data are encouraging. Nat Med. 1998;4:1341–1342.

77. Tolcher AW, Hao D, de Bono J, et al. Phase I, pharmacokinetic, and pharmacodynamic study of intravenously administered Ad5CMV-p53, an adenoviral vector containing the wild-type p53 gene, in patients with advanced cancer. J Clin Oncol. 2006;24:2052–2058.

78. Shi Y, Reiman T, Li W, et al. Targeting aurora kinases as therapy in multiple myeloma. Blood. 2007;109:3915–3921.

79. Chng WJ, Kuehl WM, Bergsagel PL, Fonseca R. Translocation t(4;14) retains prognostic significance even in the setting of high-risk molecular signature. Leukemia 2008;22(2):459–461.

80. Chng WJ, Braggio E, Mulligan G et al. The centrosome index is a powerful prognostic marker in myeloma and identifies a cohort of patients that might benefit from aurora kinase inhibition. Blood 2008;111(3):1603–1609.

Chapter 5

Cytogenetic Abnormalities in Multiple Myeloma: The Importance of FISH and Cytogenetics

Esteban Braggio, Michael Sebag, and Rafael Fonseca

Cyto-Molecular Techniques

Conventional Cytogenetics and Spectral Karyotyping

Conventional cytogenetics (CC) analysis has been employed widely in the study and clinical management of hematological malignancies, allowing the mapping of the whole genome for numeric and structural chromosomal abnormalities. Most centers, including ours, have incorporated karyotypic analysis to the baseline evaluation of multiple myeloma (MM) patients[1]. However, CC identifies abnormalities in only 10–15% of cases.[2–5] Several factors and technical restrictions are associated with this low detection rate, the most important of which is the low proliferative index (<1%) intrinsic to MM tumor cells (Table 1).[2] Additionally, while numeric and larger structural changes can be routinely identified, certain smaller structural abnormalities remain cryptic, particularly those located in subtelomeric regions, such as the t(4;14)(p16.3;q32).[6] To overcome the low proliferative index, the stimulation of bone marrow specimens with cytokines has been proposed but no consensus has been reached regarding the usefulness of this technique. Despite these limitations, a number of seminal observations have been reported using CC, which have furthered our understanding of the biology of MM as well as contributed to clinical practice.[4,7]

Karyotpic analysis has been paramount in identifying two very important MM subgroups, hyperdiploid (>46 to <76 chromosomes) and nonhyperdiploid (hypodiploid: up to 44–45 chromosomes; pseudodiploid: 44/45 to 46/47 chromosomes with gains/losses; and near tetraploid or hypotetraploid: 75 or more chromosomes), with distinct clinical courses (as discussed later in this chapter).[3,8] The separation of patients into these two genetic groups is further justified by the presence of other genetic abnormalities, which are preferentially found in the nonhyperdiploid group. Patients with the nonhyperdiploid variant of MM have a higher incidence of the three common immunoglobulin heavy chain (IgH) translocations (4p16.3, 11q13, and 16q23 regions; identified in >85%

From: *Contemporary Hematology Myeloma Therapy*
Edited by: S. Lonial © Humana Press, Totowa, NJ

of patients) than do their hyperdiploid counterparts (<30%).[3,9,10] Additionally, nonhyperdiploid MM patients have a higher frequency of chromosome 13 deletion (>70% vs 40%) and a higher proportion of structural chromosomal abnormalities (median 8.7 breaks per karyotype as compared with 4.7 breaks in hyperdiploid MM patients).[3,10] It is interesting to note that aneuploidy and IgH translocations are also seen in the very early stages of MM, suggesting that they may play a role in the initiation of this disease.[11–15] We have recently created a compendium of cytogenetic abnormalities present in MM from the Mittelman database (R Fonseca, unpublished data).

The resolution of CC can be improved using multicolor karyotypic analysis with a technique known as spectral karyotyping (SKY).[16–18] SKY allows the simultaneous visualization of all 23 human chromosome pairs in different colors in the same experiment. This approach is based on the generation of chromosome-specific probe pools, and its subsequent amplification and fluorescent labeling by degenerate oligonucleotide-primed polymerase chain reaction. The ability of SKY analysis to detect complex or equivocal chromosomal rearrangements, as well as to identify the chromosomal origins of the abnormalities, makes this a valuable tool surpassing limitations of CC and fluorescence *in situ* hybridization (FISH). However, this technique is still dependent on the presence of metaphases in MM cells and cannot identify balanced translocation as well as intrachromosomal abnormalities (Table 1).

Fluorescence *in situ* Hybridization

The introduction of FISH has resulted in an expansion in our knowledge of MM genetics and has provided us with an invaluable clinical tool.[19,20] FISH depends upon the hybridization of fluorescent DNA probes with their complementary chromosomal regions and can be performed in the absence of any

Table 1 Comparison of different methodologies utilized in chromosomal abnormatlity studies.

	Metaphase needed?	Impemented in clinical lab	Advantages	Limitations
CC	YES	YES	Grave implications for prognosis Can be done by any laboratory	Largely insensitive Misses many abnormalities
SKY	YES	NO	Higher definition of metaphase abnormalities	Still needs metaphases Unable to detect intrachromosomal abnormalities Technically demanding
FISH	NO	YES	High rate of accuracy and sensitivity Able to detect cryptic abnormalities	Not unblased Unable to analyze the whole genome
CGH	NO	NO	High ability to detect DNA copy changes	Technically demanding Difficulty in implementing in clinical laboratoy
aCGH	NO	NO	High-resolution throughput analysis	Need for analysis tools Difficult to run in a clinical laboratory Misses balanced translocations

CC conventional cytogenetics, FISH fluorescence *in situ* hybridization, SKY spectral karyotyping, CGH comparative genomic hybridization, aCGH array-based CGH.

metaphases. The probes can be target specific, thereby allowing detection of particular and recurrent chromosomal anomalies. In addition, FISH can detect cryptic translocations as well as small deletions and gains. All of these features have allowed us to overcome the limitations of CC and lead to the identification of genetic anomalies in over 90% of MM patients.[21,22]

It is important to note that clonal plasma cells (PCs) coexist with normal myeloid elements in the bone marrow, making it imperative to reliably identify anomalies in PCs and not other cell populations. This can be achieved by purifying PCs prior to FISH analysis using anti-CD 138 antibodies and magnetic bead separation. Alternatively, we have developed a technique, clg-FISH, which combines FISH with immuno-fluorescence designed to identify PCs (Fig. 1).[23] Relatively few cells are necessary to determine the presence or absence of a particular anomaly, as most genetic aberrations of interest are highly selected in the clonal PC population. Scoring few cells results in the almost perfect concordance with the standard of 100–200 cell scoring (R Fonseca, unpublished data). In cases with extensive marrow involvement the exclusion of non-PCs may not be so crucial, but this is difficult to predict *a priori* and the determination of plasmacytosis is typically unreliable.

As FISH relies on the use of specific probes, this technique is restricted to the investigation of known targets and is therefore not useful for whole genome analysis (Table 1).

Comparative Genomic Hybridization

Classic comparative genomic hybridization (CGH) is a FISH-based technique which can identify chromosomal gains, losses, and unbalanced translocations in the entire genome.[24–27] In this technique, normal metaphases are probed by the competitive hybridization of two sets of genomic DNA (tumor and reference) that have each been labeled with a different fluorochrome. The

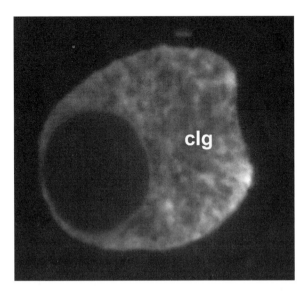

Fig. 1 Plasma cells identification by using kappa or lambda cytoplasmic immunostain (clg).

difference in fluorescence visualized along the metaphase chromosomes is the consequence of the relative amount of tumor DNA compared to reference DNA. This technique improves on the resolution of SKY and, most importantly, does not require the presence of tumoral metaphases (Table 1).

Recently, a high-resolution array-based variant of the CGH technique (aCGH) has been developed and has become a powerful molecular cytogenetic tool for mapping DNA copy number alterations.[28] Genomically mapped oligo-nucleotide probes covering the entire human genome are arrayed onto a slide to which differentially labeled tumor and normal reference DNAs are cohybridized. As in the CGH approach, differences in the relative amount of tumor and normal DNA are represented in the aCGH by variations in fluorescent intensities at the various probe sites (Fig. 2). Newer high-resolution platforms can posses up to 6 million probe sets, which represent approximately an 1 Kb average probe spatial resolution. Even higher resolutions can be achieved with custom-designed arrays. This powerful technique has the ability to quickly and reliably identify both known and unrecognized genetic anomalies in MM patient samples at an unprecedented resolution. We have recently used this technique to uncover abnormalities resulting in noncanonical NFKB pathway activation. [29]

This technique is limited principally by cost and its inability to detect balanced translocations, which are relatively common in MM (Table 1).

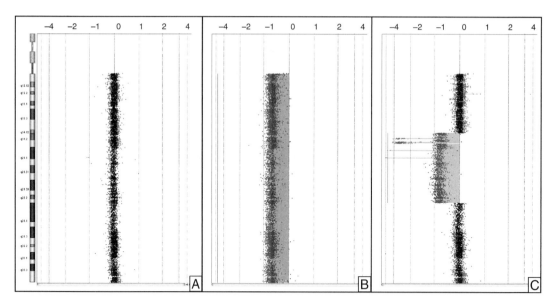

Fig. 2 Chromosome copy number abnormalities analysis by array-based comparative genomic hybridization (aCGH). Patient and reference DNAs are differentially labeled and cohybridized with an array of genomic mapped oligonucleotide probes (represented by dots) covering the entire human genome. The relative amount of tumor and reference DNA is determined from the ratio of the hybridization signal between both DNA sources. Based on this relative amount, the software assigns numerical values to each probe: values around 0 are expected when the amount of patient and reference DNA is similar (**a**); negative values are related to patient copy losses (−1 refers to 1 heterozygous deletion, −2 to −4 homozygous deletion); and positive values are related to patient copy gains (+0.5 refers to one copy gain, +1 to 2 copy gains, etc.). This strategy allows identifying entire copy losses/gains (**b**), as well as interstitial abnormalities (a monoallelic interstitial deletion with four biallelic deleted regions is boxed in (**c**). Different commercial platforms posses up to 6 million probes. The shaded region highlights the area affected by the abnormality.

Specific Chromosome Abnormalities

Chromosomal abnormalities are germane to the development and progression of MM from the premalignant monoclonal gammopathy to undetermined significance (MGUS) to more advanced stages of this disease including plasma cell leukemia (PCL).[30] It has become evident that MM is a progressive disease with distinct clinical stages: MGUS, a premalignant condition with a low tumor burden and no clinical features; smoldering MM (SMM), an asymptomatic stage with a higher tumor burden; MM, a symptomatic disease with tumor restricted to the bone marrow; PCL, an advanced stage with bone marrow-independent tumor growth. Human myeloma cell lines (HMCLs) are usually derived from the most advanced stages of MM, have the ability to grow outside the bone marrow microenvironment, and are thought to harbor the highest number and most complex genetic anomalies. The goal of identifying and characterizing chromosomal alteration in MM is to understand how this disease evolves, to classify patients into prognostic classes based on genetic subgroups as well as to potentially identify specific drug targets.

Deletion of Chromosome 13

Deletion of chromosome 13 ($\Delta13$) is one of the most recurrent abnormalities in MM; however CC detects only 15% of cases as most patients fail to demonstrate metaphases in their tumors.[5] Interphase FISH readily detects $\Delta13$ in 40–50% of newly diagnosed patients (Table 2)[31–34]. Several attempts to map the minimal common deleted region in $\Delta13$ have revealed 13q14 as the most likely affected chromosomal region.[31,34,37] This area harbors the retinoblastoma gene (*RB1*), a tumor suppressor involved in cell cycle regulation, and could therefore be a potential player in the pathogenesis of MM. However, its contribution to disease remains unclear as abnormalities, which are predicted to entirely inactivate *RB1*, such as biallelic deletions, mutations, or epigenetic silencing of the remaining allele, are rare events. Preliminary data have suggested that the commonly seen loss of one *RB1* allele (haploinsufficiency) might alone be responsible for a more aggressive MM cell (R Fonseca, unpublished data).

As $\Delta13$ seems to be clonally selected and therefore present in between 75% and over 90% of tumor clones.[34,36] In MGUS, $\Delta13$ is present at the same prevalence as in MM, indicating that it does not likely contribute to the progression

Table 2 Major chromosomal abnormalities and their respective prevalence by using CC and FISH detection methods.

Abnormality	CC(%)	FISH(%)
$\Delta13$	10–15	40–55
t(4;14)(p16.3;q32)	None	10–15
t(6;14)(p21;q32)		3–4
t(11;14)(q13;q32)	2	15–20
t(14;16)(q32;q23)	None	3–6
$\Delta17p13$	5	5–15
Hypodiploid	9–14	30–35
Hypodiploid	30	50

CC: conventional cytogenetics, FISH: fluorescence in situ hybridization from MGUS to MM,[38] as was initially proposed. While its contribution to the development of MM remains unclear, its association with poor clinical prognosis has been well characterized.[7,9,20,39-47]

Δ13 was the first chromosomal abnormality consistently associated with poor prognosis in MM.[7] To date, numerous studies have shown an association between the presence of Δ13 and a shorter event-free survival (EFS) as well as overall survival (OS).[7,9,20,39-47] This association is independent of treatment options (conventional chemotherapy, high-dose therapy, single or tandem autologous transplantation, and mini allogeneic transplant) and stage (newly diagnosed or pretreated patients). Initial studies identified the role of Δ13 in prognosis using CC alone.[7,39-42] In a cohort of 1,000 patients receiving high-dose meiphalan and stem cell support, a 5-year EFS of 0% was observed in the presence of Δ13 compared with 28% in patients without the deletion ($P < 0.0001$) and a 5-year OS of 16% and 44%, respectively ($P < 0.0001$).[39] Numerous other studies are in agreement on the role of CC-detected Δ13 as a powerful adverse prognostic factor in MM patients treated with standard chemotherapy or high-dose therapy.[7,40-43]

We and others have found that the Δ13 detected by interphase FISH (iFISH) is also an independent prognostic variable.[19,31,35,44,45] Zojer and collaborators have shown that iFISH-detected Δ13 was associated with a significantly lower response rate to conventional chemotherapy *(P = 0.009)* and shorter OS *($P < 0.005$)*[31]. In a study by the *Intergroupe Francophone du Myelome*, the Δ13 detected by iFISH was the most powerful adverse prognostic factor in patients receiving HDT as a first-line therapy.[44] This study revealed that the presence of Δ13 and a high β2m (>2.5 mg/L) are unfavorable prognostic factors, with the median OS reported in cohorts with both (median of 25.3 ± 3.2 months), one (47.3 ± 4.6 months), or no unfavorable factor (median not reached at 111.1 months; $P < 0.0001$). Another study also demonstrated increased tumor proliferation in iFISH-detected Δ13 patients treated with conventional chemotherapy as compared to those without the deletion.[35] In our cohort of 351 newly diagnosed MM patients, we determined that FISH-detected Δ13 was associated with a lower response rate to conventional chemotherapy (74 vs 63%; $P = 0.041$) and was associated with a shorter median OS (34.9 vs 51 months; $P = 0.021$).[19] Moreover, patients with Δ13 detected by iFISH can be stratified into an intermediate prognosis group (median OS of 42.3 months), and show worse prognosis than do patients with t(11;14)(q13;q32) or without abnormalities (median OS 50.5 months), but considerably better prognosis than do patients with other high-risk changes such as t(4;14)(p16.3;q32), t(14;16)(q32;q23), and/or chromosome 17p13 deletion (median OS of 24.7 months; $P < 0.00$ 1)(Fig. 3).[19]

While both CC and iFISH have been used to identify Δ13 as a marker of poor outcome, several reports have suggested that Δ13 detected by CC or metaphase FISH is associated with an even poorer prognosis than those detected by iFISH (Table 3).[43,46-48] A study directly comparing CC to iFISH has shown that the deletion detected by CC was associated with faster relapse (61% vs 38% at 3 years; $P = 0.02$).[43] Interestingly, patients with Δ13 exclusively identified in metaphase cells had poor survival (median survival of 12.7 months), whereas patients with Δ13 solely detected in interphase cells had a better survival (median survival 46.8 months; $P = 0.001$).[46] Additionally, multivariate analysis suggested that patients with Δ13 in metaphase cells have

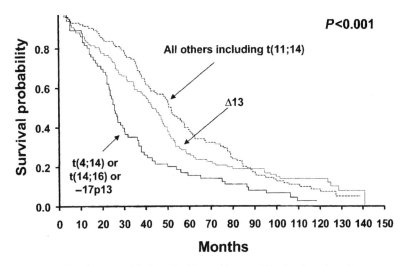

Fig. 5.3 Overall survival of patients stratified by the hierarchic classification based on the presence or absence of five specific chromosomal abnormalities by iFISH. Based on the presence of these abnormalities, it was possible to identify good, intermediate, and poor prognosis groups of patients. The poor prognosis group includes patients with Δ17p13, t(4;14)(p13;q32), and/or t(14;16)(q32;q23); the intermediate prognosis group includes those patients with Δ13 and no high-risk abnormalities; and the good prognosis group includes the remaining patients, including those with the t(11;14)(q13;q32) and none of the aforementioned abnormalities. This research was originally published in *Blood*. Fonseca R, Blood E, Rue M, et al. Clinical and biologic implications of recurrent genomic aberrations in myeloma. *Blood*. 2003;101:4569–4575. © The American Society of Hematology.

Table 3 Clinical outcome of Δ13 based on the detection method utilized.

References	CC			iFISH			N	Median follow-up (months)
	Δ13	No Δ13	P	Δ13	No Δ13	P		
[7]	29	>50	0.001		NA		155	
[39]	16	44	<0.0001		NA		993	10
[40]	19	51	<0.001		NA		984	48
[44]		NA		27±4	65–10	<0.0001	110	48
[19]		NA		35	51	0.028	325	40.5
[31]		NA		24.2	60	<0.005	97	
[45]		NA		14	60	0.0012	48	61
[47]	12.7	45	<0.001	46.8	45	NS	154	26.2
[46]	15	50	<0.001	29	47	<0.001	555–729[a]	22

[a] The numbers correspond to CC and FISH studies, respectively. CC: conventional cytogenetics, iFISH: interphase FISH.

the strongest association with poor survival, whereas all other abnormalities were associated with a better survival.[46] These findings have been supported by other reports.[45,48] In summary, the detection of Δ13 in interphase cells is not as predictive as its observation in metaphase. One reason for the difference in prognostic value is that Δ13 deletion seen in CC is an indicator of the presence of abnormal metaphases and infers a more proliferative clone and higher tumor burden. Its role as a prognostic factor, therefore, could be indirect.

The indirect role of Δ13 as a prognostic factor is further supported by observations, which suggest that it may be found in association with other high-risk abnormalities. Thus, the often seen simultaneous presence of Δ13 with the high-risk abnormalities t(4;14)(p16.3;q32), t(14;16)(q32;q23), chromosome 17p13 deletion (Δ17p13) and hypodiploidy makes the specific relationship between Δ13 and prognosis less clear.[9,20,45] As the sole abnormality, iFISH-detected Δ13 does not correlate with a shorter survival (46 vs 54 months, respectively; $P = 0.3$).[49] In addition, the 10-year survival of patients with Δ13 detected by iFISH is not different from those without the deletion.[34] Another study has shown that, in multivariate studies, Δ13 losses its prognostic value when it is not associated with the presence of t(4;14)(p16.3;q32) or Δ17p13.[20] Finally, we have noted that Δ13 does not change the prognosis of patients with either the hyperdiploid or nonhyperdiploid variants of MM.[49]

The chromosome 13 status was also analyzed in patient response and survival to specific treatment regimens such as dexamethasone and bortezomib. Studies evaluating the treatment of relapsed/refractory MM with bortezomib have reported that the overall response rates were similar in patients with or without Δ13 detected by iFISH.[50,51] Even patients in whom Δ13 has been identified by CC and who are therefore considered high risk do just as well in response to bortezomib as others, showing similar response rate, EFS, and OS.[52] Conversely, patients with CC-determined Δ13 who were treated with dexamethasone as a single agent showed worse prognosis than did patients without the deletion $(P = 0.002)$. While the duration of follow-up was not optimal in this study, it is nonetheless still compelling to conclude that bortezomib (not dexamethasone) might be useful to overcome the adverse impact of CC-detected Δ13. Furthering this conclusion, the use of bortezomib as upfront therapy (in combination with melphalan and prednisone) in elderly patients may also appear to overcome the poor prognosis conferred by Δ13[54].

IgH Translocations

Translocations involving the *IgH* gene are common events in MM pathogenesis.[54] The prevalence of this abnormality is closely related to the detection method utilized; in MGUS and MM, the IgH translocations are identified in ~10–20% by CC and in 50% by FISH (Table 2). The prevalence increases significantly in more advance stages, seen in up to 80% of PCL cases and of 90% in HMCLs.[55]

Primary immunoglobulin translocations are believed to be an initiating event in MM genesis for 50% of cases.[14,55] They are the consequence of errors in the normal process of B-cell-specific DNA modification, mostly switch recombination and occasionally somatic hypermutation.[55,56] This mechanism results in the juxtaposition of an IgH enhancer and a proto-oncogene partner, leading to the overexpression of the latter. Primary IgH translocations are clonally selected, as they are identifiable in practically all tumor cells.[19,20] In addition, they are detected with the same frequency in both MGUS and MM, supporting their role as initiating events. In contrast, secondary IgH translocations result from the genomic instability seen during the progression of MM. These are structurally complex and rarely exhibit breakpoints within the switch or J regions.[55]

The most frequent partners of primary IgH translocations in MM are 11q13 (*CCND1* gene, identified in 15% of patients); 4p16.3 (*MMSET* and *FGFR3*, 15%); 16q23 (*C-MAF*, 6%); 6p21 (*CCND3*, 3%).[57] Other regions like 20q11

(*MAF-B*) and 6q25 (IRF4/*MUM1*) are present in less than 1% of MM patients or were identified only in HMCLs. Finally, the IgH locus rearranges with unidentified partners in 20–30% of MM cases. Each of these recurrent primary translocations is associated with a distinct prognostic outcome.[19,20,58]

Cyto-molecular techniques are generally required to consistently and reliably identify IgH translocations. Depending on its partners, the subtelomeric localization of IgH makes detection of those translocations a challenge. For example, the characteristically cryptic abnormality is the t(4;14)(p16.3;q32), as both regions involved in the translocation have subtelomeric localizations (Fig. 4) and can be identified only using cyto-molecular techniques.[6] Other recurrent IgH translocations, such as t(14;16)(q32;q23) and t(6;14)(p21;q32), are only rarely detectable by CC but can be reliably identified by FISH. In the detection of IgH translocations involving unknown chromosomal partners, the dual-color break-apart FISH is a very useful approach. This strategy uses two differentially colored probes, one of which covers the entire IgH constant region while the other extends to the 3 region of *IgH* locus. Any translocation with a breakpoint within the J segments or switch regions produce separate and differentially colored signals (Fig. 5). This is the ideal detection strategy where a known breakpoint in 14q32 is associated with a number of translocation partners, some of which remain unidentified.

t(11;14)(q13;q32)

The t(11;14)(q13;q32) results in the juxtaposition of *CCND1* proto-oncogene (cyclin Dl) with the IgH locus.[58] Cyclin Dl is an important regulator of the transition from the G1 to S-phase of the cell cycle. Its presence results in the activation of cyclin-dependent kinases 4 and 6 (*CDK4/6*), which leads to the hyperphosphorylation of the RB protein, then resulting in the release of E2F transcription factors and the subsequent expression of a group of genes required for the entrance into the S-phase of the cell cycle.

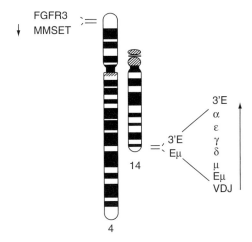

Fig. 4 The t(4;14)(p16.3;q32) is cryptic and cyto-molecular techniques are necessary for its detection. Both chromosome regions involved (p16.3 and q32) have subtelomeric localization and the translocated chromosome is unable to be detected by CC. FISH and/or RT-PCR techniques can be used in its detection. This research was originally published in Dalton et al.[59] The American Society of Hematology.

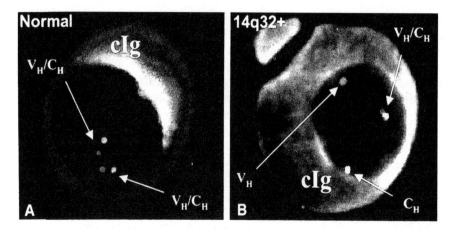

Fig. 5 Dual-color break-apart FISH. This strategy uses two differentially colored probes, one of which covers the entire IgH constant region (CH) while the other extends to the 3′ region of IgH locus (VH). Normal cells exhibit the expected two fusion signal pattern (**a**), whereas any translocation with a breakpoint within the J segments or switch regions produce separate signals (**b**). This is a useful detection strategy in MM where a known breakpoint in 14q32 is associated with a number of translocation partners, some of which remain unidentified. This research was originally published in Fonseca R et al.[37] © The American Society of Hematology.

Both techniques, CC and FISH, may be used in the detection of t(11;14) (q13;q32) in MM and result in a prevalence of 5% and 15%, respectively (Table 2).[9,19,20] Similar frequencies have been reported in MGUS, SMM.[37]

The t(11;14)(q13;q32) is found in a high proportion of MM patients with the IgM variant (90%) and light-chain amyloidosis (50%).[19,20,60–62] This translocation is associated with low plasma cell proliferation indices, low levels of cell surface CD2O expression and serum monoclonal proteins, as well as a lymphoplasmacytic or small mature PC morphology.[64,65] In addition, K-RAS mutations are also more prevalent among myeloma patients with t(11;14)(q13;q32) (50%) than in patients with the other primary IgH translocations (10%).[66]

In a cohort of 351 patients, we have shown that those who harbor only t(11;14)(q13;q32) detected by FISH have a much better prognosis than do patients with either of the other IgH translocations, Δ13 or Δl7pl3 (Fig. 3).[19] Most studies have suggested that the presence alone of t(11;14)(q13;q32) may confer a better prognosis.[9,20,65,67] However, this difference in prognosis has never reached statistical significance (i.e., probably real but of a small magnitude). In contrast, data obtained from long-period survivors have not shown a relative increase in the proportion of patients with t(11;14)(q13;q32).

The presence of t(11;14)(q13;q32) has been evaluated in a number of studies as a marker of therapeutic outcome. In patients treated with conventional or high-dose chemotherapy and stem cell support, t(11;14)(q13;q32) has not been associated with a poor EFS and OS.[9,20,67,68] Results from our cohort of 351 patients, treated with conventional chemotherapy, have suggested that patients with t(11;14)(q13;q32) have an increase in OS (50 months, CI = 37–60) compared to those without translocation (OS = 39; CI = 36–44).[19] However, this difference does not reach statistic significance *(P = 0.332)*. A similar finding was observed in the progression-free survival (PFS) data, with values of 33 (range of 28–45 months) and 27 months (25–31) in patients with and without the abnormality, respectively.[19] Patients treated exclusively with high-dose therapy show no differences in PFS (20.1 vs 15.3 months in patients with and without the translocation) and OS (36.6 vs 34.8, respectively), in a 197-patient study.[67] Finally, a French trial of 168 patients, receiving high-dose therapy with a median follow-up of 27 months, reported a trend to longer OS in patients with t(11;14)(q13;q32) (P = 0.055)[68]. At the very least, it is clear that t(11;14)(q13;q32) does not confer an unfavorable outcome following therapeutic intervention irrespective of the method used for its detection (CC or FISH).[19,20]

t(4;14)(p16.3;q32)

A t(4;14)(p16.3;q32) leads to the dysregulation of two proto-oncogenes: *MMSET* in derivative chromosome 4 (der4) and *FGFR3* in derivate chromosome 14 (der 14).[6] The t(4;14)(p16.3;q32) translocation is cryptic, and therefore impossible to detect by CC but can be detected by FISH. In addition, the breakpoints in both chromosomes were elucidated by cloning experiments in HMCLs, allowing the reverse transcription polymerase chain reaction (RT-PCR) of the IgH-MMSET hybrid transcript to be used for detection.[6]

The translocation is seen in 15% of primary MM samples and 25% of HMCLs (Table 2).[19,20,69] Its frequency in premalignant stages is still controversial, with some reports showing up to 10% in MGUS, whereas others have failed to observe it.[3,37,70] In contrast, its presence in SMM patients is well established with a reported frequency similar to that of MM.[37]

Unbalanced translocations are commonly observed, with loss of the der14 (FGFR3) seen in 25% of cases.[19,20,70] Conversely, loss of the der4 (MMSET) has yet to be reported, suggesting that MMSET may play a crucial role in the clonal expansion of t(4;14)(p16.3;q32) MM cells.[19,20,70] In contrast, the acquisition of FGFR3-activating mutations has been observed in later stages of MM progression, thus suggesting that its deregulation could be an important event in pathogenesis, as well.[6] Finally, t(4;14)(p16.3;q32) is more prevalent among patients with IgA myeloma as well as in patients with aggressive clinical features.[19,68,69]

The t(4;14)(p16.3;q32) detected by FISH is an unfavorable prognostic factor for MM patients independent of treatment type. Several studies, which include more than 1,500 patients in total, have demonstrated an association with an unfavorable prognosis and a lower OS in patients receiving diverse treatment regimens such as conventional chemotherapy, high-dose therapy, single or tandem transplant, and thalidomide.[19,20,46,67,68,69,71] A large French trial, including 936 patients (median follow-up of 40.1 months), treated with high-dose therapy and stem cell support has shown an EFS significantly shorter in patients with t(4;14)(p16.3;q32) than those without the abnormality, with values of 20.6 and 36.5 months (P < 0.001), respectively.[20] The median OS of t(4;14)(p16.3;q32) patients was 32.8 versus not reached for patients without the abnormality (expected survival at 80 months of 22.8% vs 66%; P = 0.002). In another study, including 153 patients treated with high-dose chemotherapy and stem cell support, the time to progression for patients with and without t(4;14)(p16.3;q32) was 8.2 months versus 17.8 months (P = 0.001), whereas the OS was 18.8 and 43.9 months (P = 0.001), respectively.[67] In the same study, it was shown that patients who had transplantation upfront in first response, the t(4;14)(p16.3;q32) retained its significance; thus, the median survival rates were 75 months for patients without the translocation and 29 months for those with the translocation *(P = 0.01)*. Incidentally, there have been no reports of survival differences between t(4;14)(p16.3;q32) patients with or without *FGFR3* overexpression.[68] The detection of the t(4;l4)(p16.3;q32) translocation therefore identifies high-risk patients who do not obtain benefits from conventional chemotherapy or even HDT.[67,72]

Initial results in relapsed/refractory MM patients treated with bortezomib have shown that the response rates are not statistically different in patients with or without t(4;14)(p16.3;q32).[73] This study, including 41 relapsed/refractory patients, has shown response rates of 67% and 56% in patients without and with t(4;l4)(p16.3;q32), respectively *(P = 0.68)*.[72] In addition, the differences in EFS and OS were not statistically significant in patients with and without the translocation.[73] This suggests that bortezomib may be an effective salvage therapy irrespective of the presence of genetic high-risk factors.[73] Furthermore, these results indicate that patients with t(4;l4)(p16.3;q32) may benefit most from either upfront nonconventional or investigational approaches as they seem not to benefit from conventional approaches, and have a response to "novel" therapies that is equivalent to those without t(4;14)(p16.3;q32). Finally, t(4;14)(p16.3;q32) also represents a unique opportunity to investigate the potential of targeted therapies specific to this translocation, for example, FGFR3 inhibitors.[75,76]

Other IgH Translocations

The t(14;16)(q32;q23), t(14;20)(q32;q12), and t(8;20)(q24;q12) result in the overexpression of transcription factors belonging to the MAF family.[58,77] These translocations are very difficult to detect by CC, but are identifiable by FISH in 2–5% of patients (Table 2). These abnormalities were associated with a shorter survival among patients treated with conventional or tandem transplant-based chemotherapy.[19,20,78]

The t(6;l4)(p2l;q32) is identified in only 3% of MM patients and leads to *CCND3* (cyclin D3) upregulation (Table 2)[78]. The t(6;14)(p21;q32) shares a gene expression signature with t(11;14)(q13;q32) and, as such, they may be considered as one entity for the purposes of disease biology, prognosis, and clinical outcome.[58]

17p13 Deletion

The target of the Δl7p13 is the *TP53* tumor suppressor gene p53, implicated in the regulation of cell proliferation, differentiation, and apoptosis.

Δ 17pl3 is a rare event, detected in only 5–10% of MM patients at diagnosis, but it becomes much more common in advance stages of disease.[19,20,80,81,82,83] To date, there are no reports of Δ17pl3 in MGUS. As in the case of Δl3, Δl7pl3 is generally monoallelic; however, inactivating mutations of p53 have been reported with a prevalence of 5% at diagnosis, increasing to 20–40% in advanced MM and PCL and to 60% in HMCLs (R Fonseca and M Kuehl, unpublished observations)[83]. Of note, the simultaneous presence of Δ17p13 and t(4;l4)(p16.3;q32) is unusual, suggesting that these are mutually exclusive abnormalities.[20] In one report, we found that these deletions are also cryptic as CC could identify correctly only 5 out of 9 deletions detectable by FISH (Table 2).[47]

This abnormality has been associated with development of hypercalcemia, extramedullary disease, central nervous system involvement, high-serum creatinine levels, and plasmacytomas.[19,20,67,72,84] Chromosome 17 deletions are an important negative prognostic factor, irrespective of the detection method.[47,67] Patients with this abnormality generally have a shorter PFS and OS after conventional and high-dose therapy with autologous stem cell transplantation.[19,20,47,67] In addition, patients with Δ7pl3 treated with conventional chemotherapy show a lower response rate than do those without the abnormality.[81]

In contrast, the prognostic implications of p53 mutations are not well established.[83]

1q21 Amplification

Copy number gains/amplifications of the 1q21 locus are among the most commonly reported genetic abnormalities seen in MM.[3,25,84,85] A putative target of this amplification is *CKS1B*, which promotes the degradation of p27, an inhibitor of cell cycle progression. FISH has readily detected copy number gains of 1q21 in around one third of MM patients.[88] Patients with 1q21 gains have a higher prevalence of Δ13 and t(4;14)(p16.3;q32). A recent study from the University of Arkansas has identified this region to be involved in the development of myeloma growth and survival in aggressive disease.[87] A recently published high-risk genetic signature for MM, also derived by the University of Arkansas, is highly enriched for chromosome 1 genes and includes *CKS1B*.[87] We[89] and others[90] have been unable to confirm the overriding importance of chromosome 1 abnormalities as detected by FISH in establishing the prognosis of MM patients.

Ploidy Status

Aneuploidy is frequently observed in MM and delineates this disease into two major subtypes: hyperdiploid and nonhyperdiploid.[3,8,9,91] Hyperdiploid MM patients exhibit multiple trisomies, especially of chromosomes 3, 5, 7, 9, 11, 15, 19 and 21.[3,8,9] The preferential presence of this pattern of trisomies is still unclear. For those with nonhyperdiploid disease, the most frequent changes include monosomies of chromosomes 13, 14, 16, and 22.[3,21] However, both trisomies and monosomies can be seen in both these subtypes.

Conventional cytogenetics typically fails to estimate ploidy status among MM patients. FISH strategies have been developed to identify ploidy status by employing multiple centromeric probes to detect hyperdiploidy. The probe choice is based on the most common trisomies observed in hyperdiploid MM and not all possible combinations can be practicable in each patient. Therefore, this approach can never detect all possible trisomy combinations and hyperdiploid patients; nonetheless it seems to have a high reliability in a high proportion of MM cases. This strategy was employed by our group to report the existence of hyperdiploid MGUS[11]. In contrast, the detection of hypodiploidy is more technically demanding using these same strategies.

Patients with hyperdiploid MM are more frequently older males with IgG kappa myeloma and symptomatic bone disease.[50] Hyperdiploid patients who also harbor IgH translocations appear to have a more aggressive clinical course.[50] Finally, in patients with hyperdiploid MM, the presence of Δ13 carries no significant prognostic implication, while Δ17pl3 remains an important predictor of outcome.[84]

Best Technique to Use in the Clinic?

The cytogenetic and molecular data collected in MM over the last 10 years have allowed us to stratify patients into distinct groups that differ in their biology, clinical course, and response to treatments. FISH has been incorporated successfully in clinical practice as it promises several technical advantages over CC, such as the possibility of obtaining results using interphase nuclei, the ability to more accurately determine the number of PCs with aberrations as well as to detect cryptic anomalies. On the basis of the identification of five chromosomal abnormalities by iFISH, we were able to identify three well-differentiated prognostic groups: a poor prognostic group, characterized by the presence of t(4;14)(p16.3;q32), t(14;16)(q32;q23), and/or Δl7pl3; an intermediate group with the presence of Δ13 but without any high-risk cytogenetic abnormality; and a good prognostic group, involving patients with t(l1;14)(q13;q32) or without any other high- or intermediate-risk abnormalities.The presence of any metaphase abnormality by CC or mFISH and hypodiploidy are considered to confer a poor prognosis. As such, Δ13 by CC or mFISH as well as hypodiploidy need to be added to the definition of the aforementioned poor prognostic group. While technically limited, CC still plays a role and is recommended in the evaluation of MM patients.

In summary, the detection of t(4;14)(p16.3;q32), t(14;16)(q32;q23), and Δl7pl3 by iFISH, as well as Δ13 or hypodiploidy by CC, now defines the high-risk prognostic group. The detection of high-risk abnormalities is fundamental in identifying a subgroup of patients that may not fully benefit from conventional treatment approaches and is therefore more appropriately shuttled to investigational strategies. Promising results were obtained with bortezomib as front-line therapy or in the refractory/relapsed setting, showing that the response rate is independent of the presence of high-risk abnormalities.[51-54] This approach has been published by our group in a recent article and is referred to as the mSMART approach.[92] Finally, with accurate detection of appropriate patients, clinical trials of targeted therapies, such as FGFR3 kinase inhibitors in patients with t(4;14)(p16.3;q32), can now be undertaken.[74,75]

On the basis of the available data, we recommend a combination of CC and FISH in the evaluation of all MM patients, focusing on the identification of high-risk patients with t(4;14)(p16.3;q32), t(14;16)(q32;q23), and Δ17p13 by iFISH and Δ13 and hypodiploidy by CC (Table 4). Other putative high-risk translocations, such as t(14;20)(q32;q12) and t(8;20)(q24;q12), have a very low prevalence (<2%), are generally associated with other poor prognostic abnormalities (Δ13, hypodiploidy), and are therefore not a priority for inclusion into routine testing. In the absence of high-risk abnormalities, patients are by default included in a low-risk group, irrespective of the presence of good prognosis markers such as t(6;14)(p21;q32) and t(11;14)(q13;q32) detected by iFISH and hyperdiploidy detected by CC. Therefore, detection of the latter abnormalities is optional in the routine genetic evaluation of MM patients (Table 4).

Other cytogenetic-molecular classifications have been proposed, including one which exploits the expression levels of known IgH translocation target genes and the cyclin D genes.[58] Additional techniques such as aCGH are now successfully used in the high-resolution whole genome mapping of chromosome abnormalities, and it could be implemented in the clinical lab in the

Table 4 Recommendation of the method to be used in the study of the major chromosomal abnormalities with prognostic value.

Abnormality	Prognosis	Method of detection	Priority
t(4;14)(p16.3;q32)	Poor	FISH	High
t(14;16)(q32;q23)	Poor	FISH	High
Δ17p13	Poor	FISH	High
Δ13	Poor	Karyotype	High
Hypodiploidy	Poor	Karyotype	High
Hypodiploidy	Good	FISH	Intermediate
t(11;14)(q13;q32)	Good	FISH	Intermediate
t(14;20)(q32;q12)	Poor	FISH	Low
t(8;20)(q24;q12)	Poor	FISH	Low
t(6;14)(p21;q32)	Good	FISH	Low

The level of priority to be implemented these assays in laboratorial routine is based on risk and prevalence of the abnormalities. CC: conventional cytogenetics, FISH: fluorescence *in situ* hybridization

next years, helping to design more accurate cyto-molecular classifications. However, the cytogenetic classification is still very useful in routine labs, with the advantage of being easily realized in every center by using only CC and FISH techniques.

References

1. Dispenzieri A, Rajkumar SV, Gertz MA, et al. Treatment of newly diagnosed multiple myeloma based on Mayo Stratification of Myeloma and Risk-adapted Therapy (mSMART): Consensus statement. Mayo Clin Proc. 2007;82:323–341.
2. Rajkumar SV, Fonseca R, Dewald GW, et al. Cytogenetic abnormalities correlate with the plasma cell labeling index and extent of bone marrow involvement in myeloma. Cancer Genet Cytogenet. 1999;113:73–77.
3. Debes-Marun C, Dewald G, Bryant S, et al. Chromosome abnormalities clustering and its implications for pathogenesis and prognosis in myeloma. Leukemia. 2003;17:427–436.
4. Dewald GW, Kyle RA, Hicks GA, Greipp PR. The clinical Significance of Cytogenetic Studies in 100 Patients With Multiple Myeloma, Plasma Cell Leukemia, or Amyloidosis. Blood. 1985;66:380–390.
5. Sawyer JR, Waidron JA, Jagannath S, Barlogie B. Cytogenetic findings in 200 patients with multiple myeloma. Cancer Genet Cytogenet. 1995;82:41–49.
6. Chesi M, Nardini E, Brents LA, et al. Frequent translocation t(4;l4)(p16.3;q32.3) in multiple myeloma is associated with increased expression and activating mutations of fibroblast growth factor receptor 3. Nature Genetics. 1997;16:260–264.
7. Tricot G, Barlogie B, Jagannath S, et al. Poor prognosis in multiple myeloma is associated only with partial or complete deletions of chromosome 13 or abnormalities involving 1 lq and not with other karyotype abnormalities. Blood. 1995;86:4250–4256.
8. Smadja NV, Fruchart C, Isnard F, et al. Chromosomal analysis in multiple myeloma: Cytogenetic evidence of two different diseases. Leukemia. 1998;12:960–969.
9. Fonseca R, Debes-Marun CS, Picken EB, et al. The recurrent IgH translocations are highly associated with nonhyperdiploid variant multiple myeloma. Blood. 2003;102:2562–2567.
10. Smadja NV, Leroux D, Soulier J, et al. Further cytogenetic characterization of multiple myeloma confirms that 14q32 translocations are a very rare event in hyperdiploid cases. Genes, Chromosomes & Cancer. 2003;38:234–239.

11. Chng WJ, Van Wier SA, Ahmann GJ, et al. A validated FISH trisomy index demonstrates the hyperdiploid and nonhyperdiploid dichotomy in MGUS. Blood. 2005;106:2156–2161.

12. Drach J, Angerler J, Schuster J, et al. Interphase fluorescence *in situ* hybridization identifies chromosomal abnormalities in plasma cells from patients with mono-clonalgammopathy of undetermined significance. Blood. 1995;86:3915–3921.

13. Zandecki M, Obein V, Bernardi F, et al. Monoclonal gammopathy of undetermined significance: Chromosome changes are a common finding within bone marrow plasma cells. Br. J. Haematol. 1995;90:693–696.

14. Bergsagel PL, Chesi M, Brents LA, et al. Translocations into IgH switch regions – the genetic hallmark of multiple myeloma. Blood. 1995;86:223.

15. Bergsagel PL, Chesi M, Nardini E, et al. Promiscuous translocations into immu-noglobulin heavy chain switch regions in multiple myeloma. Proc. Natl. Acad. Sci. USA. 1996;93(24):13931–13936.

16. Jalal SM, Law ME. Utility of multicolor fluorescent *in situ* hybridization in clinical cytogenetics. Genet Med. 1999;1:181–186.

17. Avet-Loiseau H, Daviet A, Brigaudeau C, et al. Cytogenetic, interphase, and mul-ticolor fluorescence *in situ* hybridization analyses in primary plasma cell leuke-mia: a study of 40 patients at diagnosis, on behalf of the Intergroupe Francophone du Myelome and the Groupe Francais de Cytogenetique Hematologique. Blood. 2001;97:822–825.

18. Rao PH, Cigudosa JC, Ning Y, et al. Multicolor spectral karyotyping identi-fies new recurring breakpoints and translocations in multiple myeloma. Blood. 1998;92:1743–1748.

19. Fonseca R, Blood E, Rue M, et al. Clinical and biologic implications of recurrent genomic aberrations in myeloma. Blood. 2003;101:4569–4575.

20. Avet-Loiseau H, Attal M, Moreau P, et al. Genetic abnormalities and survival in multiple myeloma: the experience of the Intergroupe Francophone du Myelome. Blood. 2007;109:3489–3495.

21. Tabernero D, San Miguel JF, Garcia-Sanz M, et al. Incidence of chromosome numerical changes in multiple myeloma: Fluorescence in situ hybridization analy-sis using 15 chromosome-specific probes. Am. J. Pathol. 1996;149:153–161.

22. Drach J, Schuster J, Nowotny H, et al. Multiple myeloma: High incidence of chro-mosomal aneuploidy as detected by interphase fluorescence in situ hybridization. Cancer Res. 1995;55:3854–3859.

23. Ahman GJ, Jalal SM, Juneau AL, et al. A Novel Three-Color, Clone-specific Fluorescence In situ Hybridization Procedure for Monoclonal Gammopathies. Cancer Genet Cytogenet. 1998;101:7–11.

24. Kallioniemi OP, Kallioniemi A, Sudar D, et al. Comparative genomic hybridization: A rapid new method for detecting and mapping DNA amplification in tumors. Semin Cancer Biol. 1993;4:41–6.

25. Carrasco DR, Tonon U, Huang Y, et al. High-resolution genomic profiles define distinct clinico-pathogenetic subgroups of multiple myeloma patients. Cancer Cell. 2006;9:313–325.

26. Avet-Loiseau H, Bataille R. Detection of nonrandom chromosomal changes in multiple myeloma by comparative genomic hybridization. Blood. 1998;92: 2997–2998.

27. Rao PH. Comparative genomic hybridization for analysis of changes in DNA copy number in multiple myeloma. Methods in Molecular Medicine. 2005;113:71–83.

28. Pinkel D, Segraves R, Sudar D, et al. High resolution analysis of DNA copy number variation using comparative genomic hybridization to microarrays. Nat. Genet. 1998;20:207–211.

29. Keats JJ, Fonseca R, Chesi M, et al. Promiscuous mutations activate the noncanoni-cal NF-kappaB pathway in multiple myeloma. Cancer Cell 2007;12:131–144

30. Bergsagel PL, Kuehi WM. Molecular pathogenesis and a consequent classification of multiple myeloma. J Clin Oncol. 2005;23:6333–6338.

31. Zojer N, Konigsberg R, Ackermann J, et al. Deletion of 13q14 remains an independent adverse prognostic variable in multiple myeloma despite its frequent detection by interphase fluorescence in situ hybridization. Blood. 2000;95:1925–1930.

32. Dao DD, Sawyer JR, Epstein J, et al. Deletion of the retinoblastoma gene in multiple myeloma. Leukemia. 1994;8:1280–1284.

33. Avet-Loiseau H, Daviet A, Sauner S, et al. Chromosome 13 abnormalities in multiple myeloma are mostly monosomy 13. Br J Haematol. 2000;111:1116–1117.

34. Fonseca R, Oken MM, Harrington D, et al. Deletions of chromosome 13 in multiple myeloma identified by interphase FISH usually denote large deletions of the q arm or monosomy. Leukemia. 2001;15:981–986.

35. Fonseca R, Harrington D, Oken M, et al. Biologic and prognostic significance of interphase FISH detection of chromosome 13 abnormalities (A 13) in multiple myeloma: An Eastern Cooperative Oncology Group (ECOG) Study. Cancer Research. 2002;62:715–720.

36. Avet-Loiseau H, Li JY, Morineau N, et al. Monosomy 13 is associated with the transition of monoclonal gammopathy of undetermined significance to multiple myeloma. Intergroupe Francophone du Myelome. Blood. 1999;94:2583–2589.

37. Shaughnessy J, Tian E, Sawyer J, . High incidence of chromosome 13 deletion in multiple myeloma detected by multiprobe interphase FISH. Blood. 2000;96:1505–1511.

38. Fonseca R, Bailey RJ, Ahmann GJ, et al. Genomic abnormalities in monoclonal gammopathy of undetermined significance. Blood. 2002;100:1417–1424.

39. Desikan R, Barlogie B, Sawyer J, et al. Results of high-dose therapy for 1000 patients with multiple myeloma: durable complete remissions and superior survival in the absence of chromosome 13 abnormalities. Blood. 2000;95:4008–4010.

40. Fassas AB, Tricot G. Chromosome 13 deletionlhypodiploidy and prognosis in multiple myeloma patients. Leukemia & Lymphoma. 2004;45:1083–1091.

41. Seong C, Delasalle K, Hayes K, et al. Prognostic value of cytogenetics in multiple myeloma. Br J Haematol. 1998;101:189–194.

42. Shaughnessy J, Jacobson J, Sawyer J, et al. Continuous absence of metaphasedefined cytogenetic abnormalities, especially of chromosome 13 and hypodiploidy, ensures long-term survival in multiple myeloma treated with Total Therapy I: Interpretation in the context of global gene expression. Blood. 2003;101:3849–3856.

43. Shaughnessy J, Jr., Tian E, Sawyer J, et al. Prognostic impact of cytogenetic and interphase fluorescence in situ hybridization-defined chromosome 13 deletion in multiple myeloma: early results of total therapy II. British Journal of Haematology. 2003;120:44–52.

44. Facon T, Avet-Loiseau H, Guillerm G, et al. Chromosome 13 abnormalities identified by FISH analysis and serum beta-2-microglobulin produce a powerful myeloma staging system for patients receiving high-dose therapy. Blood. 2001;97:1566–1571.

45. Perez-Simon JA, Garcia-Sanz R, Tabernero MD, et al. Prognostic value of numerical chromosome aberrations in multiple myeloma: A FISH analysis of 15 different chromosomes. Blood. 1998;91:3366–3371.

46. Chiecchio L, Protheroe RK, Ibrahim AH, et al. Deletion of chromosome 13 detected by conventional cytogenetics is a critical prognostic factor in myeloma. Leukemia. 2006;20:1610–1617.

47. Dewald GW, Therneau T, Larson D, et al. Relationship of patient survival and chromosome anomalies detected in metaphase and/or interphase cells at diagnosis of myeloma. Blood. 2005;106:3553–3558.

48. Tricot G, Sawyer JIR, Jagannath S, et al. Unique role of cytogenetics in the prognosis of patients with myeloma receiving high-dose therapy and autotransplants. J Clin Oncol. 1997;15:2659–2666.

49. Gutierrez NC, Castellanos MV, Martin ML, et al. Prognostic and biological implications of genetic abnormalities in multiple myeloma undergoing autologous stem cell transplantation: t(4; 14) is the most relevant adverse prognostic factor, whereas RB deletion as a unique abnormality is not associated with adverse prognosis. Leukemia. 2007;21:143–150.

50. Chng WJ, Santana-Davila R, Van Wier SA, et al. Prognostic factors for hyperdiploid-myeloma: effects of chromosome 13 deletions and IgH translocations. Leukemia. 2006;20:807–813.

51. Chang H, Trieu Y, Qi X, Xu W, Stewart KA, Reece D. Bortezomib therapy response is independent of cytogenetic abnormalities in relapsed/refractory multiple myeloma. Leuk Res. 2007;31:779–782.

52. Sagaster V, Ludwig H, Kaufmann H, Odelga V, Zojer N, Ackermann J, Kuenburg E, Wieser R, Zielinski C, Drach J. Bortezomib in relapsed multiple myeloma: Response rates and duration of response are independent of a chromosome 13q-deletion. Leukemia. 2007;21:164–168.

53. Jagannath S, Richardson PG, Sonneveld P, et al. Bortezomib appears to overcome the poor prognosis conferred by chromosome 13 deletion in phase 2 and 3 trials. Leukemia. 2007;21:151–157.

54. Mateos MV, Hernandez JIM, Hernandez MT, et al. Bortezomib plus melphalan and prednisone in elderly untreated patients with multiple myeloma: Results of a multicenter phase I/H study. Blood. 2006;108:2165–2172.

55. Bergsagel PL, Kuehl WM. Chromosome translocations in multiple myeloma. Oncogene. 2001;20:5611–5622.

56. Nishida K, Tamura A, Nakazawa N, et al. The Ig heavy chain gene is frequently involved in chromosomal translocations in multiple myeloma and plasma cell leukemia as detected by *in situ* hybridization. Blood. 1997;90:526–534.

57. Bergsagel PL, Kuehl WM. Critical roles for immunoglobulin translocations and cyclin D dysregulation in multiple myeloma. Immunological Reviews. 2003;194:96–104.

58. Bergsagel PL, Kuehi WM, Zhan F, et al. Cyclin D dysregulation: an early and unifying pathogenic event in multiple myeloma. Blood. 2005;106:296–303.

59. Dalton WS, Bergsagel PL, Kuehl WM, et al. Multiple Myeloma. Hematology Am Soc Hematol Educ Program. 2001;157–177.

60. Chesi M, Bergsagel PL, Brents LA, Smith CM, Gerhard DS, Kuehi WM. Dysregulation of cyclin Dl by translocation into an IgH gamma switch region in two multiple myeloma cell lines. Blood. 1996;88:674–681.

61. Fonseca R, Witzig TE, Gertz MA, et al. Multiple myeloma and the translocation t(1 1;14)(q13;q32): A report on 13 cases. Br J Haematol. 1998;101:296–301.

62. Harrison C, Mazullo H, Cheung K, et al. Chromosomal abnormalities in systemic amyloidosis. Proceedings of the VIII International Myeloma Workshop. Banff, Alberta, Canada; 2001:P18.

63. Hayman SR, Bailey RJ, Jalal SM, et al. Translocations involving heavy-chain locus are possible early genetic events in patients with primary systemic amyloidosis. Blood. 2001;98:2266–2268.

64. Garand R, Avet-Loiseau H, Accard F, et al. t(11; 14) and t(4; 14) translocations correlated with mature lymphoplasmocytoid and immature morphology, respectively, in multiple myeloma. Leukemia. 2003;17:2032–2035.

65. Fonseca R, Blood EA, Oken MM, et al. Myeloma and the t(11; 1 4)(q 13;q32); evidence for a biologically defined unique subset of patients. Blood. 2002;99:3735–3741.

66. Rasmussen T, Kuehl M, Lodahl M, Johnsen HE, Dahl IM. Possible roles for activating RAS mutations in the MGUS to MM transition and in the intramedullary to extramedullary transition some plasma cell tumors. Blood. 2005;105:317–323.

67. Gertz MA, Lacy MQ, Dispenzieri A, et al. Clinical implications of t(1 1;14)(q13;q32), t(4;14)(p16.3;q32), and -Ylpl3 in myeloma patients treated with high-dose therapy. Blood. 2005;106:2837–2840.

68. Moreau P, Facon T, Leleu X, et al. Recurrent 14q32 translocations determine the prognosis of multiple myeloma, especially in patients receiving intensive chemotherapy. Blood. 2002;100:1579–1583.

69. Keats JJ, Reiman T, Maxwell CA, et al. In multiple myeloma, t(4;14)(p16;q32) is an adverse prognostic factor irrespective of FGFR3 expression. Blood. 2003;101:1520–1529.

70. Avet-Loiseau H, Facon T, Daviet A, et al. 1 4q32 translocations and monosomy 13 observed in monoclonal gammopathy of undetermined significance delineate a multistep process for the oncogenesis of multiple myeloma. Intergroupe Francophone du Myelome. Cancer Res. 1999;59:4546–4550.

71. Fonseca R, Oken MM, Greipp PR, Eastern Cooperative Oncology Group Myeloma G. The t(4; l4.)(pl6.3;q3 2) is strongly associated with chromosome 13 abnormalities in both multiple myeloma and monoclonal of undetermined significance. Blood. 2001;98:1271–1272.

72. Chang H, Qi XY, Samiee S, et al. Genetic risk identifies multiple myeloma patients who do not benefit from autologous stem cell transplantation. Bone Marrow Transplant. 2005;36:793–796.

73. Chang H, Trieu Y, Qi X, et al. Bortezomib therapy response is independent of cytogenetic abnormalities in relapsed/refractory multiple myeloma. Leuk Res. 2006;31:779–782.

74. Mulligan G, Mitsiades C, Bryant B, et al. Gene expression profiling and correlation with outcome in clinical trials of the proteasome inhibitor bortezomib. Blood. 2007;109:3177–3188.

75. Trudel S, Li ZH, Wei E, et al. CHIR-258, a novel, multitargeted tyrosine kinase inhibitor for the potential treatment of t(4;14) multiple myeloma. Blood. 2005;105:2941–2948.

76. Trudel S, Stewart AK, Rom E, et al. The inhibitory anti-FGFR3 antibody, PRO-001 is cytotoxic to t(4;14) multiple myeloma cells. Blood. 2006;107:4039–4046.

77. Chesi M, Bergsagel PL, Shonukan OO, et al. Frequent dysregulation of the c-maf proto-oncogene at 1 6q23 by translocation to an Ig locus in multiple myeloma. Blood. 1998;91:4457–4463.

78. Zhan F, Huang Y, Colla S, et al. The molecular classification of multiple myeloma. Blood. 2006;108:2020–2028.

79. Shaughi-iessy J, Jr., Gabrea A, Qi Y, et al. Cyclin D3 at 6p2l is dysregulated by recurrent chromosomal translocations to immunoglobulin loci in multiple myeloma. Blood. 2001;98:217–223.

80. Drach J, Ackermann J, Kromer E, et al. Short survival of Patients with Multiple Myeloma and p53 gene deletion: A study by Interphase FISH. Blood. 1997;90:244a.

81. Drach J, Ackermann J, Fritz E, et al. Presence of a p53 gene deletion in patients with multiple myeloma predicts for short survival after conventional-dose chemotherapy. Blood. 1998;92:802–809.

82. Avet-Loiseau H, Li JY, Godon C, et al. P53 deletion is not a frequent event in multiple myeloma. Br J Haematol. 1999;106:717–719.

83. Chang H, Qi C, Yi QL, Reece D, Stewart AK. p53 gene deletion detected by fluorescence in situ hybridization is an adverse prognostic factor for patients with multiple myeloma following autologous stem cell transplantation. Blood. 2005;105:358–360.

84. Tiedemann RR, Gonzalez-Paz N, Kyle RA, et al. Genetic aberrations and survival in plasma cell leukemia. Leukemia. 2008; 22:1044–1052.

85. Chng WJ, Price-Troska T, Gonzalez-Paz N, et al. Clinical significance of TP53 mutation in myeloma. Leukemia. 2007;21:582–584.

86. Sawyer JR, Tricot G, Mattox S, Jagannath S, Barlogie B. Jumping translocations of chromosome 1 q in multiple myeloma: Evidence for a mechanism involving decondensation of pericentromeric heterochromatin. Blood. 1998;91:1732–1741.

87. Zhan F, Colla S, Wu X, et al. CKS1B, over expressed in aggressive disease, regulates multiple myeloma growth and survival through SKP2- and p27Kip 1-dependent and independent mechanisms. Blood. 2007;109:4995–5001.

88. Fonseca R, Van Wier SA, Chng WJ, et al. Prognostic value of chromosome 1q21 gain by fluorescent in situ hybridization and increase CKS1B expression in myeloma. Leukemia. 2006;20:2034–2040.

89. Shaughnessy JD, Jr., Zhan F, Burington BE, et al. A validated gene expression model of high-risk multiple myeloma is defined by deregulated expression of genes mapping to chromosome 1. Blood. 2007;109:2276–2284.

90. Chang H, Qi X, Trieu Y, et al. Multiple myeloma patients with CKS1B gene amplification have a shorter progression-free survival post-autologous stem cell transplantation. Br J Haematol. 2006;135:486–491.

91. Fonseca R, Barlogie B, Bataille R, et al. Genetics and cytogenetics of multiple myeloma: A workshop report. Cancer Res. 2004;64:1546–1558.

92. Stewart AK, Bergsagel PL, Greipp PR, et al. A practical guide to defining high-risk myeloma for clinical trials, patient counseling and choice of therapy. Leukemia. 2007;21:529–534.

Section 2

Historical and Cytotoxic Agent-Based Therapies for Myeloma

Chapter 6

Role of Autologous Stem Cell Transplantation in Multiple Myeloma

Jean-Luc Harousseau

Introduction

High-dose therapy (HDT) with autologous stem cell transplantation (ASCT) was introduced in the treatment of multiple myeloma (MM) 20 years ago[1,2] and its role is still controversial. The use of peripheral blood stem cells instead of bone marrow has markedly improved feasibility and for newly diagnosed MM transplant-related mortality is 1–2% in fit patients with a normal renal function and younger than 65 years. In this group of patients, randomized studies have shown the superiority of ASCT compared with conventional chemotherapy. Therefore, until now, ASCT is considered the standard of care in this population of patients. However, it is currently challenged by the introduction of novel agents such as thalidomide, bortezomib, and lenalidomide. When they are used in combination with dexamethasone or with chemotherapy, these agents appear to yield results that are comparable to those achieved with ASCT. The question is now to determine whether novel agents should replace ASCT or should be used in combination with ASCT.

Randomized Studies Comparing Conventional Chemotherapy and ASCT

The Intergroupe Francophone du Myelome (IFM) was the first to conduct a randomized trial showing the superiority of HDT with ASCT compared to conventional chemotherapy in 200 patients less than 65 years of age. In this IFM 90 trial, HDT significantly improved the response rate, event-free survival (EFS), and overall survival (OS).[3] Similar results were published 7 years later by the British Medical Research Council.[4] As a consequence of these two studies, ASCT has been proposed worldwide as part of frontline therapy, although two randomized studies have shown a longer EFS and time without symptoms, treatment, and treatment toxicity in the ASCT arm but no benefit in OS.[5,6]

Another important finding from the IFM 90 trial was the strong relationship between quality of response and OS. Patients achieving complete remission

From: *Contemporary Hematology Myeloma Therapy*
Edited by: S. Lonial © Humana Press, Totowa, NJ

(CR) or at least very good partial remission (VGPR) had a longer OS than did patients with only partial remission (PR).[3] This led to two important changes in the management of patients with MM.

CR (or at least VGPR) achievement is now considered an objective of any treatment

Response criteria have been redefined to introduce CR and VGPR, which were rarely obtained previously with conventional chemotherapy[7,8]

However, two more recent studies raised concerns due to the lack of significant survival benefit from ASCT compared to conventional chemotherapy.[9,10] In the first study from Spain, only patients whose disease responded to initial chemotherapy were randomized to undergo ASCT or further chemotherapy.[9] Although the CR rate was higher in the ASCT arm (30% vs 11%), no difference was seen in EFS and OS. Compared with other studies where randomization occurred at diagnosis, the design of this trial introduced a selection bias, and only 75% of the patients entering the study were randomized. This fact is important since ASCT is a useful salvage treatment for patients with primary refractory MM.[11,12] In the US Intergroup study, there was also a possible selection bias.[10] Since randomization occurred after induction chemotherapy, only 516 of 813 registered patients were randomized and only 424 actually underwent the assigned therapy. No difference in response rate, EFS and OS was seen between the two arms. However, while results achieved with ASCT were quite comparable to those achieved in the IFM 90 trial, results of chemotherapy were much better (Table 1). Of special interest is the CR rate achieved with conventional chemotherapy, which was much higher than that in the French trial and identical to that achieved with ASCT.

The following conclusions can be drawn from these randomized studies.

ASCT should be offered not only to patients responding to their initial chemotherapy but also to patients with primary refractory MM.

ASCT improves the outcome mostly by increasing the CR + VGPR rate.

ASCT is generally superior to standard conventional chemotherapy, but when results of conventional chemotherapy are improved, the benefit of ASCT is no more significant.

However, comparing conventional chemotherapy with ASCT is no longer a relevant question because results of ASCT have already improved compared with those achieved in the 1990s. Two different approaches have contributed to this improvement in the last few years: further dose intensification and introduction of novel agents.

The first step in improving results of ASCT was the introduction of double-intensive therapy with the objective of increasing the CR rate.[13] Arkansas developed

Table 1 Comparison of the IFM 90 trial and of the US Integroup S9321 trial.

	CR rate		7-year EFS		7-year OS	
	CC	ASCT	CC	ASCT	CC	ASCT
IFM 90[3]	5%	22%	8%	16%	27%	43%
S9321[10]	17%	17%	16%	17%	42%	37%

IFM Intergroupe Francophone du Myelome, *EFS* event-free survival, *OS* overall survival, *ASCT* autologous stem cell transplantation, *CC* Conventional chemotherapy

Table 2 Single versus double ASCT. Results of published randomized trials.

	Number of patients	EFS	OS
IFM 94[15]	399	7 years = 10% vs 20% ($p < 0.03$)	7 years 21% vs 42% ($p < 0.01$)
Bologna 96[16]	321	Median 23 months vs 35 months ($p < 0.001$)	7 years 46% vs 43% ($p = 0.90$)
Hovan 24[17]	304	Median 22 months vs 21 months 6 years 15% vs 7% ($p = 0.013$)	Median 50 months vs 55 months ($p = 0.51$)

EFS event-free survival, *OS* overall survival, *ASCT* autologous stem cell transplantation

a double ASCT program which yielded encouraging median EFS and OS of 43 months and 68 months, respectively, in newly diagnosed patients.[14]

The IFM was again the first to conduct a randomized trial comparing single and double ASCT in 599 patients up to 60 years of age. On an intent-to-treat basis, the 7-year EFS and OS were significantly improved in the double ASCT arm (20% vs 10% and 42% vs 21%, respectively).[15] The benefit in EFS but not in OS was confirmed by two other randomized studies[16,17] (Table 2).

The IFM 94 trial confirmed the feasibility of double ASCT since 75% of patients underwent the second ASCT, and the toxic death rate was less than 5%. However, many investigators considered the benefit of this approach to be marginal and were concerned by the cost and morbidity. Therefore, defining which patients benefited more from this aggressive management seemed important. In the IFM 94 trial, the only parameter to define patients who did not benefit from double ASCT was response to the first ASCT. Patients with less than 90% reduction in their M-component after one ASCT had a longer OS in the double ASCT arm, whereas patients experiencing CR of VGPR after the first ASCT had the same OS with or without the second.

Two groups tried to improve results of double ASCT by further dose-intensification. In the Arkansas Total Therapy 2 program including intensified induction and consolidation, after double ASCT patients were randomized to either receive or not receive thalidomide from initiation of treatment.[18] Comparison of 345 patients in the no thalidomide arm and 231 patients previously treated in the less intensive double ASCT Total Therapy 1 program showed that although the CR rates were identical (43% vs 41%), the 5-year probability of continuous CR (45% vs 32%; $p < .001$) and 5-year EFS (43% vs 28%; $p < 0.01$) were superior in the Total Therapy 2 program. This was translated into a trend for improved OS (62% vs 57%; $p = 0.11$). Although not randomized, this comparison favors the more intensive regimen, and particularly post-ASCT consolidation.

The IFM also proposed a more intensive regimen in the IFM 99 trial, but only for patients with poor-risk factors (high beta-2 microglobulin level + del 13 using fluorescence in situ hybridization analysis).[19] This subgroup of 219 patients underwent double ASCT with an increased dose of melphalan (220 mg/m2) before the second procedure. The CR + VGPR rate increased from 34% after one ASCT to 51% after two ASCTs, which translated into encouraging median EFS and OS (30 and 41 months, respectively). These results seemed to be superior to those achieved previously in high-risk patients.

However, in the absence of randomized trials, there is no convincing evidence that further dose intensification is superior to double ASCT.

Another possibility to improve results of ASCT is to use the three novel agents that have been introduced in the last few years in the antimyeloma armamentarium (thalidomide, bortezomib, and lenalidomide). Novel agents have been evaluated either prior to or after ASCT.

The primary objective of novel agents given in this context is to increase the CR rate not only prior to but also after ASCT. The increased CR rate could be converted into longer EFS and OS. Another interest would be to reduce the proportion of patients needing a second ASCT due to less than VGPR after the first. Thalidomide was the first novel agent to be used in this setting, either in combination with dexamethasone (TD, thalidomide–dexamethasone) compared to dexamethasone alone or to vincristine, adriamycin, and dexamethasone (VAD) or in combination with adriamycin and dexamethasone and compared to VAD. The results of these comparisons are given in Table 3.[20–23]

In all studies, TD or thalidomide, adriamycin, and dexamethasone (TAD) was superior to dexamethasone alone or VAD in terms of response rate. However, the thalidomide-based regimens did not increase the CR rate prior to ASCT and, until now, after ASCT. Moreover, these combinations with thalidomide induced a high incidence of deep-vein thrombosis.

Bortezomib has been more recently evaluated as induction treatment prior to ASCT. A number of nonrandomized studies have been performed with bortezomib combined with dexamethasone or included into multiagent combinations.[24–29] Their results are given in Tables 3 and 4.

The preliminary results show very high response rates (66–95%), an apparent increase in the CR + VGPR rate prior to ASCT (31–64%). These CR + VGPR rates are comparable to those achieved with single ASCT and could be converted into even higher CR + VGPR rates (54–81%) after ASCT. With the usual dose of 1.3 mg/m2 of bortezomib, the incidence of peripheral neuropathy is 30–48%, but grade 3 neuropathy is rare. However, only randomized trials could demonstrate the superiority of bortezomib-containing regimens compared to dexamethasone alone or VAD and are currently ongoing. In the randomized IFM 2005-01 trial, the combination of bortezomib/dexamethasone was compared to VAD as induction prior to

Table 3 Thalidomide-based regimens prior to ASCT.

	TD vs D[a]	TD vs VAD[b]	TAD vs VAD[a]	TD vs VAD[a]
Author	Rajkumar[20]	Cavo[21]	Goldschmidt[22]	Macro[23]
N	201	200	406	204
Response	RR: 69% vs 51%	RR: 76% vs 52%	RR 73% vs 60%	VGPR 35% vs 17%
Prior to ASCT	No change in CR rate	No change in CR rate	No change in CR rate	
Response After ASCT	–	–	CR 19% vs 13%	VGPR 44% vs 42%
DVT	17% vs 3%	15% vs 2%	8% vs 4%b	23% vs 7.5%

[a]Randomized studies [b]Historical control [c]Low molecular weight heparin prophylaxis [T]thalidomide, *D* dexamethasone, *V* vincristine, *A* adriamycin, *RR* response rate, *CR* complete Remission, *VGPR* very good partial emission, *DVT* deep vein thrombosis, *ASCT* autologous stem cell transplantation

Table 4 Bortezomib-based combinations prior to ASCT.

Author	Treatment	Number of patients	Response prior to ASCT	Response after ASCT	Peripheral neuropathy
Jagannath[25]	1.3 mg/m² D 1, 4,8, 11 D 40 mg D 1–2, 4–5, 8–9 <PR on cycle 2 or <CR on cycle 4	32	RR = 88% CR = 6% nCR = 19%	–	31% Grade 36%
Oakervee[26]	B 1.3 mg/m² Dl, 4, 8, 11 A escalating doses 0, 4.5 or 9 mg/m² D1–4 D 40 mg D 1–4, 8–11 and 15–18 cycle 1, D 1–4 cycles 2–4	21	RR = 95% CR = 24% nCR = 5% VGPR = 33%	CR = 43% CR + nCR = 57% CR + nCR = VGR = 81%	48% grade 35%
Popat[27]	B 1 mg/m² D 1, 4, 8, 11 AD as in 9 mg/m² D1–D4	19	RR = 89% CR = 11% nCR = 5% VGPR = 26%	RR = 100% CR + nCR = 54%	16% grade 30%
Harousseau[28]	B 1.3 mg/m² D 1,4, 8, 11 D 40 mg D 1–4, 8–11 On cycle 1–2, D 1–4 m cycles 3–4	48	RR = 66% CR + nCR = 21% VGPR = 10%	RR = 40% CR + VGPR = 54%	30% grade 6%

B bortezomib, *A* adriamycin, *D* dexamethasone, *RR* response rate, *CR* complete remission (immunofixations negative), *nCR* near complete remission (immunofixations positive), *VGPR* very good partial remission, *ASCT* autologous stem cell transplantation

Table 5 Preliminary results of the randomized trial IFM 2005-01. Intention to treat analysis.

fxl[a]

[a]Including n-CR (positive novel agents as primary treatment.

ASCT in 482 patients. The preliminary analysis on the first 162 patients appears to show a superior CR and CR + VGPR rates with bortezomib and dexamethasone, not only prior to ASCT but also after ASCT (Table 5). Combinations of bortezomib and thalidomide with either dexamethasone or chemotherapy induce rapid responses.[28,29] With these regimens, novel agents could be used at lower doses or for shorter duration to reduce the risk of toxicity, specially of peripheral neuropathy.

Lenalidomide plus dexamethasone is currently evaluated as primary treatment of MM. In patients who are candidates to ASCT, this combination appears very active as well and does not preclude stem cell collection after cyclophosphamide + G-CSF priming.[30]

Novel Agents as Maintenance After ASCT

In the IFM 99-02 trial, thalidomide was evaluated as maintenance therapy after double ASCT in patients younger than 65 years with standard prognosis (0 or 1 adverse prognostic factors defined as B2-microglobulingreater than

3 mg/L or del 13 using fluorescence in situ hybridization analysis).[31] In this three-arm study, 597 patients experiencing response to double ASCT were randomly assigned to no further treatment or pamidronate or pamidronate plus thalidomide.

The 3-year EFS was 52% in the thalidomide arm versus 36% in the control arm and 37% in the pamidronate arm ($p < 0.003$), and the 4-year OS was 87% in the thalidomide arm versus 77% and 74% in the other two arms ($p < 0.01$). While deep vein thrombosis was rare (2%) because thalidomide was used alone in low tumor burden MM, peripheral neuropathy was noted in 68% of patients and was the main reason for drug discontinuation. The median dose of thalidomide in this study was 200 mg/day and the median duration of treatment was 15 months.

These results were recently confirmed by an Australian cooperative randomized study comparing thalidomide plus prednisone versus prednisone.[32] The preliminary results also show a benefit of the thalidomide arm in terms of CR (24% vs 15%) ($p < 0.01$), 2-year EFS (66% vs 40%) ($p = 0.0005$), and 2-year OS (91% vs 80%) ($p = 0.02$).

On the contrary, in the Total Therapy 2 program, 323 patients were randomly assigned to receive thalidomide from the onset until disease progression or adverse event and were compared to 345 patients who did not receive thalidomide.[33] The thalidomide arm showed a significantly superior CR (62% vs 43%; $p < 0.001$) and a better 5-year EFS rate (56% vs 41%; $p = .01$). However, no difference was seen in the 5-year OS (65% in both groups) because of a shorter survival after relapse (median 1.1 vs 2.7 years; $p = .001$). Relapses in the thalidomide arm seemed to be more resistant than those in the control arm. Moreover, the combination of chemotherapy and thalidomide during induction treatment induced a high incidence of deep vein thrombosis (30%), and a peripheral neuropathy grade greater than 2 was observed in 27% of patients.

These results raise the question of the optimal dose and duration of thalidomide in this setting. In the IFM 95-02 and in the Australian studies, thalidomide was given only after ASCT, while in the Arkansas study, thalidomide was also given prior to ASCT. In the Australian study, the daily dose of thalidomide was 200 mg. In the American and French studies, the initial dose was 400 mg/day.

It is of interest to note that in the IFM 99-02 trial, the benefit from thalidomide maintenance was significant only in patients who were not CR or VGPR after the second ASCT, and was therefore mostly caused by an increase in the CR + VGPR (from 50% after two ASCTs to 68%). This could mean that post-ASCT thalidomide is mostly useful by increasing the CR rate. If confirmed by other studies, this could encourage us to use thalidomide just as a post-ASCT consolidation treatment (for a limited period of time since responses to thalidomide are usually rapid).

Ongoing studies are evaluating the impact of bortezomib and lenalidomide in this setting.

Which Patients Benefit from ASCT?

Randomized studies showing the superiority of ASCT compared to conventional chemotherapy (CC) have been performed in patients aged 65 years or less and with a normal renal function. Although ASCT is feasible in selected patients over 65 years of age,[34] the usual preparative regimen (melphalan 200 mg/m^2) may be too toxic, specially over 70.[35]

Palumbo et al. showed that two to three courses of melphalan 100 mg/m2 supported by ASCT were feasible in patients up to 75 years of age[36] and were superior to conventional chemotherapy using the classical regimen melphalan–prednisone (MP).[37] However, the IFM group failed to confirm this finding.[38] In the three-arm, randomized IFM 99-06 trial for patients aged 65–75 years, this regimen gave a higher CR rate than MP, but progression-free survival and OS were not significantly superior. Moreover, the combination of MP plus thalidomide was significantly superior. Results of this IFM study do not support the use of ASCT in older patients out of a clinical trial.

Although ASCT is feasible in patients with renal failure, preparative regimen is more toxic and no randomized trial has evaluated the impact of ASCT compared to conventional chemotherapy.[39–41] Therefore, ASCT should not be performed in patients with end-stage renal failure out a clinical trial.

A number of prognostic factors have been defined in the context of ASCT including biological characteristics and cytogenetic abnormalities.[42,43] While patients with a low beta-2 microglobulin level and without deletion 13 have prolonged EFS,[44–46] patients with a high beta-2 microglobulin level and unfavourable cytogenetics (deletion 13 or hypodiploidy) have a poor outcome even with double ASCT.[44,46,47]

Prognostic impact of cytogenetic abnormalities in the context of ASCT has been recently reevaluated. Besides chromosome 13 deletion/monosomy, two other frequent abnormalities are associated with a poor prognosis, t(4;14) and del(17p), which are found in 14–15% and 10–11% of cases, respectively. Patients with these abnormalities have significantly shorter EFS and OS despite HDT and ASCT.[48–51] Interestingly, t(4;14) and del(17p) are often associated with del(13) and it appears that most of the negative impact of del(13) is related to t(4;14) and del(17p)[52]. In multivariate analysis of the IFM 99 trials (with double transplantation for all patients), del(13) was not found to be an independent prognostic factor and in patients without t(4;14) and del(17 p), there was no statistically significant difference between patients with or without del(13).

Finally, the combination of beta-2 microglobulin level or International Strategy System and assessment of t(4;14) and del(17p) appeared to be the most important prognostic factor.[52] Patients with both a high 132 microglobulin level and one of these abnormalities had a very poor outcome even with double ASCT. In these patients, novel approaches are clearly needed and the role of bortezomib and lenalidomide is currently evaluated in this subgroup of patients.

Are Novel Agents Going to Replace ASCT?

The IFM and the Italian group have compared MP with the same combination plus thalidomide in patients over the age of 65 years.[38,53] In both studies the response rate (including CR rate) and EFS were superior in the thalidomide arm. The OS was also longer in the thalidomide arm, although the difference was not yet significant at the time of publication in the Italian study. The logical consequence of these studies is that MP should not be considered any longer the standard of care for older patients. But these results also raise again the question of the interest of ASCT because MP–thalidomide used in older

Table 6 Combinations including novel agents as primary treatment.

Author	Regimen	Number of patients	Age (Years)	CR	CR + VGPR	CR + PR	EFS
Facon[38]	MPT	125	65–75	16%	50%	81%	Median 28 months
Palumbo[53]	MPT	129	60–85	16%	36%	76%	54% at 2 years
Mateos[54]	MPV	60	>65	32%	43%	89%	82% at 16 months
Palumbo[55]	MPR	54	Median 71	24%	48%	81%	87% at 16 months
Lacy[56]	RD	34	Median 34	18%	56%	91%	59% at 2 years

M melphalan, *P* prednisone, *T* thalidomide, *V* velcade, *R* Revlimid®, *CR* complete remission, *VGPR* very good partial remission, *PR* partial remission, *EFS* event-free survival

Table 7 Comparison of results achieved with MPT and with ASCT.

	MPT Palumbo	MPT Facon	IFM 99 trials A vet-Loiseau	TTz Barlogie (thalidomide arm)
CR	16%	16%	32%a	62%
EFS	54% at 2 years	Median 28 months	Median 39 months	56% at 5 years
OS	80% at 3 years	NR at 56 months	62% at 5 years	65% at 5 years

aCR + nCR

IFM Intergroupe Francophone du Myelome, *EFS* event-free survival, *OS* overall survival, *MPT* melphalan–prednisone–thalidomide, *ASCT* autologous stem cell transplantation, *CR* complete remission, *nCR* near complete remission

patients yielded CR rate and EFS that are comparable to those achieved in younger patients with HDT + ASCT.

Other combinations with bortezomib (MPV) or with lenalidomide (MPR or RD) also yield very high CR rates and encouraging short-term EFS (Table 6).

However these results do not necessarily mean that ASCT will be abandoned as primary treatment of MM, for a number of reasons:

1. In the last, the arguments against ASCT were morbidity and cost. Since the combinations using novel agents have been given for at least 9 months, they have induced toxicities (peripheral neuropathy, infections, and thrombosis) and are expensive as well.
2. Quality of life is an important aspect of modern treatments; while ASCT, as a "single short" treatment, induces a severe impairment of quality of life during the short period following HDT, prolonged treatment with novel agents could also induce a delayed quality of life impairment.
3. More important, the results of combination including novel agents are generally compared to the results achieved in the 1990s with single ASCT. But results of ASCT have recently improved, specially with double ASCT and with introduction of novel agents (Table 7).

Therefore, rather than comparing ASCT and novel agents, it should be more useful to combine ASCT with novel agents to further increase the CR rate, to reduce the need for a second ASCT, and to prolong remission duration. Another possibility could be to compare novel agents plus early versus late ASCT.

References

1. Barlogie B, Hall R, Zander A et al. High-dose melphalan with autologous bone marrow transplantation for multiple myeloma. Blood 1986; 67: 1298–1301.
2. Barlogie B, Alexanian R, Dicke KA et al. High-dose chemoradiotherapy and autologous bone marrow transplantation for resistant multiple myeloma. Blood 1987; 70: 869–872.
3. Attal M, Harousseau JL, Stoppa AM et al. For the Intergroupe Français du Myelome. A prospective, randomized trial of autologous bone marrow transplantation and chemotherapy in multiple myeloma. N Engl J Med 1996; 335: 91–97.
4. Child JA, Morgan GJ, Davies FE et al. Medical research council adult leukemia working party: High-dose chemotherapy with hematopoietic stem-cell rescue for multiple myeloma. N Engl J Med 2003; 348: 1875–1883.
5. Fermand JP, Ravaud P, Chevret S et al. High-dose therapy and autologous peripheral blood stem cell transplantation in multiple myeloma: Up-front or rescue treatment? Results of a multicenter sequential randomized trial. Blood 1998; 92: 3131–3136.
6. Fermand JP, Katsahian S, Divine M et al. High-dose therapy and autologous blood stem cell transplantation compared with conventional treatment in myeloma patients aged 55 to 65 years: Long-term results of a randomized control trial from the Groupe Myelome-Autogreffe. J Clin Oncol 2005; 23: 9227–9233.
7. Blade J, Samson D, Reece D et al. Criteria for evaluating disease response and progression in patients with multiple myeloma treated by high-dose therapy and haematopoietic stem cell transplantation. Myeloma Subcommittee of the EBMT. European Group for Blood and Marrow Transplant. Br J Haematol 1998; 102: 1115–1123.
8. Durie BG, Harousseau JL, Miguel JS et al. International uniform response criteria for multiple myeloma. Leukemia 2006; 20: 1467–1473.
9. Blade J, Rosinol L, Sureda A et al. High-dose therapy intensification compared with continued standard chemotherapy in multiple myeloma patients responding to the initial chemotherapy: Long-term results from a prospective randomized trial from the Spanish cooperative groupe PETHEMA. Blood 2005; 106: 3755–3759.
10. Barlogie B, Kyle RA, Anderson KC et al. Standard chemotherapy compared with high dose chemoradiotherapy for multiple myeloma: Final results of phase III US Intergroup Trial S9321. J Clin Oncol 2006; 24: 929–936.
11. Alexanian R, Dimopoulos MA, Hester J et al. Early myeloablative therapy for multiple myeloma. Blood 1994; 84: 4278–4282.
12. Kumar S, Lacy MQ, Dispenzieri A et al. High-dose therapy and autologous stem cell transplantation for multiple myeloma poorly responsive to initial therapy. Bone Marrow Transplant 2004; 34: 161–167.
13. Harousseau JL, Milpied N, Laporte JP et al. Double-intensive therapy in high-risk multiple myeloma. Blood 1992; 79: 3131–3136.
14. Barlogie B, Jagannath S, Desikan KR et al. Total therapy with tandem transplants for newly diagnosed multiple myeloma. Blood 1999; 93: 55–65.
15. Attal M, Harousseau JL, Facon T et al. Intergroupe Francophone du Myelome: Single versus double autologous stem cell transplantation for multiple myeloma. N Engl J Med 2003; 349: 2495–2502.
16. Cavo M, Tosi P, Zamagni E et al. Prospective randomized study of single compared with double autologous stem cell transplantation for multiple myeloma: Bologna 96 clinical study. J. Clin Oncol 2007; 25: 2434–2441.
17. Sonneveld P, Van Der Holt B, Segeren CM et al. Intermediate-dose melphalan compared with myeloablative treatment in multiple myeloma: Long-term follow-up of the Deutch Cooperative Group HOVaN 24 trial. Haematologica 2007; 92: 928–935.

18. Barlogie B, Tricot G, Rabmussen E et al. Total therapy 2 without thalidomide in comparison with total therapy 1: Role of intensified induction and post-transplantation consolidation therapies. Blood 2006; 107: 2633–2638.

19. Moreau P, Hullin C, Garban F et al. Tandem autologous stem cell transplantation in high risk de novo multiple myeloma: Final results of the prospective and randomized IFM 99-04 protocol. Blood 2006; 107: 397–403.

20. Rajkumar V, Blaad E, Vesole D et al. Phase III clinical trial of Thalidomide plus Dexamethasone compared with Dexamethasone alone in newly diagnosed multiple myeloma: A clinical trial coordinated by the Eastern Cooperative Oncology Group. J Clin Oncol 2006; 24: 431–436.

21. Cava M, Zamagni E, Tosi P et al. Superiority of thalidomide and dexamethasone over vincristine-doxorubicine-dexamethasone (VAD) as primary therapy in preparation for autologous transplantation for multiple myeloma. Blood 2005; 106: 35–39.

22. Goldschmidt H, Sonneveld P, Breitkreuz I et al. HOVON 50/GMMG-HD3 trial: Phase III study on the effect of thalidomide combined with high-dose melphalan in myeloma patients up to 65 years. Blood 2005; 106: 128a (abstract).

23. Macro M, Divine M, Uzunban Y et al. Dexamethasone + thalidomide compared to VAD as pre-transplant treatment in newly diagnosed multiple myeloma: A randomized trial. Blood 2006; 108: 22a (abstract).

24. Jagannath S, Durie B, Wolf J et al. Bortezomib therapy alone and in combination with dexamethasone for previously untreated symptomatic multiple myeloma. Br J Haematol 2005; 129: 776–783.

25. Oakervee HE, PoHat R, Curry N et al. PAD combination therapy (PS34l, doxorubicin and dexamethasone) for untreated multiple myeloma. Br J Haematol 2005; 755–762.

26. Popat R, Oakervee HE, Curry N et al. Reduced dose PAD (PS 341, adriamycin and dexamethasone) for previously untreated patients with multiple myeloma. Blood 2005; 106: 717a (abstract).

27. Harousseau JL, Attal M. Bortezomib plus dexamethasone as induction treatment prior to autologous stem cell transplantation in patients with newly diagnosed multiple myeloma. Haematologica 2006; 91: 1498–1505.

28. Barlogie B, Tricot G, Rasmussen E et al. Total therapy incorporating Velcade into upfront management of multiple myeloma: Comparison with TT2+thalidomide. Blood 2005; 106: 337a (abstract).

29. Wang M, Delaballe K, Giralt S et al. Rapid control of previously untreated multiple myeloma with bortezomib-thalidomide-dexamethasone followed by early intensive therapy. Blood 2005; 106: 231a (abstract).

30. Rajkumar SV, Hayman SR, Lacy MQ et al. Combination therapy with lenalidomide plus dexamethasone for newly diagnosed myeloma. Blood 2005; 106: 4050–4053.

31. Attal M, Harousseau JL, Leyvras S et al. Maintenance therapy with thalidomide improves survival in multiple myeloma patients. Blood 2006; 15: 3289–3294.

32. Spencer A, Prince M, Roberts AW et al. First analysis of the Australian leukaemia and lymphoma group trial of thalidomide and alternate day prednisone following autologous stem cell transplantation for patients with multiple myeloma. Blood 2006; 108: 22a (abstract).

33. Barlogie B, Tricot G, Anaissie E et al. Thalidomide and hematopoietic cell transplantation for multiple myeloma. N Engl J Med 2006; 354: 1021–1030.

34. Siegel DS, Desikan KR, Nehta J et al. Age is not a prognostic variable with autotransplants for multiple myeloma. Blood 1999; 93: 51–54.

35. Badros A, Barlogie B, Siegel E et al. Autologous stem cell transplantation in elderly multiple myeloma patients over the age of 70 years. Br J Haematol 2001; 114: 600–607.

36. Palumbo A, Triolo S, Argentin C. Dose intensive melphalan with stem-cell support is superior to standard treatment in elderly myeloma patients. Blood 1999; 94: 1248–1253.

37. Palumbo A, Bringhen S, Petrucci MT et al. Intermediate-dose Melphalan improves survival of myeloma patients aged 50–70: Results of a randomized controlled trial. Blood; 2004: 3052–3057.

38. Facon T, Mary JY, Hulin C et al. Melphalan and prednisone plus thalidomide versus melphalan and prednisone alone or reduced-intensity autologous stem cell transplantation in elderly patients with multiple myeloma (IFM 99–06): a randomised trial. Lancet 2007; 370: 1209–1218

39. Badros A, Barlogie B, Siegel E et al. Results of autologous stem cell transplant in multiple myeloma patients with renal failure. Br J Haematol 2001; 114: 822–829.

40. Tosi P, Zamagni E, Ronconi S et al. Safety of autologous hematopoietic stem cell transplantation in patients with multiple myeloma and renal failure. Leukemia 2000; 14: 1310–1313.

41. San Miguel J, Lahuerta JJ, Garcia-Sanz R et al. Are myeloma patients with renal failure candidate for autologous stem cell transplantation. Hematol J 2000; 1: 28–36.

42. Barlogie B, Jagannath S, Desikan KR et al. Total therapy with tandem transplants for newly diagnosed multiple myeloma. Blood 1999; 93: 66–75.

43. Vesole D, Tricot G, Jagannath S et al. Autotransplant in multiple myeloma: What have we learned? Blood 1996; 88: 838–847.

44. Facon T, A vet-Loiseau H, Guillerm G et al. Chromosome 13 abnormalities identified by Fish analysis and serum B2 microglobulin produce powerful myeloma staging system for patients receiving high-dose therapy. Blood 2001; 97: 1566–1571.

45. Tricot G, Spencer T, Sawyer J et al. Predicting long-term (~5 years) event-free survival in multiple myeloma patients following planned tandem autotransplant. Br J Haematol 2002; 116: 211–217.

46. Shaughnessy J, Jacobson J, Sawyer J et al. Continuous absence of metaphase-defined cytogenetic abnormalities especially of chromosome 13 and hypodiploidy ensures long-term survival in multiple myeloma treated with Total Therapy I: Interpretation in the context of global gene expression. Blood 2003; 101: 3849–3856.

47. Fassas AT, Spencer T, Sawyer J et al. Both hypodiploidy and deletion of chromosome 13 independently confer poor prognosis in multiple myeloma. Br J Haematol 2002; 118: 1041–1047.

48. Chang H, Sloan S, Li D et al. The t(4;14) is associated with poor prognosis in myeloma patients undergoing autologous stem cell transplant. Br J Haematol 2004; 125: 64–68.

49. Gertz M, Lacy MQ, Dispenzieri A et al. Clinical implications of t(11;14) (q13;q32), t(4;14) (p16.3;q32), and 17p13 in myeloma patients treated with high-dose therapy. Blood 2005; 106: 2837–2840.

50. Jaksic W, Trudel S, Chang H et al. Clinical outcomes in t(4;14) multiple myeloma: A chemotherapy-sensitive disease characterized by rapid relapse and alkylating agent resistance. J Clin Oncol 2005; 23: 7069–7073.

51. Chang H, Qi C, Yi QL et al. p53 gene deletion detected by fluorescence in situ hybridisation is an adverse prognostic factor for patients with multiple myeloma following autologous stem cell transplantation. Blood 2005; 105: 358–360.

52. A vet-Loiseau H, Attal M, Moreau P et al. Genetic abnormalities and survival in multiple myeloma: The experience of the Intergroupe Francophone du Myelome. Blood 2007; 109: 3489–3495.

53. Palumbo A, Bringhen S, Caravita T et al. Oral Melphalan and prednisone chemotherapy plus thalidomide compared with melphalan and prednisone alone in elderly patients with multiple myeloma: Randomised controlled trial. Lancet 2006; 367: 825–831.

54. Mateos MV, Hernandez JM, Gutierrez WC et al. Bortezomib plus melphalan and prednisone in elderly untreated patients with multiple myeloma: Results of a multicenter phase l/II study. Blood 2006, online.

55. Palumbo A, Falco P, Falcone A et al. Oral revlimid plus melphalan and prednisone for newly diagnosed multiple myeloma: Results of a multicenter phase I/II study. Blood 2006; online.
56. Lacy M, Gertz M, Dispenzieri A et al. Lenalidomide plus dexamethasone in newly diagnosed myeloma: Response to therapy, time to progression and survival Lancet 2006; 367: 825–831.

Chapter 7

Maintenance Therapy in Multiple Myeloma

Jonathan L. Kaufman, Ronald Mihelic, and Sagar Lonial

Introduction

Maintenance therapy has long been an essential component of treatment for patients with hematologic malignancies. Maintenance therapy is defined as prolonged therapy delivered at regular intervals after remission induction.[1] The goals of maintenance therapy are dependent on the underlying disease. Multidrug, long-term conventional chemotherapy as maintenance has been well established as an integral part of therapy to increase the cure rate in patients with acute lymphoblastic leukemia.[2] However, the goal of maintenance therapy is different in patients with follicular lymphoma. In patients with follicular lymphoma, a disease characterized by long median survival and invariable relapse, the goal of maintenance therapy is to prolong disease-free survival while minimizing the toxicity of the maintenance therapy.[3] The goal of maintenance therapy for myeloma should, at a minimum, be to prolong remission duration with minimal toxicity. But the ultimate goal of maintenance therapy should be to also prolong overall survival (OS). That is, an optimal maintenance therapy will result in better outcomes compared to that same therapy delivered at relapse in patients who have not had maintenance therapy. As outlined in other chapters of this volume, some patients with myeloma have a clinical course characterized by prolonged remissions followed by indolent relapse, whereas other patients have a more aggressive disease with short remission durations and aggressive relapse. These differences in clinical course are the result of underlying differences of myeloma biology. Defining the optimal maintenance strategy will depend on defining risk groups based on cytogenetics and remission status. The following represents a review of previously tested maintenance strategies, current research in the field as well as potential future maintenance approaches.

Conventional Therapy

Prolongation of conventional chemotherapy has been evaluated in well-designed randomized clinical trials, and this was reviewed recently.[4] In one study, patients who responded to the combination of melphalan and prednisone

From: *Contemporary Hematology Myeloma Therapy*
Edited by: S. Lonial © Humana Press, Totowa, NJ

and were in plateau phase were randomized to no further therapy versus continued (maintenance) melphalan and prednisone. While patients in the maintenance therapy armhad an improvement in progression-free survival (PFS), the median OS was not different between the two arms. Several other studies with similar designs had the same conclusion.[4] Given the known toxicity of prolonged melphalan use, conventional chemotherapy as maintenance is not recommended.

Interferon

Interferon (IFN) has been studied extensively as maintenance following both conventional therapy and high-dose therapy.[1] A meta-analysis on the use of IFN both as maintenance and as part of the induction therapy was reported by the Myeloma Trialists' Collaborative Group. PFS (27% vs 19% at 3 years, $p < 0.00001$) and response duration were improved compared to no maintenance.[5] However, OS was actually poorer for patients receiving IFN as maintenance therapy ($p = 0.007$). The magnitude of benefit of IFN was greatest in smaller trials, with no clear benefit from the larger trials. In a separate analysis by Ludwig and Fritz, 1,615 patients from 13 different trials were evaluated. In their analysis, there was a small benefit in both PFS and OS for those receiving IFN as maintenance therapy with moderate toxicity.[6] Based on the marginal data in terms of efficacy, and the toxicity and expense associated with IFN, it is not routinely recommended for use outside of a clinical trial.

Corticosteroids

Corticosteroids are an integral part of treatment for patients with myeloma, both as induction and in the relapsed setting. Several investigators have subsequently assessed the role of steroids as maintenance.[1] The strongest data to date comes from the Southwest Oncology Group (SWOG) 9210 clinical trial.[7] Patients were originally randomized to receive vincristine, doxorubicin (Adriamycin), and dexamethasone (VAD) plus prednisone versus VAD plus prednisone and quinine. After remission, induction patients were randomized to either 10 or 50 mg prednisone, both administered every other day. Therapy was continued until disease progression. There was no difference in response rate, PFS, or OS between the two induction schedules. Of the 250 patients originally on this trial, only 126 participated in the second randomization. In subjects receiving 50 mg of prednisone every other day, PFS (14 vs 5 months, $p = 0.003$) and OS (37 vs 26 months, $p = 0.05$) were significantly longer when compared to those receiving 10 mg every other day. The toxicities at these schedules were not severe and comparable, with only one patient in the high-dose prednisone group who had therapy discontinued early and similar grade 3 or worse toxicity (21% for the 10 mg schedule and 26% for the 50 mg schedule). Of note, there was no information regarding the treatment of patients at relapse. As accrual ended in December 1997, it is unlikely that a significant number of subjects had access to thalidomide.[7] This raises several questions regarding the clinical utility of this study in the modern era. First, few clinicians used VAD as induction therapy and second, no patients had access to bortezomib or lenalidomide, therapies that are known to prolong survival in patients with relapsed myeloma. With that said, this study has formed the justification for trials testing the benefit of maintenance steroids following either high-dose therapy or standard therapy for myeloma.

Thalidomide

As outlined in other chapters in this volume, thalidomide has a role in the treatment of patients with myeloma whether used as part of induction therapy or in the relapsed setting. Given its ease of administration and potential use over prolonged periods of time, thalidomide represents an excellent option for clinical investigation in the maintenance setting after both conventional therapy or high-dose therapy and autologous hematopoietic stem cell transplantation (AHSCT). Alexanian and colleagues assessed the role of thalidomide with dexamethasone for patients in a stable partial remission after AHSCT. An improvement in response from proliferation (PR) to at least a very good partial response was noted in 57% of the patients. Toxicity of the regimen was manageable and included the expected toxicities of thalidomide including constipation, fatigue, and neuropathy.[8] To assess the optimal dose of thalidomide when used after high-dose therapy and AHSCT, Stewart performed and randomized phase II (MY-9) study comparing thalidomide at 200 mg to 400 mg, both administered with prednisone 50 mg every other day. The primary outcome was to assess the proportion of patients discontinuing therapy or reducing the dose of therapy due to treatment-related toxicity observed within 6 months of commencing maintenance treatment.[9] After a median follow-up of 36.8 months, 31% of patients in the 200 mg arm and 69% in the 400 mg arm either dropped out or had a dose reduction due to side effects. Patients remaining on maintenance therapy after 18 months were 76% in the 200 mg versus 41% in the 400 mg arm. Neuropathy was the most common reason for discontinuation of thalidomide in both treatment groups. Grade 3 or 4 nonhematological toxicities were observed in 36% and 27% of patients in the 400 and 200 mg dose arms, respectively. The occurrence of symptomatic venous thrombosis was 7.5% for all patients with no difference between the groups. There was no difference between the two arms in the frequency or rate of discontinuation of prednisone during the study. While there was no formal comparison of PFS, the median PFS posttransplant for both arms combined was 32.3 months. The authors concluded that 200 mg was the recommended dose for a randomized phase III trial comparing thalidomide and prednisone to placebo as maintenance after transplant.[9]

To determine the optimal dose of single-agent thalidomide as maintenance therapy after AHSCT, the Medical Research Council (MRC) performed a pilot study comparing different dose levels of thalidomide. The main end point for this study was toxicity and duration of remission post-AHSCT. The long-term tolerance of thalidomide was assessed at five dose levels: 50, 100, 200, 250, and 300 mg. With a median follow-up of 6 months, 21% (18/84) of patients discontinued thalidomide, 7 due to progression of disease and 11 due to secondary to toxicities.[10] With early follow-up, the authors concluded that an apparent increase in toxicity-related dropout was seen in doses above 200 mg/day, with only 58% of patients remaining on study drug as compared to 82% patients taking 200 mg or less. In this study of single-agent thalidomide, only one thrombotic event (1%) was seen despite lack of prophylactic antico-agulation. This is in contrast to the 7.5% thrombosis rate when thalidomide was combined with prednisone as maintenance.[9] Longer follow-up of this study has defined a subgroup of patients who derive the greatest benefit from single-agent thalidomide maintenance. Those patients who achieve a complete response (CR) after initiation of thalidomide have a prolonged PFS.[11]

In a retrospective analysis by Brinker et al., a total of 112 patients were evaluated who received maintenance therapy with IFN, thalidomide, or obser-vation, following high-dose chemotherapy and AHSCT.[12] Patients who received thalidomide at any point after transplant had improved median survival (79.6 months) compared to patients who did not (39.6 months). In a multivari-ate analysis of this patient group taking into account response to transplant, stem cell source, and other factors that may influence outcomes following transplant, the significant predictors for OS were age, and the use of thalido-mide anytime after transplant ($p = 0.09$). While this analysis only indirectly addresses maintenance therapy (one half of the thalidomide group was treated as maintenance with the rest receiving thalidomide at the time of relapse), patients who received maintenance thalidomide had an improved OS compared to patients treated with thalidomide at the time of relapse ($p = 0.05$).

The Intergroupe Francophone du Myelome (IFM) 99-02 study was the first randomized study to compare single-agent thalidomide to no maintenance after high-dose therapy and AHSCT (Tables 1 and 2). The trial was initiated to assess the impact of thalidomide maintenance on duration of response post-AHSCT in patients with zero or one risk factor as defined by the IFM of an elevated beta-2 microglobulin (β_2M) or deletion 13 by fluorescence in situ hybridization (FISH) analysis. Seven hundred and eighty patients less than 65 years old were enrolled to receive VAD induction followed by tandem autolo-gous transplant prepared with melphalan (first transplant 140 mg/m^2, second transplant 200 mg/m^2). Patients with stable disease or better 2 months after

Table 1 Efficacy of thalidomide as maintenance after high-dose therapy and autologous hematopoietic stem cell transplantation in randomized trials.

Title	Ref	Design	N	PFS	p value	OS	p value
IFM 99 02	13	Tandem AHSCT	597	3 years	0.003	4 years	0.04
		Arm 1: No maintenance	200	38%		77%	
		Arm 2: Pamidronate	196	39%		74%	
		Arm 3: Thal 400 mg and pamidronate	201	51%		87%	
ALLG MM6	14,15	Single AHSCT	243	3 years	0.0003	3 years	0.02
		Arm 1: Thal 200 mg/Pred	114	35%		86%	
		Arm 2: Pred	129	25%		75%	
NCIC MY 9	9	Single AHSCT	67	Median 32 months		4 years 75%	
		Arm 1: Thal 200 mg/Pred	45	nr		nr	
		Arm 2: Thal 400 mg/Pred	22	nr		nr	

Ref reference number, *Thal* thalidomide, *Pred* prednisone 50 mg every other day, *nr* not reported, *AHSCT* autologous hematopoi-etic stem cell transplantation, *OS* overall survival, *PFS* progression-free survival, *IFM* Intergroupe Francophone du Myelome, *ALLG* Australian Leukaemia and Lymphoma Group

Table 2 Toxicity of thalidomide as maintenance after high-dose therapy and autologous hematopoietic stem cell transplantation in randomized trials.

Title	Ref	Design	N	Thal dose	Thrombosis (%)	Neuropathy (%) (% grade 3–4)
IFM 99 02	13	Tandem AHSCT	597			
		Arm 1: No maintenance	200	na	2	8 (1)
		Arm 2: Pamidronate	196	na	1	15 (2)
		Arm 3: Thal 400 mg and pamidronate	201	200 mg (mean)	4	68 (7)
ALLG MM6	14,15	Single AHSCT	243		nr	nr
		Arm 1: Thal 200 mg/Pred[5]	114	100 mg (median)	nr	nr
		Arm 2: Pred	129	na	nr	nr
NCIC MY 9	9	Single AHSCT	67		7.5	54 (25)
		Arm 1. Thal 200 mg/Pred	45	133 mg		
(median)	nr	24% grade3/4				
		Arm 2: Thal 400 mg/Pred	22	320 mg (median)	nr	27% grade3/4

Ref reference number, *Thal* thalidomide, *na* not applicable, *nr* not reported, *Pred* prednisone 50 mg every other day, *AHSCT* autologous hematopoietic stem cell transplantation, *IFM* Intergroupe Francophone du Myelome, *ALLG* Australian Leukaemia and Lymphoma Group

the second transplant were randomized to one of three maintenance therapy arms. At the time of final analysis, 593 of the 780 patients were randomized to receive (1) observation, (2) pamidronate 90 mg/month, or (3) thalidomide 100 mg/day plus pamidronate 90 mg/month as maintenance therapy. At ~29 month median follow-up from randomization (2 months after second transplant), patients randomized to thalidomide had improvement in event-free survival compared to those patients randomized to no treatment or pamidronate alone (arm 3: 52% vs arm 1: 36% and arm 2: 37%, $p = 0.002$).[13] In addition, there was a substantial improvement in OS for the patients randomized to receive maintenance thalidomide compared to the other two arms (arm 3: 87% vs arm 1: 77% and arm 2: 74%, $p = 0.04$). Importantly, the survival after relapse was not different between the three arms, suggesting that maintenance thalidomide does not result in resistant disease. While the population as a whole had an improvement in event-free survival, relapse-free survival, and OS, there were two subsets of patients who did not benefit from maintenance thalidomide. Patients with deletion 13 (as determined by FISH, fluorescence in situ hybridization) and patients who had achieved a very good PR, as defined by a 90% reduction in the paraprotein from baseline, derived no improvement in event-free survival when randomized to maintenance thalidomide. In fact, the lack of benefit for the patients with deletion 13 was independent of response. This data further supports the ongoing investigation of maintenance thalidomide, but suggests that separate maintenance strategies need to be developed for patients with deletion 13. This study also questions the role of maintenance thalidomide as a single agent in patients who have achieved a very good or better PR following high-dose therapy.

Table 3 Ongoing trials assessing the role of IMIDs (immunomodulatory drugs) as maintenance after high-dose therapy and autologous hematopoietic stem cell transplantation.

Title	Study design	Control arm	Experimental arm
NCIC/ECOG MY10	Single AHSCT Melphalan 200 mg/m^2	No maintenance	Thalidomide 200 mg and prednisone 50 mg every other day
BMT CTN 0102	Tandem AHSCT Melphalan 200 mg/m^2 twice	No maintenance	Thalidomide 200 mg and dexemethasone 40 mg for 1–4 days in a 28-day cycle
MRC Myeloma IX	Single AHSCT Melphalan 200 mg/m^2	No maintenance	Thalidomide 50–100 mg
CALGB 100104	Single AHSCT Melphalan 200 mg/m^2	No maintenance	Lenalidomide 10 mg daily
IFM 2005-02	Single AHSCT Melphalan 200 mg/m^2 VGPR or better	No maintenance	Lenalidomide

VGPR very good partial response, *AHSCT* autologous hematopoietic stem cell transplantation, *MRC* Medical Research Council, *IFM* Intergroupe Fran

The Australian Leukemia and Lymphoma Group (ALLG) recently reported results from a randomized trial of thalidomide starting at 200 mg/day in combination with prednisone 50 mg every other day (arm 1, $n = 114$) compared with prednisone 50 mg every other day alone (arm 2, $n = 129$).[14,15] Thalidomide was administered for at most 12 months and prednisone was administered until progression in both arms. In the Australian Leukemia and Lymphoma Group, MM6 trial patients were randomly assigned to one of the two arms after high-dose therapy and AHSCT. The percentage of patients in an immunofixation CR was similar between the two arms (arm 1–9% vs arm 2–11%). The percentage of patients maintaining a PR or better at 12 months was improved in arm 1 compared to arm 2 (83% vs 53%, $p<0.01$). PFS was improved for arm 1 compared to arm 2 at 1 year (91% vs 69%), 2 years (65% vs 36%), and 3 years (35% vs 25%) after randomization. In addition, OS at 3 years was improved for patients receiving thalidomide in addition to prednisone compared to prednisone alone (86% vs 75%, $p = 0.02$).[15] The full report of this study including toxicity is pending. In addition, subgroup analysis by response or cytogenetics was not reported.

Clearly, further studies are needed to address the overall role of maintenance thalidomide, both as a single agent and in combination with corticosteroids. Detailed analysis of these studies with subgroup analysis incorporating depth of remission, stage at diagnosis, and cytogenetics are critical. Ongoing studies including these will be critical in understanding the role of thalidomide as maintenance (Table 3).

Future Directions

In addition to thalidomide, several investigators are actively assessing the role of other novel therapeutics as maintenance therapy after both conventional and high-dose therapy. Single-agent bortezomib administered at a dose of 1.3 mg/m^2 once weekly, 4 out of 5 weeks post single AHSCT has been studied. In this small trial, long-term efficacy data is not available. The investigators did note a 39% varicella-zoster reactivation rate.[16] In a phase I/II study, bortezomib was administered at doses of 1.0, 1.3, and 1.6 mg/m² once weekly, 3 out of 4 weeks. The maximum tolerate dose was 1.3 mg/m². Efficacy results are pending. The main toxicities were diarrhea, fatigue, nausea, peripheral neuropathy, and again varicella-zoster reactivation.[17] A third group also assessed bortezomib at dose of 1.0 and 1.3 mg/m². Two of the twenty patients had a conversion of response from very good partial response to CR during treatment. Again, varicella-zoster reactivation was noted. Investigators modified the protocol to include prophylaxis with acyclovir.[18] More studies are needed to determine the optimal dose and long-term response of bortezomib as maintenance. Clearly, prophylactic use of acyclovir is needed to prevent varicella-zoster reactivation. Low-dose lenalidomide is being tested by the Cancer and Leukemia Group B (CALGB) and the IFM in posttransplant randomized placebo-controlled maintenance trials. As myelosuppression is one of the major toxicities of lenalidomide, careful monitoring of posttransplant patients will be critical. Ongoing clinical trials assessing the role of these novel therapeutics in the maintenance setting are necessary in improving outcomes for patients with myeloma.

Conclusion

The Food and Drug Administration (FDA) and the American Society of Hematology held a workshop to define end points in clinical trials for patients with myeloma. The maintenance therapy workshop recommended the following triad as the optimal goals of clinical trials evaluating maintenance therapies: (1) improvement in CR rate, (2) improved PFS, and (3) acceptable toxicity profile as measured by quality-of-life parameters. Current evidence does not support the use of IFN as maintenance therapy due to its lack of significant improvement in survival and unacceptable toxicity. The scant data that is available does not justify the recommendation of corticosteroids as maintenance therapy for all patients. Conflicting evidence exists for the use of thalidomide as maintenance treatment. Current data is promising, but further randomized trials are needed to verify its effectiveness and those who will most likely benefit from maintenance thalidomide.

The discovery of targets in myeloma and the development of novel therapeutics are rapidly changing the treatment options for patients with myeloma. Building treatment programs that maximize survival while maintaining quality of life remain the goal of maintenance treatments for patients with myeloma.

References

1. Mihelic R, Kaufman JL, Lonial S. Maintenance therapy in multiple myeloma. Leukemia. 2007;21(6):1150–1157.
2. Faderl S, Jeha S, Kantarjian HM. The biology and therapy of adult acute lymphoblastic leukemia. Cancer. 2003;98:1337–1354.
3. Berinstein NL. Principles of maintenance therapy. Leuk Res. 2006;30(Suppl. 1): S3–S10.
4. Dispenzieri A, Rajkumar SV, Gertz MA, et al. Treatment of newly diagnosed multiple myeloma based on Mayo stratification of myeloma and risk-adapted therapy (mSMART): Consensus statement. Mayo Clin Proc. 2007;82:323–341.
5. Interferon as therapy for multiple myeloma: An individual patient data overview of 24 randomized trials and 4012 patients. Br J Haematol. 2001;113:1020–1034.

6. Fritz E, Ludwig H. Interferon-alpha treatment in multiple myeloma: Meta-analysis of 30 randomised trials among 3948 patients. Ann Oncol. 2000;11:1427–1436.

7. Berenson JR, Crowley JJ, Grogan TM, et al. Maintenance therapy with alternate-day prednisone improves survival in multiple myeloma patients. Blood. 2002;99: 3163–3168.

8. Alexanian R, Weber D, Giralt S, Delasalle K. Consolidation therapy of multiple myeloma with thalidomide-dexamethasone after intensive chemotherapy. Ann Oncol. 2002;13:1116–1119.

9. Stewart AK, Chen CI, Howson-Jan K, et al. Results of a multicenter randomized phase II trial of thalidomide and prednisone maintenance therapy for multiple myeloma after autologous stem cell transplant. Clin Cancer Res. 2004;10:8170–8176.

10. Feyler S, Graham J, Rawstron A, EL-Sherbiny Y, Snowden J, Johnson R. Thalidomide maintenance following high dose therapy in multiple myeloma: A UK Myeloma Forum Phase 2 Study. Blood. 2003;102:Abstract #2558.

11. Feyler S, Rawstron A, Jackson G, Snowden J, Hawkins K, Johnson RJ. Thalidomide maintenance following high dose therapy in multiple myeloma: a UK Myeloma Forum phase 2 study. ASH Annual Meeting Abstracts. Blood. 2003;106:641–691a.

12. Brinker BT, Waller EK, Leong T, Heffner LT, Redei I, Langston AA, Lonial S. Maintenance therapy with thalidomide improves overall survival after autologous hematopoietic progenitor cell transplantation for multiple myeloma. Cancer. 2006;106:2171–2180.

13. Attal M, Harousseau JL, Leyvraz S, et al. Maintenance therapy with thalidomide improves survival in patients with multiple myeloma. Blood. 2006;108:3289–3294.

14. Spencer A, Prince M, Roberts AW, Bradstock KF, Prosser IW. First analysis of the Australasian Leukaemia and Lymphoma Group (ALLG) trial of thalidomide and alternate day prednisolone following autologous stem cell transplantation (ASCT) for patients with multiple myeloma (ALLG MM6). ASH Annual Meeting Abstracts. 2006;108:58–77a.

15. Spencer AP, Prince M, Roberts AW, Bradstock KF, Prosser IW. Thalidomide improves survival when used following ASCT. Haematologica. 2007;92:41–42.

16. Peles S, Fisher NM, Devine SM, Tomasson MH, DiPersio JF, Vij R. Bortezomib (Velcade) when given pretransplant and once weekly as consolidation therapy following high dose chemotherapy (HDCT) leads to high rates of reactivation of Varicella Zoster Virus (VZV). ASH Annual Meeting Abstracts. 2005;106:3237–905a.

17. Schiller GJ, Sohn JP, Malone R, et al. Phase I/II Trial of Bortezomib maintenance following autologous peripheral blood progenitor cell transplantation as treatment for intermediate- and advanced-stage multiple myeloma. ASH Annual Meeting Abstracts. 2006;108:5433–453b.

18. Knop S, Hebart H, Kunzmann V, Angermund R, Einsele H. Bortezomib once weekly is well tolerated as maintenance therapy after less than a complete response to high-dose melphalan in patients with multiple myeloma. ASH Annual Meeting Abstracts. 2006;108:5099–364b.

Chapter 8

Therapy for Patients not Eligible for Autologous Transplant

Bringhen Sara and Palumbo Antonio*

Introduction

High-dose therapy supported by autologous stem cell transplant is considered a category 1 recommendation for newly diagnosed multiple myeloma (MM) patients.[1] Currently, MM is the most common indication for autologous transplant, with ~ 4,500 transplants performed yearly in North America (Center for International Blood and Marrow Transplant Research [CIBMTR] data) and 5,300 in Europe.[2] Therefore, one of the first steps in choosing an initial therapy for symptomatic MM patients is to determine whether they would be candidates for stem cell transplant. The criteria to define eligibility for stem cell transplant include comorbidities, age, and performance status. Abnormal cardiac, pulmonary, renal, and liver functions are generally considered exclusion criteria for transplant protocols. Sixty-five years of age is commonly the higher limit age used to define eligible patients. However, it should be noted that advanced age and renal dysfunction are not absolute contraindications for transplant. In a recent study on 678 consecutive patients who underwent autologous transplant, age did not affect outcome, whereas patients with high creatinine levels had a shorter duration of overall survival (OS). The authors concluded that transplant could be offered to selected patients either older than 65 years of age or with elevated creatinine levels.[3] In contrast, transplant rates for patients aged 65 years and under have ranged between 43% and 63%.[4,5]

The primary reasons for (non-inclusion) in high-dose therapy are comorbidity (34%) and patient decision (10%). High-risk patients may be worth discussing in a separate chapter. Patient prognosis is based on the International Staging System[6] and on the cytogenetic abnormalities that are detected either by routine karyotyping or by fluorescence in situ hybridization analysis. Chromosome 13 deletion is the most commonly reported prognostic abnormality for MM.[7,8] The negative prognostic role of specific chromosomal translocations, such as

*Palumbo Antonio has received scientific advisory board and lecture fees from Pharmion, Celgene, and Janssen-Cilag. The other author declares no conflicts of interest.

t(4;14) and t(14;16), or deletion of 17q13 has been established.[7,9] The negative impact of these chromosomal abnormalities on outcome has not been overcome by autologous transplant.[10] These data indicate that novel therapeutic approaches may be required for this subgroup of patients.

In conclusion, almost two thirds of myeloma patients are older than 65 years of age and approximately half of those younger than 65 years of age did not proceed to transplant; thus, ~80% of all MM patients at diagnosis were not candidates for high-dose therapy. This chapter will provide a comprehensive review of the induction therapies available for those patients.

Conventional Chemotherapy

Oral melphalan and prednisone (MP) have historically been considered the standard treatment for patients who are not eligible for high-dose therapy, with a response rate of ~50% and a median OS duration of 2–3 years.[11] Several alkylating agent combinations have been used without a significant impact on survival. An overview of 6,633 patients showed a response rate of 60% from combination chemotherapy versus 53.2% from the simpler and less toxic oral MP combination ($p < 0.001$), while no significant differences in survival were observed.[12] High-dose dexamethasone is one of the most active agents both alone and in combination with chemotherapy.[13,14] A randomized trial compared the combination of melphalan and dexamethasone (MD) with the standard MP treatment; a higher proportion of complete response (CR) was observed in the MD treatment group, but no differences in survival were observed.[15] Facon et al. recently confirmed these findings in a randomized trial involving patients aged 65–75 years.[16] Patients were randomized into four different treatment regimens: MP, MD, high-dose dexamethasone, or high-dose dexamethasone plus interferon-α. MD treatment induced a significantly higher response rate than did the other regimens. The median time to progression was almost doubled after MP and MD treatments, while high-dose dexamethasone and high-dose dexamethasone plus interferon-α did not influence remission duration. OS was similar among the four treatment groups. Dexamethasone-based regimens were additionally associated with a greater risk of severe toxicity, including pulmonary infections and septicemia. These results indicate that oral melphalan should be considered the standard of care and incorporated into all induction treatments for patients who are not candidates for autologous transplant.

Induction Therapy with New Drugs

During the last 5 years, novel antimyeloma therapies have expanded nontransplant options and improved conventional chemotherapy. The most recently approved new drugs – thalidomide, bortezomib, and lenalidomide – either alone or in combination with conventional chemotherapy, have expanded the therapeutic options available to patients; thalidomide showed improvement in the rate of event-free survival, but a substantial improvement in OS rate was observed in the French trial only.

Thalidomide in Newly Diagnosed Myeloma

Thalidomide was used in the 1960s both as a hypnotic sedative and for the treatment of leprosy. During the last decade, it has been used to treat malignant

Table 1 Thalidomide-based regimens at diagnosis.

Therapy	Number of patients	Median age (range)	>65 years (%)	≥PR (%)	CR (%)	Progression-free survival	Overall survival	References
T	28	ND	ND	36	0	50% at 4 months	ND	Weber et al.[18]
TD	103	65 (38–83)	ND	63	4	50% at 22 months	72% at 2 years	Rajkumar et al.[19]
MPT	129	72 (60–85)	59[a]	76	16	54% at 2 years	80% at 3 years	Palumbo et al.[21]
MPT	124	ND (65–75)	100	76	13	50% at 28 months	50% at 51 months	Facon et al.[22]
ThaDD	50	71 (65–75)	64[a]	88	34	60% at 3 years	74% at 3 years	Offidani et al.[23]
CTD	15	ND	ND	60	27[b]	ND	ND	Sidra et al.[24]

PR partial response, *CR* complete response, *T* thalidomide, *TD* thalidome + dexamethasone, *ND* not determinate, *MPT* mephalan + prednisone + thalidomide, *ThaDD* thalidomide + dexamethasone + pegylated lyposomal doxorubicin, *CTD* cyclophosphamide + thalidomide + dexamethasone

[a]>70 years

[b]Very good partial response

diseases, particularly MM. The major clinical trials involving thalidomide as an induction therapy are summarized in Table 1.

Thalidomide Alone and with Dexamethasone

Two phase II studies showed that thalidomide alone showed significant activity in indolent or smoldering[17] as well as asymptomatic MM patients,[18] with partial responses (PRs) of 38% and 36%, respectively. The association of thalidomide with dexamethasone (TD) increased response rates to 72%, including a CR rate of 16%.[18] The combination of thalidomide and dexamethasone was compared with high-dose dexamethasone in a phase III trial. TD consisted of thalidomide at a dose of 200 mg/day and dexamethasone at a dose of 40 mg/day on days 1–4, 9–12, and 17–20 every 4 weeks. TD significantly increased both the PR rate compared with high-dose dexamethasone alone (63% vs 41%, $p = 0.0017$) and the 2-year time to progression ($p > 0.001$), although survival was similar in both groups.[19] It should be noted, however, that this trial was a 4-month induction trial and, as such, not intended for long-term follow-up. Grades 3–4 adverse events were more common in patients on TD and were seen in 67% of patients. The most common side effects were thrombosis, neuropathy, constipation, and skin toxicity. The combination of TD was also compared with standard MP in a phase III trial. Thalidomide was initiated at a dose of 200 mg/day and dexamethasone at a dose of 40 mg on days 1–4 and 15–18 (only odd cycles). Thalidomide was dosed up to 400 mg/day. An interim analysis of the first 125 patients enrolled showed a significantly higher PR rate in the thalidomide treatment group (52% vs 37%, $p = 0.05$). The toxicity profile was similar to that described by Rajkumar et al.[20]

Thalidomide with Chemotherapeutic Agents

Thalidomide Plus MP: Two independent, prospective randomized trials which compared oral MP plus thalidomide (MPT) with MP alone were conducted in elderly patients who were not candidates for autologous transplant.[21,22] In the Italian trial, patients older than 65 years of age or younger who were ineligible for high-dose therapy were randomly assigned to receive either MPT or MP. MPT therapy consisted of the oral administration of melphalan at a dose of 4 mg/m^2 on days 1 through 7 and oral prednisone at a dose of 40 mg/m^2 on days 1 through 7. Each cycle was repeated every 4 weeks for a total of six cycles. Thalidomide was administered at a dose of 100 mg/day continuously during the six cycles and then at 100 mg/day, as maintenance therapy, until progression. Combined CR and PR rates were 76% for MPT and 48% for MP alone; combined near-CR (nCR) and CR rates were 27.9% and 7.2%, respectively. The 2-year event-free survival rates were 54% for MPT and 27% for MP ($p = 0.0006$). The 3-year survival rates were 80% for MPT and 64% for MP ($p = 0.19$). [21] The second phase III trial that compared MPT with MP was performed by the French Cooperative Group and included a third arm with an intermediate dose of melphalan at a dose of 100 mg/m^2 and autologous stem cell transplant. The MPT schedule was slightly different from that in the Italian study, consisting of the oral administration of MP every 6 weeks for a total of 12 cycles and of thalidomide up to a dose of 400 mg/day continuously during the 12 cycles. No maintenance therapy with thalidomide was planned. In the final analysis of this study, a higher overall PR rate in both the MPT and the intermediate-dose melphalan groups compared with the MP group was observed (76% vs 65% vs 35%, respectively). Similarly, the CR rates were significantly higher after both MPT and autologous transplant only. Otherwise, progression-free survival was superior in the MPT patients compared with both MP ($p < 0.0001$) and autologous transplant ($p = 0.0002$) groups. Survival was also significantly improved in the MPT group compared with both MP ($p = 0.0006$) and autologous transplant ($p = 0.027$) groups.[22]

In both studies, MPT was associated with a higher risk of severe toxicity; at least one grades 3–4 adverse event was observed in ~40% of MPT patients. The most common side effects were infections, thromboembolic complications, peripheral neuropathy, constipation, and cardiac events. In the Italian trial,[21] the introduction of enoxaparin prophylaxis significantly reduced the rate of thromboembolism from 20% to 3% ($p = 0.005$). The risk of venous thromboembolism is particularly high in the first 4–6 months of therapy. Infections and cardiac events are more frequent in patients older than 70 years of age.

Together, these results provide a clear indication that MPT should be considered the standard of care in newly diagnosed patients who are not candidates for autologous transplant.

Thalidomide Plus Other Chemotherapeutic Agents: Currently, drug combinations of thalidomide with other chemotherapeutic agents have been tested only in small phase II studies. The more promising associations appear to be those with pegylated liposomal doxorubicin and with cyclophosphamide. Thalidomide plus pegylated liposomal doxorubicin in newly diagnosed patients older than 65 years of age showed a PR rate of 88%, including a CR rate of 34%. The main grades 3–4 adverse events were neutropenia, infections, and thromboembolism.[23] Thalidomide combined with cyclophosphamide as induction therapy showed a PR rate of 60%, including a very good PR (VGPR) rate of 26.7%.[24]

Prognostic Factors and Thalidomide

Thalidomide may reduce the impact of β2-microglobulin by an unknown mechanism. Data presented by Barlogie et al. from Total Therapy II showed that the probability of event-free survival was significantly lower in patients with high levels of β2-microglobulin. However, this parameter failed to predict OS by multivariate analysis.[25] In the Italian MPT study, no significant differences in OS were observed between patients with either high or low β2-microglobulin levels in the MPT group; at 18 months, the OS rates were 80% and 84%, respectively. By contrast, in the MP group, β2-microglobulin remained a prognostic factor.[26] In a recent study, β2-microglobulin did not predict outcome in patients treated at relapse with thalidomide and dexamethasone.[27] The majority of these studies were not designed to evaluate prognostic factors and precautions are mandatory; however, there is growing evidence that β2-microglobulin may have a lesser impact on OS after thalidomide treatment. This evidence calls for a better identification of newer prognostic factors that may better define patient subcategories that will more likely benefit from these regimens.

Lenalidomide in Newly Diagnosed Myeloma

The need to limit the toxicity of thalidomide and improve its efficacy led to the development of a more potent and less toxic analog, CC-5013 (lenalidomide). The major clinical trials of lenalidomide, as induction therapy, are summarized in Table 2.

Lenalidomide with Dexamethasone

One phase II study tested the association of lenalidomide with dexamethason (RD) in 34 newly diagnosed MM patients. Lenalidomide was administered orally at a dose of 25 mg/day on days 1–21 of a 28-day cycle; dexamethasone was administered orally at a dose of 40 mg/day on days 1–4 and 17–20 of each cycle. The PR rate was 91%, including a CR plus VGPR rate of 56%. In 13 patients, autologous transplant was performed after four induction cycles of RD and the 2-year progression-free survival was 83%. The RD

Table 2 Lenalidomide-based regimens at diagnosis.

Therapy	Number of patients	Median age (range)	>65 years (%)	≥PR (%)	CR (%)	Progression-free survival	Overall survival	References
RD	34	64 (32–78)	ND	91	18	59% at 2 years	90% at 2 years	Lacy et al.[29]
MPR	53	71 (57–77)	96	81	24	92% at 1 year	100% at 1 year	Palumbo et al.[31]

PR partial response, *CR* complete response, *RD* lenalidomide + dexamethasone, *ND* not determinate, *MPR* melphalan + prednisone + lenalidomide induction regimen was administered for a prolonged period of time without a subsequent autologous transplant in 21 patients and the 2-year progression-free survival was 59%. Grade 3 adverse events included neutropenia, pneumonia, and cutaneous rash. Deep vein thrombosis was present in only 3% of patients, with prophylactic aspirin during treatment.[28,29] A randomized phase III trial of lenalidomide plus high-dose dexamethasone versus lenalidomide plus low-dose dexamethasone (40 mg; days 1, 8, 15, and 22) was recently reported; however, efficacy data are not available. The dexamethasone dose reduction allowed a significant reduction in the incidence of adverse events; early deaths were reduced from 5% to 0.5%, infections were reduced from 16% to 9%, and deep-vein thrombosis was reduced from 22% to 7%.[30]

Lenalidomide with Chemotherapeutic Agents
The available efficacy data of RD combination therapy support the incorporation of melphalan in induction treatments of myeloma patients. One phase I/II study that evaluated both safety and efficacy of different doses of lenalidomide in combination with oral melphalan and prednisone (MPR) for nine cycles was conducted in the authors' institution. Four different dose levels were tested: (1) 0.18 mg/kg melphalan plus 5 mg/day lenalidomide; (2) 0.25 mg/kg melphalan plus 5 mg/day lenalidomide; (3) 0.18 mg/kg melphalan plus 10 mg/day lenalidomide; and (4) 0.25 mg/kg melphalan plus 10 mg/day lenalidomide. Prednisone (2 mg/kg) and melphalan were administered for 4 days and lenalidomide was administered for 21 days every 4 weeks. All patients received ciprofloxacin and aspirin prophylactically. Fifty-three newly diagnosed patients were enrolled with a median age of 71 years. The maximum tolerated dose was 0.18 mg/kg melphalan plus 10 mg/day lenalidomide. At this dose, the PR rate was 81%, including a VGPR of 48% and a CR rate of 24%. The event-free survival and OS rates at 1 year were 92% and 100%, respectively.[31] These data favorably compared with those of MPT patients. Major grades 3–4 adverse events included hematological toxicities, primarily neutropenia and thrombocytopenia, cutaneous rash, infections, and thromboembolic events. These observations provided the basis for the ongoing large international randomized trial comparing MP with MPR treatments followed by lenalidomide maintenance treatment.

Prognostic Factors and Lenalidomide
Few data are available on the role of lenalidomide therapy in poor-risk patients, although preliminary data have emerged from the Italian MPR study. Fluorescence in situ hybridization data on chromosome 13q deletion and on t(4;14) translocation revealed no differences in response rates and progression-free survival between patients with or without these chromosomal abnormalities.[31]

Bortezomib in Newly Diagnosed Myeloma

Bortezomib represents a new antitumor drug that interrupts an intracellular, multicatalytic protease complex known as the proteasome, which is responsible for the degradation of cellular products, including short-lived proteins, regulatory cyclins, and cyclin-dependent kinase inhibitors that control cell-cycle progression. The major clinical trials of bortezomib as induction therapy are summarized in Table 3.

Table 3 Bortezomib-based regimens at diagnosis.

Therapy	Number of patients	Median age (range)	>65 years (%)	≥PR (%)	CR (%)	Progression-free survival	Overall survival	References
V	32	60 (45–84)	ND	40	3	ND	87% at 1 year	Jagannath et al.[32]
VD	22	60 (45–84)	ND	88	6	ND	87% at 1 year	Jagannath et al.[32]
VMP	60	75 (65–85)	100	89	32	83% at 16 months	90% at 16 months	Mateos et al.[33]
PAD	21	55 (37–66)	ND	95	24	ND	ND	Oakervee et al.[34]

PR partial response, *CR* complete response, *VD* bortezomib + dexamethasone, *ND* not determinate, *VMP* bortezomib + melphalan + prednisone, *PAD* bortezomib + doxorubicin + dexamethasone

Bortezomib Alone and with Dexamethasone

Bortezomib as a single agent and in combination with dexamethasone (VD) was evaluated in 32 untreated patients. Bortezomib was administered by intravenous bolus at a dose of 1.3 mg/m^2 on days 1, 4, 8, and 11 for a maximum of six 3-week cycles; 40 mg dexamethasone on the day of and on the day after bortezomib infusion was added if suboptimal responses were achieved (<PR after two cycles or <CR after four cycles). All 32 patients received the first two cycles, obtaining a PR of 40% and a CR of 3%. Dexamethasone therapy was added to the regimens of 22 patients, with 13 patients beginning steroids at cycle 3 and 9 patients beginning steroids at cycle 5. This approach improved the suboptimal responses in 68% of patients. After the addition of dexamethasone, the PR rate was 88%, including a CR of 6% and an nCR of 19% with a median time to response of 2 months.[32] The most common grades 3–4 adverse events included sensory neuropathy, myalgia, and neutropenia. Sensory neuropathy greater than or equal to grade 2 was reversible within a median time of 3 months in five out of ten patients.

Bortezomib with Chemotherapeutic Agents

The combination of bortezomib and standard MP (VMP) was evaluated in a large phase I/II study of 60 untreated myeloma patients more than 65 years of age (of whom half were older than 75 years).[33] The VMP regimen consisted of four 6-week cycles followed by maintenance therapy with five 5-week cycles. Bortezomib was infused at two dose levels (1.0 and 1.3 mg/m^2) on days 1, 4, 8, 11, 22, 25, 29, and 32 for the first four cycles and on days 1, 8, 15, and 22 for the last five cycles. Oral melphalan at a dose of 9 mg/m^2 and prednisone at a dose of 60 mg/m^2 were administered on days 1–4 for nine cycles. The maximum tolerated dose was 1.3 mg/m^2 bortezomib. Seven patients did not complete the first cycle and were not evaluated. The best response after a median of seven cycles was a PR rate of 89%, including a CR rate of 32%. The event-free survival rate was 83% at 16 months, and the OS rate was 90% at 16 months. In historical controls treated only with MP, the 16-month event-free survival and OS rates were 51% and 62%, respectively. Even without a randomized comparison, the VMP combination appeared to be significantly superior to MP therapy. Grades 3–4 adverse events included thrombocytopenia, neutropenia, peripheral neuropathy, infection, and diarrhea. Side effects were more evident during early cycles and in patients more than 75 years of age. A large international randomized phase III study has recently compared this VMP regimen with MP.

Combinations of bortezomib with other chemotherapeutic agents have been tested only in small phase I/II studies. The most promising association appears to be combination therapy with doxorubicin, resulting in a PR rate of 95%, including a CR rate of 24%. The most frequent severe adverse events were infections and peripheral neuropathy.[34]

Prognostic Factors and Bortezomib

The role of prognostic laboratory parameters and chromosomal abnormalities in patients treated with bortezomib has recently been studied in a limited number of patients. Jagannath et al. demonstrated that response and survival of relapsed or refractory patients treated with bortezomib alone were comparable in those with or without the chromosomal 13 deletion and in those with either high or low β2-microglobulin levels.[8] Similarly, Sagaster et al. showed that response, response duration, and OS did not differ between patients with or without the chromosomal 13 deletion and those with either high or low β2-microglobulin levels. Patients who did not respond to bortezomib as a single agent and subsequently had a short time to progression and OS were identified by low-serum albumin plus the chromosomal 13 deletion.[35] In the Spanish VMP trial, all patients with the chromosomal 13 deletion responded to therapy, and there was no difference in progression-free survival and OS between patients with or without this cytogenetic alteration.[33] In conclusion, bortezomib appears to overcome the poor prognosis conferred by the chromosomal 13 deletion and by high β2-microglobulin levels. Given the small sample size reported in these studies, further investigation is clearly needed to better define the role of well-known prognostic factors in bortezomib-treated patients.

Management of the Most Common New Drug-Related Side Effects

Thalidomide-Related Side Effects

Teratogenicity is the most feared adverse event that occurs when thalidomide is administered between days 27 and 40 of gestation. The use of thalidomide in pregnancy is absolutely contraindicated and prescription safety programs must be followed to prevent such teratogenic effects.[36] Thromboembolism, peripheral neuropathy, constipation, and somnolence are the most common adverse events in thalidomide-based regimens. The risk of thrombosis is low when thalidomide is administered alone, but increases to 12–26% in association with dexamethasone and to 28% in combination with chemotherapy such as doxorubicin. The risk of venous thromboembolism is particularly high in the first 4–6 months of therapy. At present, while there is no clear best prophylactic regimen for such patients, some type of antithrombotic prophylaxis, such as low-molecular weight heparin, warfarin, or aspirin, is recommended.[37] The incidence of peripheral neuropathy after long-term use of thalidomide

(>6 months) is ~70%. Peripheral neuropathy appears to be dose dependent and is correlated with preexisting neuropathy, age, dose of thalidomide, and duration of treatment. To minimize this risk, neurological evaluation should be performed prior to thalidomide treatment, prompt thalidomide dose reduction should be instituted for any grade 2 or greater neurological adverse events observed, and therapy should be limited to less than 6-month duration.[38]

Lenalidomide-Related Side Effects

The major toxicities of lenalidomide include myelosuppression (primarily neutropenia and thrombocytopenia) and venous thromboembolism. The incidence of thromboembolic events in relapsed patients who received lenalidomide and dexamethasone ranged from 8% to 18%. The addition of aspirin markedly reduced the risk of thromboembolic events in newly diagnosed patients treated with lenalidomide. Although the optimal prophylactic strategy has not yet been identified, aspirin appears to be the preferred choice.[37]

Bortezomib-Related Side Effects

The most common adverse events observed were thrombocytopenia, infections, and peripheral neuropathy. Thrombocytopenia was transient, cyclic, and more frequent in thrombocytopenic patients at baseline.[39] In patients receiving bortezomib in combination with chemotherapy, a higher incidence of infections, especially herpes zoster virus reactivation, was observed.[40] Prophylactic antiviral medication is highly recommended in patients with a history of herpes infection. Peripheral neuropathy occurred in ~35% of patients. The risk of neuropathy increased progressively during the first five cycles of bortezomib and subsequently reached a plateau, consistent with a cumulative, dose-related adverse effect. Neuropathy is more frequent in patients with preexisting neuropathy or those who previously received neurotoxic therapy.[41] The current recommendations for management of neuropathy focus on dose reduction according to the severity of symptoms; the discontinuation of bortezomib usually resolves bortezomib-related neuropathy.

Maintenance Therapy

Several compounds, such as interferon-α, glucocorticoids, as well as low doses of new drugs, have been tested as maintenance therapies for MM with the objective to prolong OS. The role of maintenance therapy in MM has been extensively reviewed by Mihelic et al.[42] Unfortunately, the majority of these studies have been performed in a post-transplant setting, and few trials have focused on patients who are not eligible for high-dose therapy. In the last decade, two meta-analyses on the use of interferon as maintenance therapy were reported.[43,44] The first one noted only a limited improvement in clinical outcome.[43] The second meta-analysis showed that the effect of interferon was not significantly related to the dose or duration of interferon or to patient characteristics.[44] Progression-free survival was improved by interferon treatment, but survival benefit, if any, was small and needs to be balanced against both cost and toxicity. The use of two different doses of prednisone (50 mg or 10 mg every other day) was evaluated in a large randomized Southwest Oncology Group (SWOG) trial.[45] After a median follow-up period of 53 months, there were no differences in either progression-free survival or OS. However, from the time of maintenance randomization, progression-free survival and OS were both significantly improved in patients who received 50 mg prednisone compared with 10 mg prednisone every other day. Either observation alone or dexamethasone, at a daily dose of 40 mg for 4 days every month as maintenance therapy, was evaluated in previously untreated MM patients after induction therapy with either MP or MD. With a median follow-up period of 35.3 months, no benefit in OS was observed. Progression-free survival was found to be superior in patients who were randomized to receive dexamethasone.[46] No data are available on maintenance with new drugs in patients who are not candidates for autologous transplant. Two different trials evaluated the role of thalidomide as maintenance after autologous transplant and yielded conflicting results.[25,47] In both studies, patients who were randomized to receive thalidomide showed improvement in the rate of event-free survival, but a substantial improvement in OS rate was observed in the French trial only.

Conclusion

Approximately 80% of myeloma patients are not candidates for autologous transplant due to advanced age or concomitant pathologies. The outcomes of these patients after conventional chemotherapy have not dramatically changed since 1960 when MP was first introduced, suggesting the need for further treatment options. The data available from the most recent studies suggest that the combination of conventional chemotherapy with new drugs has the potential to improve patient outcomes in patients who are ineligible for high-dose therapy. It now seems appropriate to consider MPT as the new standard of care, since two independent randomized trials demonstrated more rapid and higher response rates and improved progression-free survival compared with standard MP therapy.[21,22] In the future, new schemes, such as MPR or VMP, which were recently tested in phase I/Il trials and are now under evaluation in large international randomized phase III studies, might show similar advantages. MPR[31] might prove to possess a better toxicity profile and show a similar or improved efficacy profile than MPT. VMP appears to be equally attractive with a higher CR rate, but it also results in a higher incidence of adverse events.[33] When melphalan was omitted from induction therapy, such as in the TD[19] or RD[28] regimens, a shorter progression-free survival was observed. Thromboembolism, peripheral neuropathy, and cardiac abnormalities were the most frequently reported adverse events in the thalidomide-based regimens. Neutropenia, as well as thromboembolism, is specific to drug combinations including lenalidomide, while thrombocytopenia and peripheral neuropathy are often side effects of bortezomib-containing regimens. International Staging System and cytogenetic abnormalities, such as the deletion of chromosomes 13 and 17 as well as the translocations t(4;14) and t(14;16), are considered to be the major negative prognostic factors for MM.[6-10] In MPT patients, no significant differences in OS were observed between patients with either high or low β2-microglobulin levels.[26] In VMP patients,[33] as well as in a smaller

Table 4 Novel induction therapies including oral melphalan and prednisone.

Regimen	Schedule	Timing	Reference
MPT	Melphalan 4 mg/m^2 orally on days 1–7	Six 4-week cycles	Palumbo et al.[21]
	Prednisone 40 mg/m^2 orally on days 1–7	Six 4-week cycles	
	Thalidomide 100 mg orally each day	Continuously	
MPT	Melphalan 0.25 mg/Kg orally on days 1–4	Twelve 6-week cycles	Facon et al.[22]
	Prednisone 2 mg/Kg orally on days 1–4	Twelve 6-week cycles	
	Thalidomide up to 400 mg orally each day	Twelve 6-week cycles	
MPR	Melphalan 0.18 or 0.25 mg/kg orally on days 1–4	Nine 4-week cycles	Palumbo et al.[31]
	Prednisone 2 mg/kg orally on days 1–4	Nine 4-week cycles	
	Lenalidomide 5 or 10 mg orally on days 1–21	Continuously	
VMP	*Induction:* Melphalan 9 mg/m^2 orally on days 1–4	Four 6-week cycles	Mateos et al.[33]
	Prednisone 60 mg/m^2 orally on days 1–4		
	Bortezomib 1.0 or 1.3 mg/m^2 intravenously on days 1, 4, 8, 11, 22, 25, 29, and 32		
	Maintenance: Melphalan 9 mg/m^2 orally on days 1–4	Five 5-week cycles	
	Prednisone 60 mg/m^2 orally on days 1–4		
	Bortezomib 1.0 or 1.3 mg/m^2 intravenously on days 1, 8, 15, and 22		

MPT melphalan + prednisone + thalidomide, *MPR* melphalan + prednisone + lenalidomide, *VMP* bortezomib + melphalan + prednisone

cohort of MPR patients,[31] the event-free survival of patients with a chromosome 13 deletion or a chromosomal translocation (4:14) was not significantly different from those who did not show such genetic abnormalities. The differences in both safety profiles and the roles of prognostic factors among different new drug regimens might suggest the correlation of a particular combination to a preexisting co-morbidity and/or risk feature. Preexisting peripheral neuropathy or cardiac abnormalities may indicate lenalidomide treatment, while a previous episode of deep-vein thrombosis may indicate bortezomib therapy. Cytogenetic abnormalities may indicate treatment with either lenalidomide or bortezomib, while high levels of β2-microglobulin may indicate thalidomide therapy. The use of maintenance therapy after induction therapy remains an open question, especially in patients who are not candidates for autologous transplant. Owing to the paucity of data in this subset of patients, it is not possible to recommend the use of a specific compound at present. Hopefully, future trials will evaluate the validity of these hypotheses and treatment algorithms, and bring us closer to a personalized approach for MM that is likely to optimize patient outcome. The schedules for novel induction therapies, including oral MP, are listed in Table 4.

Acknowledgment: Supported in part by the Università degli Studi di Torino, Fondazione Neoplasie Sangue Onlus, Associazione Italiana Leucemie, Compagnia di S Paolo, Fondazione Cassa di Risparmio di Torino, Ministero dell'Università e della Ricerca (MIUR), and Consiglio Nazionale delle Ricerche (CNR), Italy.

References

1. Anderson KC, Alsina M, Bensinger W, et al. National Comprehensive Cancer Network(NCCN). Multiple myeloma. Clinical practice guidelines in oncology. J Natl Compr Canc Netw 2007;5:118–47.
2. Gratwohl A, Baldomero H, Frauendorfer K, Urbano-lspizua A. EBMT activity survey2004 and changes in disease indication over the past 15 years. Bone Marrow Transplant 2006;37: 1069–85.
3. Gertz MA, Lacy MQ, Dispenzieri A, et al. Impact of age and serum creatinine value onoutcome after autologous blood stem cell transplantation for patients with multiple myeloma. Bone Marrow Transplant 2007;39:605–11.
4. Lenhoff S, Hjorth M, Holmberg E, et al. Impact of survival of high-dose therapy with autologous stem cell support in patients younger than 60 years with newly diagnosed multiple myeloma: A population-based study. Blood 2000;95:7–11.
5. Morris TCM, Velangi M, Jackson G, Marks DI, Ranaghan L. Less than half of patientsaged 65 years or under with myeloma proceed to transplantation: Results of a two region population-based survey. Br J Haematol 2005;128:510–12.
6. Greipp PR, San Miguel J, Dune BG, et al., International staging system for multiple myeloma. J Clin Oncol 2005;23:3412–20.
7. Chng WJ, Santana-Davila R, Van Wier SA, et al. Prognostic factors for hyper-diploidmyeloma: Effects of chromosome 13 deletions and IgH translocations. Leukemia 2006;20:807–13.
8. Jagannath S, Richardson PG, Sonneveld P, et al. Bortezomib appears to overcome the poor prognosis conferred by chromosome 13 deletion in phase 2 and 3 trials. Leukemia 2007;21:151–57.
9. Jaksic W, Trudel S, Chang H, et al. Clinical outcomes in t(4;14) multiple myeloma: A chemotherapy-sensitive disease characterized by rapid relapse and alkylating agent resistance. J Clin Oncol 2005;23:7069–73.
10. Avet-Loiseau H, Attal M, Moreau P, et al. Genetic abnormalities and survival in multiple myeloma: The experience of the lntergroupe Francophone du Myelome. Blood 2007; 109:3489–95.
11. Alexanian R, Haut A, Khan AU, et al. Treatment for multiple myeloma. Combination chemotherapy with different melphalan dose regimens. JAMA 1969;208:1680–85.
12. GROUP MTC. Combination chemotherapy versus MP as treatment of multiple myeloma: An overview of 6,633 patients from 27 randomised trials. J Clin Oncol 1998; 16:3832–42.
13. Alexanian R, Dimopoulos MA, Delasalle K, Barlogie B. Primary dexamethasone treatment of multiple myeloma. Blood 1992;80:887–90.
14. Segeren CM, Sonneveld P, Van Der Holt B, et al. Vincristine, doxorubicin and dexam-ethasone (VAD) administered as rapid intravenous infusion for first-line treatment in untreated multiple myeloma. Br J Haematol 1999;105:127–30.
15. Hernandez JM, Garcia-Sanz R, Golvano E, et al. Randomized comparison of dexamethasone combined with melphalan versus melphalan with prednisone in the treatment of elderly patients with multiple myeloma. Br J Haematol 2004; 127:159–164.
16. Facon T, Mary JY, Pegourie B, et al. Dexamethasone-based regimens versus mel-phalan-prednisone for elderly multiple myeloma patients ineligible for high-dose therapy. Blood 2006;107:1292–98.
17. Rajkumar SV, Dispenzieri A, Fonseca R, et al. Thalidomide for previously untrea-tedindolent or smoldering multiple myeloma. Leukemia 2001;15:1274–76.
18. Weber D, Rankin K, Gavino M, Delasalle K, Alexanian R. Thalidomide alone or with dexamethasone for previously untreated multiple myeloma. J Clin Oncol 2003;21:16–19.
19. Rajkumar SV, Blood E, Vesole D, Fonseca R, Greipp PR. Eastern Cooperative Oncology Group. Phase Ill clinical trial of thalidomide plus dexamethasone compared

with dexamethasone alone in newly diagnosed multiple myeloma: A clinical trial coordinated by the Eastern Cooperative Oncology Group. J Clin Oncol 2006;24:431–36.

20. Ludwig H, Drach J, Tothová E, et al. Thalidomide-dexamethasone versus melphalan-prednisolone as first line treatment in elderly patients with multiple myeloma: An interim analysis. Blood 2005;106:782a.

21. Palumbo A, Bringhen S, Caravita T, et al. Oral melphalan and prednisone chemotherapy plus thalidomide compared with melphalan and prednisone alone in elderly patients with multiple myeloma: Randomised controlled trial. Lancet 2006;367:825–31.

22. Facon T, Mary J, Hulin C, et al. Melphalan and prednisone plus thalidomide versus melphalan and prednisone alone or reduced-intensity autologous stem-cell transplantation in elderly patients with multiple myeloma (IFM 99-06): a randomised trial. Lancet 2007;370:1209–18.

23. Offidani M, Corvatta L, Piersantelli MN, et al. Thalidomide, dexamethasone, and pegylated liposomal doxorubicin (ThaDD) for patients older than 65 years with newly diagnosed multiple myeloma. Blood 2006:108:2159–64.

24. Sidra G, Williams CD, Russet NH, Zaman S, Myers B, Byrne JL. Combination chemotherapy with cyclophosphamide, thalidomide and dexamethasone for patients with refractory, newly diagnosed or relapsed myeloma. Haematologica 2006;91:862–63.

25. Barlogie B, Tricot G, Anaissie E, et al. Thalidomide and hematopoietic-cell transplantation for multiple myeloma. N EngI J Med 2006;354:1021–30.

26. Palumbo A, Bringhen S, Liberati AM, et al. Oral melphalan, prednisone, thalidomide in elderly patients with multiple myeloma: up-dated results of a randomized, controlled trial. Blood 2008;doi:10.1182/Blood-2008-04-149427.

27. Palumbo A, Bringhen S, Falco P, et al. Time to first progression, but not ~2-microglobulin, predicts outcome in myeloma patients who receive thalidomide as salvage therapy. Cancer 2007; 110:824–29.

28. Rajkumar SV, Hayman SR, Lacy MQ, Combination therapy with lenalidomide plus dexamethasone (Rev/Dex) for newly diagnosed myeloma. Blood 2005;106:4050–53.

29. Lacy M, Gertz M, Dispenzieri A, et al. Long term results of response to therapy, time to progression, and survival with lenalidomide plus dexamethasone in newly diagnosed myeloma. Mayo Clin Proc 2007;82:1179–84.

30. Rajkumar V, Jacobus S, Callander N, et al. A randomized phase III trial of lenalidomide plus high-dose dexamethasone versus lenalidomide plus low-dose dexamethasone in newly diagnosed multiple myeloma (E4A03): A trial coordinated by the Eastern Cooperative Oncology Group. Blood 2006;108:799a.

31. Palumbo A, Falco P, Corradini P, et al. Melphalan, prednisone, and lenalidomide treatment for newly diagnosed myeloma: a report from the GIMEMA-Italian Multiple Myeloma Network. J Clin Oncol 2007;25:4459–65.

32. Jagannath S, Dune BC, Wolf J, et al. Bortezomib therapy alone and in combination with dexamethasone for previously untreated symptomatic multiple myeloma. Br J Haematol 2005;129:776–83.

33. Mateos MV, Hernandez JM, Hernandez MI, et al. Bortezomib plus melphalan and prednisone in elderly untreated patients with multiple myeloma: results of a multicenter phase I/Il study. Blood 2006;108:2165–72.

34. Oakervee HE, Popat R, Curry N, et al. PAD combination therapy (PS-341/bortezomib, doxorubicin and dexamethasone) for previously untreated patients with multiple myeloma. Br. J. Haematol 2005; 129:755–62.

35. Sagaster V, Ludwig H, Kaufmann H, et al. Bortezomib in relapsed multiple myeloma: response rates and duration of response are independent of a chromosome 13q-deletion. Leukemia 2007;21:164–68.

36. Zeldis JB, Williams BA, Thomas SD, Elsayed ME. S.T.E.P.S.: A comprehensive program for controlling and monitoring access to thalidomide. Clin Ther 1999;21:319–30.

37. Bennet CL, Angelotta C, Yarnold PR, et al. Thalidomide- and lenalidomide-associated thromboembolism among patients with cancer. JAMA 2006;296:2558–60.
38. Dimopoulos MA, Eleutherakis-Papaiakovou V. Adverse effects of thalidomide administration in patients with neoplastic diseases. Am J Med 2004; 117:508–15.
39. Lonial S, Wailer EK, Richardson PG, et al. SUMMIT/CREST investigators risk factors and kinetics of thrombocytopenia associated with bortezomib for relapsed, refractory multiple myeloma. Blood 2005; 106:3777–84.
40. Palumbo A, Ambrosini MT, Benevolo G, et al. Bortezomib, melphalan, prednisone and thalidomide for relapsed multiple myeloma. Blood 2007;109:2767–72.
41. Richardson PG, Briemberg H, Jagannath S, et al. Frequency, characteristics, and rever-sibility of peripheral neuropathy during treatment of advanced multiple myeloma with bortezomib. J Clin Oncol 2006;24:3113–20.
42. Mihelic R, Kaufman JL, Lonial S. Maintenance therapy in multiple myeloma. Leukemia 2007;21:1150–57.
43. Fritz E, Ludwig H. Interferon-{alpha} treatment in multiple myeloma: Meta-analysis of 30 randomised trials among 3948 patients. Ann Oncol 2000;11:1427–36.
44. The Myeloma Trialists' Collaborative Group. Interferon as therapy for multiple myeloma: an individual patient data overview of 24 randomized trials and 4012 patients. Br J Haematol 2001;113:1020–34.
45. Berenson JR, Crowley JJ, Grogan TM, et al. Maintenance therapy with alternate-day prednisone improves survival in multiple myeloma patients. Blood 2002;99:3163–68.
46. Shustik C, Belch A, Robinson S, et al. Dexamethasone (dex) maintenance versus observation (obs) in patients with previously untreated multiple myeloma: A National Cancer Institute of Canada Clinical Trials Group Study: MY.7. J Clin Oncol 2004;22 (Suppl 15): 651 Oa.
47. Attal M, Harousseau JL, Leyvraz S, et al. Maintenance therapy with thalidomide improves survival in patients with multiple myeloma. Blood 2006;108:3289–94.

Chapter 9

Current Role of Anthracyclines in the Treatment of Multiple Myeloma

Sikander Ailawadhi and Asher Chanan-Khan

Introduction

Anthracyclines are an important class of antineoplastic drugs that have undergone extensive preclinical and clinical evaluation in various neoplastic disorders including multiple myeloma (MM). They remain an important ingredient in various therapeutic regimens for several hematologic cancers with major impact as part of combination chemotherapy regimens. In MM, anthracyclines (doxorubicin) remain an integral part of the frontline VAD (vincristine, doxorubicin, and dexamethasone) regimen, which is one of the most common antimyeloma regimens used worldwide. This chapter will thus focus on the current role of anthracyclines in the management of patients with MM.

Pharmacology

Anthracyclines are naturally occurring antibiotics that are derived from actinobacteria S*treptomyces peucetius* var. *caesius*. Daunorubicin was the first agent to be discovered in this category that demonstrated antitumor activity in murine model system of human cancers. Further development of this class of anticancer agents resulted in the discovery of doxorubicin, epirubicin, idarubicin, valrubicin, and most recently, pegylated liposomal doxorubicin (PLD). Of all these agents, doxorubicin, a hydroxylated derivative of daunorubicin, has the most diverse antitumor activity with clinical activity observed in various hematologic malignancies (Hodgkin's and non-Hodgkin's lymphoma, MM), and nonhematologic cancers (lung, ovary, stomach, bladder, thyroid, breast, and sarcoma) as well as several pediatric cancers.[1]

All anthracyclines share a quinone-containing rigid planar aromatic ring structure bound by a glycosidic bond to an amino sugar, daunosamine.[2] Modest structural changes from the parent compound have led to the formation of different agents in this category. This complex structure is also responsible for the unique cardiac toxicity profile of this class of anticancer drugs; enzymatic electron reduction of doxorubicin by a variety of oxidases, reductases, and dehydrogenases generates highly reactive species including the hydroxyl free radical OH−. This free radical formation is implicated in doxorubicin cardiotoxicity by means of Cu (II) and Fe (III) reduction at the cellular level.

Recently, a new formulation of doxorubicin (PLD, Doxil®) has been made available. In PLD, doxorubicin hydrochloride is encapsulated in long-circulating Stealth® liposomes. Liposomes are microscopic vesicles composed of a phospholipid bilayer that are capable of encapsulating active drugs. The Stealth® liposomes of PLD are formulated with surface-bound methoxypolyethylene glycol (pegylation) which protects liposomes from detection by the mononuclear phagocyte system increasing drug circulation time. This increases the half-life and allows PLD to penetrate the altered and often compromised vasculature of tumors more effectively, resulting in enhanced tumor exposure to the drug.[3,4] First- and second-phase half-lives of PLD are ~5 h and 55 h, respectively, compared with ~10 min and 30 h, respectively, for conventional doxorubicin. Thus, PLD may be administered at a lower dose than the conventional formulation, potentially reducing the incidence of anthracycline-induced toxicities, especially cardiac toxicity.[5] Since myeloma cells have a low proliferative index, the increased drug exposure time can potentially overcome drug resistance and enhance tumor cell killing.[5,6]

Mechanism of Action and Resistance

Anthracyclines inhibit the topoisomerase IIα enzyme.[7] They form "cleavable complexes" with DNA and topoisomerase IIα to create uncompensated DNA helix torsional tension that leads to DNA breaks and cell death. This seems to be the primary though not the only mechanism of anthracycline-mediated antitumor activity. As the pattern of cleavable complex formation by different anthracyclines varies, it may suggest additional proapoptotic mechanisms involved,[8] such as transcription inhibition through inhibition of DNA-dependent RNA polymerase. Furthermore, cell structure studies on treatment with doxorubicin have demonstrated rapid cell penetration and perinuclear chromatin binding, rapid inhibition of mitotic activity and nucleic acid synthesis, and induction of mutagenesis and chromosomal aberrations.

All anthracyclines are substrates for the P-glycoprotein-mediated drug efflux pump, and thus MDR-1-associated pleiotropic drug resistance may be an important determinant of clinical drug sensitivity. Other drug efflux pumps such as breast cancer resistance protein (BCRP) can also reduce intracellular anthracycline accumulation and may further contribute to clinical resistance to anthracyclines.[9] In addition, drug resistance resulting from topoisomerase IIα point mutations or from downregulation of the enzyme has been characterized in preclinical in vitro investigations, although the significance of these in humans remains undetermined.

Anthracyclines in Multiple Myeloma

Doxorubicin has been used for many years as part of the standard induction treatment in the VAD regimen.[10] Clinical responses reported with VAD regimen in treatment naïve MM patients range between 55% and 84% in various studies,[10,11] although experts argue that the most potent ingredient in VAD regimen is dexamethasone and not doxorubicin. Nevertheless, VAD continues to be the most commonly employed therapeutic regimen worldwide especially in countries where novel molecules such as immunomodulatory drugs (IMIDs) or bortezomib are not readily available. The use of doxorubicin in VAD is associated with several disadvantages such as prolonged continuous intravenous infusion often requiring hospitalization, requirement of a central line access as well as cumulative cardiac toxicity. Over the last few years, the availability of IMIDs (oral formulation) and other effective and more patient-convenient regimens (with steroids, chemotherapy, or both) have resulted in a significantly decreased use of VAD regimen as primary therapy in the United States.

Interestingly, the availability of PLD with improved pharmacokinetics has renewed interest in the use of anthracyclines in patients with MM. PLD overcomes the inconveniences of the standard doxorubicin while maintaining the clinical efficacy of the compound. Thus, clinical investigations have focused on its clinical impact when substituted for doxorubicin in the VAD and other regimens against MM.

Previously Untreated MM

Hussein et al. investigated the efficacy of PLD in the VAD-like regimen in a phase II clinical trial. The regimen consisted of vincristine (2 mg on day 1), PLD (40 mg/m^2 on day 1), and low-dose oral or intravenous dexamethasone (40 mg/day for 4 days) – the DVd regimen. A total of 33 previously untreated MM patients were enrolled.[5] Overall response rate (ORR) was 88% with a 12% complete remission (CR) rate with overall survival (OS) reported at 3 years to be 67%. None of the patients discontinued treatment due to adverse events. Myelosuppression was manageable and the most common toxicities were palmar–plantar erythrodysesthesia, mucositis, and neutropenia. The incidence of cardiotoxicity was very low, with only one patient observed to have cardiotoxicity. Based on these encouraging results, a multicenter, randomized phase III clinical trial was initiated comparing the VAD regimen versus the DVd regimen.[12] Final results of this study were reported by Rifkin et al. and demonstrated no advantage in efficacy of substitution of PLD in the DVd regimen over the VAD regimen. Of note, the DVd regimen was associated with improved safety and convenience to patients. Also, patients receiving the DVd regimen had less neutropenia and growth factor requirement, decreased frequency of alopecia, and fewer toxicity-related hospitalizations. In addition, PLD use in this trial was associated with shorter duration of hospital stay, less frequent catheter use, and shorter duration of drug administration.[12] Results of this and other studies using anthracycline-based regimens in previously untreated MM are summarized in Table 1.

Zervas et al. investigated addition of thalidomide to the DVd regimen. Oral thalidomide (200 mg/day) was given continuously with DVd (DVd-T).[13] Among the 39 patients with untreated MM enrolled in this study, an ORR of 74% with a CR rate of 10% was reported. In a similar effort to further optimize the clinical responses to induction regimen, Offindani in a phase II clinical trial investigated addition of PLD to the dexamethasone/thalidomide regimen in patients older than 65 years with newly diagnosed MM.[14] Overall this regimen was noted to be very efficacious and well tolerated with an ORR of 98%, of which 14% patients achieved a CR. Time to progression (TTP), event-free

Table 1 Anthracycline-based regimens in previously untreated multiple myeloma.

Regimen	ORR (%)	Reference
Vincristine + doxorubicin + dexamethasone (VAD)	55–84	Alexanian et al.,[10] Samson et al.[11]
Vincristine + PLD + dexamethasone (DVd)	88	Hussein et al.[5]
Vincristine + PLD + dexamethasone + thalidomide (DVd-T)	74	Zervas et al.[13]
Thalidomide + PLD + dexamethasone (ThalDD)	98	Offidani et al.[14]
Vincristine + PLD + dexamethasone + low-dose thalidomide (DVd-T)	80	Deauna-Limayo et al.[15]
PLD + bortezomib	79	Orlowski et al.[19]
Bortezomib + PLD + dexamethasone (VDD)	89	Jakubowiak et al.[21]

ORR overall response rate, *PLD* pegylated liposomal doxorubicin

survival, and projected OS at 3 years were 60%, 57%, and 74%, respectively. The toxicity profile was favorable in this elderly population cohort, which usually has several preexisting comorbidities.[14] A variation of the DVd-T regimen has been a lower dose of thalidomide (100 mg) that was studied in patients with previously untreated MM. Responses similar to the previous DVd-T regimen were noted and there was no adverse impact on stem cell harvest associated with this therapy. Major responses were achieved rapidly, and patients were taken for early stem cell harvest and autologous transplant after two cycles of therapy.[15]

Resistance to DNA-damaging agents including anthracyclines can be mediated by an NF-κB-driven antiapoptotic mechanism, involving the Bcl-2 and inhibitor of apoptosis protein families, which has been shown to be blocked by proteasome inhibition.[16] There has been other preclinical data supporting the fact that bortezomib (Velcade®), a proteasome inhibitor, enhances the sensitivity of MM cells to conventional chemotherapeutic agents including anthracyclines.[17,18] Orlowski et al. reported the combination of bortezomib with PLD. This was conducted as a Cancer and Leukemia Group B (CALGB) cooperative study in previously untreated MM patients.[19] Preliminary response data were reported in 57 patients, of whom 16% achieved a CR or near-CR (nCR), while 58% attained at least a partial response (PR). Final response data were reported for 29 patients who completed their study-directed therapy and among these the CR + nCR rate was 28%, with an ORR of 79%. This steroid-free regimen was well tolerated, and those patients who were planned to get an autologous peripheral blood stem cell transplant were not noticed to have any compromise in stem cell collection due to this induction regimen.[19]

Attempts have been made to improve upon the existing regimens to better the response rates and tolerability. After the encouraging results from the combination of bortezomib and PLD, another regimen reported as phase II data is bortezomib and dexamethasone with PLD (VDD). This was initially studied in the relapsed/refractory setting,[20] but was recently reported as induction regimen in previously untreated MM patients.[21] Forty patients were enrolled, of which 37 were evaluable at the time of the reported data. After induction treatment with VDD, patients were given either maintenance bortezomib or stem cell transplant. A PR rate of 89%, very good partial response rate (>75% reduction in monoclonal protein) of 50%, and a CR/nCR rate of 37% was reported with the induction regimen. The treatment was well tolerated with no grade 4 hematological toxicities reported. The authors conducted correlative studies demonstrating that apoptotic pathways in the cellular milieu of these patients were upregulated more when PLD was added to bortezomib or bortezomib plus dexamethasone, suggesting the integral role of anthracyclines in treatment combinations.[21]

Relapsed/Refractory MM

Anthracyclines have also been investigated and used as a part of several salvage treatment regimens among patients with relapsed or refractory disease (Table 2). Barlogie et al. initially reported response rates of 50–70% with VAD regimen in patients with relapsed or refractory myeloma.[22] Subsequent studies with anthracyclines had less impressive results, with as little as an ORR of 20% with VAD and only 8% and 9% with epirubicin with ifosfamide and vincristine, doxorubicin with prednisone (VAP) regimens, respectively.[23]

More recently, Hussein et al. investigated the clinical efficacy of the DVd-T regimen in patients with relapsed/refractory MM.[24] In this study, PLD (40 mg/m^2 intravenous, day 1), vincristine (2 mg intravenous, day 1), and dexamethasone (40 mg orally, days 1–4) were given with thalidomide (dose escalated ≤ 400 mg/day) to patients with relapsed/refractory MM. After the initial treatment, patients were maintained on prednisone 50 mg orally every other day plus the individual's maximum tolerated dose (MTD) of thalidomide till toxicity or disease progression. Data on 35 patients were reported for efficacy and toxicity. Overall, 74% of patients demonstrated a response to therapy using the

Table 2 Anthracycline-based regimens in relapsed/refractory multiple myeloma.

Regimen	ORR (%)	Reference
Vincristine + doxorubicin + dexamethasone (VAD)	50–70	Barlogie et al.,[22] Palva et al.[23]
Vincristine + PLD + dexamethasone + thalidomide (DVd-T)	74	Hussein et al.[24]
Bortezomib + PLD + thalidomide (VDT)	65	Chanan-Khan et al.[28]
PLD + bortezomib (phase I)	73	Orlowski et al.[26]
Vincristine + PLD + dexamethasone + lenalidomide (DVd-R)	83	Baz et al.[25]
Bortezomib + PLD + dexamethasone (VDD)	83	Jakubowiak et al.[20]
Melphalan + PLD + bortezomib (MVD)	NR	Chari et al.[31]
Bortezomib + PLD + dexamethasone + thalidomide (VDD-T)	75	Ciolli et al.[30]
PLD + bortezomib (phase III)	44	Orlowski et al.[27]

NR not reported

Southwest Oncology Group (SWOG) response criteria ($\geq 50\%$ decreases in myeloma protein). Three patients (9%) achieved CRs and another 13 patients (37%) achieved nCRs. The median time to initial response was 1 month (range, 0.7–5.6 months) and the median time to best response was 2.7 months (range, 0.9–6.3 months). This study provided for supportive precautionary measures including antimicrobials, G-CSF or GM-CSF, acetylsalicylic acid for antiplatelet activity, and erythropoietin analogues, which reduced grade 3/4 toxicities to a minimum.[24] Results from these data suggested that the addition of thalidomide to anthracycline-based regimens improved the response rate and quality of response of the traditional anthracycline-based regimens VAD or DVd, possibly by overcoming resistance to chemotherapy in patients with relapsed/refractory MM.

Lenalidomide (CC-5013, Revlimid®) is a thalidomide analogue and pre-clinical data have shown it to be more potent than thalidomide in stimulating T-cell proliferation and augmenting IL-2 and IFN-γ production. A modification of the DVd-T regimen is DVd with lenalidomide (DVd-R) which has been reported as a phase II trial in relapsed/refractory MM patients.[25] PLD (40 mg/m^2) and vincristine (2 mg) were administered intravenously on day 1, dexamethasone (40 mg) orally daily for 4 days, and lenalidomide at 10 mg daily for 21 days in each 28-day cycle. Of the 45 evaluable patients, 13% had CR and 83% were noted to have some degree of response. Interestingly, 67% of the patients had previously received and were refractory to thalidomide-based regimens. Grade 3 or greater toxicities were noted, but no treatment-related deaths or discontinuation of the regimens was reported.[25]

In a novel clinical trial, Orlowski et al. investigated for the first time a combination of bortezomib with PLD in a dose-escalation phase I study in patients with relapsed/refractory MM.[26] Bortezomib was administered at 0.9–1.5 mg/m^2 on days 1, 4, 8, and 11, while PLD was administered at 30 mg/m^2 on day 4. Among 22 evaluable patients, the ORR was 73% with a CR/nCR rate of 36%. Interestingly, some patients with previously anthracycline-resistant disease demonstrated clinical response to the combination regimen, possibly hinting on the ability of bortezomib to restore in vivo sensitivity to doxorubicin. The pioneering work conducted by Orlowski et al. led to a more rigorous investigation of PLD in patients with MM. A recently completed multicenter, randomized phase III clinical trial compared the efficacy of bortezomib/PLD combination with bortezomib alone in relapsed or refractory MM. A total of 646 patients were enrolled with at least one prior therapy.[27] Bortezomib (standard dose and schedule) was given for eight treatment cycles to both groups of patients. PLD was given at 40 mg/m^2 on day 4 to all patients randomized to the combination arm and patients received a total of eight cycles of the combination regimen. The primary endpoint of this study was TTP. Recently published results of this study demonstrated that there was no statistical difference in ORR (41% and 44%, $p = 0.043$) and the CR rate (11% and 13%) in the bortezomib versus bortezomib/PLD arm, respectively. Interestingly, there was significant improvement in the duration of response (0.2 vs 7 months, $p = 0.0008$) and the TTP (9.3 vs 6.5 months, $p = 0.000004$) in the combination versus single-agent bortezomib arm, respectively. This benefit in TTP was noted in all patients irrespective of markers of high-risk disease such as elevated β2-microglobulin and advance age or previous treatments such as prior stem cell transplantation or IMID therapy. Based on improvement in these clinical parameters, PLD recently secured approval from the FDA for treatment of relapsed or refractory MM in combination with bortezomib.

To further improve upon the efficacy of this combination, a phase II clinical trial was conducted combining bortezomib/PLD with continuous dosing of thalidomide (VDT) at Roswell Park Cancer Institute. This allowed targeting the tumor microenvironment concurrently with the tumor cell. A total of 23 patients with stage III relapsed or refractory MM were enrolled.[28] Bortezomib was administered at a dose of 1.3 mg/m^2 on days 1, 4, 15, and 18, along with PLD 20 mg/m^2 on days 1 and 15 and daily low-dose (100 mg) thalidomide. Evaluable patients ($n = 21$) showed a PR or better response in 65% of the cases and a CR in 23% of the cases. The median progression-free survival was 10.9 months with a median OS of 15.7 months. No significant nonhematologic grade 3/4 toxicities were seen. The impressive clinical result of this steroid-free regimen has prompted to look at its efficacy in previously untreated MM patients. This phase II clinical trial by the same group of investigators is ongoing.

Jakubowiak et al. reported the phase II data on VDD in patients with relapsed/refractory MM.[20] CR/nCR was noted in 33% out of the 18 evaluable patients. An ORR of 83% was reported. The same group of authors recently reported a subanalysis of the efficacy and tolerability of this PLD and bortezomib combination regimen in previously treated older (≥ 65 years) individuals.[29] They noted that the response rates and toxicity profile of this combination was similar in older patients when compared to the younger patients. Also, in either group of patients, efficacy improved when PLD was added to bortezomib.[29] Using the same rationale of combining novel agents with anthracycline-based regimens, a regimen including bortezomib, PLD, dexamethasone, and thalidomide (VDD-T) is being studied in the setting of refractory MM.[30] Recently reported preliminary data included 28 patients, of which 35% achieved a CR or nCR and 75% had some overall response to treatment. Median TTP and OS had not been reached after a median follow-up of 9 months at the time of this report.

Melphalan is one of the long-established agents with antimyeloma activity. Attempts have been made to study the efficacy of melphalan in combination with anthracyclines and newer agents. Chari et al. reported a dose-escalation study of PLD, melphalan, and bortezomib in relapsed/refractory MM to determine the MTD and dose-limiting toxicity of this combination.[31] Only the first five patients on this trial were reported so far, with no dose-limiting toxicities. Dose escalation is continuing to determine the MTD.

Conclusion

Anthracyclines have been used in the treatment of MM for several decades. Among these the most common formulation used was doxorubicin. Recent development of a more convenient pegylated formulation of doxorubicin, PLD, has demonstrated antimyeloma activity in combination with bortezomib. The approval of PLD by the FDA is encouraging and demonstrates an important and continued role played by the anthracycline group of drugs in myeloma patients.

Several novel agents are demonstrating promising antimyeloma activity in preclinical model systems. Future clinical investigation will focus on how these new molecules can be safely and effectively incorporated with the currently available drugs such as the PLD.

References

1. Chu E, DeVita VC. Physician's cancer chemotherapy drug manual. Sudbury, MA: Jones and Bartlett; 2006.
2. Robert J. Anthracyclines. In: A clinician's guide to chemotherapy pharmacokinetics and pharmacodynamics. Vol. 93 (3rd edition). Baltimore, MD: Williams 8 Wilkins; 1983.
3. Sharpe M, Easthope SE, Keating GM, et al. Polyethylene-glycol-liposomal doxorubicin: A review of its use in the management of solid and hematological malignancies and AIDS-related kaposi's sarcoma. Drugs. 2002;62:2089–2126.
4. Gabizon AA. Pegylated liposomal doxorubicin: Metamorphosis of an old drug into a new form of chemotherapy. Cancer Invest. 2001;19:424–436.
5. Hussein MA, Wood L, Hsi E, et al. A phase II trial of pegylated liposomal doxorubicin, vincristine, and reduced-dose dexamethasone combination therapy in newly diagnosed multiple myeloma patients. Cancer. 2002;95:2160–2168.
6. Lee CC, Gillies ER, Fox ME, et al. A single dose of doxorubicin-functionalized bow-tie dendrimer cures mice bearing C-26 colon carcinomas. PNAS. 2006;103:16649–16654.
7. Tewey KM, Rowe TC, Yang L, et al. Adriamycin-induced DNA damage mediated by mammalian DNA topoisomerase II. Science. 1984;226:466.
8. Doroshow JH. Anthracyclines and anthracenediones. In: Cancer chemotherapy and biotherapy: Principles and practice. Vol. 500 (3rd edition). Philadelphia, PA: Lippincott Williams 8 Wilkins; 2001.
9. Doyle LA, Ross DD. Multidrug resistance mediated by the breast cancer resistance protein BCRP (ABCG2). Oncogene. 2003;22:7340.
10. Alexanian R, Barlogie B, Tucker S. VAD-based regimens as primary treatment for multiple myeloma. Am J Hematol. 1990;33:86–89.
11. Samson D, Gaminara E, Newland A, et al. Infusion of vincristine and doxorubicin with oral dexamethasone as first-line therapy for multiple myeloma. Lancet. 1989;2: 882–885.
12. Rifkin RM, Gregory SA, Mohrbacher A, et al. Pegylated liposomal doxorubicin, vincristine, and dexamethasone provide significant reduction in toxicity compared with doxorubicin, vincristine, and dexamethasone in patients with newly diagnosed multiple myeloma. Cancer. 2006;106:848–858.
13. Zervas K, Dimopoulos MA, Hatzicharissi E, et al. Primary treatment of multiple myeloma with thalidomide, vincristine, liposomal doxorubicin and dexamethasone (T-VAD doxil): A phase II multicenter study. Ann Oncol. 2004;15:134–138.
14. Offidani M, Corvatta L, Piersantelli M, et al. Thalidomide, dexamethasone, and pegylated liposomal doxorubicin (ThaDD) for patients older than 65 years with newly diagnosed multiple myeloma. Blood. 2006;108:2159–2164.
15. Deauna-Limayo D, Aljitawi O, Mayo M, et al. Pegylated liposomal doxorubicin (Doxil®), dexamethasone and low dose thalidomide (DDt) as therapy for newly diagnosed multiple myeloma. Blood. 2005;106:Abstract 5164.
16. Orlowski RZ, Baldwin AS Jr. NF-kappa B as a therapeutic target in cancer. Trends Mol Med. 2002;8:385–389.
17. Ma MH, Yang HH, Parker K, et al. The proteasome prohibitor PS-341 markedly enhances sensitivity of multiple myeloma tumor cells to chemotherapeutic agents. Clin Cancer Res. 2003;9:1136–1144.
18. Mitsiades N, Mitsiades CS, Richardson PG, et al. The proteasome inhibitor PS-341 potentiates sensitivity of multiple myeloma cells to conventional chemotherapeutic agents: Therapeutic applications. Blood. 2003;101:2377–2380.

19. Orlowski RZ, Peterson BL, Sanford B, et al. Bortezomib and Pegylated Liposomal Doxorubicin as Induction Therapy for adult patients with symptomatic multiple myeloma: Cancer and leukemia group B study 10301. Blood. 2006;108:Abstract 797.

20. Jakubowiak AJ, Brackett L, Kendall T, et al. Combination therapy with Velcade, Doxil, and Dexamethasone (VDD) for patients with relapsed/refractory multiple myeloma (MM). Blood. 2005;106:Abstract 5179.

21. Jakubowiak A, Al-Zoubi A, Kendall T, et al. Combination therapy with bortezomib(Velcade®), Doxil®, and dexamethasone(VDD) in newly diagnosed myeloma: updated results of phase II clinical trial. Haematologica. 2007;92:Abstract PO-721.

22. Barlogie B, Smith L, Alexanian R. Effective treatment of advanced multiple myeloma refractory to alkylating agents. N Engl J Med. 1984;310:1353–1356.

23. Palva IP, Ahrenberg P, Ala Harja K, et al. Intensive chemotherapy with combinations containing anthracyclines for refractory and relapsing multiple myeloma. Finnish leukaemia group. Eur J Haematol. 1990;44:121–124.

24. Hussein MA, Elson P, Tsoe EA, et al. Doxil (D), vincristine (V), decadron (d) and thalidomide (T) (DVd-T) for relapsed/refractory multiple myeloma (RMM). Blood [abstract]. 2002;100:403a.

25. Baz R, Choueiri TK, Abou Jawde R, et al. Doxil (D), Vincristine (V), reduced frequency Dexamethasone (d) and Revlimid(R) (DVd-R) results in a high response rate in patients with refractory multiple myeloma (RMM). Blood. 2005;106: Abstract 2559.

26. Orlowski RZ, Voorhees PM, Garcia RA, et al. Phase I trial of the proteasome inhibitor bortezomib and pegylated liposomal doxorubicin in patients with advanced hematological malignancies. Blood. 2005;105:3058–3065.

27. Orlowski RZ, Zhuang SH, Parekh T, et al. The combination of pegylated liposomal doxorubicin and bortezomib significantly improves time to progression of patients with relapsed/refractory multiple myeloma compared with bortezomib alone: results from a planned interim analysis of a randomized phase III study. Blood. 2006;108: Abstract 404.

28. Chanan-Khan AA, Padmanabhan S, Miller KC, et al. Final results of a phase II study of bortezomib (Velcade) in combination with liposomal doxorubicin (Doxil) and thalidomide (VDT) demonstrate a sustained high response rate in patients (pts) with relapsed (rel) or refactory (ref) multiple myeloma. Blood. 2006;108:Abstract 3539.

29. San-Miguel JF, Hajek R, Nagler A, et al. Doxil®+Velcade® in previously treated ≥65y myeloma pts. Haematologica. 2007;92:PO-620.

30. Ciolli S, Leoni F, Casini C, et al. Liposomal doxorubicin (Myocet®) enhance the efficacy of bortezomib, dexamethasone plus thalidomide in refractory myeloma. Blood. 2006;108:Abstract 5087.

31. Chari A, Kaplan L, Linker C, et al. Phase I/II study of bortezomib in combination with liposomal doxorubicin and melphalan in relapsed or refractory multiple myeloma. Blood. 2005;106:Abstract 5182.

Section 3

Immune-Based Therapies

Chapter 10

Allogeneic Transplantation for Multiple Myeloma

Fengrong Wang and Edmund K. Waller

Introduction

Autologous hematopoietic stem cell transplantation (HSCT) is currently considered part of the standard care in the management of patients with newly diagnosed multiple myeloma (MM). Autologous transplantation has extended overall survival and progression-free survival by 1–1.5 years compared to conventional dose chemotherapy in randomized clinical studies[1–3] in patients up to 65 years of age. Unfortunately, long-term survival for patients treated with autologous HSCT is rare, and virtually all patients relapse. Allogeneic (Allo-) HSCT can induce long-term molecular remission and is possibly the only curative treatment for MM based on the graft-versus-tumor (GVT) or graft-versus-myeloma (GVM) effects mediated by the allogeneic donor immune cells, particularly donor T-cells. Advantages of allogeneic HSCT in comparison to autologous HSCT are a tumor-free stem cell source and the GVM effect. Current clinical research is trying to define the clinical outcomes of patients allocated to allogeneic transplantations based on the availability of human leukocyte antigen (HLA)-matched donor versus patients without a suitable donor who undergo one or two autologous transplantations.[4,5] Recent publications indicated that durable engraftment and less regimen-related toxicity can be obtained in allogeneic transplantation using reduced intensity conditioning (RIC) regimen that do not result in myeloablation.[6–8] Despite reduced early mortality, significant rates of graft-versus-host (GVH) disease and late relapse remain problems following RIC regimens, highlighting the need for novel strategies to enhance and target the GVM effect in allogeneic transplantation. This chapter will highlight the antigenic targets for GVM and review the clinical experience with donor leukocyte infusions, myeloablative transplants, nonmyeloablative conditioning regimens, and the use of tandem auto-allo transplants for this disease.

Myeloma as an Antigen-Presenting Cell

MM is a clonal B-cell malignancy characterized by an excess of mature plasma cells in the bone marrow in association with a monoclonal protein in serum and/or urine, and decreased levels of normal immunoglobulin (Ig).

From: *Contemporary Hematology Myeloma Therapy*
Edited by: S. Lonial © Humana Press, Totowa, NJ

B cells function as antigen-presenting cells and, as such, may function to initiate activation of donor 7-cells following allogeneic HSCT and serve as the target for immune-mediated GVM effects. After antigen has bound to Ig on B cell, the B cell internalizes the antigen, partially degrades it, and subsequently presents a fragment of the degraded antigen on its surface to a T cell, activating the T cell, leading in turn to B-cell activation. B cells also express an array of immune-regulating molecules on their cell surface, which play a role in the B cell's interactions with T cells, such as MHC class II molecules, B7, and CD40.

The success of myeloma to immunotherapeutic strategies is presently being explored by vaccine strategies using dendritic cells, genetically modified tumor cell preparations, as well as myeloma-expressed DNA and proteins.[9–11] Thus, the curative potential of allogeneic HSCT in the treatment of myeloma is based on the recognition of myeloma cells by activated donor T cells, a phenomenon that is termed the GVM effect.[12–14] The GVM effect can be augmented by using donor lymphocyte infusion (DLI) to treat relapse and to eradiate minimal residual disease (MDR) after allo-HSCT.[15]

Clinical Evidence for the Efficacy of Immune-Mediated Antimyeloma Therapy in HSCT

Several studies compared the results of autologous and allogeneic HSCT in relatively large cohorts of patients and demonstrated that allogeneic GVM effect results in significant and durable antimyeloma activity. These data had shown that there was no difference in the complete remission (CR) rate after transplantation between allogeneic and autologous groups, but disease progression and recurrence was more frequent after auto-HSCT compared to allo-HSCT at 4–5 years (66–70% vs 46–50%).[12,16,17] In one study focused on MRD after transplantation, 7 of 14 (50%) patients became PCR negative after allo-HSCT while only 17% (5 of 30 patients) became negative in the autologous group. In addition, for the PCR positive population, 14% experienced clinical relapse after allo-HSCT compared to 40% of patients who relapsed after auto-HSCT.[17] Taken together, these studies provide evidence for the presence of a clinically significant GVM effect after allo-HSCT.

The most direct evidence for an effective immune-mediated therapy for myeloma has been the clinical regression of disease observed following infusion of lymphocytes from an allogeneic HSCT donor.[18] DLI was developed as a form of T cell-adoptive therapy for patients with CML relapsed after allo-HSCT using allogeneic lymphocytes from the original HSCT donor. Results from a collection of small series of myeloma patients treated with allogeneic donor lymphocytes are shown in Table 1. Initial documentation of the GVM effect came from several individual cases reports. In 1996, Tricot et al. described one patient with progressive disease after T-cell-depleted allo-HSCT, who responded to 1.2×10^6 donor T cells/kg infusion.[27] At the same time, another report from Europe showed that two patients relapsed after T-cell-depleted BMT achieved complete response after DLI, T cell doses of 1.1×10^8/kg and 3.3×10^8/kg, respectively.[28] The response rates in two large studies comfirmed the efficacy of DLI in relapsed myeloma patients (Table 1). Fourteen of 27 (52%) and 10 of 25 (40%) patients with active and measurable myeloma following allogeneic HSCT have responses

Table 1 Result of DLI as treatment or prophylaxis in MM patients after transplantation.

Study	No. of patients	Type of transplant (No.)	Additional therapy	DLI as prophylaxis	CD3 cell dose (×10⁶/kg) median (range)	Response rate (%)		% with GVHD (≥ grade 2) acute/chronic	TRM (%)	Outcome (years)	Follow-up median (months)
						CR	PR				
Lockhorse et al. 1997, Urecht, NE[18]	13	Sib, TCD	–		19,2 (1–330)	31	31	66/56	15	OS 77%	18
Lockhorse et al. 2004, Urecht, NE[19]	54	Sib, TCD (50)	–		NA (1–500)	17	35	46/47	5	OS ca. 40% (2)	
Salama et al. 2000, Dallas, USA[20]	25	Sib (24)	INF α (4)		100 (2–220)	28	12	52/44	12	OS 48% (1)	13
Kroger, et al. 2004, Hamburg, Germany[21]	18	VUD (1) Sib/VUD RIC (17) Standard(1)	Thalidomide		Escalating dose	22	45	0/33	0	OS 100% PFS 84% (2)	24
Van der Donk et al. 2006, European[22]	63	NA	Thalidomide/ bortezomib		NA	19	19	38/43	11	OS 68.3%	14
Alyea et al. 2001, Boston, USA[23]	14	Sib, TCD	–	Y	NA (10–30) CD4⁺	43	29	50ᵃ	7	OS 83% PFS 65% (2)	28
Badros et al. 2001, Little Rock, USA[24]	14	Sib	–	Y	Escalating dose 200 (120–220)	36	50	71/50	0 d100	OS 64% (1)	
Peggs et al. 2003, London, UK[25]	14	Sib/MUD, RIC	Campath	Y			50ᵇ	21/14	–	OS 71%	
Peggs et al. 2004, London, UK[26]	19	Sib RIC (12) MUD RIC (7)	Campath	Y	NA (1–300)	5	42	47ᵃ	26	PFS 30% (2) OS 53%	NA
Total	**177**					27ᶜ	40ᶜ		10ᶜ		

ATG antithymocyte globulin, *CR* complete remission, *DLI* donor lymphocyte infusion, *GVHD* graft versus host disease, *MM* multiple myeloma, *OS* overall survival, *PFS* progression-free survival, *PR* partial remission, *RIC* reduced intensity conditioning, *TCD* T cell depletion, *TRM* transplant-related mortality, *VUD* volunteer unrelated donor, *Y* yes, *NA* not available, *MUD* matched unrelated donor.
ᵃBoth acute and chronic GVHD.
ᵇTotal response after DLI.
ᶜWeighted average form reported studies.

to DLI, ~25% achieved a CR, 21% achieved a PR. Total CD3[+] T cell ranged from 1×10^6/kg to 330×10^6/kg body weight. However, responses were mostly detected after relatively high T-cell doses achieved following multiple DLIs.[19,20] One study by Salama et al.[20] involved the use of chemotherapy before DLI or DLI combined with INF α treatment. Interferon (IFN) α, as an immunological modulator, may enhance the GVM effect by increasing the expression of cell-surface molecules that are necessary for the activation of immune effector cells, or by a direct antimyeloma effect.

In addition to treating relapsed MM patients after HSCT, prophylactic DLI has been used as part of allogeneic transplantation strategy in order to reduce disease recurrence.[23,24] Alyea et al.[23] reported a study in the Dana-Farber Cancer Institute of CD6 T-cell-depleted allogeneic HSCT combined with CD4+ donor T lymphocyte prophylactic infusion in MM patients. Twenty-four patients with matched sibling donors and chemotherapy-sensitive disease enrolled in this study. Only five patients had more than grade 2 acute graft-versus-host disease (aGVHD) after HSCT. Although significant GVM responses were noted after DLI in 10 of 11 patients with persistent disease (CR 6, PR 4), only 58% (14 of 24) patients were able to receive DLI due to toxicity of the myeloablative conditioning regimen and/or GVHD. Two-year current progression-free survival (PFS) was superior (65%) in these 14 patients compared to historical patients who did not receive DLI. Taken together, the GVM activity of DLI supports the curative potential of allogeneic HSCT in myeloma, but points out regimen-related toxicity and GVHD as significant limitations in the overall clinical effectiveness of myeloablative conditioning.

Reduced intensity or nonmyeloablative allo-HSCT can effectively reduce treatment-related toxicity, but is associated with higher frequencies of disease recurrence, especially in relapsed or refractory MM patients. Therefore, in the past few years, some groups have used an RIC regimen and allo-HSCT combined with prophylactic DLI posttransplantation to promote GVM activity.[25,26,29,30] Peggs et al. reported 14 patients treated with reduced-intensity transplantation with in vivo T-cell depletion and adjuvant dose-escalation DLI. The overall response post DLI was 42.8% (14% in CR). Two-year OS and PFS rates were 71% and 30%, respectively.[25] Another report from the same group including additional patients showed 58% (11 of 19) patients alive and progression free after 2.2 years follow-up.[26]

These studies indicate that DLI following allo-transplantation is a valuable strategy for relapsed or persistent disease. However, the major disadvantage of the treatment model remains that the effect of GVM seems ineluctably bound up with the development of GVHD and durable remissions can be achieved only in a small part of patients.

More recently, it has been shown that some new chemotherapeutic agents, such as thalidomide and bortezomib, given along with DLI can improve response rates with very promising OS and PFS rates of 100% and 84%, respectively, at 2 years and only minimal risk of GVHD.[21,22]

Antigen Targets for Antimyeloma Immunotherapy

Despite the widespread use of allo-HSCT and DLI in MM patients to treat or prevent relapse, the outcomes demonstrate the lack of durability of responses in the majority of cases and the difficulty in separating GVM from GVHD with current approaches. To find target antigens expressed on myeloma cells but not on nonmalignant cells would be of major interest to induce myeloma-specific donor T-cells in vitro for adoptive transfer and therefore improving the safety and efficiency of allogeneic HSCT and DLI.

Myeloma is derived from a single expanded B cell clone; it expresses an Ig with a unique idiotype (Id) (the variable regions of Ig), which had been examined as a tumor-associated antigen (TAA) in B-cell malignancies including myeloma.[11,31] Although using tumor-derived Id as an immunogen to elicit antitumor immunity against B-cell malignancies is an attractive idea, the broader use of idiotypic vaccines has been hampered by the fact that autologous Id is not only a weakly immunogenic self antigen but also patient-specific so that the vaccine must be individually prepared for each patient.[32] Secondly, myeloma cells secrete large amounts of soluble Ig that may lead to tolerance. Kwak et al. reported that one MM patient received allo-HSCT from the donor who was immunized by the patient-specific monoclonal Ig, and that the anti-idiotype cellular immune response was detectable in both the donor and the patient.[33]

Other possible antigens present on MM cells, such as MUC-1, PRAME, and MAGE family, may also be recognized as TAAs by activated CD8$^+$ cytotoxic[34] or CD4$^+$ T cells[35] that can inhibit tumor growth and eradicate cancer cells. MUC-1 is an immunogenic epithelial mucin present in a hypoglucosylated form on breast, pancreatic, and ovarian cancer.[36] Myeloma cells express underglycosylated MUC-1 recognized by cytotoxic T cells in an HLA-unrestricted manner.[37] Vaccine strategies that have been used in breast and ovarian cancer patients may be applicable to myeloma patients. PRAME is frequently expressed in several tumor types including MM. It is an attractive candidate for immunotherapy trials, as several PRAME epitopes are presented by different HLA molecules to specific CTL that lyse various tumor cells expressing PRAME.[38] Another category of target antigens frequently present on MM cells is encoded by cancer germline-specific genes (MAGE, BAGE, GAGE, LAGE-1, NY-ESO-1). These genes are frequently expressed in many tumor types but are silent in normal tissues except testis and placental trophoblast cells, both lacking HLA expression and therefore being unable to present antigenic peptides to CTL.

Analysis of the MM gene expression database supplemented by immuno-histochemistry for protein expression indicated that the cancer-testis antigen NY-ESO-1 is expressed in >60% of newly diagnosed and 100% of relapsed poor prognosis MM characterized by abnormal cytogenetics.[39,40] When examining the sera of MM patients, NY-ESO-1-specific antibodies were detected in 2/11 NY-ESO-1-positive and 1/21 NY-ESO-1-negative patients.[39] These and other data indicate the high immunogenicity of NY-ESO-1 and other cancer-testis antigens, which present a potential target for donor-derived T cells after allogeneic HCT.

Although T cells clearly play a critical role in the development of the GVM effect, several lines of evidence suggest that antitumor immunity in vivo represents a coordinated immune response involving B cells as well as T cells. Using patient serum to screen recombinant cDNA expression libraries derived from different tumor (SEREX, serological identification of antigens by recombinant expression cloning), investigators have reported the identification of a large number of serologically defined TAAs. NY-ESO-1 and MAGE-1 were also identified by this method.[40,41] By using this method, Belluci et al. identified a panel of 13 gene products (including BCMA), reactive with post-DLI serum but negative with pre-DLI and pre-HSCT serum. Antibodies to these proteins were absent or minimal in patients who underwent allogeneic transplantation without DLI and in normal donors.[42,43] Post-DLI serum was able to induce complement-mediated lysis and ADCC of transfected cells and primary myeloma cells expression BCMA. These results demonstrated that the GVM effect is associated with the MM-specific antibody responses, and antibody responses to BCMA and other myeloma TAAs may contribute directly to tumor rejection in vivo.[43]

Myeloablative Conditioning Regimens

Allogeneic HSCT following a standard myeloablative regimen has a limited role in MM due to unacceptably high rates of regimen-related toxicity. Only a few MM patients can receive this treatment with typical age limits of 55 years in patients with HLA identical sibling donors. Even in younger patients, treatment related mortality (TRM) remain high due to GVHD and infection.

Standard myeloablative regimens are mostly based on alkylating agents such as busulfan, melphalan (Mel), and cyclophosphamide (Cy) in combination with total body irradiation (TBI) as shown in Table 2. The long-term DFS after myeloablative allo-HSCT varied from 13% to 40%. A retrospective multicenter study by the British Society for Blood and Marrow Transplantation (BSBMT) showed that the type of conditioning has a major effect on the transplantation outcome.[53] The Mel/TBI group had a significantly better OS and PFS compared to the Cy/TBI group (44% vs 28% and 36% vs 13%, respectively), but no significant difference could be detected in TRM between these two groups. The major benefit of Mel/TBI was in its greater antitumor activity, as demonstrated by the higher CR rate (65% vs 47%) and lower relapse risk (5-year relapse/progression rate was 37% vs 81%, respectively).

Although data from the European Group for Blood and Marrow Transplantation (EBMT) suggested that results could be improved by performing earlier transplantation,[49] TRM and relapse remain the major factors that influence the OS after allo-HSCT. The Seattle group reported a 100-day TRM of 44% using HLA-matched sibling donors and much higher TRM (65%) for patients who received transplants from unrelated or mismatched related donors. Of note, 4.5-year PFS was only 20% in this study.[45] The EBMT group reported a TRM rate close to 50% after matched sibling-donor transplantation for MM.[44] Recently, the EBMT compared MM patients who received allogeneic transplantation from matched sibling donors during 1983–93 and 1994–98, and found a significant reduction in TRM, 38% and 21% at 6 months, and 46% and 30% at 2 years, for earlier and later periods, respectively.[49] More recent studies using related donors and myeloablative dose conditioning regimens have reported 100-day TRM rates of 16–42% (see Table 2).[16, 48–50, 52–54] In a large number of reports, utilizing unrelated donor transplant facilitated by the NMDP, the 100-day TRM rate was 42%, with the most common cause of TRM being infection, and the 5-year estimated OS was only 9% ± 7%.[52] The incidence of aGVHD reported after sibling transplants for MM ranged from 34% to 72%, contributing the high rates of TRM observed, following myeloablative

Table 2 Results of myeloablative allogeneic transplantation results in MM.

Study	Number of patients	Type of transplant (No.)	Conditioning	GVHD Acute (≥Grade2)	GVHD Chronic	TRM % (months)	OS % (years)	PFS % (years)	Follow-up median (months)
Gahrton et al. 1995, EBMT[44]	162	Sib	Variety of regimens; Cy-TBI commonest	63%	NA	25	32 (4)	34 (6)	
Bensinger et al. 1996, Seattle, USA[45]	80	Sib (71)	Bu-Cy ± TBI	34%	41%	44 (3)	24 (4.5)	20 (4.5)	
Mehta et al. 1998, Little Rock, USA[46]	42	MUD (9) Sib (35) MUD (7) TCD (14)	Majority Bu-Cy	NA	NA	43 (12)	29 (3)	20 (3)	20
Kulkarni et al. 1999, UK[47]	33	Sib	Majority Mel-TBI			54 (12)	36 (3)	39 (3)	
Le Blanc et al. 2001, Montreal, Canada[48]	37	Sib	Majority Cy-TBI	39%	41%	16 (4)	32 (3.3)	47 (3.3)	
Gahrton et al. 2001, EBMT[49]	1983–1993: 334 1994–1998 BM: 223 1994–1998 PBPC: 133	Sib	Variety of regimens; Cy-TBI and Mel-TBI used in approximately 1/3 of cases in each cohort	46% 40% 48%	27% 11% 17%	38 (6) 21 (6) ca. 20 (6)	28 (5) 50 (4) 57 (3)		7 19 15
Kroger et al. 2003, Hamburg, Germany[50]	18	Sib (17) MUD (1)	Bu/Cy/TBI (ATG)	35%	27%	22 (3)	77 (6)	31 (6)	
Alyea et al. 2003, Boston, USA[13]	66	Sib, TCD	Cy-TBI	NA	NA	24 (48)	39 (4)	23 (4)	
Lockhorst et al. 2003, HOVON 24 center[51]	53	Sib, TCD	Cy-TBI	45%	43%	34 (12)	ca. 50 (2)		38
Ballen et al. 2005, Boston, USA[52]	71	MUD	TBI based	47%	NA	42 (3)	27 (2)	21 (2)	
Hunter et al. 2005, London, UK[53]	39 78	Sib TCD (9) Sib	Cy-TBI Mel-TBI	68% 60%	NA NA	32 (12) 35 (12)	28 (5) 44 (5)	13 (5) 36 (5)	
Kuruvilla et al. 2007, Vancouver, Canada[54]	72	Sib (58) MUD (14)	Mel based 70% TBI based 18%	72%	68%	22 (12)	48 (5)	33 EFS (5)	
Total	1441			49%[a]	27%[a]	31[a]	39[a] (4)	29[a] (4)	

ATG antithymocyte globulin, *BM* bone marrow, *Bu* busulphan, *CR* complete remission, *Cy* cyclophosphamide, *EFS* event-free survival, *GVHD* graft versus host disease, *Mel* melphalan, *MM* multiple myeloma, *OS* overall survival, *PBPC* peripheral blood progenitor cell, *PFS* progression-free survival, *PR* partial remission, *Sib* sibling donor, *TBI* total body irradiation, *TCD* T cell depletion, *TRM* transplant-related mortality, *VUD* volunteer unrelated donor.

[a] Weighted average form reported studies.

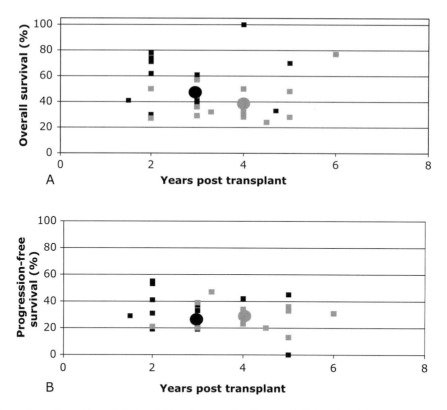

Fig. 1 Comparison of overall survival (panel A) and progression-free survival (panel B) following myeloablative conditioning (grey symbols) and nonmyeloablative conditioning (black symbols) and allogeneic HSCT in patients with multiple myeloma. The large circles represent a weighted average for the survival data presented in individual studies.

conditioning.[53,54] A summary of the reported outcomes following myeloablative conditioning regimens is presented in Table 2, and the rates of overall and progression-free survival following this approach are shown in Fig. 1. Of note, the weighted average for overall survival (at an average reported follow-up of 4 years) was 39%, with a weighted average for progression-free survival of 29%, so that ~20% of recipients of myeloablative conditioning and allogeneic transplant alive at 4 years are predicted to have persistent disease.

One way to control TRM is to reduce the incidence and severity of GVHD by T cell depletion, but this strategy to reduce GVHD has been associated with a higher incidence of disease relapse. Lokhorst et al.[51] reported the result of a multicenter study involving 53 patients who received TCD allo-grafts from HLA identical sibling donors. aGVHD developed in 43% of patients; only 19% achieved CR; and the median OS was 25 months. Another multicenter study of TCD allotransplantation reported similar results: among 71 patients who received transplants from matched unrelated donors (including 39% of whom received TCD grafts), 2-year OS rate was only 27%, and the incidence of aGVHD was 47%.[52] However, the presence of GVHD, which has been shown to correlate with a decreased risk of relapse in some studies, did not correlate with a lower relapse rate in this study. In a very recent report from the EBMT, the use of alemtuzumab, as an in vivo method of TCD, was significantly associated with an increased relapse risk (HR 1.6).[55]

Nonmyeloablative Conditioning Regimens

The need to explore new strategies reducing treatment-related toxicity while maintaining the GVT effect in allogeneic HSCT has led to the development of reduced-intensity conditioning/nonmyeloablative transplantation. These conditioning regimens are primarily immunosuppressive and facilitate engraftment by donor stem cells that establish donor-derived hematopoiesis and donor immune cells that eliminate host hematopoietic cells, converting the transplant recipient to full donor chimerism. However, tumor recurrence rate is higher, when using RIC, especially in patients with refractory/relapse disease. So, RIC has often been used as part of tandem myeloablative conditioning autologous and nonmyeloablative conditioning allogeneic transplantations. Pilot studies of RIC allogeneic HSCT in patients with advanced disease have confirmed a lower toxic death rate, and the feasibility of the procedure in patients more than 60 years of age with sibling donor,[6,8,56–58] or with unrelated donors.[59]

The most widely used nonmyeloablative conditioning prior to allo-graft was developed using the Seattle canine transplant model. A combination of low-dose (200 cGy) TBI conditioning and postgrafting immunosuppression including mycophenolate mofetil (MMF) and cyclosporine (CSP) allowed stable allogeneic engraftment.[60] In their pilot study, eight MM patients received this regimen before allo-transplantation; all of them had initial engraftment, including six with sustained engraftment.[17] However, low-dose TBI (200 cGy), as the sole conditioning agent, was reported to be associated with a high risk of graft failure in MM patients who had never received intensive therapy. When given within 3–9 months of high-dose melphalan as part of a tandem autologous-allogeneic transplant maneuver, this regimen resulted in consistent and durable donor cell engraftment.

Purine analog-based RIC also demonstrated feasibility and acceptable toxicity in patients considered ineligible for myeloablative high-dose chemotherapy and allo-HSCT either because of age or morbidity. Conditioning regimens included mostly melphalan 100–140 mg/m^2 and fludarabine with or without 2Gy TBI, or fludarabine in combination with cyclophosphamide or low-dose busulfan. Recently, antithymocyte globulin (ATG)[60,61] or anti-CD52 antibody alemtuzumab[23,55,62] (CAMPATH 1H) has been incorporated in nonmyeloablative conditioning regimens, in order to deplete both host and donor T lymphocytes in vivo, enhancing engraftment and reducing the incidence of aGVHD at the same time. However, the reduction in rates of GVHD may translate into a higher relapse rate, and inferior outcomes due to disease progression. In the multicenter reports from the EBMT, the use of any form of TCD was associated with a higher relapse rate, and OS, PFS, and relapse rates were inferior in patients receiving alemtuzumab.[17,55,63] Although there is currently no consensus on the superiority of any particular regimen in terms of toxicity or efficacy, caution should be taken in the use of ex vivo or in vivo TCD in patients with myeloma undergoing allogeneic HSCT.

Initial studies of RIC in MM patients have been encouraging with nonrelapse mortality (NRM) of 2–19%, rates of grades 2–4 aGVHD of 40–46%, and OS and PFS rates close to 70%.[56,59,63,64] With longer follow-up reported 1 year, NRM was increased to 10–40%, with relapse rates around 32–54%, and OS and PFS rates of 31–45% and 21–37%, respectively (Table 3). In a very recent

Table 3 Results of non-myeloablative allogeneic transplantation results in MM.

Study	Number of patients (VUD)	Conditioning regimen	Age Median (range)	Number of tandem auto	GVHD (%) Acute GvHD (≥Grade 2)	CGvHD	Early mortality d100d/1Y	Response rate (%) CR	PR	Rel	% OS (years)	% PFS (years)	Follow-up (months)
Bactros et al. 2000, Little Rock USA[56]	31(6)	Mel 100, TBI, Flu	56 (38–69)	0	58	41	10%/30%	39	22	71(1)		31 (2)	6
Giralt et al. 2002, Houston, USA[58]	22 (9)	Flu, HDM	51 (45–64)	0	46	27	19%/40%	32	4		30 (2)	19 (2)	15
Kroger et al. 2002, Hamburg, Germany[59]	21 (21)	HDM100-140, Flu, ATG	50 (32–61)	9	38	37	10%/26%	40	50		74 (2)	53 (2)	13
Maloney et al. 2003, Seattle[63]	54 (0)	TBI 2Gy, Flu	52 (29–71)	54	39	60	2%/10%	57	26		78 (2)	55 (2)	
Motty et al. 2004, Marseille, France[61]	41	Bu,Flu,ATG	52 (35–61)	0	36	41	NA/17%	24	27	51	62 (2)	41 (2)	13
Gerull et al. 2005, Heidelberg, Germany[65]	52 (20)	TBI 2 Gy, Flu	52 (36–68)	0	37	70	NA/17%	27		56	41 (1.5)	29 (1.5)	18
Crawley et al. 2005, Cambridge EBMT [62]	229	Flu based	52 (32–66)	NA	31	50	10%/22%	25	48	41	41 (3)	21 (3)	28
Martino et al. 2006, Italy[66]	15	Flu, Cy	51 (40–57)	15	13	40	0%	47	53	0	100 (4)	42 (4)	44

Majolino et al. 2007, Rome, Italy[67]	53 (0)	Thioteopa, Flu, Mel	52 (38–68)	21	45	64	13%	62		32	45 (3)	37 (3)	22
Crawley et al. 2007, EBMT[55]	320 (49)	Flu + TBI/Mel/Bu (60%TCD)	51 (31–66)	part	36	50	11%/24% (2 years)	37	47	54	38 (3)	19 (3)	
Georges et al. 2007, Seattle[68]	24 (24)	TBI 2 Gy, Flu	50 (29–66)	13	67	75	21% (3 years)	42	17	21	61 (3)	33 (3)	36
Garban et al. 2006, Nantes, France[4]	46 (0)	Bu,Flu,ATG	54 (36–65)	46	24	43	2% (2)/13% (1)	33	48	56	33 (7)	0 (5)	56
Bruno et al 2007, Turin, Italy[5]	58 (0)	TBI 2 Gy	55 (34–65)	58	43	32	10% (2 years)	55	31	14	70 (5)	45 (5)	46
Total	966				37[a]	47[a]		44	37	37	47[a] (3)	26[a] (3)	

ATG antithymocyte globulin, *Bu* busulphan, *CR* complete remission, *Cy* cyclophosphamide, *GVHD* graft versus host disease, *HDM* high-dose melphalan, *Mel* melphalan, *MM* multiple myeloma, *OS* overall survival, *PFS* progression-free survival, *Rel* relapse, *TBI* total body irradiation, *TCD* T cell depletion, *TRM* transplant-related mortality, *VUD* volunteer unrelated donor.

[a] Weighted average from reported series.

retrospective study from the EBMT, outcomes of 320 patients who received RIC regimens were compared with 196 recipients of traditional myeloablative conditioning. These data confirm that RIC had a significantly lower nonrelapse mortality at 2 years, 24% versus 37%, $p = 0.002$, but survival was inferior due to an increased relapse rate after RIC. OS was similar comparing RIC to myeloablative conditioning, 38.1% versus 50.8% (no significant difference), with lower PFS seen in the RIC group, 18.9% versus 34.5% ($p = 0.001$), respectively.[55] The outcome of RIC is also closely related to the extent of the disease, with an improved OS associated with a CR or PR prior to transplantation and very high relapse rates in patients transplanted with end-stage MM.

Tandem Autologous/Reduced Intensity Conditioning Regimens

Recently, the M.D. Anderson Cancer Center had reported its result of RIC allografting as salvage therapy for myeloma patients who relapsed after first autografting. IT compared second autologous transplantation to RIC allografting. Fourteen patients received a second autograft whereas 26 patients underwent a RIC allo-transplantation, with the median interval between the first and second transplants being 25 and 17 months, respectively. The two groups had similar response rates (64% and 69%, respectively) and day 100 nonrelapse mortalities (7% vs 11%), but overall nonrelapse mortality was lower in the tandem auto transplant group due to GVHD following RIC and allogeneic HSCT (14% vs 27%). Disease progression remained the major cause of treatment failure, with median PFS of 6.8 versus 7.3 months and median OS of 29 versus 13 months in autologous and allogeneic groups, respectively.[69]

In the past few years, a strategy combining tumor-burden reduction with high-dose chemotherapy plus ASCT and RIC allo-HSCT has been widely used. Patients are given high-dose melphalan 200 mg/m2 and autologous stem cell rescue, then, 2–6 months later, after recovery, patients receive an RIC regimen and allo-HSCT from a sibling donor[63,67] or a volunteer unrelated donor (VUD).[55,66,70]

One of the largest studies using this approach reported on 52 patients who received a tandem auto-allo transplant. All patients had sustained donor-derived hematopoitic engraftment, 38% developed aGVHD, and only 8% had grades 3–4 severe aGVHD. With a median follow-up of 4 years after allografting, OS and PFS rates were 69% and 45%, respectively.[8,63] Similar data, shown in Table 3, demonstrate that this strategy is highly effective, with complete response rates of over 50%, and short-term OS and PFS are encouraging. A more recent study from Seattle also confirmed that it is an effective treatment approach even in patients with poor-risk, relapsed or refractory MM. In their study, patients who received tandem autologous-unrelated donor allogeneic transplantation had a superior 3-year OS and PFS (77% and 51%) compared with patients proceeding directly to RIC-unrelated donor transplantation (44% and 11%).[68] But with longer follow-up, it appeared that late relapses can occur and chronic GVHD remains a frequent complication (with a reported incidence of more than 75%)[71] that can add late morbidity and impair quality of life, contributing to a 1-year nonrelapse TRM of 10–20%.

The outcome from RIC for advanced disease and heavily pretreated patients is disappointing. The patients who had failed prior autologous transplants had worse results compared to patients who received planned tandem autologous-mini-allotransplantation. In Lee et al.'s study, 45 patients received RIC allotransplant after one or more autografts, including 14 chemosensitive versus 31 chemoresistant. Although the CR plus near-CR rate was high (64%), even in refractory disease, overall survival at 3 years was poor, only 36%. There was a significantly better survival for patients transplanted as part of the planned tandem strategy than among patients who had progressive disease following autografts, with 3-year OS of 80% versus 19% and EFS of 80% versus 0%, respectively.[71] Kroger et al.[64] reported the results of 120 patients treated with RIC and allogeneic HSCT and found that relapse from a prior autologous transplantation was the most significant risk factor for TRM, relapse, and death. Data from the EBMT confirmed that chemoresistance ($p = 0.001$), patients in greater than first remission ($p = 0.001$), two or more prior autografts ($p = 0.02$) were all adverse risk factors for shorter PFS on univariate analysis.[19] It seems that heavily pretreated patients and patients with progressive disease do not achieve long-term disease control following RIC and allogeneic HSCT, despite the encouraging low TRM. A summary of the reported outcomes following RIC regimens is presented in Table 3, and the rates of overall and progression-free survival following this approach are shown in Fig. 1. Of note, the weighted average for overall survival (at an average reported follow-up of 3 years) was 47%, but progression-free survival was only 26%, indicating the significance of late relapses following RIC and allogeneic transplantation in this disease.

Results of and Future Directions for Clinical Trials of Allogeneic HSCT in the Management of Patients with Multiple Myeloma

Result of nonrandomized studies comparing tandem auto-allo HSCT (IFM99-03 trial) versus tandem auto-auto HSCT (IFM99-04 trial) has been published recently.[4] This study recruited newly diagnosed high-risk MM patients between 2000 and 2004 (with ß2-microglobulin level greater than 3 mg/L and chromosome 13 deletion at diagnosis). After registration, patients received an induction regimen consisting of vincristine, adriamycin (doxorubicin), and dexamethasone (VAD) followed by high-dose melphalan conditioning (200 mg/m²) and autologous stem cell transplantation. Then, according to the availability of an HLA-identical sibling donor, patients received either an RIC allogeneic stem cell transplantation using busulfan, fludarabine, and ATG (IFM99-03 trial) or a second auto-HSCT that followed high-dose melphalan conditioning (220 mg/m²) with or without anti-IL-6 monoclonal antibody (IFM99-04 protocol). Two hundred eighty-four patients entered and finished at least on course of VAD, 65 in the IFM99-03 trial and 219 in the IFM99-04 trial, respectively. The IFM99-03 strategy was relatively safe with day 100 TRM of only 4% and overall TRM of 10.9% compared to 5% for the IFM99-04. The combined rates of CR and very good PR were 51% and 62%, respectively, for IFM99-03 and IFM99-04. However, the promising response rates and low TRM rates did not translate into long-term survival, with estimated

5-year EFS of 0% for patients who underwent the tandem auto-allo transplant maneuver. There was no significant difference in OS or EFS between the tandem auto-auto HSCT and tandem auto-allo HSCT on the basis of intent-to-treat, and with median OS of 35 versus 41 months, and EFS was 25 versus 30 months, respectively. The outcome results were among patients who actually finished the protocols, and with a trend for a better OS in patients treated with tandem auto-auto HSCT (median, 47.2 versus 35 months; $p = 0.07$). Overall, these results suggest that tandem ASCT followed by RIC allograft is not superior to the tandem ASCT in de novo high-risk patients. The negative impact of part or whole deletion of chromosome 13 had already been shown by Fassas[72] and Kroger.[73] For this group of high-risk patients, new therapeutic strategies remain to be determined.

More recently, another multicenter study, including patients from Italy, compared the tandem auto-allo HSCT with tandem auto-auto HSCT in newly diagnosed myeloma.[5] One hundred and sixty-two patients who had at least one sibling who underwent HLA typing were enrolled. Patients received VAD induction followed by high-dose melphalan and autologous stem-cell rescue, with treatment allocation to a second autologous transplant or an allogeneic transplant, following an RIC regimen determined by the availability of a HLA-matched related donor, similar to the protocol of IFM9903-04. There was no significant difference in treatment-related mortality between two groups, but a significantly higher disease-related mortality was found in the tandem auto-auto HSCT group, 43% versus 7%, $p < 0.001$. After a median follow-up of 45 months, the median OS and EFS were longer in 80 patients allocated to the tandem auto-allo HSCT group compared to 82 patients allocated to tandem auto-auto HSCT group (median OS of 80 vs 54 months, $p = 0.01$, and median EFS of 35 versus 29 months, $p = 0.02$, respectively). Interestingly, in their study, neither chromosome 13 abnormalities nor ß2-microglobulin level appeared to affect the outcome after allografting. These results suggest that tandem auto-allo HSCT has a superior survival in newly-diagnosed myeloma patients versus tandem auto-auto HSCT.

The different results of these two studies, especially in the high-risk patient group, may be related to the different reduced-intensity regimens prior to allo-HSCT, the use of pretransplantation immunosuppression, and the lower doses of melphalan used in the tandem auto-auto study by Bruno et al.[5] Using high-dose ATG among patients who received tandem auto-allo HSCT in the French experience may have prevented GVM activities by in vivo T cell depletion.[74]

Currently, large prospective multicenter trials comparing tandem autologous transplantations and tandem autologous/RIC allogeneic transplantations are in follow-up phase in the United States and Europe. The allocation of treatment with the tandem autologous or allogeneic transplant is based on whether patients have an available HLA identical sibling donor. The results of these ongoing studies will help address the role of tandem auto-allo HSCT in the management of MM. New strategies to decrease the posttransplantation relapse rate by using different regimens, modulating immunosuppressive drugs, or combining chemotherapy with novel "targeted" agents will likely be necessary to successfully treat patients with poor risk or refractory MM using allogeneic HSCT. Improvement in the overall results of allogeneic transplantation in the management of MM will likely require methods to selectively enhance donor T-cell-mediated antimyeloma activity through pre- or posttransplant vaccination.[33,36,37]

References

1. Attal M, Harousseau JL, Stoppa AM, et al. A prospective, randomized trial of autologous bone marrow transplantation and chemotherapy in multiple myeloma. Intergroupe Francais du Myeloma. N Engl J Med 1996; 335:91–97.

2. Child JA, Morgan GJ, Davies FC, et al. High-dose chemotherapy with hematopietic stem cell rescue for multiple myeloma. N Engl J Med 2003; 348:1875–1883.

3. Palumbo A, Bringhen S, Petrucci MT, et al. Intermediate-dose melphalan improves survival of myeloma patients aged 50–70: results of a randomized controlled trial. Blood 2004; 104:3052–3057.

4. Garban F, Attal M, Michallet M, et al. Prospective comparison of autologous stem cell transplantation followed by dose-reduced allograft(IFM99-03 trial) with tandem autologous stem cell transplantation(IFM99-04 trial) in high-risk de novo multiple myeloma. Blood 2006; 107:3474–3480.

5. Bruno B, Rotta M, Patriarca F, et al. A comparison of allografting with autografting for newly diagnosed myeloma. N Engl J Med 2007; 356:1110–1120.

6. McSweeney PA, Niederwieser D, Shizuru JA, et al. Hematopoietic cell transplantation in older patients with hematologic malignancies: replacing high-dose cytotoxic therapy with graft-versus-tumor effects. Blood 2001; 97:3390–3400.

7. Barlogie B, Shaughnessy J, Tricot G, et al. Treatment of multiple myeloma. Blood 2004; 103:20–32.

8. Bensiger WI. The current status of reduced-intensity allogeneic hematopoietic stem cell transplantation for multiple myeloma. Leukemia 2006; 20:1683–1689.

9. Liso A, Stockerl-Goldsteim KE, Auffermann-Gretzinger S, et al. Idiotype vaccination using dendritic cells after autologous peripheral blood progenitor cell transplantation for multiple myeloma. Biol Blood Marrow Transplant 2000; 6:621–627.

10. Hansson L, Abdalla AO, Mosfegh A, et al. Long-term idiotype vaccination combined with IL-12 or IL-12 and GM-CSF, in early stage multiple myeloma patients. Clin Cancer Res 2007; 13:1503–1510.

11. Ruffini PA, Neelapu SS, Kwak L, . Idiotypic vaccination for B-cell malignancies as a model for therapeutic cancer vaccines: from prototype protein to second generation vaccines. Haematologica 2002; 87:989–1001.

12. Harrison SJ, Cook G, Nibbs R. Immunotherapy of multiple myeloma: the start of a long and tortuous journey. Expert Rev Anticancer Ther 2006; 6:1769–1785.

13. Alyea E, Weller E, Schlossman R, et al. Outcome after autologous and allogeneic stem cell transplantation for patients with multiple myeloma: impact of graft-versus-myeloma effect. Bone Marrow Tansplant 2003; 32:1145–1151.

14. Huff CA, Fuchs EJ, Noga SJ, et al. Long-term follow-up of T cell-depleted allogeneic bone marrow transplantation in refractory multiple myeloma: importance of allogeneic T cells. Biol Blood Marrow Transplant 2003; 9:312–319.

15. Zeiser R, Bertz H, Spyridonidis A, et al. Donor lymphocyte infusions for multiple myeloma: clinical results and novel perspectives. Bone Marrow Transplant 2004; 34:923–928.

16. Bjorkstrand B, Ljungman P, Svensson H, et al. Allogeneic bone marrow transplantation versus autologous stem cell transplantation in multiple myeloma: a retrospective case-matched study form the European group for Blood and Marrow Transplantation. Blood, 1996; 88:4711–4718.

17. Martinelli G, Terragna C, Zamagni E, et al. Molecular remission after allogeneic or autologous transplantation of hematopoietic stem cells for multiple myeloma. J clin Oncol 2000; 18:2273–2281.

18. Lokhorst HM, Schattenberg A, Cornelissen JJ, et al. Donor leukocyte infusions are effective in relapsed multiple myeloma after allogeneic bone marrow transplantation. Blood 1997; 90:4206–4211.

19. Lokhorst HM, Wu K, Verdonck LF, et al. The occurrence of graft-versus-host disease is the major predictive factor for response to donor lymphocyte infusions in multiple myeloma. Blood 2004; 103:4362–4364.

20. Salama M, Nevill T, Marcellus T, et al.. Donor leukocyte infusions for multiple myeloma. Bone Marrow Tansplant 2000; 26:1179–1184.
21. Kroger N, Shimoni A, Zagrivnaja M, et al. Low-dose thalidomide and donor lymphocyte infusions adoptive immunotherapy after allogeneic stem cell transplantation in patients with multiple myeloma. Blood 2004; 104:3361–3363.
22. Van de Donk NWCJ, Kroger N, Hegenbart U, et al. Remarkable activity of novel agents bortezomib and thalidomide in patients not responding to donor lymphocyte infusions following nonmyeloablative allogeneic stem cell transplantation in multiple myeloma. Blood 2006; 107:3415–3416.
23. Alye E, Weller E, Schlossman R, et al. T-cell depleted allogeneic bone marrow transplantation followed by donor lymphocyte infusion in patients with multiple myeloma: induction of graft-versus-myeloma effect. Blood 2001; 98:934–939.
24. Badros A, Barlogie B, Morris C, et al. High response rate in refractory and poor-risk multiple myeloma after allotransplantation using a nonmyeloablative conditioning regimen and donor lymphocyte infusions. Blood 2001; 97:2574–2575.
25. Peggs KS, Mackinnon S, Williams CD, et al. Reduced intensity transplantation with in vivo T-cell depletion and adjuvant dose-escalation donor lymphocyte infusions for chemotherapy-sensitive myeloma: limited efficacy of graft-versus-tumor activity. Biol Blood Marrow Transplant 2003; 9:257–265.
26. Peggs KS, Thomson K, Hart DP, et al. Dose-escalated donor lymphocyte infusions following reduced intensity transplantation: toxicity, chimerism, and disease responses. Blood 2004; 103:1548–1556.
27. Tricot G, Vesole DH, Jagannath S, et al. Graft versus myeloma effect: proof of principle. Blood 1996; 87:1196–1198.
28. Verdonck L, Lokhorst H, Dekker A, et al. Graft-versus-myeloma effect in two cases. Lancet 1996; 347:800–801.
29. Bellucci R, Alyea EP, Weller E, . Immunologic effects of prophylactic donor lymphocyte infusion after allogeneic marrow transplantation for multiple myeloma. Blood 2002; 99:4610–4617.
30. Bethge WA, Hegenbart U, Stuart M, et al. Adoptive immunotherapy with donor lymphocyte infusions after allogeneic hematopoietic cell transplantation following nonmyeloablative conditioning. Blood 2004; 103:790–795.
31. Coscia M, Mariani S, Battaglio S, et al. Long-term follow-up of idiotype vaccination in human myeloma as a maintenance therapy after high-dose chemotherapy. Leukemia 2004; 18:138–145.
32. Kofler DM, Mayr C and Wendtner CM. Current status of immunotherapy in B cell malignancies. Current Drug Targests 2006; 7:1372–1374.
33. Kwak LW, Taub DD, Duffey PL, . Transfer of myeloma idiotype-specific immunity from an actively immunized marrow donor. Lancet 1995; 345:1016.
34. Rosenberg SA. A new era for cancer immunotherapy based on the genes that encode cancer antigens. Immunity 1999; 10:282–287.
35. Wang RF. The role of MHC class II-restricted tumor antigens and CD4+ T cells in antitumor immunity. Trends Immunol 2001; 22:269–276.
36. Barratt-Boyes SM. Making the most of mucin: a novel target for tumor immunotherapy. Cancer Immunol Immunother 1996; 43:142–151.
37. Takahashi T, Makiguchi Y, Hinoda Y, et al. Expression of MUC-1 on myeloma cells and induction of HLA-unrestricted CTL against MUC-1 form a multiple myeloma patient. J Immunol 1994; 152:2102–2112.
38. Zeiser R, Bertz H, Spyridonidis A, et al. Donor lymphocyte infusions for multiple myeloma: clinical results and novel perspectives. Bone Marrow Transplant 2004; 34:923–928.
39. Szmania SM, Pomtree M, Batchu RB, Pre-existent humoral and cellular immunity to NY-ESO-1. Blood 2003; 102(suppl 1):3464a.
40. van Rhee F, Szmania SM, Zhan F, NY-ESO-1 is highly expressed in poor-prognosis multiple myeloma and induces spontaneous humoral and cellular immune responses. Blood 2005; 106; 3939e–3944e.

41. Chen Y, Scanlan MJ, Sahin U, et al. A testicular antigen aberrantly expressed in human cancers detected by autologous antibody screening. Proc Natl Acad Sci 1997; 94:1914–1918.

42. Bellucci R, Wu CJ, Chiaretti S, et al. Completed response to donor lymphocyte infusion in multiple myeloma is associated with antibody responses to highly expressed antigens. Blood 2004; 103:656–663.

43. Bellucci R, Alyea EP, Chiaretti S, et al. Graft-versus-tumor response in patients with multiple myeloma is associated with antibody responses to BCMA, a plasma-cell membrane receptor. Blood 2005; 105:3945–3950.

44. Gahrton G, Tura S, Ljungman P, et al. Prognostic factors in allogeneic bone marrow transplantation for multiple myeloma. J Clin Oncol 1995; 13:1312–1322.

45. Bensinger WI, Buckner CD, Nansetti C, et al. Allogeneic marrow transplantation for multiple myeloma: an analysis of risk factors on outcome. Blood 1996; 88:2787–2793.

46. Mehta J, Tricot G, Jagannath S, et al. Salvage autologous or allogeneic transplantation for multiple myeloma refractory to or relapsing after a first-line autograft? Bone Marrow Transplant 1998; 21:887–892.

47. Kulkarni S, Powles RL, Treleaven JG, et al. Impact of previous high-dose therapy on outcome after allografting for multiple myeloma. Bone Marrow Transplant 1999; 23:675–680.

48. Le Blanc R, Montminy-Métivier S, Bélanger R, et al. Allogeneic transplantation for multiple myeloma: further evidence for a GVHD-associated graft-versus-myeloma effect. Bone Marrow Transplant 2001; 28:841–848.

49. Gahrton G, Svensson H, Cava M, et al. Progress in allogeneic bone marrow and peripheral blood stem cell transplantation for multiple myeloma: a comparison between transplants performed 1983–93 and 1994–98 at European Group for Blood and Marrow Transplantation centres. Br J Haematol 2001; 113:209–216.

50. Kroger N, Einsele H, Wloff D, et al. Myeloablative intensified conditioning regimen with in vivo T-cell depletion(ATG) followed by allografting in patients with advanced multiple myeloma. A phase I/II study of the German Study-group Multiple Myeloma(DSMM). Bone Marrow Transplant 2003; 31:973–979.

51. Lokhorst HM, Segeen CM, Verdonck LF, et al. Partially T-cell depleted allogeneic stem-cell transplantation for first-line treatment of multiple myeloma: a prospective evaluation of patients treated in the phase III study Hovon 24 MM. J Clin Oncol 2003; 21:1728–1733.

52. Ballen KK, King R, Carston M, et al. Outcome of unrelated transplants in patients with multiple myeloma. Bone Marrow Transplant 2005; 35:675–681.

53. Hunter HM, Peggs K, Powles R, Analysis of outcome following allogeneic haemo-poietic stem cell transplantation for myeloma using myeloablative conditioning--evidence for a superior outcome using melphalan combined with total body irradiation. Br. J Haematol 2005; 128:496–502.

54. Kuruvilla J, Shepherd JD, Sutberland HJ, et al. Long-term outcome of myeloablative allogeneic stem cell transplantation for multiple myeloma. Biol Blood Marrow Transplant 2007; 9:257–265.

55. Crawley C, Lacobelli S, Bjorkstrand B, et al. Reduced-intensity conditioning for myeloma: lower nonrelapse mortality but higher relapse rates compared with myeloablative conditioning. Blood 2007; 109:3588–3594.

56. Badros A, Barlogie B, Spegel E, et al. Improved outcome of allogeneic transplantation in high-risk multiple myeloma patients after non myeloablative conditioning. J Clin Oncol 2002; 20:1295–1303.

57. Einsele H, Shafer HJ, Hebart H, et al. Follow-up of patients with multiple myeloma undergoing allografts after reduced-intensity conditioning. Br J Haematol 2003; 121:411–418.

58. Giralt S, Aleman A, Anagnostopoulos A, et al. Fludarabine/melphalan conditioning for allogeneic transplantation in patients with multiple myeloma. Bone Marrow Transplant 2002;30:367–373.

59. Kroger N, Sayer HG, Schwerdtfeger R, et al. Unrelated stem cell transplantation in multiple myeloma after reduced intensity conditioning with pretransplantation antithymocyte globulin is highly effective with low transplantation-related mortality. Blood 2002; 100:3919–3924.

60. Storb R, Yu C, Zaucha JM, et al. Stable mixed hematopoietic chimerism in dog given antigen, CTLA4Ig and 100 cGy total body irradiation before and pharmacologic immunosuppression after marrow transplant. Blood 1999; 94:2523–2529.

61. Mohty M, Boiron JM, Damaj G, et al. Graft-versus-myeloma effect following antithymocyte globulin-based reduced intensity conditioning allogeneic stem cell transplantation. Bone Marrow Transplant 2004; 34:77–84.

62. Crawley C, Lalancette M, Szydlo R, et al. Outcomes for reduced-intensity allogeneic transplantation for multiple myeloma: an analysis of prognostic factors from the Chronic Leukemia Working Party of the EBMT. Blood 2005; 105:4532–4539.

63. Maloney DG, Molina AJ, Sahebi F, et al. Allografting with nonmyeloablative conditioning following cytoreductive autografts for the treatment of patients with multiple myeloma. Blood 2003; 102:3447–3454.

64. Kroger N, Perez-Simon JS, Myint H, et al. Relapse to prior autograft and chronic graft-versus-host disease are the strongest prognostic factors for outcome of melphalan/fludarabine-based dose-reduced allogeneic stem cell transplantation in patients with multiple myeloma. Biol Blood Marrow Transplant 2004; 10:698–708.

65. Gerull S, Goerner M, Benner A, et al. Long-term outcome of nonmyeloablative allogeneic transplantation in patients with high-risk multiple myeloma. Bone Marrow Transplant 2005; 36:963–969.

66. High-dose therapy and autologous peripheral blood stem cells transplantation followed by a very low reduced intensity regimen with fludarabine+cyclophosphamide and allograft improve complete remission rate in de novo multiple myeloma patients. Am J Hematol 2006; 81:973–978.

67. Majolino I, Davoli M, Carnevalli E, et al. Reduced intensity conditioning with thiopa, fludarabine and melphalan is effective in advanced multiple myeloma. Leuk Lymphoma 2007; 48:759–766.

68. Georges GE, Maris MB, Maloney DG, et al. Nonmyeloablative unrelated donor hematopoietic cell transplantation to treat patients with poor-risk, relapsed, or refractory multiple myeloma. Biol Blood Marrow Transplant 2007; 13:423–432.

69. Qazilbash MH, Saliba R, De Lima M, et al. Second autologous or allogeneic transplantation after the failure of first autograft in patients with multiple myeloma. Cancer 2006; 106:1084–1089.

70. Kroger N, Schwerdtfeger R, Kiehl M, et al. Autologous stem cell transplantation followed by a dose-reduced allograft induces high complete remission rate in multiple myeloma. Blood 2002; 100:755–760.

71. Lee CK, Badros A, Barlogie B, et al. Prognostic factors in allogeneic transplantation for patients with high-risk multiple myeloma after reduced intensity conditioning. Exp Hematol 2003; 31:73–80.

72. Fassas ABT, Spencer R, Sawyer J, et al. Both hypodipliody or deletion of chromosome 13 independently confer post prognosis in multiple myeloma. Br J Haematol 2002; 118:1041–1047.

73. Kroger N, Schilling G, Einsele H, et al. Deletion of chromosome b and 13q14 as detected by fluorescence in situ hybridization is a prognostic factor in patients with multiple myeloma who are receiving allogeneic dose-reduced stem cell transplantation. Blood 2004; 103:4056–4061.

74. Waller EK, Langston AA, Lonial S, et al. Pharmacokinetics and pharmacodynamics of anti-thymocyte globulin in recipients of partially HLA-matched blood hematopoietic progenitor cell transplantation. Biol Blood Marrow Transplant 2003; 9:460–471.

Chapter 11

Immunobiology and Immunotherapy of Multiple Myeloma

Madhav V. Dhodapkar

Clinical Heterogeneity of Myeloma

Multiple myeloma (MM) is a common B-cell malignancy characterized by clonal expansion of transformed plasma cells in the bone marrow.[1] Natural history of MM is characterized by disease progression, and the development of anemia, lytic bone disease, and infections. However, although clonal expansion of transformed plasma cells is an essential prerequisite for the development of MM, the most common clinical outcome of such expansions in vivo in humans is not MM, but the development of monoclonal gammopathy of undetermined significance (MGUS). MGUS has been estimated to occur in up to 1–3% of the elderly population, and is commonly viewed as a preneoplastic state. However, most patients with MGUS will generally remain stable throughout their life, and only a small proportion (estimated at about 1% per year) will develop MM.[2] Another clinically distinct subset is patients with asymptomatic MM, who also have a relatively indolent course, but much higher risk for transformation to symptomatic MM.[3] Recent application of interphase cytogenetics and genomic technologies has yielded the surprising finding that many of the cytogenetic and genomic changes in tumor cells initially identified in MM can now also be detected in the tumor cells in MGUS.[4,5] In many instances, genetic lesions such as deletion of chromosome 13 that seem to impart an adverse outcome in MM do not do so in MGUS. These findings therefore suggest the possibility that clinical outcome in MM depends not only on the properties of the tumor cells themselves but also on changes in the host tumor microenvironment and their interactions with the tumor cells. An important component of this microenvironment is the cells of the immune system.[6] Therefore, improved understanding of the immune microenvironment in MM might provide newer approaches for therapy and prevention of this disease. Below, I will first briefly discuss some of the general principles underlying the mechanisms of immune control and escape of tumors, and then describe the current studies about the status of immune cells in MM and MGUS. Understanding the status of the host immune response is an essential first step for optimal development of therapeutic approaches targeting the immune system in MM.

From: *Contemporary Hematology Myeloma Therapy*
Edited by: S. Lonial © Humana Press, Totowa, NJ

Basic Principles of Cancer Immunobiology

Mechanisms of Immune Control and Surveillance of Tumors

The fact that nearly all tumors (and their "preneoplastic" counterparts) express antigenic determinants that can be potentially recognized by the immune system is now well established.[7–9] Molecular basis of this has come in part from the understanding that genetic instability of tumors leads to a tremendous array of genetic and cellular alterations in each tumor cell.[9] Surprisingly, in some instances (such as melanoma), when the specificity of T cells infiltrating tumors was determined, the immune response was found to be directed against nonmutated tissue differentiation antigens also expressed by normal tissue counterparts.[10] Nonetheless, although tumors are derived from "self" tissues, they appear to be sufficiently "foreign" or "altered" to allow their potential recognition by the immune system.[11] Indeed, recent attempts to sequence the genome in human cancers have provided evidence that common human tumors have much higher numbers of genomic mutations than initially anticipated.[12] While this may serve as a challenge for developing targeted chemotherapies, it also provides several targets for the immune system. The inability of the immune system to protect against tumors thus seems largely not due to the lack of antigenic targets but due to the inability of the host to mount a protective immune response.

The immune system has several components that can theoretically be recruited to protect from tumors.[13] CD4+ and CD8+ T cells are the adaptive arms of cell-mediated immunity, able to differentiate upon antigen encounter to produce cytokines and lytic products, to clonally expand, and to establish memory. Natural killer (NK) and NKT cells have innate functions, already prepared to kill and produce cytokines upon tumor recognition. NK and NKT cells do grow upon exposure to cytokines like IL-2, but they are not known to establish memory with either expanded cell numbers or improved function. Finally, antibodies or humoral immune system may kill tumor cells either directly or by recruiting innate effector mechanisms such as complement- or antibody-dependent cytotoxicity. Recent studies in mice have demonstrated the role of interferon-γ and lymphocytes in protection against spontaneous and carcinogen-induced tumors in mice.[14] Interactions of the immune system with the developing tumors might lead to "editing" of these tumors in vivo. Evidence has now emerged for the role of both adaptive and innate lymphocytes (NK or NKT) cells in this process. It is important to appreciate that the immune system can serve as a two-edged sword, capable of both promoting and inhibiting cancer.[15]

Mechanisms of Tumor Immune Escape

The mechanisms by which antigenic tumors might be able to grow in vivo and evade the immune system have largely been studied using transplantable tumors in mice.[16–18] Several hypotheses have been proposed to help explain the natural ability of growing tumors to evade the immune system. Because tumors are poor antigen-presenting cells (APCs), it has been suggested that the generation of antitumor CD8+ T cell response requires the acquisition and presentation of tumor antigens by a bone marrow-derived APC.[19]

The most likely candidate for such a cell at present is the dendritic cell (DC).[20] DCs can acquire exogenous antigen from tumor cells and present it to elicit both CD4 and CD8+ T cell immunity.[20] Other studies have argued that tumors may grow because tumors or their antigens do not gain access to the lymphoid organs, and hence the immune system largely remains "ignorant" of the growing tumor.[21] An evolving concept in immunology is that the balance between immunity and tolerance may be regulated at the level of the APC.[22] Thus, the presentation of antigen by DCs in the steady state can lead to the induction of tolerance, while an activated DC can efficiently elicit immunity in vivo.[22] Experimental evidence to support this hypothesis has now begun to emerge.[23,24] It has therefore been suggested that tumors may lead to the induction of tolerance or anergy of tumor-specific T cells.[25,26] Even if a T-cell response is elicited, it may be weak, allowing tumor growth to essentially outpace the immune system.[27] Yet another possibility is that the immune effectors in tumor-bearing patients may be dysfunctional. Immune escape may also be due to inadequacy of tumor cells as targets, due to downregulation of major histocompatibility complex (MHC) molecules, tumor antigens, or loss of antigen-processing machinery on tumor cells.[28] Even if tumor-reactive T cells are generated in the periphery, they may fail to home to the tumor, or be susceptible to inhibitory cytokines (such as TGF-β or IL-10) in the tumor microenvironment, or to apoptosis inducing signals derived from tumor cells.[28] Other elements that might suppress tumor immunity include myeloid-derived suppressor cells that may recruit several biochemical pathways for immune suppression.[29] Finally, antitumor effector function in the tumor bed may be silenced by other immune cells such as regulatory T cells in the tumor bed.[30]

It is important to recognize that many of these hypotheses have largely been developed with transplantable tumors in mice. While elegant, these models do have some limitations in that they may not fully replicate the natural state of spontaneous tumor development, which in humans takes several years. Importantly, the growth of tumor in humans often occurs in specific tissue microenvironments (e.g., bone marrow in the case of myeloma). Direct study of the issue of immune escape in patients has thus far been limited, due to difficulties in isolating tumor and immune cells directly from the tumor microenvironment in patients.

Immune Microenvironment in MM

A key feature of MM is the multifocal nature of involvement of the bone marrow, while sparing most other lymphoid tissues. The multifocal pattern of involvement is indeed responsible for the term "multiple" to describe the tumor, and suggests that tumor growth in vivo may depend on specialized niches in the tumor microenvironment. It is now increasingly clear that tumors not only modify the microenvironment they grow in but also actively recruit elements of the microenvironment required for their growth, metastasis, and survival.[31] This may apply not only to the immune and myeloid components of the tumor bed but also to other cells such as bone cell and angiogenesis. The focus in this chapter is on the immune component of this microenvironment. As MM is a tumor of an immune cell (plasma cell), it stands to reason that the tumor cells have a greater likelihood of direct interactions with other immune cells, compared to epithelial tumors.

CD4 and CD8[+] T Cells

Both CD4[+] and CD8[+] T cells play a central role in immune-mediated protection from tumors in mice.[9] Therefore, understanding the nature of antitumor T-cell response is critical to understanding tumor immune interactions in MM.[32] Unfortunately, the lack of knowledge about antigenic targets of tumor-specific T cells in most patients has limited this assessment. Patients with advanced myeloma may have an altered distribution of CD4[+] and CD8[+] lymphoid subsets as compared to healthy controls.[33,34] These reports suggest that the decline in T cells is predominantly in CD4[+]/CD45RA[+] cells.[35–37] Some have argued an increase in B7[+] T cells as evidence for chronic antigenic stimulation in myeloma.[38] In some studies, the levels of immune T cells were reported to carry prognostic significance.[36] Several studies suggest that T cells from blood or bone marrow of patients with newly diagnosed myeloma remain functional, even in patients with advanced disease.[39,40] Immunity to viral antigens measured using assays to detect antigen-specific interferon-γ production appears to be relatively intact in these patients, when compared to healthy controls.[40,41] However, one report suggested that influenza-specific T cells in patients with myeloma may have a reduced proliferative response to antigen stimulation in vitro.[42] T cells within the bone marrow mononuclear cell fraction of patients with myeloma were shown to have an increased proliferative response to anti-CD3 monoclonal antibody (mAb) stimulation, as compared to healthy controls.[43] In some studies, increased antiplasma cell activity of both blood and bone marrow cells was suggested, although this required high effector:target ratios.[44] Although the studies discussed above suggested that T cells in myeloma are generally functionally competent, others have reported abnormalities in signaling molecules and enhanced susceptibility to apoptosis resulting from increased surface Fas expression and reduced bcl-2 levels.[45,46]

Nearly all of the focus for immunity to defined antigens in myeloma has to date been on the detection of T-cell responses to circulating immunoglobulins (Igs). These studies have utilized high doses of Igs and required in vitro culture for the detection of responses.[47–50] Nonetheless, T-cell clones generated after stimulation with IL-2 and F(ab')[2] fragments of autologous Ig could produce IL-2, interferon-γ, and IL-4 after stimulation with autologous Ig.[51] Both CD4[+] and CD8[+] idiotype-reactive T cells using such assays can be detected particularly in patients with low tumor burden, although the clinical significance of their detection remains unclear.[52] Recently, it was shown that idiotype-reactive T cells could recognize and kill autologous tumor cells, although it required multiple cycles of selection and stimulation.[50] T cells from donors immunized with idiotype proteins from the recipients released T helper-1-type cytokines when stimulated with recipient myeloma cells in an MHC-I-restricted fashion.[53] T cell receptor (TCR) variable region repertoire analyses from peripheral blood or marrow have shown oligoclonal T-cell expansions.[54,55] However, whether this represents tumor-specific immune activation or bystander proliferation is not known. Indeed, when reactivity to idiotype was tested in some of these studies, it resided in the nonexpanded populations.[56] At present, only limited information exists about cellular immune response of patients with myeloma to tumor antigens other than tumor-derived Ig, especially using quantitative assays.[57] These studies should pay attention to not just CD8[+] killer T cells but CD4[+] T cells as well.

One approach to address antitumor immunity in myeloma is to measure immunity to autologous tumor, either directly or via loading these tumor cells onto DCs ex vivo. In this regard, myeloma actually represents a useful model system for tumor immunology, as one can readily purify autologous tumor cells, without the need for ex vivo culture, or enzyme treatments. In studies with newly diagnosed patients with myeloma, we observed that freshly isolated T cells from blood or marrow of these patients do not react detectably to autologous tumor.[40] However, this was not due to tumor-induced deletion of antitumor immune effectors as T cells from even the tumor bed (marrow) of these patients could be readily expanded using tumor-loaded DCs to yield antitumor killer T cells.[40] Interestingly, this reactivity was largely specific for autologous tumor, and not directed against tumor-derived Ig. Other groups have similarly documented the presence of tumor-specific killer T cells in the blood and/or bone marrow of patients with progressive myeloma.[58,59] Thus, disease progression in MM is not due to the deletion of antitumor immune T cells from the tumor bed, or immune escape by downregulation of MHC-I or tumor antigens, but likely due to lack of appropriate activation of these immune T cells, or suppression of these responses in vivo.

Another important insight about the functional aspects of antitumor T cells in MM has come from the study of immune T cells against tumor cells in preneoplastic gammopathy (MGUS). In contrast to earlier studies in MM, freshy isolated T cells from the marrow in MGUS are enriched for antitumor interferon-γ producers.[60] Analogous to the results with MM, these T cells are again specific for autologous preneoplastic cells. The immune response consists of both CD4 and CD8+ T cells. Thus, the immune system is capable of recognizing preneoplastic states. The pattern of antigens against which an immune response is elicited in MGUS may differ from that in overt MM. A proportion of patients with MGUS develop naturally occurring T cell and humoral immunity to an embryonal stem cell marker, Sox2.[61] Development of this immune response seems to correlate with improved clinical outcome. Improved understanding of antigenic targets of immune recognition in MGUS may provide insights into the nature of possible rejection antigens in MM.

Humoral Immunity

In contrast to T-cell immunity, marked defect in humoral immunity is commonplace in myeloma. Indeed, a prominent clinical feature of active disease is the suppression of uninvolved polyclonal Igs. Patients with myeloma also have low levels of antibody titers against pneumococcus, tetanus, and diptheria toxoids, and have a poor response to immunizations.[62,63] Both functional and phenotypic abnormalities of B cells, such as a reduction in B cells and an increase in pre-B cells, have been described.[64,65] Some studies have found a correlation between the presence of increased numbers of CD5+ B cells and humoral immunosuppression.[66] Macrophages from patients with myeloma have been shown to inhibit the production of polyclonal Ig in vitro.[67] This may be due to the secretion of a suppressive factor by macrophages in response to myeloma cells.[68] The number of circulating CD19+ B cells was shown to be of prognostic import in a recent study.[36] Another example of potential importance of humoral immunity to tumor control is the finding that patients who achieve complete responses to donor lymphocyte infusions develop antibody responses to antigens expressed on tumor cells.[69] Further study is needed to understand the role of these antibodies in immune protection, as they may help provide novel targets for immune therapy in myeloma.

Innate Lymphocytes

In addition to conventional αβ T cells, other cells such as γδ T cells and NKT cells also play important roles in immune surveillance of tumors in mice.[70,71] These "innate" lymphocytes are capable of rapid activation and cytokine release. Thus, these cells represent a major source of early induction of interferon-γ, a key cytokine for protection against tumors.[14] Interferon-γ may, in principle, also mediate antimyeloma effects by nonimmune mechanisms such as anti-angiogenesis, modulation of signal transducer and activator of transcription (STAT3) signaling on tumor cells, and receptor activator of nuclear factor kappa B ligand (RANKL) signaling in osteoclasts.[72–74] γδ T cells recognize and respond to phosphate antigens such as isoprenylpyrophosphate.[75] Although very few systematic studies of γδ T cells in myeloma have been reported, interest in these cells as antimyeloma effectors increased when it was noted that aminobisphosphonates commonly used in the clinical care in MM are recognized by these cells.[75,76]

NKT cells are distinct lymphocytes that recognize glycolipid ligands in the context of CD1 family of antigen-presenting molecules. Upon antigen recognition, NKT cell can secrete large amounts of cytokines, such as interferon-γ or IL-4, generally 100 times greater than an antigen-specific T cell.[70] NKT cells also cause effective downstream activation of other effectors such as NK cells and T cells, as well as DCs.[70] Recent studies have shown that NKT cells in several patients with advanced cancer including in myeloma are defective in their ability to secrete interferon-γ upon ligand-mediated activation.[77] However, this defect is reversible, at least in vitro, and NKT cells can recognize and kill myeloma cells in a CD1d-dependant fashion. Therefore, there is interest in attempts to target NKT cells in myeloma for therapeutic benefit. It should be recognized, however, that in mice, NKT cells can both promote and inhibit tumors. The former has been ascribed to IL-13-producing NKT cells, which, in turn, promote the secretion of transforming growth factor (TGF)-β by Gr1+ CD11b+ myeloid cells.[70] Further studies are needed to understand the role of NKT cells in myelomagenesis.

Another component of the innate immune system implicated in immune regulation in myeloma is the Fcγ receptor system. Hoover et al. reported an increase in CD16-expressing T cells in patients with IgG myeloma.[78] These T cells often also express CD56, and were not increased in non-IgG myeloma, consistent with isotype dependency. Others have found a stage-dependent increase in soluble CD16 in patients with myeloma.[79] Further studies are needed to understand the role of Fc receptor- expressing cells in myeloma.

Natural Killer Cells

Natural killer (NK) cells are innate effectors involved in the immune defense against viral infections and tumor cells. Triggering of NK cells depends largely on natural cytotoxicity receptors (NCRs) and members of lectin-like receptors (e.g., NKG2D). Studies looking at NK cells in myeloma and monoclonal gammopathies have found both increase and decrease in cells with NK-associated markers and NK function in these patients, both in the blood and in the bone marrow.[80–83] A recent study reported reduced MHC I expression (and reciprocally increased MHC class I-related protein A [MIC-A, a ligand for NKG2D]) in myeloma cell lines obtained from the bone marrow versus those obtained from pleural effusions.[84] These studies also suggested that autologous NK cells can recognize primary myeloma cells, and support further evaluation and targeting of NK cells for antimyeloma effects.

Myeloid Cells Including DCs

Myeloma lesions are highly enriched for cells of myeloid origin. Perhaps the best known of these are osteoclasts, which are central to the development of lytic bone disease. However, MM lesions are also highly enriched for DCs, which are likely actively recruited to these lesions by chemokines secreted by tumor cells.[85,86] Because of their central role in antigen presentation, several studies have tried to characterize the nature of the circulating DC compartment in MM. It was shown that circulating DCs in myeloma are numerically normal but functionally defective, in that they fail to upregulate CD80 expression after CD40 ligand stimulation because of inhibition by TGF β and IL-10.[87] Cytokines such as IL-6 or VEGF may contribute to the observed dysfunction of DCs in the blood of patients with myeloma.[88,89] It has been suggested that this defect can be reversed, at least in vitro by cytokines such as IL-12.[90] Infection of DCs in myeloma with Kaposi Sarcoma-associated herpesvirus (KSHV) was demonstrated in some studies, but not in others.[91,92] Even studies that detected the KSHV virus in patient DCs did not find clear evidence for DC dysfunction as a result of the viral infection.[93,94] Further studies are needed to dissect the nature of DC dysfunction in myeloma and the immunologic outcome of this interaction.

The role of DCs in human MM is likely not restricted to its effects on antitumor immunity. Indeed, two studies have now documented that the interactions of DCs with tumor cells may promote clonogenic growth and survival of tumor cells.[86,95] Kukreja et al. have demonstrated that DC-mediated enhancement of tumor clonogenicity in human MM is mediated by Baff/APRIL and RANK–RANKL-mediated mechanisms.[95] Interestingly, tumor–DC interactions are associated with induction of BCL6, a transcription factor normally silenced in plasma cells, suggesting that the differentiation state of tumor cells in MM may be plastic. Myeloid cells including DCs may be an important component of the tumor bed in MM.

Regulatory Cells

The finding that antitumor T cells can be detected in the tumor bed in MM and yet fail to control tumor has encouraged the study of regulatory pathways that control T-cell immunity. An important element of homeostatic regulatory networks is T regulatory cells. Several subsets of these cells have been described, and the best studied of these are $CD4^+$, $CD25^+$, and $FoxP3^+$ T_{regs}, which play an essential role in the maintenance of immune tolerance. Recent studies have suggested an increase in $FoxP3^+$ Tregs in MM, although their significance, function, and antigen specificity remain to be clarified.[96,97] Functional properties of Tregs may depend on the nature of APCs and in some setting may increase after vaccination.[98] Understanding the balance of induction of effector versus regulatory T cells may be critical for effective recruitment of immune system to treat cancer.[99]

Antigenic Targets in Myeloma

As discussed earlier, most tumors including myeloma express several antigens that may be targets of the immune system. It is likely that this list will grow, as the genomic changes in the myeloma tumor cells are better understood. An unresolved issue in myeloma, as with most other tumors, is to identify which of these potential antigenic targets will be true rejection antigens, and valuable for immune targeting in the clinic (Table 1).

Tumor-Derived Immunoglobulin

The best-studied tumor-associated antigen in myeloma and B-cell tumors to date is the tumor-derived Ig, wherein idiotypic determinants may serve as tumor-specific antigens that are unique for each patient.[100,101] The initial evidence for idiotype-specific immune regulation was obtained in the MOPC-315 plasmacytoma model, wherein this has been extensively characterized by several groups.[100,102–104] In view of its tumor specificity, the tumor-derived idiotype is an attractive antigen for immune therapy. However, in contrast to lymphoma, the tumor cells in myeloma secrete rather than express the intact Ig on their cell surface.[104] Thus, the idiotype is not available on the cell surface in a form that would be a target for an antiidiotype antibody response, which appears to be an important component of tumor protection in the lymphoma experiments. Moreover, high levels of circulating Ig in myeloma may interfere with an antiidiotype antibody response and may in fact promote deletion of specific T cells.[105] These considerations also raise concern about whether T cell repertoire reacting to the idiotype will be of sufficiently high affinity to be biologically important in patients with myeloma. Much of the evidence supporting the role of idiotype in myeloma still comes from the MOPC315 plasmacytoma model, wherein idiotype-specific tumor resistance can be produced by idiotype vaccination and by adoptive transfer of idiotype-specific CD4+ T cell clones.[106,107] It was also shown that an idiotype-specific peptide derived from the third hypervariable region (amino acids 91–101 of the $\lambda 2^{315}$ light chain presented by I-E^d class II molecule) was recognized by idiotype-specific CD4+ T cells.[104] Although idiotype-specific T cells can protect against challenges by small numbers of MOPC315 tumor cells, they become deleted in progressive plasmacytomas.[104] The MOPC315 plasmacytoma cells, however, are MHC class II negative and therefore cannot present antigen to idiotype-specific CD4+ T cells.[108] It was shown that the DCs isolated from these tumors can acquire

Table 1 Some of the antigenic targets/preparations in human myeloma.

- Tumor-derived immunoglobulin/idiotype (several publications)
- Cancer–testis antigens[122–125]
- Muc-1[129]
- h-TERT[130]
- WT1[196]
- DKK-1[131]
- Survivin[197]
- HM1.24[132]
- Whole tumor cells, tumor-derived RNA[198]
- Tumor-derived heat shock proteins[139]
- Tumor stem cell-associated antigens[61]

antigen from these plasmacytomas and activate idiotype-specific transgenic T cells.[109] These APCs can also phagocytose Ig-coated beads and present Ig-derived peptides to idiotype-specific T cells.[110] Recent studies in patients with myeloma have established the proof of concept that T cells expanded using idiotype-pulsed DCs can recognize and kill primary myeloma cells.[53,111] However, the current studies to harness the idiotype-reactive T cell response in the clinic have been disappointing, even using DCs as APCs.[112–114]

Cancer–Testis Antigens

Cancer–testis (C–T) antigens are of interest, as they are expressed only on the tumor and germ cells (which lack MHC expression), and therefore are relatively tumor specific.[115] The expression of several members of this family can be detected using reverse transcriptase polymerase chain reaction (RT-PCR) in primary myeloma cells and cell lines.[116–118] Recently, we examined the expression of these antigens in myeloma tumor cells at the protein level. These data confirmed the presence of several members of this family of antigens in myeloma. Comparisons of gene expression profiles between normal and malignant plasmablasts have also pointed to dysregulation of expression of C–T antigens in myeloma.[119] However, the expression of these antigens on tumor cells is highly heterogeneous, and high level of expression at the protein level is detectable by immnohistochemistry in only a proportion (generally <25%) of tumor cells from most patients.[120] Of the panel of C–T antigens that we examined, MAGE-A3 and MAGE-C1/CT-7 were the most commonly expressed antigens.[120] Another C–T antigen being targeted in clinical studies in many other tumors is NY-ESO-1.[121] However, the expression of this antigen at the protein level in myeloma is less impressive than in solid tumors.[120] Expression of C–T antigens in myeloma seems to correlate with the presence of high-risk features.[122–124] Expression of these antigens also appears to be higher in extramedullary plasmacytomas and myeloma cell lines.[120] Other cancer testis-type antigens described in myeloma include PASD1 and SSX family of antigens.[125] At present there are no systematic or comprehensive studies about the immunity to these antigens in patients with myeloma. Development of newer methods to study immunity to tumor antigens irrespective of the human leukocyte antigen (HLA) haplotype will likely facilitate understanding the nature of host response to these antigens in myeloma and may provide the basis for rational development of approaches for immune targeting of these antigens in these patients.

Mucin-1

Mucin-1 (muc-1) is a glycosylated transmembrane protein normally expressed on the luminal surfaces of secretory glands. Overexpression of an underglycosylated form of muc-1 has been found in several solid and hematologic tumors.[126] Muc-1 core protein is expressed on the surface of myeloma cells but is not tumor specific in that it is also expressed on normal B cells.[127] Immunity to muc-1 has been shown to mediate the regression of muc-1-bearing tumors in mice. These considerations have prompted attempts to harness immunity to muc-1 in myeloma. However, patients with myeloma often have high levels of soluble muc-1, which again might promote tolerance to this antigen.[128] A recent study found increased frequency of muc-1-specific MHC tetramer-binding T cells in the blood and marrow of patients with patients.[129] Although the frequency of tetramer-positive T cells was similar between blood and marrow, the ability of these T cells to secrete interferon-Γ was higher in marrow-derived T cells from some but not all patients. These data support the hypothesis that muc-1 may be a target of spontaneously occurring antitumor T-cell response in patients with myeloma.

Other Antigens

Myeloma cells also express several antigens that are also commonly expressed in other tumors, hence, the term universal tumor antigens.[130] One such antigen is the catalytic subunit of human telomerase (h-TERT).[130] There is evidence that epitopes derived from this protein can be recognized by human T cells. This has led to novel approaches to boost immunity to this antigen in tumor-bearing patients including in myeloma. A recent study proposed the wnt antagonist DKK1 as a target for T cell-based immune therapy[131]; however, DKK1 is not unique to MM and also overexpressed in other inflammatory states. Another antigen under study is the myeloma-associated antigen HM1.24, which can also be targeted by a mAb.[132–134]

Patient-Specific Undefined Antigens

Another possibility is that each patient's tumor expresses a multitude of heterogeneously expressed potential antigenic targets. In some cases, this may include antigens shared between tumors, such as the ones discussed above. However, the net picture is shaped by a number of factors including intraclonal heterogeneity and gene expression profiles of these subclones within the bulk tumor population. For example, chromosomal translocations leading to aberrant gene products may provide specific immunologic targets, unique to each patient. This would create a situation wherein the antigenic profile of each patient's bulk tumor is relatively unique, at least with reference to the frequency of cells overexpressing a certain antigen. Indeed, when bulk CD138 + tumor cells in myeloma have been used as a source of antigen to stimulate autologous T cells (using DCs pulsed with tumor-derived lysates, antibody-coated tumor cells, or tumor-derived RNA), the elicited T-cell response appears to be directed largely toward antigens derived from autologous tumor cells.[40,59,118,135–135] These considerations have encouraged the use of autologous tumor cells as sources of antigens in immune-based therapies in myeloma. Another approach being considered is to load DCs with heat shock protein (hsp) (gp96) derived from tumor cells,[139] as a way to immunize against hsp-chaperoned proteins.

Tumor Microenvironment in Immune Escape

Tumor microenvironment also presents several obstacles to effective antitumor immunity. Tumor cells produce a number of immunosuppressive factors that are enriched in the immediate vicinity of the tumor. TGF-β is a potent immunomodulatory cytokine that can inhibit T-cell responses. High levels of TGF-β were found in patients with advanced myeloma,[140] and both tumor cells and bone marrow stromal cells have been implicated in the secretion of TGF-β.[141–143] In contrast to its effects on normal B cells, TGF-β does not decrease the proliferation of myeloma cells in vitro, and may even augment IL-6 secretion and related proliferation.[144] Tumor-derived TGF-β can inhibit IL-2-induced T-cell proliferation and phosphorylation of STAT-3 and STAT-5, which is reversed by IL-15.[145] Tumor microenvironment in myeloma may also be rich in IL-10, which can inhibit T-cell responses, and promote the induction of regulatory T cells.[146] Vascular endothelial growth factor (VEGF) is also produced in large amounts by tumor cells, and in addition to its role in promoting angiogenesis, VEGF may inhibit maturation of DCs, which can lead to inhibition of T-cell responses.[147] IL-6 is a key growth factor in myeloma, which may also impair DC development.[148] Elevated levels of beta 2 microglobulin were implicated as contributing to immune dysfunction in one study.[149] Metabolic pathways recruited by myeloid suppressor cells such as arginase or inducible nitric oxide synthase may also be operative in MM, and a target for therapeutic targeting.[150] Finally, some investigators have shown that tumor cells in myeloma express both Fas and Fas ligand.[151] It has been postulated that the expression of FasL by tumor cells may be a mechanism of immune escape, by the induction of apoptosis in Fas + T cells. Thus, several hypotheses have been postulated to explain the obstacles to effective antitumor immunity in the tumor bed. Direct and systematic study of adequate cohorts of patients with myeloma using quantitative assays that take advantage of improved understanding of antigen presentation and T-cell stimulation is needed to dissect the relative importance of each of these putative mechanisms of immune escape.

Approaches to Harness Immunity in MM

Rationale for Immunotherapy in MM

The therapy for MM has changed considerably in the last decade and excellent responses can be achieved in most patients with current regimens.[152] However, the net impact on survival is relatively modest and current therapies are not considered to be curative. Although there are several new targets which could be targeted by newer agents, most of these targets and agents are not tumor specific, and therefore do carry a risk for toxicity. Harnessing the immune system has the potential advantage of tumor specificity, relatively low toxicity, and the potential to recruit immunologic memory. In spite of considerable advances, we have only begun to scratch the understanding of tumor–immune interactions in MM. The most compelling arguments about the potential utility of immune-based approaches in MM stem from the responses to donor lymphocyte infusions and allogeneic transplantation, responses to immune modulatory drugs (e.g., Revlimid), and newer insights about immune recognition in MGUS. However, much more work is needed to translate these insights into improvements in specific immunotherapy of MM (Table 2).

Allogeneic Transplantation (HSCT) and Donor Lymphocyte Infusions

The observation that patients who survive allogeneic-HSCT have a lower relapse rate than do patients treated with autologous-HSCT supports the existence of a graft versus myeloma (GVM) effect.[153] However, improvements in disease control were achieved at the cost of higher treatment-related mortality, prompting the consideration of nonmyeloablative transplants. Donor lymphocyte infusion (DLI) provides a direct demonstration of GVM, but is

Table 2 Some approaches to potentially harness antitumor immunity in myeloma.

- Allogeneic stem cell transplantation
- Donor lymphocyte infusions
- Immunomodulatory drugs (e.g., lenalidomide)
- Immunogenic chemotherapy (e.g., bortezomib)
- Antitumor monoclonal antibodies
- Tumor-specific vaccination (e.g., antigen-loaded dendritic cells)
- Adoptive T, NK, or NKT therapy

also associated with high rates of graft versus host (GVH) disease.[154,155] Active vaccination of the donor with myeloma idiotype has been attempted to boost the GVM effect.[156] A major challenge is to be able to separate GVH from GVM to fully harness the potential for this therapy. A recent study described antimyeloma T cells against an activation-induced minor histocompatibility gene in a patient treated with DLI.[157] Another recent study demonstrated that the development of immune responses to NY-ESO1 was associated with durable survival in recipients of allogeneic HSCT.[158] Such targets may allow enhancement of antimyeloma effects without enhancing GVH.

Immune Modulatory Therapies

A major advance in current MM therapy was the recognition of clinical activity of thalidomide.[159] The discovery that thalidomide enhances costimulation of T cells[160] led to the development of immune modulatory derivatives (ImiDs), of which lenalidomide has been most extensively tested in MM. The ability of these agents to enhance T-cell costimulation has also been extended to MM.[161] Thalidomide and lenalidomide may also have effects on innate lymphocytes, such as NK cells, although the mechanism of NK activation appears to be mediated indirectly by T cell-derived cytokines.[162] Lenalidomide also leads to enhancement of ligand-dependent activation of CD1d-restricted NKT cells.[163] Therefore, lipid-reactive T cells may also be a proximal target of these agents. Together these data support combining lenalidomide with antigen-specific immune therapeutic approaches for potentially enhancing the efficacy of either approach.

Immunogenic Chemotherapy

The goal of most antitumor therapies is to induce death of tumor cells. Recent studies have shown that the mode of induction of cell death has major effects on the immune system.[164,165] In particular, cell death induced by some of the agents may be immunogenic.[166] A common emerging theme from these studies is that one of the mechanisms of immunogenic forms of cell death is the exposure of hsps on the surface of dying cells.[167–169] For example, induction of cell death by bortezomib, a proteasome inhibitor, leads to the exposure of hsp90 on the surface of dying cells and enhances DC-mediated induction of antitumor immunity.[167,168] Therefore, agents like bortezomib may be useful agents for harnessing immune resistance in MM. Agents like cyclophosphamide may also serve as useful immune adjuncts, as it is effective in depleting regulatory T cells.[170] It is also worth noting that cure of bulky plasmacytomas in mice by melphalan also requires an intact immune system,[171,172] although the role of the immune system in durability of responses to melaphalan-based therapy in patients has not been systematically evaluated.

Antitumor Monoclonal Antibodies

In spite of the remarkable success of anti-CD20 mAb (Rituxan) in lymphoma, the clinical or preclinical data for mAb-based therapy in MM is limited.[173] Studies have examined targeting CD138, CD38, CD54, CD40, VEGF, and HM1.24 as targets, with limited success.[174,175] To date, the experience with Rituxan in MM is limited as less than 20% of MM tumor cells express CD20.[176,177] However, this is being revisited because of the possibility of expression of CD20 on the putative MM clonogenic progenitors.[178] Development of mAb therapy in MM may benefit both from identification of newer targets and from application of recent advances in understanding of effector and immune mechanisms recruited by these mAbs.[179,180]

Antitumor Vaccines

Several studies have tried to test tumor-specific vaccination in MM. Nearly all of the studies to date have focused on tumor-derived Ig (termed as idiotype or Id) as an antigen. Several approaches have been tested to generate an effective Id vaccine. These include the use of DNA, purified whole Id protein, light or variable heavy chain regions linked to keyhole limpet hemocyanin (KLH), cytokines (such as IL12, IL2, or GMCSF), toxins, or bacterial DNA.[181–185] Others have tried to immunize patients with Id-pulsed monocyte-derived DCs, either alone or with IL2.[114,186,187] In another DC-based approach, blood-derived DCs loaded with Id protein fused with GMCSF (Mylovenge, Dendreon Corporation, Seattle) have been tested in a phase II trial. Some of these studies were able to document an increase in Id-specific immunity; however, the published clinical results to date have been generally disappointing. This may, however, relate in part to patient selection, as many of these studies involved patients with prior extensive chemotherapy or with significant tumor burden, with high levels of circulating tumor-associated Ig. More recent studies have begun to evaluate this in patients with earlier-stage disease.[188,189] Other approaches that are being tried and reported in preliminary fashion include the injection of DCs loaded with tumor lysates and DC–tumor fusion.[59,138,190] It is hoped that application of recent insights in immunobiology of MM will translate to real improvement in design and testing of tumor-specific immune-based approaches in this tumor.

Adoptive Immune Therapy

There is evidence that chemotherapy leads to severe and sustained disruption of TCR diversity in patients with myeloma.[191] As MM is commonly found in elderly individuals who have limited thymic function, it is likely that the effects of chemotherapy on immune reconstitution are long lasting. The presence of a restricted TCR repertoire has been associated with adverse outcome in MM.[191,192] These observations have prompted attempts to enhance immune reconstitution by adoptive transfer of ex vivo-expanded T cells.[193] The feasibility of this approach has been demonstrated in the context of recovery of T cells against pathogens and now needs to be extended toward enhancement of T-cell immunity to tumors. Another approach under study involves adoptive transfer of NK cells or NKT cells based on the premise that these cells can mediate cytotoxicity against human myeloma cells.[194,195]

Summary

Myeloma is an attractive tumor for the study of tumor–immune interactions because in this tumor, both the tumor cells and the infiltrating immune cells are readily accessible for study. Emerging data point to a role for the immune system in control of myeloma cell growth. With progressive disease, these patients acquire several defects in both innate and adaptive components of the immune system. However, many of these defects appear to be reversible, at least in vitro. The ability of the immune system to control myeloma in the clinic is illustrated by the responses to infusions of donor lymphocytes after allogeneic transplantation, as well as immune modulatory drugs. However, refinement in our current understanding of host immune response is needed before specific approaches targeting the enhancement of the immune system as a therapeutic or preventive approach in myeloma.

Acknowledgment: MVD was supported in part by funds from the National Institutes of Health, Dana Foundation, and Damon Runyon Cancer Research Fund.

References

1. Mitsiades CS, Mitsiades N, Munshi NC, Anderson KC. Focus on multiple myeloma. Cancer Cell 2004;6(5):439–44.
2. Kyle RA, Therneau TM, Rajkumar SV, et al. A long-term study of prognosis in monoclonal gammopathy of undetermined significance. N Engl J Med 2002;346(8):564–9.
3. Kyle RA, Remstein ED, Therneau TM, et al. Clinical course and prognosis of smoldering (asymptomatic) multiple myeloma. N Engl J Med 2007;356(25):2582–90.
4. Zhan F, Hardin J, Kordsmeier B, et al. Global gene expression profiling of multiple myeloma, monoclonal gammopathy of undetermined significance, and normal bone marrow plasma cells. Blood 2002;99(5):1745–57.
5. Fonseca R, Barlogie B, Bataille R, et al. Genetics and cytogenetics of multiple myeloma: a workshop report. Cancer Res 2004;64(4):1546–58.
6. Munshi NC. Immunoregulatory mechanisms in multiple myeloma. Hematol Oncol Clin North Am 1997;11(1):51–69.
7. Boon T, Van Der Bruggen P. Human tumor antigens recognized by T lymphocytes. J Exp Med 1996;183:725–9.
8. Gilboa E. The makings of a tumor rejection antigen. Immunity 1999;11(3):263–70.
9. Pardoll D. Does the immune system see tumors as foreign or self? Annu Rev Immunol 2003;21:807–39.
10. Houghton AN, Gold JS, Blachere NE. Immunity against cancer: lessons learned from melanoma. Curr Opin Immunol 2001;13(2):134–40.
11. Houghton AN. Cancer antigens: immune recognition of self and altered self. J Exp Med 1994;180:1–4.
12. Sjoblom T, Jones S, Wood LD, et al. The consensus coding sequences of human breast and colorectal cancers. Science 2006;314(5797):268–74.
13. Sogn JA. Tumor immunology: the glass is half full. Immunity 1998;9(6):757–63.
14. Dunn GP, Bruce AT, Ikeda H, Old LJ, Schreiber RD. Cancer immunoediting: from immunosurveillance to tumor escape. Nat Immunol 2002;3(11):991–8.

15. Bui JD, Schreiber RD. Cancer immunosurveillance, immunoediting and inflammation: independent or interdependent processes? Curr Opin Immunol 2007;19(2):203–8.

16. Marincola FM, Jaffee EM, Hicklin DJ, Ferrone S. Escape of human solid tumors from T-cell recognition: molecular mechanisms and functional significance. Adv Immunol 2000;74:181–273.

17. Zinkernagel RM. Immunity against solid tumors? Int J Cancer 2001;93(1):1–5.

18. Pardoll D. T cells and tumors. Nature 2001;411:1010–2.

19. Huang AYC, Golumbek P, Ahmadzadeh M, Jaffee E, Pardoll D, Levitsky H. Role of bone marrow-derived cells in presenting MHC class I-restricted tumor antigens. Science 1994;264:961–5.

20. Heath WR, Carbone FR. Cross-presentation, dendritic cells, tolerance and immunity. Annu Rev Immunol 2001;19:47–64.

21. Ochsenbein A, Sierro S, Odermatt B, et al. Roles of tumor localization, second signals and cross priming in cytotoxic T cell induction. Nature 2001;411:1058–64.

22. Mellman I, Steinman RM. Dendritic cells: specialized and regulated antigen processing machines. Cell 2001;106(3):255–8.

23. Hawiger D, Inaba K, Dorsett Y, et al. Dendritic cells induce peripheral T cell unresponsiveness under steady state conditions in vivo. J Exp Med 2001;194(6):769–79.

24. Liu K, Iyoda T, Saternus M, Kimura Y, Inaba K, Steinman RM. Immune tolerance after delivery of dying cells to dendritic cells in situ. J Exp Med 2002;196(8):1091–7.

25. Sotomayor EM, Borrello I, Rattis FM, et al. Cross-presentation of tumor antigens by bone marrow-derived antigen-presenting cells is the dominant mechanism in the induction of T-cell tolerance during B-cell lymphoma progression. Blood 2001;98(4):1070–7.

26. Staveley-O'Carroll K, Sotomayor E, Montgomery J, et al. Induction of antigen-specific T cell anergy: an early event in the course of tumor progression. Proc Natl Acad Sci 1998;95:1178–93.

27. Hanson HL, Donermeyer DL, Ikeda H, et al. Eradication of established tumors by CD8 + T cell adoptive immunotherapy. Immunity 2000;13(2):265–76.

28. Gilboa E. How tumors escape immune destruction and what we can do about it. Cancer Immunol Immunother 1999;48(7):382–5.

29. Herber DL, Nagaraj S, Djeu JY, Gabrilovich DI. Mechanism and therapeutic reversal of immune suppression in cancer. Cancer Res 2007;67(11):5067–9.

30. Terabe M, Berzofsky JA. Immunoregulatory T cells in tumor immunity. Curr Opin Immunol 2004;16(2):157–62.

31. Bissell MJ, Radisky D. Putting tumours in context. Nat Rev Cancer 2001;1(1):46–54.

32. Dhodapkar MV. Harnessing host immune responses to preneoplasia: promise and challenges. Cancer Immunol Immunother 2005;54(5):409–13.

33. Serra HM, Mant MJ, Ruether BA, Ledbetter JA, Pilarski LM. Selective loss of CD4 + CD45R + T cells in peripheral blood of multiple myeloma patients. J Clin Immunol 1988;8(4):259–65.

34. San Miguel JF, Garcia-Sanchez R, Gonzales A. Lymphoid subsets and prognostic factors in multiple myeloma. Br J Hem 1992;80:305–9.

35. Kay N, Leong T, Kyle RA, et al. Altered T cell repertoire usage in CD4 and CD8 subsets of multiple myeloma patients, a Study of the Eastern Cooperative Oncology Group (E9487). Leuk Lymphoma 1999;33(1–2):127–33.

36. Kay NE, Leong TL, Bone N, et al. Blood levels of immune cells predict survival in myeloma patients: results of an Eastern Cooperative Oncology Group phase 3 trial for newly diagnosed multiple myeloma patients. Blood 2001;98(1):23–8.

37. Kay NE, Leong T, Bone N, et al. T-helper phenotypes in the blood of myeloma patients on ECOG phase III trials E9486/E3A93. Br J Haematol 1998;100(3):459–63.

38. Brown R, Murray A, Pope B, et al. B7 + T cells in myeloma: an acquired marker of prior chronic antigen presentation. Leuk Lymphoma 2004;45(2):363–71.

39. Yi Q, Dabadgao S, Osterborg A, Bergenbrant S, Holm G. Myeloma bone marrow plasma cells: evidence for their capacity as antigen presenting cells. Blood 1997;5:1960–7.

40. Dhodapkar MV, Krasovsky J, Olson K. T cells from the tumor microenvironment of patients with progressive myeloma can generate strong tumor specific cytolytic responses to autologous tumor loaded dendritic cells. Proc Natl Acad Sci 2002;99:13009–13.

41. Brander C, Raje N, O'Connor PG, et al. Absence of biologically important Kaposi sarcoma-associated herpesvirus gene products and virus-specific cellular immune responses in multiple myeloma. Blood 2002;100(2):698–700.

42. Maecker B, Anderson KS, von Bergwelt-Baildon MS, et al. Viral antigen-specific CD8 + T-cell responses are impaired in multiple myeloma. Br J Haematol 2003;121(6):842–8.

43. Massaia M, Attisano C, Peola S, et al. Rapid generation of antiplasma cell activity in the bone marrow of myeloma patients by CD3-activated T cells. Blood 1993;82(6): 1787–97.

44. Paglieroni TG, MacKenzie MR. In vitro cytotoxic response to human myeloma plasma cells by peripheral blood leukocytes from patients with multiple myeloma and benign monoclonal gammopathy. Blood 1979;54:226–37.

45. Bianchi A, Mariani S, Beggiato E, et al. Distribution of T-cell signalling molecules in human myeloma. Br J Haematol 1997;97(4):815–20.

46. Massaia M, Borrione P, Attisano C, et al. Dysregulated Fas and Bcl-2 expression leading to enhanced apoptosis in T cells of multiple myeloma patients. Blood 1995;85(12):3679–87.

47. Osterborg A, Henriksson L, Mellstedt H. Idiotype immunity (natural and vaccine-induced) in early stage multiple myeloma. Acta Oncol 2000;39(7):797–800.

48. Osterborg A, Yi Q, Bergenbrant S, Holm G, Lefvert AK, Mellstedt H. Idiotype-specific T cells in multiple myeloma stage I: an evaluation by four different functional tests. Br J Haematol 1995;89(1):110–6.

49. Wen T, Mellstedt H, Jondal M. Presence of clonal T cell populations in chronic B lymphocytic leukemia and smoldering myeloma. J Exp Med 1990;171(3):659–66.

50. Wen YJ, Barlogie B, Yi Q. Idiotype-specific cytotoxic T lymphocytes in multiple myeloma: evidence for their capacity to lyse autologous primary tumor cells. Blood 2001;97(6):1750–5.

51. Osterborg A, Masucci M, Bergenbrant S, Holm G, Lefvert AK, Mellstedt H. Generation of T cell clones binding F(ab')2 fragments of the idiotypic immunoglobulin in patients with monoclonal gammopathy. Cancer Immunol Immunother 1991;34(3):157–62.

52. Yi Q, Osterborg A, Bergenbrant S, Mellstedt H, Holm G, Lefvert AK. Idiotype-reactive T-cell subsets and tumor load in monoclonal gammopathies. Blood 1995;86(8):3043–9.

53. Li Y, Bendandi M, Deng Y, et al. Tumor-specific recognition of human myeloma cells by idiotype-induced CD8(+) T cells. Blood 2000;96(8):2828–33.

54. Lim SH, Badros A, Lue C, Barlogie B. Distinct T-cell clonal expansion in the vicinity of tumor cells in plasmacytoma. Cancer 2001;91(5):900–8.

55. Halapi E, Werner A, Wahlstrom J, et al. T cell repertoire in patients with multiple myeloma and monoclonal gammopathy of undetermined significance: clonal CD8 + T cell expansions are found preferentially in patients with a low tumor burden. Eur J Immunol 1997;27(9):2245–52.

56. Yi Q, Eriksson I, He W, Holm G, Mellstedt H, Osterborg A. Idiotype-specific T lymphocytes in monoclonal gammopathies: evidence for the presence of CD4 + and CD8 + subsets. Br J Haematol 1997;96(2):338–45.

57. Romero P, Cerottini JC, Waanders GA. Novel methods to monitor antigen-specific cytotoxic T-cell responses in cancer immunotherapy. Mol Med Today 1998;4(7):305–12.

58. Noonan K, Matsui W, Serafini P, et al. Activated marrow-infiltrating lymphocytes effectively target plasma cells and their clonogenic precursors. Cancer Res 2005;65(5):2026–34.
59. Wen YJ, Min R, Tricot G, Barlogie B, Yi Q. Tumor lysate-specific cytotoxic T lymphocytes in multiple myeloma: promising effector cells for immunotherapy. Blood 2002;99(9):3280–5.
60. Dhodapkar MV, Krasovsky J, Osman K, Geller MD. Vigorous premalignancy specific effector T cell response in the bone marrow of patients with preneoplastic gammopathy. J Exp Med 2003;198:1753–7.
61. Spisek R, Kukreja A, Chen LC, et al. Frequent and specific immunity to the embryonal stem cell-associated antigen SOX2 in patients with monoclonal gammopathy. J Exp Med 2007;204(4):831–40.
62. Pilarski LM, Andrews EJ, Mant MJ, Ruether BA. Humoral immune deficiency in multiple myeloma patients due to compromised B-cell function. J Clin Immunol 1986;6(6):491–501.
63. Hargreaves RM, Lea JR, Griffiths H. Immunologic factors and risk of infection in plateau phase myeloma. J Clin Path 1995;48:260–9.
64. Pilarski LM, Mant MJ, Ruether BA. Pre-B cells in peripheral blood of multiple myeloma patients. Blood 1985;66(2):416–22.
65. Pilarski LM, Mant MJ, Ruether BA, Belch A. Severe deficiency of B lymphocytes in peripheral blood from multiple myeloma patients. J Clin Invest 1984;74(4):1301–6.
66. Paglieroni T, MacKenzie MR, Caggiano V. Abnormalities in immunoregulatory CD5 + B cells precede the diagnosis of multiple myeloma. Ann N Y Acad Sci 1992;651:486–7.
67. Broder S, Humphrey R, Durm M, et al. Impaired synthesis of polyclonal (non-paraprotein) immunoglobulins by circulating lymphocytes from patients with multiple myeloma. Role of suppressor cells. N Engl J Med 1975;293(18):887–92.
68. Ullrich S, Zolla-Pazner S. Immunoregulatory circuits in myeloma. Clin Haematol 1982;11(1):87–111.
69. Bellucci R, Wu CJ, Chiaretti S, et al. Complete response to donor lymphocyte infusion in multiple myeloma is associated with antibody responses to highly expressed antigens. Blood 2004;103(2):656–63.
70. Smyth MJ, Crowe NY, Hayakawa Y, Takeda K, Yagita H, Godfrey DI. NKT cells—conductors of tumor immunity? Curr Opin Immunol 2002;14(2):165–71.
71. Girardi M, Oppenheim DE, Steele CR, et al. Regulation of cutaneous malignancy by gammadelta T cells. Science 2001;294(5542):605–9.
72. Coughlin CM, Salhany KE, Gee MS, . Tumor cell responses to IFNgamma affect tumorigenicity and response to IL-12 therapy and antiangiogenesis. Immunity 1998;9(1):25–34.
73. Catlett-Falcone R, Landowski TH, Oshiro MM, et al. Constitutive activation of Stat3 signaling confers resistance to apoptosis in human U266 myeloma cells. Immunity 1999;10(1):105–15.
74. Takayanagi H, Ogasawara K, Hida S, et al. T-cell-mediated regulation of osteoclastogenesis by signalling cross-talk between RANKL and IFN-gamma. Nature 2000;408(6812):600–5.
75. Wilhelm M, Kunzmann V, Eckstein S, et al. Gammadelta T cells for immune therapy of patients with lymphoid malignancies. Blood 2003;102(1):200–6.
76. Kunzmann V, Bauer E, Feurle J, Weissinger F, Tony HP, Wilhelm M. Stimulation of gammadelta T cells by aminobisphosphonates and induction of antiplasma cell activity in multiple myeloma. Blood 2000;96(2):384–92.
77. Dhodapkar MV, Geller MD, Chang DH, et al. A reversible defect in natural killer T cell function characterizes the progression of premalignant to malignant multiple myeloma. J Exp Med 2003;197(12):1667–76.

78. Hoover RG, Lary C, Page R, et al. Autoregulatory circuits in myeloma. Tumor cell cytotoxicity mediated by soluble CD16. J Clin Invest 1995;95(1):241–7.

79. Mathiot C, Galon J, Tartour E, et al. Soluble CD16 in plasma cell dyscrasias. Leuk Lymphoma 1999;32(5–6):467–74.

80. Nielsen H, Nielsen HJ, Tvede N, et al. Immune dysfunction in multiple myeloma. Reduced natural killer cell activity and increased levels of soluble interleukin-2 receptors. APMIS 1991;99(4):340–6.

81. Uchida A, Yagita M, Sugiyama H. Strong natural killer (NK) cell activity in bone marrow of myeloma patients: accelerated maturation of bone marrow NK cells and their interaction with other NK cells. Int J Cancer 1984;34:375–81.

82. Osterborg A, Nilsson B, Bjorkholm M, Holm G, Mellstedt H. Natural killer cell activity in monoclonal gammopathies: relation to disease activity. Eur J Haematol 1990;45(3):153–7.

83. Garcia-Sanz R, Gonzalez M, Orfao A. Analysis of natural killer associated antigens in the peripheral blood and bone marrow of multiple myeloma patients: prognostic implications. Br J Hematology 1996;93:81–9.

84. Carbone E, Neri P, Mesuraca M, et al. HLA class I, NKG2D, and natural cytotoxicity receptors regulate multiple myeloma cell recognition by natural killer cells. Blood 2005;105(1):251–8.

85. Said JW, Rettig MR, Heppner K, et al. Localization of Kaposi's sarcoma-associated herpesvirus in bone marrow biopsy samples from patients with multiple myeloma. Blood 1997;90(11):4278–82.

86. Bahlis NJ, King AM, Kolonias D, et al. CD28-mediated regulation of multiple myeloma cell proliferation and survival. Blood 2007;109(11):5002–10.

87. Brown RD, Pope B, Murray A, et al. Dendritic cells from patients with myeloma are numerically normal but functionally defective as they fail to up-regulate CD80 (B7–1) expression after huCD40LT stimulation because of inhibition by transforming growth factor-beta1 and interleukin-10. Blood 2001;98(10):2992–8.

88. Ratta M, Fagnoni F, Curti A, et al. Dendritic cells are functionally defective in multiple myeloma: the role of interleukin-6. Blood 2002;100(1):230–7.

89. Podar K, Anderson KC. The pathophysiological role of VEGF in hematological malignancies: therapeutic implications. Blood 2005;105(4):1383–1395.

90. Brown R, Murray A, Pope B, et al. Either interleukin-12 or interferon-gamma can correct the dendritic cell defect induced by transforming growth factor beta in patients with myeloma. Br J Haematol 2004;125(6):743–8.

91. Rettig MB, Ma HJ, Vescio RA, et al. Kaposi's sarcoma-associated herpesvirus infection of bone marrow dendritic cells from multiple myeloma patients. Science 1997;276(5320):1851–4.

92. Yi Q, Ekman M, Anton D, et al. Blood dendritic cells from myeloma patients are not infected with Kaposi's sarcoma-associated herpesvirus (KSHV/HHV-8). Blood 1998;92(2):402–4.

93. Raje N, Kica G, Chauhan D, et al. Kaposi's sarcoma-associated herpesvirus gene sequences are detectable at low copy number in primary amyloidosis. Amyloid 2000; 7(2):126–32.

94. Raje N, Gong J, Chauhan D, et al. Bone marrow and peripheral blood dendritic cells from patients with multiple myeloma are phenotypically and functionally normal despite the detection of Kaposi's sarcoma herpesvirus gene sequences. Blood 1999;93(5):1487–95.

95. Kukreja A, Hutchinson A, Dhodapkar K, et al. Enhancement of clonogenicity of human multiple myeloma by dendritic cells. J Exp Med 2006;203(8): 1859–65.

96. Prabhala RH, Neri P, Bae JE, et al. Dysfunctional T regulatory cells in multiple myeloma. Blood 2006;107(1):301–4.

97. Beyer M, Kochanek M, Giese T, et al. In vivo peripheral expansion of naive CD4 + CD25high FOXP3 + regulatory T cells in patients with multiple myeloma. Blood 2006;107(10):3940–9.

Chapter 11 Immunobiology and Immunotherapy **161**

98. Banerjee D, Dhodapkar MV, Matayeva E, Steinman RM, Dhodapkar K. Expansion of FOXP3high regulatory T cells by human dendritic cells (DCs) in vitro and after DC injection of cytokine matured DCs in myeloma patients. Blood 2006;108(8):2655–2661.

99. Zhou G, Drake CG, Levitsky HI. Amplification of tumor-specific regulatory T cells following therapeutic cancer vaccines. Blood 2006;107(2):628–36.

100. Lynch RG, Graff RJ, Sirisinha S, Simms ES, Eisen HN. Myeloma proteins as tumor-specific transplantation antigens. Proc Natl Acad Sci USA 1972;69(6):1540–4.

101. Kwak LW, Thielemans K, Massaia M. Idiotypic vaccination as therapy for multiple myeloma. Semin Hematol 1999;36(1 Suppl 3):34–7.

102. Milburn GL, Lynch RG. Immunoregulation of murine myeloma in vitro. II. Suppression of MOPC-315 immunoglobulin secretion and synthesis by idiotype-specific suppressor T cells. J Exp Med 1982;155(3):852–62.

103. Abbas AK. T lymphocyte-mediated suppression of myeloma function in vitro. I. Suppression by allogeneically activated T lymphocytes. J Immunol 1979;123(5):2011–8.

104. Bogen B, Malissen B, Haas W. Idiotope-specific T cell clones that recognize syngeneic immunoglobulin fragments in the context of class II molecules. Eur J Immunol 1986;16(11):1373–8.

105. Bogen B. Peripheral T cell tolerance as a tumor escape mechanism: deletion of CD4 + T cells specific for a monoclonal immunoglobulin idiotype secreted by a plasmacytoma. Eur J Immunol 1996;26(11):2671–9.

106. Lynch RG, Graff RJ, Sirisinha S. Myeloma proteins as tumor specific transplantation antigens. Proc Natl Acad Sci USA 1972;69:1540–4.

107. Daley MJ, Gebel HM, Lynch RG. Idiotype specific transplantation resistsnce to MOPC315: abrogation by post-immunization thymectomy. J Immunol 1978;120:1620–4.

108. Lauritzsen GF, Bogen B. The role of idiotype-specific, CD4 + T cells in tumor resistance against major histocompatibility complex class II molecule negative plasmacytoma cells. Cell Immunol 1993;148(1):177–88.

109. Dembic Z, Schenck K, Bogen B. Dendritic cells purified from myeloma are primed with tumor-specific antigen (idiotype) and activate CD4 + T cells. Proc Natl Acad Sci USA 2000;97(6):2697–702.

110. Dembic Z, Rottingen JA, Dellacasagrande J, Schenck K, Bogen B. Phagocytic dendritic cells from myelomas activate tumor-specific T cells at a single cell level. Blood 2001;97(9):2808–14.

111. Wen YJ, Barlogie B, Yi Q. Idiotype-specific cytotoxic T lymphocytes in multiple myeloma: evidence for their capacity to lyse autologous primary tumor cells. Blood 2001;97(6):1750–5.

112. Yi Q, Desikan R, Barlogie B, Munshi N. Optimizing dendritic cell-based immunotherapy in multiple myeloma. Br J Haematol 2002;117(2):297–305.

113. Wen YJ, Ling M, Bailey-Wood R, Lim SH. Idiotypic protein-pulsed adherent peripheral blood mononuclear cell-derived dendritic cells prime immune system in multiple myeloma. Clin Cancer Res 1998;4(4):957–62.

114. Reichardt VL, Milazzo C, Brugger W, Einsele H, Kanz L, Brossart P. Idiotype vaccination of multiple myeloma patients using monocyte-derived dendritic cells. Haematologica 2003;88(10):1139–49.

115. Chen YT, Old LJ. Cancer-testis antigens: targets for cancer immunotherapy. Cancer J Sci Am 1999;5(1):16–7.

116. van Baren N, Brasseur F, Godelaine D, et al. Genes encoding tumor-specific antigens are expressed in human myeloma cells. Blood 1999;94(4):1156–64.

117. Pellat-Deceunynck C, Mellerin MP, Labarriere N, et al. The cancer germ-line genes MAGE-1, MAGE-3 and PRAME are commonly expressed by human myeloma cells. Eur J Immunol 2000;30(3):803–9.

118. Dhodapkar K, Krasovsky J, Williamson B, Dhodapkar M. Anti-tumor monoclonal antibodies enhance cross presentation of cellular antigens and the generation of tumor specific killer T cells by dendritic cells. J Exp Med 2002;195:125–33.

119. Tarte K, Zhan F, De Vos J, Klein B, Shaughnessy J. Gene expression profiling of plasma cells and plasmablasts: toward a better understanding of the late stages of B-cell differentiation. Blood 2003;102(2):592–600.

120. Dhodapkar MV, Osman K, Teruya-Feldstein J, et al. Expression of cancer/testis (CT) antigens MAGE-A1, MAGE-A3, MAGE-A4, CT-7, and NY-ESO-1 in malignant gammopathies is heterogeneous and correlates with site, stage and risk status of disease. Cancer Immun 2003;3:9.

121. Batchu RB, Moreno AM, Szmania S, et al. High-level expression of cancer/testis antigen NY-ESO-1 and human granulocyte-macrophage colony-stimulating factor in dendritic cells with a bicistronic retroviral vector. Hum Gene Ther 2003;14(14):1333–45.

122. Dhodapkar MV, Osman K, Feldstein J, et al. Expression of cancer-testis antigens (MAGE-A1, -A3, -A4, CT-7 and NY-ESO-1 in malignant gammopathies is heterogeneous and correlates with site, stage and risk status of disease. Cancer Immun 2003;3:9–16.

123. van Rhee F, Szmania SM, Zhan F, et al. NY-ESO-1 is highly expressed in poor-prognosis multiple myeloma and induces spontaneous humoral and cellular immune responses. Blood 2005;105(10):3939–44.

124. Jungbluth AA, Ely S, Diliberto M, et al. The Cancer-Testis antigens CT7 (MAGE-C1) and MAGE-A3/6 are commonly expressed in multiple myeloma and correlate with plasma cell proliferation. Blood 2005;106(1):167–174.

125. Sahota SS, Goonewardena CM, Cooper CD, et al. PASD1 is a potential multiple myeloma-associated antigen. Blood 2006;108(12):3953–5.

126. Brossart P, Schneider A, Dill P, et al. The epithelial tumor antigen MUC1 is expressed in hematological malignancies and is recognized by MUC1-specific cytotoxic T-lymphocytes. Cancer Res 2001;61(18):6846–50.

127. Treon SP, Mollick JA, Urashima M, . Muc-1 core protein is expressed on multiple myeloma cells and is induced by dexamethasone. Blood 1999;93(4):1287–98.

128. Mileshkin L, Prince HM, Seymour JF, Biagi JJ. Serum MUC-1 as a marker of disease status in multiple myeloma patients receiving thalidomide. Br J Haematol 2003;123(4):747–8; author reply 8.

129. Choi C, Witzens M, Bucur M, et al. Enrichment of functional CD8 memory T cells specific for MUC1 in bone marrow of multiple myeloma patients. Blood 2005;105(5):2132–2134.

130. Vonderheide RH, Hahn WC, Schultze JL, Nadler LM. The telomerase catalytic subunit is a widely expressed tumor-associated antigen recognized by cytotoxic T lymphocytes. Immunity 1999;10(6):673–9.

131. Qian J, Xie J, Hong S, et al. DKK1 is a widely expressed and potent tumor-associated antigen in multiple myeloma. Blood 2007;110(5):1587–1594.

132. Rew SB, Peggs K, Sanjuan I, et al. Generation of potent antitumor CTL from patients with multiple myeloma directed against HM1.24. Clin Cancer Res 2005;11(9):3377–84.

133. Jalili A, Ozaki S, Hara T, et al. Induction of HM1.24 peptide-specific cytotoxic T lymphocytes by using peripheral-blood stem-cell harvests in patients with multiple myeloma. Blood 2005;106(10):3538–45.

134. Hundemer M, Schmidt S, Condomines M, et al. Identification of a new HLA-A2-restricted T-cell epitope within HM1.24 as immunotherapy target for multiple myeloma. Exp Hematol 2006;34(4):486–96.

135. Dhodapkar MV, Krasovsky J, Osman K, Geller MD. Vigorous premalignancy-specific effector T cell response in the bone marrow of patients with monoclonal gammopathy. J Exp Med 2003;198(11):1753–7.

136. Milazzo C, Reichardt VL, Muller MR, Grunebach F, Brossart P. Induction of myeloma-specific cytotoxic T cells using dendritic cells transfected with tumor-derived RNA. Blood 2003;101(3):977–82.

137. Hayashi T, Hideshima T, Akiyama M, et al. Ex vivo induction of multiple myeloma-specific cytotoxic T lymphocytes. Blood 2003;102(4):1435–42.

138. Raje N, Hideshima T, Davies FE, et al. Tumour cell/dendritic cell fusions as a vaccination strategy for multiple myeloma. Br J Haematol 2004;125(3):343–52.

139. Qian J, Wang S, Yang J, et al. Targeting heat shock proteins for immunotherapy in multiple myeloma: generation of myeloma-specific CTLs using dendritic cells pulsed with tumor-derived gp96. Clin Cancer Res 2005;11(24 Pt 1):8808–15.

140. Jiang X, Kanai H, Hiromura K, Sawamura M, Yano S. Increased intra-platelet and urinary transforming growth factor-beta in patients with multiple myeloma. Acta Hematol 1995;94:1–6.

141. Matthes T, Werner-Farve C, Tang H, Zang X, Kindler V, Zubler RH. Cytokine gene expression during in vitro response of human B lymphocytes: kinetics of B cell tumor necrosis factor alpha, interleukin-6, interleukin-10, and transforming growth factor-beta 1 mRNAs. J Exp Med 1993;178:521–8.

142. Cook G, Campbell JD, Carr CE, Boyd KS, Franklin IM. Transforming growth factor beta from multiple myeloma cells inhibits proliferation and IL-2 responsiveness in T lymphocytes. J Leukoc Biol 1999;66(6):981–8.

143. Cook G, Campbell JD. Immune regulation in multiple myeloma: the host-tumour conflict. Blood Rev 1999;13(3):151–62.

144. Urashima M, Ogata A, Chauhan D, et al. Transforming growth factor-beta1: differential effects on multiple myeloma versus normal B cells. Blood 1996;87(5):1928–38.

145. Campbell JD, Cook G, Robertson SE, et al. Suppression of IL-2-induced T cell proliferation and phosphorylation of STAT3 and STAT5 by tumor-derived TGF beta is reversed by IL-15. J Immunol 2001;167(1):553–61.

146. Ameglio F, Alvino S, Trento E. Serum interleukin-10 levels in patients affected with multiple myeloma: correlation with the monoclonal component and disease progression. Int J Oncol 1995;6:1189–92.

147. Gabrilovich DI, Chen HI, Girgis KR, et al. Production of vascular endothelial growth factor by human tumors inhibits the functional maturation of dendritic cells. Nat Med 1996;2:1096–103.

148. Chomarat P, Banchereau J, Davoust J, Palucka AK. IL-6 switches the differentiation of monocytes from dendritic cells to macrophages. Nat Immunol 2000;1(6):510–4.

149. Xie J, Wang Y, Freeman ME, 3rd, Barlogie B, Yi Q. Beta 2-microglobulin as a negative regulator of the immune system: high concentrations of the protein inhibit in vitro generation of functional dendritic cells. Blood 2003;101(10):4005–12.

150. Serafini P, Meckel K, Kelso M, . Phosphodiesterase-5 inhibition augments endogenous antitumor immunity by reducing myeloid-derived suppressor cell function. J Exp Med 2006;203(12):2691–702.

151. Villunger A, Egle A, Marschitz I, et al. Constitutive expression of Fas (Apo-1/CD95) ligand on multiple myeloma cells: a potential mechanism of tumor-induced suppression of immune surveillance. Blood 1997;90(1):12–20.

152. Barlogie B, Shaughnessy J, Tricot G, et al. Treatment of multiple myeloma. Blood 2004;103(1):20–32.

153. Bruno B, Rotta M, Patriarca F, . A comparison of allografting with autografting for newly diagnosed myeloma. N Engl J Med 2007;356(11):1110–20.

154. Tricot G, Vesole DH, Jagannath S, Hilton J, Munshi N, Barlogie B. Graft-versus-myeloma effect: proof of principle. Blood 1996;87(3):1196–8.

155. Lokhorst HM, Schattenberg A, Cornelissen JJ, . Donor lymphocyte infusions for relapsed multiple myeloma after allogeneic stem-cell transplantation: predictive factors for response and long-term outcome. J Clin Oncol 2000;18(16):3031–7.

156. Kwak LW, Taub DD, Duffey PL, et al. Transfer of myeloma idiotype-specific immunity from an actively immunised marrow donor. Lancet 1995;345(8956):1016–20.

157. van Bergen CA, Kester MG, Jedema I, et al. Multiple myeloma-reactive T cells recognize an activation-induced minor histocompatibility antigen encoded by the ATP-dependent interferon-responsive (ADIR) gene. Blood 2007;109(9):4089–96.

158. Atanackovic D, Arfsten J, Cao Y, . Cancer-testis antigens are commonly expressed in multiple myeloma and induce systemic immunity following allogeneic stem cell transplantation. Blood 2007;109(3):1103–12.

159. Singhal S, Mehta J, Desikan R, et al. Antitumor activity of thalidomide in refractory multiple myeloma. N Engl J Med 1999;341(21):1565–71.

160. Haslett PA, Corral LG, Albert M, Kaplan G. Thalidomide costimulates primary human T lymphocytes, preferentially inducing proliferation, cytokine production, and cytotoxic responses in the CD8 + subset. J Exp Med 1998;187(11): 1885–92.

161. LeBlanc R, Hideshima T, Catley LP, et al. Immunomodulatory drug costimulates T cells via the B7-CD28 pathway. Blood 2004;103(5):1787–90.

162. Davies FE, Raje N, Hideshima T, et al. Thalidomide and immunomodulatory derivatives augment natural killer cell cytotoxicity in multiple myeloma. Blood 2001;98(1):210–6.

163. Chang DH, Liu N, Klimek V, et al. Enhancement of ligand dependent activation of human natural killer T cells by lenalidomide: therapeutic implications. Blood 2006;108(2):618–621.

164. Lake RA, Robinson BW. Immunotherapy and chemotherapy—a practical partnership. Nat Rev Cancer 2005;5(5):397–405.

165. Lake RA, van der Most RG. A better way for a cancer cell to die. N Engl J Med 2006;354(23):2503–4.

166. Casares N, Pequignot MO, Tesniere A, et al. Caspase-dependent immunogenicity of doxorubicin-induced tumor cell death. J Exp Med 2005;202(12):1691–701.

167. Spisek R, Dhodapkar MV. Towards a better way to die with chemotherapy: role of heat shock proteins on dying tumor cells. Cell Cycle 2007;6(16):1962–1965.

168. Spisek R, Charalambous A, Mazumder A, Vesole DH, Jagannath S, Dhodapkar MV. Bortezomib enhances dendritic cell (DC) mediated induction of immunity to human myeloma via exposure of cell surface heat shock protein 90 on dying tumor cells: therapeutic implications. Blood 2007;109(Jun 1):4839–45.

169. Obeid M, Tesniere A, Ghiringhelli F, et al. Calreticulin exposure dictates the immunogenicity of cancer cell death. Nat Med 2007;13(1):54–61.

170. North RJ, Awwad M. T cell suppression as an obstacle to immunologically-mediated tumor regression: elimination of suppression results in regression. Prog Clin Biol Res 1987;244:345–58.

171. Barker E, Mokyr MB. Importance of Lyt-2 + T-cells in the resistance of melphalan-cured MOPC- 315 tumor bearers to a challenge with MOPC-315 tumor cells. Cancer Res 1988;48(17):4834–42.

172. Barker E, Mokyr MB. Some characteristics of the in vivo antitumor immunity exhibited by mice cured of a large MOPC-315 tumor by a low dose of melphalan. Cancer Immunol Immunother 1987;25(3):215–24.

173. Maloney DG, Donovan K, Hamblin TJ. Antibody therapy for treatment of multiple myeloma. Semin Hematol 1999;36(1 Suppl 3):30–3.

174. Ono K, Ohtomo T, Yoshida K, et al. The humanized anti-HM1.24 antibody effectively kills multiple myeloma cells by human effector cell-mediated cytotoxicity. Mol Immunol 1999;36(6):387–95.

175. Stevenson GT. CD38 as a therapeutic target. Mol Med 2006;12(11–12):345–6.

176. Lim SH, Zhang Y, Wang Z, Varadarajan R, Periman P, Esler WV. Rituximab administration following autologous stem cell transplantation for multiple myeloma is associated with severe IgM deficiency. Blood 2004;103(5):1971–2.

177. Musto P, Carella AM, Jr., Greco MM, et al. Short progression-free survival in myeloma patients receiving rituximab as maintenance therapy after autologous transplantation. Br J Haematol 2003;123(4):746–7.

178. Matsui W, Huff CA, Wang Q, et al. Characterization of clonogenic multiple myeloma cells. Blood 2004;103(6):2332–6.

179. Clynes R. Antitumor antibodies in the treatment of cancer: Fc receptors link opsonic antibody with cellular immunity. Hematol Oncol Clin North Am 2006;20(3):585–612.

180. Dhodapkar KM, Dhodapkar MV. Recruiting dendritic cells to improve antibody therapy of cancer. Proc Natl Acad Sci USA 2005;102(18):6243–4.

181. Osterborg A, Yi Q, Henriksson L, et al. Idiotype immunization combined with granulocyte-macrophage colony-stimulating factor in myeloma patients induced type I, major histocompatibility complex-restricted, CD8- and CD4-specific T-cell responses. Blood 1998;91(7):2459–66.

182. Rasmussen T, Hansson L, Osterborg A, Johnsen HE, Mellstedt H. Idiotype vaccination in multiple myeloma induced a reduction of circulating clonal tumor B cells. Blood 2003;101(11):4607–10.

183. King CA, Spellerberg MB, Zhu D, et al. DNA vaccines with single-chain Fv fused to fragment C of tetanus toxin induce protective immunity against lymphoma and myeloma. Nat Med 1998;4(11):1281–6.

184. Stritzke J, Zunkel T, Steinmann J, Schmitz N, Uharek L, Zeis M. Therapeutic effects of idiotype vaccination can be enhanced by the combination of granulocyte-macrophage colony-stimulating factor and interleukin 2 in a myeloma model. Br J Haematol 2003;120(1):27–35.

185. Coscia M, Mariani S, Battaglio S, et al. Long-term follow-up of idiotype vaccination in human myeloma as a maintenance therapy after high-dose chemotherapy. Leukemia 2004;18(1):139–45.

186. Reichardt VL, Brossart P. Dendritic cells in clinical trials for multiple myeloma. Methods Mol Med 2005;109:127–36.

187. Liso A, Stockerl-Goldstein KE, Auffermann-Gretzinger S, . Idiotype vaccination using dendritic cells after autologous peripheral blood progenitor cell transplantation for multiple myeloma. Biol Blood Marrow Transplant 2000;6(6):621–7.

188. Abdalla AO, Hansson L, Eriksson I, et al. Idiotype protein vaccination in combination with adjuvant cytokines in patients with multiple myeloma—evaluation of T-cell responses by different read-out systems. Haematologica 2007;92(1):110–4.

189. Hansson L, Abdalla AO, Moshfegh A, et al. Long-term idiotype vaccination combined with interleukin-12 (IL-12), or IL-12 and granulocyte macrophage colony-stimulating factor, in early-stage multiple myeloma patients. Clin Cancer Res 2007;13(5):1503–10.

190. Vasir B, Borges V, Wu Z, et al. Fusion of dendritic cells with multiple myeloma cells results in maturation and enhanced antigen presentation. Br J Haematol 2005;129(5):687–700.

191. Mariani S, Coscia M, Even J, et al. Severe and long-lasting disruption of T-cell receptor diversity in human myeloma after high-dose chemotherapy and autologous peripheral blood progenitor cell infusion. Br J Haematol 2001;113(4):1051–9.

192. Brown RD, Yuen E, Nelson M, Gibson J, Joshua D. The prognostic significance of T cell receptor beta gene rearrangements and idiotype-reactive T cells in multiple myeloma. Leukemia 1997;11(8):1312–7.

193. Rapoport AP, Stadtmauer EA, Aqui N, et al. Restoration of immunity in lymphopenic individuals with cancer by vaccination and adoptive T-cell transfer. Nat Med 2005;11(11):1230–7.

194. Frohn C, Hoppner M, Schlenke P, Kirchner H, Koritke P, Luhm J. Anti-myeloma activity of natural killer lymphocytes. Br J Haematol 2002;119(3):660–4.

195. Luhm J, Brand JM, Koritke P, Hoppner M, Kirchner H, Frohn C. Large-scale generation of natural killer lymphocytes for clinical application. J Hematother Stem Cell Res 2002;11(4):651–7.

196. Azuma T, Otsuki T, Kuzushima K, Froelich CJ, Fujita S, Yasukawa M. Myeloma cells are highly sensitive to the granule exocytosis pathway mediated by WT1-specific cytotoxic T lymphocytes. Clin Cancer Res 2004;10(21):7402–12.

197. Grube M, Moritz S, Obermann EC, et al. CD8 + T cells reactive to survivin antigen in patients with multiple myeloma. Clin Cancer Res 2007;13(3):1053–60.
198. Dhodapkar KM, Krasovsky J, Williamson B, Dhodapkar MV. Antitumor monoclonal antibodies enhance cross-presentation of cellular antigens and the generation of myeloma-specific killer T cells by dendritic cells. J Exp Med 2002;195(1):125–33.

Chapter 12

Antibody and Other Immune-Based Therapies for Myeloma

Nikhil C. Munshi and Yu-Tzu Tai

Introduction

Antibodies against tumor-associated markers are increasingly recognized as important biological agents for the detection and treatment of cancer.[1] After almost three decades of studies and advancement in production methods, monoclonal antibodies (mAbs) are now established as an important therapeutic modality in various malignancies. Since the first approval of rituximab targeting CD20 by the US Food and Drug Administration (US FDA) for the treatment of B-cell non-Hodgkin's lymphoma (NHL) in 1997, at least one anticancer mAb has been approved each year.[2] However, because of the heterogenicity in myeloma with a wide variety of genetic aberrations, the complexity of bone marrow (BM) microenvironment influences, and the lack of universal multiple myeloma (MM) markers specifically expressed on malignant MM cells, there is still no mAb-based therapy approved for treatment of MM. By 2000, there were relatively few surface antigens on the plasma cells (PCs) suitable for mAb-directed treatment. Possible molecules include CD19, CD20, HM1.24, CD38, ICAM (CD54), CD40, CD45, and syndecan-1. Studies in early 2000 showed that rituximab and anti-CD38 antibodies had minimal clinical activity in MM.[3–9] Despite disappointing beginning with these two mAbs, more than ten potential mAb candidates targeting MM cells (CD40, CD20, CS1, IL-6R, HM1.24, IGF-1R, CD74, and CD38) have entered clinical development in recent years. This is mainly accredited to better understanding of MM biology and identification of antigen expression pattern by expression profiling, as well as flow cytometric analysis of proteins expressed on the cell surface of the majority of patient MM cells. Furthermore, the advancement in the success of mAbs engineering as well as better understanding of mechanisms by which mAbs elicit tumor-killing activities are improving prospect for their clinical applications in MM.

Mechanisms of Action for mAbs as Therapeutic Agents

Antibodies, most commonly, IgG, are unique proteins with dual functionality. All naturally occurring antibodies are multivalent, with IgG having two binding

From: *Contemporary Hematology Myeloma Therapy*
Edited by: S. Lonial © Humana Press, Totowa, NJ

"arms." They are composed of two identical heavy chains, each composed of variable domains and constant domains (Fig. 1). Antigen-binding specificity is encoded by three complementarity-determining regions (CDRs) on each variable chain, while the Fc-region on each constant chain is responsible for binding to serum proteins (e.g., complement) or cells, as well as maintaining constant concentrations of IgG in the circulation. An Ab itself is usually not responsible for killing target cells, but instead marks the cells that other components or effector cells of the immune system should attach, antibody-dependent complement-mediated cytotoxicity (CDC), or it can initiate signaling mechanism in the targeted cell that leads to the cell's self-destruction, antibody-dependent cellular cytotoxicity (ADCC). ADCC involves the recognition of the Ab by immune cells that engage the Ab-marked cells and either through their direct action or through the recruitment of other cell types lead to the tagged-cell's death. CDC is a process where a cascade of different complement proteins become activated, usually when several IgGs are in close proximity to each other, with either direct cell lysis or by attracting other immune cells for effector cell function. Abs, when bound to the cell surface molecule, can induce signaling mechanisms in cells to undergo growth inhibition or apoptosis. For example, when rituximab binds to two CD20 molecules, this triggers signals that can induce apoptosis.[10,11] If rituximab is cross-linked by other Abs, the apoptotic signal is intensified.[12] This cross-linking could also occur when the Ab is bound by another immune cell through its Fc-gamma receptors (FcγR). Because cells frequently have alternative pathways for critical functions, interrupting a single signaling pathway alone might not be sufficient to ensure cell death. From this perspective, antibody is often best used in combination

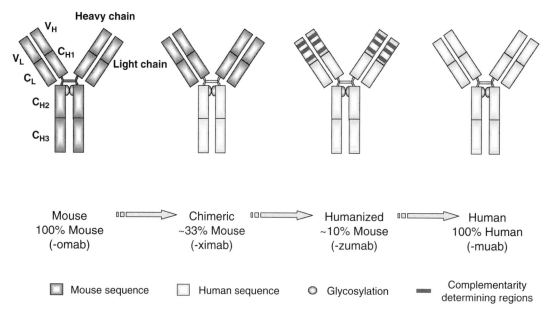

Fig. 1 A schematic representation of the process involved in engineering murine mAbs to reduce their immunogenecity. A chimeric antibody (*Ab*) splices the variable light (V_L) and variable heavy (V_H) portions of the murine IgG to a human IgG. A humanized Ab splices only the complementarity determining region (*CDR*) portions from the murine monoclonal antibody (*mAb*), along with some of the adjacent "framework" regions to help maintain the conformational structure of the *CDRs* (*see* Plate 3).

with chemotherapy and radiation therapy to augment their antitumor effects. Abs also can block molecules associated with cell adhesion, thereby inhibiting tumor metastasis.[13–16] With such diverse mechanisms of action, there are a number of opportunities for Ab-based therapeutics.

Abs may exert antitumor effects by inducing apoptosis, interfering with ligand–receptor interactions, or preventing the expression of proteins that are critical to the neoplastic phenotype. In addition, Abs have been developed that target components of the tumor microenvironment, perturbing vital structures such as the formation of tumor-associated vasculature. Some Abs target receptors, whose ligands are growth factors, thus inhibit natural ligands stimulating cell growth from binding to target tumor cells.

Natural killer (NK) cells are an important component of the innate immune system. mAbs rely on NK cell cytotoxicity for their effectiveness via Fc receptor FcgammaRIIIa (FcGR3 or CD16). By unraveling the molecular basis for Ab cytotoxicity, not only more effective Abs can be designed but also a more rational approach for combination of agents can be developed. For example, interleukin-2 (IL-2) and interleukin-12 (IL-12) were demonstrated to increase CD3-CD16$^+$ NK cell number and function, conferring increased ADCC against targets cells.[17–22] Immunomodulatory reagents, such as thalidomide and lenalidomide, could induce secretion of IL-2 and IL-15 from peripheral blood mononuclear cells from patients with MM, which, in turn, enhances ADCC to lyse target MM cell lines and patient MM cells induced by rituximab[23] and anti-CD40 mAbs (SGN-40 and HCD122).[24]

Limitations of Antibody Therapy

Experiences from early clinical trials as well as advancement in molecular engineering techniques have overcome some of the problems to successful mAb-based therapy (Table 1). Molecular engineering techniques have overcome the problem of immunogenicity by grafting critical sequences in the human heavy chain backbone onto the xenogeneic murine antibody structure or producing human antibodies directly from XenoMouse ® (Abgenix). It is now possible to create fully human immunoglobulin (Ig) that does not induce human antimouse Ab (HAMA). In addition, some tumor antigens are shed or secreted, thus limiting the amount of unbound Ab available to bind to the tumor. The difficulty of Ab distribution within tumor includes heterogeneity of antigen distribution within tumors. Barriers impeding Ab distribution within tumors would limit Ab reaching their targets, although this is more critical in solid tumors rather than hematological cancers such as MM. Evidence that

Table 1 Obstacles to effective antibody therapy.

Immunogenicity of xenogeneic antibodies
Shedding of antigen into circulation
Heterogeneity of antigen on tumor surface
Limited numbers of effector cells at tumor
Immunosuppressive tumor microenvironment
Disordered vasculature in tumors
Expression of CD55, CD59, and CD46 on tumor cells

Abs can efficiently mediate ADCC in vivo is limited since sufficient numbers of effector cells, such as macrophages, NK cells, or cytotoxic T cells, must be present in the tumor. In addition, myeloma may secret factors that downregulate the immune response (i.e., TGF-β, FasL, vascular endothelial growth factor, and Muc-1).[25,26] Despite these obstacles, preclinical and clinical data with improved Abs continue to support Ab-based therapy as an important component in MM treatments.

Characteristics of Antibody Targets

Protein/Receptor molecules on the surface of cancer cells are potential candidates for Ab-directed therapies. Targets differentially expressed at higher levels by MM cells than by normal cells are considered to be most clinically useful candidates. Antibodies targeting these molecules will selectively affect MM cells and induce potent cytotoxicity. Receptors on the surface of MM cells are particularly attractive targets for therapeutic antibodies if binding of the receptor perturbs a downstream signaling event, or blocks the binding of ligand to its receptor, thereby inhibiting signaling pathways essential for MM cell growth and survival. As for antibodies conjugated with radioactive substance, immunotoxin, or chemotherapeutic agents, it maximizes the effectiveness by internalization and release of the toxic drugs specifically in MM cells. Monoclonal antibodies are selected for immunotoxin conjugation based on their reactivity toward cell surface receptors or antigens that are preferentially expressed on malignant cells. After mAb-mediated internalization, the toxin portion of an immunotoxin traffics into the cytosol, where the enzymatic activity innate to the toxin catalytically inhibits protein synthesis and results in cell death. The use of these chimeric or humanized mAb-based immunoconjugates that are relatively nonimmunogenic with high affinity for tumor-associated antigens and that are efficiently internalized into cells once they bind to the target antigen has the potential to both improve antitumor efficacy and reduce the systemic toxicity of therapy.

MM Target Antigens

Several mAbs directed against MM cell surface are being investigated as potential therapy in MM. Listed below are mAbs against receptor antigens that are currently under clinical development or investigation in MM (Table 2).

Limited Clinical Benefit from Rituximab Trials in MM

Rituximab (the chimeric anti-CD20 mAb) is the first chimeric Abs to be approved by the US FDA for the treatment of B-cell NHL in 1987. It is perhaps the most prominent example of a highly successful paradigm of Ab therapy. The experience and subsequent introduction of rituximab into the treatment of NHL can be credited for the expanded interest in unconjugated Abs for cancer therapy (Fig. 2).

CD20 is expressed on MM cells in less than 20% of patients, and a CD20[+] phenotype is associated with the t(11;14)(q13;q32) translocation.[27] In general, myeloma cells either lack the CD20 antigen or express it very weakly in the large majority of patients.[28] Thus, although occasional clinical responses have

Table 2 Antigens targeted by antibodies in multiple myeloma in different stages of preclinical/clinical development.

Target	Brand name	Company/Sponsor	Type of mAb (conjugate)	Indication	Reference	Phase	Remarks
CD138	B-B4-DM1	ImmunoGen	The maytansinoid immunoconjugate mouse IgG1 mAb B-B4	Decreased growth and survival of MM cells in cell cultutre and in mice models	Tassone et al.[66, 67]	Preclinical	
HM1.24	Humanized HM1.24	Chugai Pharmaceutical Co. Ltd.	Humanized	Induced ADCC that is enhanced by cytokine stimulation of effector cells	Ozaki et al.[128]	Preclinical	
HLA-DR	1D09C3	GPC Biotech, AG	Human	Fully human anti-HLA-DR antibody induces cell death; its anti-mm activity is enhanced by IFN-gamma	Carlo-Stella et al.[164]	Preclinical	
CD74	IMMU-110	Immunomedics, Inc.	Humanized; doxorubicin conjugated	Humanized mAb conjugated with doxorubicin and targeted to CD74 to induce MM cell death	Sapra 2005[172]	Preclinical	
Kininogen	C11C1	Temple University School of Medicine	Mouse	Monoclonal antibody to kininogen may improve the efficacy of conventional MM treatment with minimal side effects	Sainz et al.[167]	Preclinical	
HLA class I	2D7-DB	Chugai Pharmaceutical Co. Ltd.	Converted from mouse IgG2b	Single-chain Fv diabody	Sekimoto et al.[165]	Preclinical	
β2-microglobulin	Anti-B2M mAbs	MD Anderson Cancer Center	Mouse	Strong apoptotic effect on myeloma cells supports potential use as therapeutic agents	Yang 2006[174]	Preclinical	
CD38	MOR202	MorphoSys AG	Human	This mAb induce ADCC and CDC against MM cells and block MM cell growth in vivo	Stevenson et al.[98]	Preclinical	

(continued)

Table 2 (continued)

Target	Brand name	Company/ Sponsor	Type of mAb (conjugate)	Indication	Reference	Phase	Remarks
CD32B	MGA321	MacroGenics	Humanized	mAb against low-affinity Fc receptor for use in the treatment of hematologic cancers by cell-depleting, functional, and adjuvant strategies	Rankin 2006[173]	Preclinical	Blood. 2006;108: 2384–2391.
FGFR3	PRO-001	Prochon Biotech Ltd.	Human	Anti-FGFR3 neutralizing antibody that is cytotoxic to t(4;14)-positive MM cells	Trudel et al.[139]	Preclinical	
mAb, ICAM-1	UV3	Abiogen	Mouse	UV3 significantly prolonged the survival of mice with either early or advanced stages of disease	Coleman 2006[175]	Preclinical	
BLyS	BLyS/rGel	Targa Therapeutics	Fusion protein of an antibody tethered to a toxin	The potential treatment of myeloma and autoimmune diseases	Nimmanapalli 2007[176]	Preclinical	
DKK	Anti-DKK1	UAMS	Mouse	DKK1 neutralizing antibodies reduce osteolytic bone resorption, increase bone formation, and help control myeloma growth in lab mice	Yaccoby et al.[149]	Preclinical	
CD20	Rituxan	NCI	Chimeric	High-dose cyclophosphamide in combination with rituximab in patients with primary refractory, high-risk, or relapsed myeloma; FOR being studied for the treatment of peripheral neuropathy in patients with MGUS	NCT0258206	II (Ongoing trial)	Three small phase II studies have evaluated rituximab in myeloma, each with conflicting results. (1) Treon et al.[28] conducted a phase II study of 19 patients with previously treated myeloma, treated with rituximab At 3 months, 32% had partial

response or stable disease; of these, all had CD20+ bone marrow plasma cells. Median time to treatment failure was 5.5 months. . (2) Zojer et al.[29] performed a phase II study of 10 patients (1 patient had CD20 expression on (10% of bone marrow plasma cells, another patient had CD20+ on 50% of marrow plasma cells) At 6 months, no patients had an objective response; 2 patients had stable disease, and 5 withdrew early for progressive disease. Rituximab treatment resulted in decrease in circulating B cells and IgM levels but no effect on bone marrow plasma cells, suggesting an effect of rituximab on normal B cells but not on malignant myeloma cells. (3) Moreau et al. conducted a phase II study of 14 patients with myeloma (7 stage I never pretreated, 7

(continued)

Table 2 (continued)

Target	Brand name	Company/ Sponsor	Type of mAb (conjugate)	Indication	Reference	Phase	Remarks
							stage III previously treated), in which 33% of bone marrow plasma cells were CD20[+], treated with rituximab.[31] One patient had partial response through 18 months of rituximab treatment. Five patients had stable disease at follow-ups ranging from 3 to 12 months. Three patients had stable disease at 3 months but progressed at 10–15 months. Five patients had no response despite partial clearance of CD20[+] plasma cells in the bone marrow.
CD20	Zevalin(yttrium Y 90 ibritumomab tiuxetan)	NCI	Mouse IgG1 antibody ibritumomab in conjunction with the chelator tiuxetan, to which a radioactive isotope yttrium-90 is added	Studying the side effects and best dose of yttrium Y 90 ibritumomab tiuxetan when given together with rituximab, melphalan, and autologous peripheral stem cell transplant in treating patients with previously treated MM.	NCT00477815	I (Ongoing trial)	
CD40	SGN-40	Seatle Genetics	Humanized	Multi-dose study of SGN-40 in patients with refractory or recurrent MM; SGN-40, lenalidomide (Revlimid®), and dexamethasone in MM patients started in August 2007	Tai et al.[81,157]	I (Ongoing trial)	

Target	Antibody	Company	Type	Reference	Indication	Phase	Comments
CD40	HCD122	Norvatis	Human	Tai et al.[89]	To determine the highest tolerated dose, safety, and activity of HCD122 in relapsed MM patients	I (Ongoing trial)	
CD20	Bexxar (131 I tositu-momab)	GlaxoSmithKline	Radioactive iodine 131 attaching to anti-CD20;mu IgG2a (131I)	NCT00135200	Consolidation treatment with iodine I 131 tositumomab	II (Ongoing trial)	
CD56 (NCAM)	huN901-DM1(BB-10901)	Immunogen, Vernalis	hz IgG$_1$ (maytansine DM1)	Chanan-Khan et al.115; NCT00346255	Relapsed and refractory CD56-positive MM	I (Ongoing trial)	
OPG osteo-protegerin	AMG162 Denosumab	Amgen	Human	Body et al.[147]	For the treatment of patients with relapsed or plateau-phase MM	II (Ongoing trial)	Body et al.[147] studied 29 patients with breast cancer and 25 patients with myeloma with bone lesions, who were treated with varying doses of denosumab versus pamidronate Serum and urine markers of bone turnover decreased with both treatments. Denosumab conferred a prolonged, dose-dependent duration of 84 days at higher doses.
VEGF	Avastin becacizumab	Genentech	Humanized	NCT00482495; Roche ML18704; NCT00473590	Given in combination with Velcade to patients with relapsed/refractory MM	II (Trial NCT00482495 of bevacizumab monotherapy was suspended, trial ML18704	Somlo et al.[171] studied 12 patients with stages I–III refractory myeloma who were randomized to bevacizumab +/− thalidomide. For bevacizumab monotherapy,

(continued)

Table 2 (continued)

Target	Brand name	Company/Sponsor	Type of mAb (conjugate)	Indication	Reference	Phase	Remarks
							of bevacizumab monotherapy is ongoing, trial NCT00473590 of bevacizumab and bortezomib is ongoing)	median time-to-progression was 2 (range 1-4) months. For bevacizumaband thalidomide, median progression-free survival was 9 (range 6-over 30) months. Study was closed because of slow accerual
CD52	Campath-1H(alemtuzumab)	NCI and Fred Hutchinson Cancer Research Institute	Humanized	Used before allogeneic transplant to prevent GVHD	ClinicalTrials.gov identifier NCT00040846	II (Ongoing trial NCT00040846 of alemtuzumab, total body irradiation, and fludarabine followed by allogeneic stem cell transplant)	A flow cytometry study by Kumar et al.[106] reported 52% of plasma cells isolated from patients with myeloma were positive for CD52, predominantly in the CD38+ CD45+ plasma cell fraction. A separate flow cytometry study by Westermann et al.[108] reported only a small fraction of CD52+ cells among the CD38+ CD45+ myeloma plasma cell population . Another study by Rawstron et al.[109] found only low levels of CD52 expression on myeloma plasma cells. A study by Kroger et al.[169] compared antithymocyte globulin (ATG) versus alemtuzu mab in 73 patients with myeloma treated with reduced conditioring with

| IL-6 | CNTO 328 | Centocor | Given in combination with Velcade to patients with relapsed/refractory MM | I (Ongoing trial NCT00412321 of CNTO 328 in non-Hodgkin's lymphoma, myeloma, or Castleman,s disease), II (ongoing trial NCT00401843 of bortezomib +/– CNTO 328 in relapsed or refractory myeloma) | Trikha et al.[62]; NCT00412321; NCT00401843 | Clinical studies have been done using both anti-IL6 murine mAb (BE-8) and the chimeric human–mouse anti-IL6 antibody (CNTO 328). Bataille et al.[58] conducted a phase I trial of BE-8 in 10 patients with myeloma and found antiproliferative effects in the bone marrow, along with a 30% reduction in tumor mass in 1 patient, but no clinically significant effects . van Zaanen et al.[61] conducted a phase I dose-escalating study of CNTO 328 in 12 patients with myeloma and found decreases in CRP below the level of detection in 11 patients but not clinically |

melphalan/fludarabine, followed by allogeneic stem cell transplant; alemtuzumab, as compared to ATG, had similar 2-year overall survival (54% vs 45%) and progression-free survival (30% vs 36%), lower incidence of GVHD, but higher probability of relapse (hazard ratio 2.37).

(continued)

Table 2 (continued)

Target	Brand name	Company/ Sponsor	Type of mAb (conjugate)	Indication	Reference	Phase	Remarks
							significant responses. Moreau et al.[56] studied the combination of BE-8[+] dexamethasone followed by high-dose melphalan as a conditioning regimen for autologous stem cell transplant in 16 patients with advanced myeloma and found a high CR rate . Moreau et al.[162] reported a subsequent study of 166 patients with myeloma who had high levels of beta-2-microglobulin and a chromosome 13 deletion, who underwent tandem autologous stem cell transplantation in which the conditioning regimen for the first transplant was melphalan, and that for the second transplant was melphalan+ dexamethasone +/– BE-8. This study showed no difference in overall survival or event-free survival with addition of BE-8 to the conditioning regimen.
IL-6R	MRA(Tocilizumab)	Roche Pharmaceuticals	Humanized anti–IL-6R	Specifically blocks IL-6 actions and ameliorates the diseases with IL-6 overproduction, thus, blockade of IL-6R may prove effective in limiting MM cell growth.	Nishimoto et al.[63]	I	

Target	Drug name	Company	Type	Description	Reference	Phase
TRAIL–R1	Mapatumumab(TRM-1)	Human Genome Sciences	Human	Binds to TRAIL, a TNF; Cleared by FDA for Phase I trial. Mapatumumab in combination With bortezomib (Velcade) and bortezomib alone	Menoret et al.[135]; NCT00315757	II (NCT00315757 ongoing Phase II trial of bortezomib +/- mapatumumab in relapsed or refractory myeloma)
EGFR	Erbitux(EMMA-1)	Imclone:Bristol Meyers-Squibb	Chimerized	Trial is open to all stages of myeloma; patient must have had at least one prior treatment with disease progression, +/- dexamethasone	NCT00368121	II (Ongoing trial)
CS1	HuLuc63	PDL Biopharma	Human	Multicenter, open-label, dose-escalation study of HuLuc63 in subjects with advanced MM	NCT00425347	I (Ongoing trial)
MUC-1(CD227)	Brevarex	Altarex	Murine	Treon et al.[4] reported that MUC-1 is expressed on myeloma cells . In a separate study, BrevaRex mAb was shown to induce B- and T-cell anti-neoplastic responses to MUC-1 in a phase I study of 17 patients with advanced solid tumors.[170] A phase II study of Brevarex, and a phase I/II study of NM-3 (another agent that downregulates MUC-1 expression), are underway.		I/II (Ongoing trial)

MM multiple myeloma, mA6 monoclonal antibody, DKK Dickkopf, ADCC antibody-dependent cellular cytotoxicity, FGFR fibroblast growth factor receptors, VEGF Vascular endothelial growth factors, EGFR epidermal growth factor receptor.

Every effort has been made to obtain reliable data from multiple sources (company and other web sites, [Glennie and van de Winkel 2003][176]), but accuracy cannot be guaranteed.

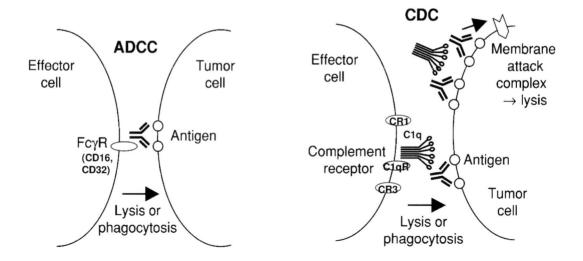

Fig. 2 Mechanisms of action associated with unconjugated antibodies (*Abs*). If antibodies are positioned closely together, they are chemo-attractants for immune effector cells and stimulate blood flow. *Ab*-dependent cellular cytotoxicity (*ADCC*) is triggered by interactions between the Fc region of an *Ab* bound to a tumor cell and Fc receptors, particularly FcRI and FcRIII, on immune effector cells such as neutrophils, macrophages, and natural killer cells. The tumor cell is eradicated by phagocytosis or lysis, depending upon the type of mediating effector cell. In the case of complement-mediated cytotoxicity (*CDC*), recruitment of C1q by IgG bound to the tumor cell surface is an obligatory first step. This triggers a proteolytic cascade that leads to generation of the effector molecule, C3b, and then to formation of a membrane attack complex that kills the target cell by disrupting its cell membrane. Alternatively, C3b can bind to complement receptors such as C1qR, CR1 (CD35), and CR3 (CD11b/CD18) expressed on effector cells such as granulocytes, macrophage, and natural killer cells. This can trigger cell-mediated tumor cell lysis or phagocytosis, depending upon the type of effector cell.

been reported in selected patients with CD20[+] myelomatous PCs,[28] MM is usually not considered as a disease suitable for anti-CD20 therapy. However, it has been also suggested that circulating CD20[+] clonotypic B cells could act as precursors or "neoplastic stem cells" in patients with MM, representing the proliferative compartment of the disease, able to play a role in determining relapse after effective treatments.[28] Thus, its clinical role in this setting remains uncertain.[29] It has been studied as a single agent,[3,30–32] with modest results and in combination with melphalan/prednisone, also with equivocal results. These studies concluded that rituximab treatment yielded significant reductions in circulating B cells and serum IgM levels but had no beneficial clinical anti-MM effect. Rituximab was investigated as a useful maintenance therapy in MM after autologous hematopoietic stem cell transplantation (HSCT).[33] Although the number of patients was too low to draw definitive conclusions, in this study, the use of rituximab as maintenance therapy after PBSCT was associated with an unexpectedly high rate of early relapses in patients with MM.[33] Most recently, rituximab was studied specifically in CD20[+] MM with t(11;14).[31] A single patient (out of 14) experienced an ongoing minor response, 18 months after rituximab therapy. The resistance of MM against rituximab therapy could be due to the low level of CD20 expression, dissociated action of CDC and ADCC, polymorphism in FcGR3 (CD16) receptor, and inadequate dose schedule.

Targeting IL-6/IL-6R Pathway

IL-6 in MM Cell Growth and Survival

IL-6 is a major growth and survival signal in MM with both autocrine and paracrine effects.[34–36] Serum IL-6 levels correlate with the proliferative fraction of MM cells, and high levels are associated with a poor prognosis.[37,38] IL-6 is predominantly secreted by BM stromal cells (BMSCs), and secretion is augmented by direct binding of MM cells to BMSCs, as well as by additional cytokines, such as tumor necrosis factor alpha (TNFβ), vascular endothelial factor (VEGF), and transforming growth factor beta (TGFβ), within the BM microenvironment. In addition, soluble IL-6R (sIL-6R) plays a role in the pathogenesis of MM by forming complexes with IL-6, thus producing a tenfold increase in the sensitivity of human IL-6-dependent cell lines.[39,40] The presence of high levels of sIL-6R in the serum of patients with MM, independent of tumor cell mass and disease status, suggests that this circulating protein has an important functional role in the pathogenesis of monoclonal gammopathy.[40,41]

IL-6 activates several major signaling cascades, including the Ras/Raf/MEK/ERK, the JAK2/STAT3, and the PI3K/Akt cascades, which mediate cell proliferation, survival, and drug resistance, respectively.[42–44] The initial step in the activation of these pathways involves the binding of IL-6 to its low-affinity receptor (IL-6Rα/gp80) and the subsequent homodimerization of signal transducer, gp130.[45,46] Notably, gp130 has no IL-6-binding capacity by itself, but activation by the IL-6/IL-6R complex results in homodimerization and phosphorylation of tyrosine residues in the intracellular domain of gp130 by the JAK family of enzymes.[47,48]

Molecular targets regulating IL-6-protective effects on MM cells have been recently identified, including the induction of proapoptotic Bcl-2-related protein Mcl-1, at both mRNA and protein levels and STAT3-associated survival pathway.[49–51] In addition, blocking Mcl-1 induced MM cell apoptosis.[52] Using the model of overexpression of Mcl-1 in myeloma cells showed that IL-6 is primarily a survival factor and not a proliferation factor for myeloma cells.[53] These studies support targeting IL-6/IL-6R pathway in MM and potential combined use of IL-6 inhibitors and chemotherapy.

Monoclonal Antibodies Against IL-6/IL-6R Function

Antibody Against IL-6: Various therapeutic agents able to block IL-6-mediated effects have been evaluated including IL-6-conjugated mAbs directed against IL-6 and IL-6R. Initial studies were performed with mouse mAb to IL-6 (murine BE-4 and BE-8),[54,55] which could suppress the proliferation of myeloma cells in vitro. These studies demonstrated the potential of mAb therapy directing against IL-6, resulting in a transient tumor cytostasis and reduction in IL-6-related toxicities from IL-6. Moreau et al.[56] investigated the potential of combination therapy, including a murine mAb to IL-6 (BE-8; 250 mg), dexamethasone (49 mg/day), and high-dose melphalan (220 mg/m^2 [HDM220]), followed by autologous SCT in the treatment of 16 patients with advanced MM. IL-6 activity was strongly inhibited, as indicated by reduced C-reactive protein (CRP) levels. Overall, 13 out of 16 patients (81.3%) exhibited a response, with a complete response (CR) seen in 6 patients (37.5%) without any toxic or allergic reactions. But a higher incidence of thrombocytopenia and neutropenia was observed. The results of a recent study by Rossi et al.[57] showed that (i) BE-8 was able to fully neutralize IL-6 activity in vivo before and after melphalan (HDM: 140 mg/m^2) as shown by inhibition of CRP production; (ii) there was no occurrence of hematological toxicity; (iii) there was a significant reduction in mucositis and fever; along with (iv) a median event-free survival (EFS) of 35 months and an overall survival (OS) of 68.2% at 5 years with a median follow-up of 72 months; and (v) the overall daily IL-6 production progressively increased on and after 7 days post-HDM, with the increased serum CRP levels. In the 5 out of 24 patients with uncontrolled CRP production, a large IL-6 production was detected (320 µg/day) that could not possibly be neutralized by BE-8. These data showed the feasibility to neutralize IL-6 in vivo with BE-8 in the context of HDM. Another study by Lu et al.[58] demonstrated that BE-8 could not efficiently block daily production of IL-6 at a level greater than 18 µg/day. This particular study observed an inverse correlation between clinical response and daily production of IL-6 during treatment if production exceeded 18 µg/day. This confirmed the importance of evaluating this particular parameter for optimizing an anti-IL-6 dosing strategy. Furthermore, Moreau et al.[59] recently showed that in high-risk patients with MM, the dose intensity of melphalan at 220 mg/m^2 led to encouraging results, but the addition of BE-8 to the second conditioning regimen, however, did not improve progression-free survival (PFS)/EFS or OS. One limitation is the amount of BE-8 that can be injected due to its short half-life (3–4 days) and the continuous production of IL-6 in vivo. Therefore, it was suggested that the chimeric Ab CNTO 328 with an 18-day half-life may be beneficial for chronic administration.

More recently, the chimeric mouse mAb to IL-6 CNTO 328 (Centocor) has been investigated in a phase I clinical trial in patients with MM at end-stage, progressive MM resistant to second-line therapy.[60,61] CNTO 328 therapy normalized endogenous IL-6 production but did not affect the IL-6 production associated with infection. Subsequently, in a second report,[61] three additional patients were enrolled in CNTO 328 dose-escalation study. Overall, disease stabilized in 11 out of 12 patients; the 12th patient with progressive disease responded to the second course of treatment. Despite stabilization of disease, none of the patient had a clinically significant response (e.g., a reduction in the level of M protein greater than 50%). Moreover, immune response to chimeric anti-IL-6 mAb was not observed, CRP levels became undetectable in 11 out of 12 patients, and life-threatening side effects were not associated with CNTO 328 therapy. Pharmacokinetic measurements indicated that the circulating mAb had a long half-life (17.8 days). The lack of clinically meaningful response in this end-stage patients may be related to the presence of IL-6-independent immature myeloma cells in end-stage MM,[61] which cannot be targeted by a mAb to IL-6. Treatment with mAb to IL-6 normalizes endogenous IL-6 production, probably by blocking a positive feedback loop in MM-associated IL-6 production. Overall analysis of data from six structured clinical trials of various mAbs to IL-6 in the treatment of human malignancies has shown a number of interesting observations. Monoclonal antibodies were well tolerated and exhibited a decrease in cancer-related symptoms (i.e., fever, cachexia, and pain). Administration of anti-IL-6 mAbs resulted in inhibition of CRP production below detection limits as well as neutralization of IL-6 production in vivo, transiently inhibiting MM cell proliferation. However, patients with severe disease produce huge amounts of IL-6, making anti-IL-6 mAb unable to completely and/or efficiently neutralize them. Considering the risk of immunization against the murine anti-IL-6 mAb, humanized anti-IL-6 mAb might prove useful, especially for treatment of patients with earlier stage disease.[62] Because IL-6 blocks dexamethasone-induced apoptosis, a main issue in MM will be to use anti-IL-6 mAb therapy to potentiate tumor killing by various drugs, including dexamethasone or high-dose chemotherapy.[62]

Antibody Against IL-6R

An alternate approach is to target the IL-6 receptor (gp80). A humanized anti-IL-6R mAb tocilizumab (rhPM-1, IgG1 class) is currently tested in phase I/II trials in patients with MM[63] (see next paragraph). Other approaches include the combination of anti-IL-6 or anti-IL-6R mAbs that shorten the half-life of the IL-6–IL-6R complexes (from 4 days to less than 20 min) in vivo, in addition to the formation of polymeric complexes instead of monomeric complexes, a situation compatible with increased clearance of these IL-6–IL-6R complexes.[64] Honemann et al.[65] analyzed the effect of the IL-6R antagonist SANT-7 on the growth and survival of the IL-6-dependent MM cell lines as well as primary MM cells from seven patients. SANT-7, when tested as a single agent, did not induce major growth inhibition if MM cells were cocultured with primary human BMSCs. However, when dexamethasone or a trans retinoic acid (ATRA) was given in combination with SANT-7, strong growth inhibition was achieved in cell lines and primary MM cells. This effect was due to cell cycle arrest and induction of apoptosis. Thus, combining SANT-7 with additional drugs could be a useful approach in the treatment of MM. Tassone et al.[66,67] have shown that SANT-7 significantly enhanced growth inhibition and apoptosis in both MM cell lines in vitro and in vivo murine model, as well as patient MM cells.[66,68] In the novel murine model[67] of human MM in which IL-6-dependent INA-6 MM cells were directly injected into human BM implants in severe combined immunodeficient (SCID) mice (SCID-hu), inhibition of IL-6 signaling by SANT-7 significantly potentiated the therapeutic action of dexamethasone against MM cells.

Tocilizumab (MRA, atlizumab, Roche Pharmaceuticals) is a humanized antihuman IL-6R antibody (rhPM-1, IgG1 class).[69–71] Tocilizumab specifically blocks IL-6 actions and ameliorates the diseases with IL-6 overproduction. Besides Castleman's disease and reumatitis arthritis (RA), tocilizumab has been shown to be effective for patients with juvenile idiopathic arthritis and Crohn's disease.[72] Tocilizumab treatment is generally well tolerated and safe. It is being evaluated in open-label phase I (US) and phase II (France) trials to assess its safety and efficacy in MM.

NRI, a new receptor inhibitor of IL-6 by genetically engineering tocilizumab, is under preclinical evaluation.[71] NRI consists of VH and VL of tocilizumab in a single-chain fragment format dimerized by fusing to the Fc portion of human Ig G1. The binding activity to the IL-6 receptor and the biological activity of the purified NRI were found to be similar to those of parental tocilizumab. Because NRI is encoded on a single gene, it is easily applicable to a gene delivery system using virus vehicles. An adenovirus vector encoding NRI was administered to mouse intraperitoneally (i.p.) and monitored the serum NRI level and growth reduction property on IL-6-dependent MM cell line S6B45, in vivo.[71] Adequate amount of the serum NRI level to exert anti-IL-6 action could be obtained, and this treatment significantly inhibited the in vivo S6B45 cell growth.

Targeting IGF-1/IGF-1R Signaling Cascades

The IGF-1 signaling pathway is implicated in cellular mitogenesis, angiogenesis, tumor cell survival, and tumorigenesis in MM.[36,73,74] Inhibition of this pathway results in decreased cell growth, inhibition of tumor formation in animal models, and increased apoptosis in cells treated with cytotoxic chemotherapy.[75] Strategies targeting IGF-1 and IGF-1 receptor (IGF-1R) may therefore be important to develop efficient anti-MM therapeutics. Tai et al. reported a functional association of IGF-IR and β1 integrin in mediating MM cell homing, providing the preclinical rationale for novel treatment strategies targeting IGF-1/IGF-1R in MM.[76] Recent studies showed that IGF-1R tyrosine kinase (IGF-1RTK) inhibitors NVP-ADW742[73] or picropodophyllin (PPP)[74,77] produced significant antitumour activity. A mAb targeting IGF-1R, CP-751,871, has been investigated in phase I/II clinical trial in patients with relapsed and refractory MM. CP-751,871, a fully human anti-type 1 IGF-R IgG2 Ab, both as a single agent and in combination with adriamycin, 5-fluorouracil, or tamoxifen, showed marked antitumour activity in vivo and blocked the binding of IGF-1 to its receptor, IGF-1-induced receptor autophosphorylation, and induced downregulation of IGF-1R in vitro and in tumor xenografts.[78]

Targeting CD40/CD40L Therapy

Biological Sequelae of CD40 Activation in MM Cells

CD40 is expressed on the majority of primary MM cells and is engaged in the critical nuclear factor-κB pathway of cell survival.[79–82] Triggering human MM cells via CD40 also induces increased homotypic and heterotypic cell adhesion,[83] upregulation of various cell surface markers,[83,84] translocation of Ku86/Ku70 to the cell surface,[84,85] and increased interleukin 6 (IL-6)[83] and TGF-β1.[86] Upregulation of MM cell adhesion to BMSCs, upon CD40 activation, in turn, triggers the transcription and secretion of IL-6 in BMSCs. Ligation of CD40 with sCD40L or an agonistic anti-CD40 mAb (G28.5) also induces vascular endothelial growth factor[87] and urokinase-type plasminogen activator,[88] suggesting its role in MM homing and migration. These studies support inhibition of the CD40L/CD40 pathway as a novel therapeutic strategy.

Humanized/Human Anti-CD40 mAbs

Novel mAbs targeting CD40 activation in MM cells, SGN-40 (Seatle, Genetics) and HCD122 (Norvatis), have been investigated by Tai et al.[81,89] In preclinical studies, SGN-40, a humanized IgG1 mAb, mediates cytotoxicity against CD40-expressing MM cell lines and patient MM cells via suppression of IL-6-induced proliferative and antiapoptotic effects, as well as antibody-dependent cell-mediated cytotoxicity. SGN-40 also induced significant anti-tumor activity in xenograft mouse models of human MM and lymphoma.[90] HCD122 (Norvatis), a novel, fully human, IgG1 antagonistic mAb, specifically blocked CD40L-induced adhesion, cytokine secretion, and survival of MM, as well as induced marked ADCC against CD40+ MM cells. In vivo anti-MM activity by HCD122 was demonstrated in a xenograft model of 12BM MM plasmacytoma in mice. Both anti-CD40 mAbs are currently under clinical investigations in MM.

SGN-40 was evaluated in a phase I, multi-dose, single-agent, dose-escalation study for patients with relapsed or refractory MM.[91] This single-arm trial was designed to evaluate safety, pharmacokinetics, immunogenicity, and antitumor activity. Thirty-two patients were treated at five clinical sites. The schedule was well tolerated at 0.5, 1.0, and 2.0 mg/kg/week; however, two out of three patients experienced toxicities following the first dose at 4 mg/kg. Both had headache with aseptic meningitis (grade 3); both patients fully recovered after symptom management. There was neither recurrence of grade 3 neurotoxicity nor evidence of cumulative toxicity. Pharmacokinetic analysis demonstrates dose-proportional changes in Cmax and AUC with a relatively short terminal half-life, similar to that seen in nonhuman primates. Further dose escalation with modified infusion schedule is ongoing. Although in vivo depletion of B cells was observed and several patients demonstrated decreased M protein and improvement in subjective symptoms, no patient has yet met criteria for objective response. Five patients (16%) had stable disease at the time of restaging. Some patients with advanced myeloma appeared to derive some clinical benefit from therapy, and further development of this antibody, either as monotherapy or in combination with other antimyeloma therapies, is indicated.

The phase 1 study of HCD122 to determine the maximum tolerated dose (MTD) of this mAb in patients with MM who were relapsed or refractory after at least one prior therapy is ongoing.[92] Planned dose levels are 1, 3, and 10 mg/kg administered intravenously once weekly for 4 weeks. Of the six patients at 3 mg/kg, one had partial response (PR) at week 9 and was confirmed at week 15, one had SD for more than 5 weeks, and four had pharmacodynamics at week 5. Preliminary studies showed that HCD122 was safe and well tolerated to date at doses of 1 mg/kg and 3 mg/kg weekly for four doses with preliminary evidence of antimyeloma activity. Enrollment is continuing to determine the MTD.

Since ADCC is induced by both clinical-grade anti-CD40 mAbs to kill MM cells, Tai et al. have further studied the effects of an immunomodulatory drug (IMiD), lenalidomide, on SGN-40-induced ADCC,[24] since IMiDs could upregulate IL-2 secretion, thereby promoting NK cell function.[93] Pretreatment of effector cells with lenalidomide augmented SGN-40-induced MM cell lysis, associated with an increased number of CD56$^+$ CD3$^-$ NK cells expressing CD16 and LFA-1. Importantly, pretreatment with lenalidomide or lenalidomide and SGN-40 markedly enhanced NK-cell-mediated lysis of autologous patient MM cells triggered by SGN-40. These studies show that the addition of lenalidomide to SGN-40 enhances cytotoxicity against MM cells, providing the framework for a clinical study combining lenalidomide and SGN-40 to both directly target MM cells and induce immune effectors against MM.

Targeting CS1 by HuLuc63 mAb in MM

Using subtractive hybridization of naïve B-cell cDNA from memory B/PC cDNA, CS1 (CD2 subset-1, CRACC, SLAMF7, CD319), a member of the signaling lymphocyte activating-molecule (SLAM)-related receptor (RR) family 18, was one of the genes that appeared to be highly expressed in PCs.[94–96] This molecule is characterized by two or four extracellular Ig-like domains and an intracellular signaling domain with immune receptor tyrosine-based switch motifs (ITSM) with the consensus amino acid sequence TxYxxV/I. CS1 expression was restricted to NK cells, as previously published, as well as a subset of T-cells, activated monocytes and activated dendritic cells, and was not expressed in any major body organs. The restricted expression profile of CS1 in normal cells and tissues, as well as the high uniform expression of CS1 in MM, provides the rationale to target the antigen with specific mAb. CS1 mRNA and protein are universally expressed in CD138-purified primary tumor cells from the majority of patients with MM (>97%). CS1 was expressed at adhesion-promoting uropod membranes of polarized MM cells, and short interfering RNA (siRNA) targeted to CS1 inhibited MM cell adhesion to BMSCs. A novel humanized anti-CS1 mAb HuLuc63 was selected because of its potent tumor-killing activity in vivo and in vitro.[97] HuLuc63 inhibited MM cell binding to BMSCs[96] and significantly induced ADCC against MM cells in dose-dependent and CS1-specific manners.[94–97] Importantly, HuLuc63 triggered autologous ADCC against primary MM cells resistant to conventional or novel therapies, including bortezomib and HSP90 inhibitor; and pretreatment with conventional or novel anti-MM drugs markedly enhanced HuLuc63-induced MM cell lysis.[96] Administration of HuLuc63 resulted in significant dose-dependent tumor regression in xenograft models of human MM using MM1S, OPM2, and L363 MM cells. These results thus define the functional significance of CS1 in MM and provide the preclinical rationale for testing HuLuc63 in clinical trials, either alone or in combination. A phase I study of HuLuc63 is currently underway in MM.

Targeting CD38 in Multiple Myeloma

Early Studies Using Anti-CD38 mAb with or Without Immunotoxin(ricin)
The CD38 molecule is expressed on cell surfaces in majority of lymphoid tumors, notably MM, AIDS-associated lymphomas, and posttransplant lymphoproliferative disease. Therefore, this molecule is a promising target for antibody-based therapy. In an early assessment, the chimeric mouse Fab directed against CD38 (from OKT10 clone)-human Fc(human IgG1) efficiently mediates ADCC against CD38-expressing lymphoid cell line using human blood mononuclear effector cells.[7] Although CD38 is expressed on all NK cells, the major effector population in the assay did not impair their effector function. Goldmacher et al.[8] have further reported the in vitro cytotoxic properties of a conjugate of the anti-CD38 mAb HB7 with ricin that has been chemically modified so that its galactose-binding sites of the B chain are blocked by covalently attached affinity ligands (blocked ricin). HB7-blocked ricin was 100-fold to 500-fold more sensitive in inhibiting MM cells compared to the normal BM cells. However, these early investigations have not led to useful clinical applications.

Human Anti-CD38 mAbs
Most recently, a human anti-CD38 IgG1, HuMax-CD38 (Genmab), was raised after immunizing transgenic mice possessing human, but not mouse, Ig genes. Preclinical studies indicated that HuMax-CD38 was effective in killing primary CD38$^+$ CD138$^+$ patient MM cells and a range of MM/lymphoid cell lines by both ADCC and CDC. In SCID mouse animal models, using sensitive bioluminescence imaging, treatment with HuMax-CD38 inhibited CD38$^+$ tumor cell growth in both preventive and therapeutic settings. In addition, HuMax-CD38 inhibits the CD38 ADP-ribosyl cyclase activity in target cells, which may contribute to the effectiveness of HuMax-CD38 in killing both primary MM and PC leukemia cells.

Similarly, MOR202 (MorphoSysAG), a fully human anti-CD38 IgG1 mAb, also efficiently triggers ADCC against CD38$^+$ MM cell lines and patient MM cells in vitro as well as in vivo in a xenograft mouse model.[98] One practical problem in applying anti-CD38 therapy is the wide expression on lymphoid, myeloid, and epithelial cells, especially following cell activation.

Targeting CD52 Using Therapeutic mAb CamPath-1H in MM

Another therapeutic antibody that has the potential for use in MM is alemtuzumab (CamPath-1H, Berlex; Genzyme), a humanized mAb directed against the CD52 cell surface protein.[99] CD52, a glycopeptide, is abundantly expressed on T- and B-lymphocytes and has been found on a subpopulation (<5%) of granulocytes but not on erythrocytes, platelets, or hematopoietic stem cells. Alemtuzumab can cause cell lysis and growth inhibition of primary cells and malignant cells via a variety of mechanisms, including complement fixation and antibody-dependent cell-mediated cytotoxicity.[100–102] Alemtuzumab has been utilized to treat patients with a number of lymphoid malignancies including advanced chronic lymphocytic leukemia, T-prolymphocytic leukemia, and low-grade NHL with response rates of 40–90%.[103–105] Recent studies have found that CD52 is expressed at variable levels on MM cells.[106–109] It has also been demonstrated that cross-linking the CD52 receptor with alemtuzumab can induce direct growth inhibitory and apoptotic effects in myeloma cell lines and primary MM cells and may have a modest effect as a single agent in treating patients with MM.[107] As in other settings involving alemtuzumab administration, it will be necessary to observe patients closely for cytopenias and provide prophylaxis against opportunistic infections. If alemtuzumab is found to be safe and have clinical activity in patients with MM, then it may be used to treat MM either alone or in combinations with chemotherapeutic agents, biologic agents, or other therapeutic antibodies either before or after autologous or allogeneic transplantation. In allogeneic transplants, alemtuzumab treatment in the peritransplant period may also help to prevent GVHD [110–112] and graft rejection as well as reduce the MM tumor burden.

Targeting CD56 with Immunotoxin-Conjugated mAb

Preclinical Studies of huN901-DM1

CD56, identified as neuronal cell adhesion molecule (NCAM), is a membrane glycoprotein belonging to the Ig superfamily. In the hematopoietic compartment, CD56 expression is restricted to NK cells and a subset of T lymphocytes. The expression of CD56 has also been detected on a variety of cancer cells, including MM. Although normal PCs do not express CD56, it is expressed by a subset of PCs in patients with monoclonal gammapathy of undetermined significance and strongly expressed on MM cells from a majority of patients.[113] A recent study demonstrated CD56 expression in 22 out of 28 patients (79%).[114] HuN901 is a humanized mAb that binds with high affinity to CD56. HuN901 conjugated with the maytansinoid N2′-deacetyl-N2′-(3-mercapto-1-oxopropyl)-maytansine (DM1), a potent antimicrotubular cytotoxic agent, may provide targeted delivery of the drug to CD56-expressing tumors. HuN901-DM1 induced specific cytotoxicity against CD56+ but not CD56-MM cell lines. HuN901-DM1 treatment selectively decreased survival of CD56+ MM cell lines and depleted CD56+ MM cells from mixed cultures with a CD56 cell line or adherent BMSCs. HuN901-DM1 treatment further inhibited serum paraprotein secretion and tumor growth and increased survival in a xenograft model of CD56+ OPM2 human MM cells. These data demonstrated that huN901-DM1 has significant in vitro and in vivo anti-MM activity at doses that are well tolerated in a murine model.

Clinical Trial of huN901-DM1 in MM

The initial phase I clinical study of huN901-DM1 (BB-10901) in MM is aimed at determining the MTD, the dose-limiting toxicities , and pharmacokinetics of the drug given on a weekly schedule. Relapsed or relapsed/refractory patients with MM who have failed at least one prior therapy and have CD56-expressing myeloma received a single IV infusion of BB-10901 on two consecutive weeks every 3 weeks. Subjects are enrolled in cohorts of three at each dose level. The starting dose was 40 mg/m^2/week based on experience from a prior phase I trial in solid tumors. Five patients have received BB-10901, three at 40 mg/m^2/week and two at 60 mg/m^2/week. No patient has experienced serious adverse events related to study. Immunohistochemistry performed on marrow aspirates about 24 h after huN901-DM1 infusion at 40 mg/m^2 confirmed the presence of huN901-DM1 on myeloma cells in the marrow. Two patients treated at 60 mg/m^2/week and who had failed multiple prior therapies including bortezomib, thalidomide, and/or lenalidomide demonstrated antitumor response with a decrease in M proteins of 90% and 33%, respectively.[115] This phase I study provides preliminary evidence of the safety and clinical activity of BB-10901 in patients with CD56-positive MM who have failed established MM treatments. The MTD is not yet defined.

Targeting CD138 with Toxin-Conjugated Murine mAb B-B4

Biological Role of CD138 in MM Cells

Syndecans act as coreceptors for heparin-binding growth factors (HBGFs) and may increase local concentration of these ligands, allowing enhanced receptor activation even at low ligand concentrations. Sundecan-1 (CD138) is widely expressed on patient MM cells and mediates hepatocyte growth factor binding and promotes Met signaling in MM cells.[116] Syndecan-1 (CD138) mediates myeloma cell adhesion, and loss of syndecan-1 from the cell surface may contribute to myeloma cell proliferation and dissemination and influence the prognosis in patients with MM.[117–121] Soluble syndecan-1 level is an independent prognostic factor both at diagnosis and at plateau phase.[122,123] These studies support CD138 as a potential target for MM.

Preclinical Evaluation of B-B4-DM1 in MM

Tassone et al. demonstrated the in vitro and in vivo antitumor activity of the maytansinoid DM1 covalently linked to the murine mAb B-B4 targeting syndecan-1 (CD138).[124] B-B4-DM1 selectively decreased the growth and survival of MM cell lines, patient MM cells, and MM cells adherent to BMSCs. Tumor regression and improvement in OS and reduction in levels of circulating human paraprotein were observed in mice bearing myeloma treated with B-B4-DM1. Although immunohistochemical analysis demonstrated restricted CD138 expression in human tissues, the lack of B-B4 reactivity with mouse tissues precludes evaluation of its toxicity in these models. The study concluded that B-B4-DM1 is a potent anti-MM agent that kills cells in an antigen-dependent manner in vitro and mediates in vivo antitumor activity, providing the rationale for clinical trials of this immunoconjugate in MM.

Targeting HM1.24 on MM Cells

HM1.24 (CD137) was originally identified as a cell surface protein differentially overexpressed on MM cells[125] and later was found to be identical to bone stromal cell antigen 2 (BST-2). A role of HM1.24 in trafficking and signaling between the intracellular and cell surface of MM cells was suggested since it is one of the important activators of the NF-kappaB pathway.[126] The humanized anti-HM1.24 antibody (IgG1/kappa, AHM, Chugai Pharmaceutical Co., Ltd.) is able to effectively induce ADCC against some human myeloma cells in the presence of human peripheral blood mononuclear cells (PBMCs) as effectively as a chimeric anti-HM1.24 antibody.[125,127,128] Single intravenous injection of AHM significantly inhibited tumor growth in both orthotopic and ectopic human MM xenograft models.[129] In addition, HM1.24-specific cytotoxic T lymphocytes (CTLs) could be generated and these specifically activated CD8[+] CTLs are able to lyse HM1.24-expressing MM cell lines.[130–132] AHM will be evaluated in a phase I clinical trial in MM in UK.

Targeting TRAIL Death Signaling Pathway

Tumor necrosis factor-related apoptosis-inducing ligand (TRAIL), a member of the TNF ligand superfamily, induces apoptosis through the activation of TRAIL-R1 (DR4) and TRAIL-R2 (DR5) death signaling receptors. TRAIL induces the death of cancer cells but spares normal cells, supporting it as an attractive targeted cancer therapy. MM cells are TRAIL sensitive and may be dependent on the ratio of c-FLIP and caspase 8.[133,134] A recent report showed that myeloma cells are widely sensitive to TRAILR triggering and induction of cleavage of key MM survival molecule Mcl-1 is followed.[135] Two human mAbs directed against TRAILR1 (HGS-ETR1, TRM-1) and TRAILR2 (HGS-ETR2) killed 68% and 45% of MM cell lines, respectively.[135] Only 18% of MM cell lines are resistant to either antibody. There is no correlation between TRAILR expression level and sensitivity to TRAIL-R1 or TRAIL-R2 triggering. Both the extrinsic (caspase 8, Bid) and the intrinsic (caspase 9) pathways are activated by anti-TRAIL mAbs. These studies encourage clinical trials of anti-TRAILR1 mAb in MM.

The mapatumumab targeting TRAIL-R1 (TRM-1, fully human TRAIL-R1 mAb, Human Genome Sciences, Inc.) is being evaluated in a phase I, open-label, dose-escalation trial in MM to assess the safety, tolerability, immunogenicity, and pharmacokinetics. A randomized phase II study combining TRM-1 with bortezomib (Velcade®) and compared with bortezomib alone in patients with relapsed or refractory MM recently started in mid-2006.

Targeting FGFR3 in t(4;14) MM

The t(4;14)(p16.3;q32) translocation, which occurs in ~15–20% of MM tumors, results in the dysregulated expression of two putative oncogenes, MMSET and fibroblast growth factor receptor 3 (FGFR3). Studies indicate that FGFR3 may play a significant, albeit not a singular, role in myeloma oncogenesis, thus making this receptor tyrosine kinase (RTK) an attractive target for therapeutic intervention.[136] Activation of wild-type FGFR3 promotes proliferation of myeloma cells and is weakly transforming in a hematopoietic mouse model.[137] Subsequent acquisition of activating mutations of FGFR3 in some MM is associated with disease progression and is strongly transforming in several experimental models.[136,138] PRO-001, a highly specific anti-FGFR3-neutralizing antibody, binds to FGFR3, inhibits downstream ERK1/2 phosphorylation, and induces apoptosis of primary t(4;14)[+] MM cells.[139]

Inhibition of viability was observed when cells were cocultured with stroma or in the presence of IL-6 or IGF-1. Additional testing of (PRO-001) in combination with other therapies, such as cytotoxic chemotherapy, and novel agents, such as bortezomib and lenalidomide, and development of highly specific cytotoxic-conjugated antibodies, is warranted to further optimize anti-FGFR3 antibody-based treatments.

Antibodies Targeting MM Cells in the Bone Marrow Microenvironment

Since myeloma grow and survive, as well as develop drug resistance by interacting with BM microenvironment, there is a need to develop mAb-based targeted therapies to inhibit growth and survival advantages provided by their interaction.

MM-Induced Bone Lesion

One of the hallmarks of MM is lytic bone lesions, causing intractable bone pain and pathological fractures. The formation of osteolytic lesion occurs through hyperactivation of bone-resorbing osteoclasts through the action of cytokines that are secreted by the MM cells. Targeting these interactions may provide both anti-MM effects and improvement in bone disease with consequent improvement in quality of life.

Targeting RANK/RANKL/OPG Axis Using Denosumab for MM-Associated Bone Destruction

Receptor activator of nuclear factor-kappaB ligand (RANKL) is a cytokine member of the tumor necrosis factor family that is the principal mediator of osteoclastic bone resorption.[140] RANKL binds to RANK on preosteoclasts and mature osteoclasts, and mediates the differentiation, function, and survival of osteoclasts.[141] Osteoprotegerin, a natural soluble decoy receptor of RANKL, modulates the effect of RANKL[141] and is able to prevent excessive bone resorption in the normal state. RANKL expression is elevated in patients with MM.[142,143] Denosumab (AMG 162, Amgen, Inc., Thousand Oaks, CA) is an investigational fully human mAb with a high affinity and specificity for RANKL in a way that mimics the natural bone-protecting actions of Osteoprotegerin (OPG)[140,144] It was developed to treat patients with skeletal diseases mediated by osteoclasts, such as bone metastasis, MM, and hormone ablation-induced bone loss in patients with cancer. Denosumab is a human IgG2 molecule with a long circulatory residence time and a rapid and sustained decrease in bone resorption in healthy postmenopausal women following a single subcutaneous dose.[145,146] By inhibiting the action of RANKL, denosumab reduces the differentiation, activity, and survival of osteoclasts, thereby slowing the rate of bone resorption. A phase 1 clinical trial[147] in patients with MM ($n = 25$) or breast carcinoma with bone metastases ($n = 29$) showed that following a single s.c. dose of denosumab (0.1, 0.3, 1.0, or 3.0 mg/kg), levels of urinary and serum N-telopeptide decreased within 1 day, and this decrease lasted through 84 days at the higher denosumab doses. Mean half-lives of denosumab were 33.3 and 46.3 days for the two highest dosages. Larger trials are underway to investigate the effect of denosumab for the treatment of cancer-induced bone disease and other bone loss disorders.

Targeting the Wnt inhibitor Dickkopf-1 (DKK-1)

Dickkopf-1 (DKK1), a soluble inhibitor of wingless (Wnt) signaling secreted by MM cells, contributes to osteolytic bone disease by inhibiting the differentiation of osteoblasts. Tian et al.[148] have observed that secretion of an inhibitor of the canonical Wnt signaling pathway, DKK1, by MM cells strongly correlated with the severity of osteolytic lesions. Given that signaling by the canonical Wnt pathway is critical for the differentiation of progenitors into osteoblasts, the bone repair deficit in MM lies in the osteoinhibitory properties of DKK1. The effect of anti-DKK1 mAb on bone metabolism and tumor growth in a SCID-rab system where rabbit bones and fresh human MM cells were co-implanted into immunocompromised mice has been evaluated.[149] The implants of control animals showed signs of MM-induced resorption, whereas mice treated with anti-DKK1 antibodies blunted resorption and improved the bone mineral density of the implants. Histologic examination revealed that myelomatous bones of anti-DKK1-treated mice had increased numbers of osteocalcin-expressing osteoblasts and reduced number of multinucleated Tartarate-resistant acid phosphatase (TRAP)-expressing osteoclasts. The bone anabolic effect of anti-DKK1 was associated with reduced MM burden ($P < .04$). Anti-DKK1 also significantly increased the Bone mineral density (BMD) of the implanted bone and murine femur in nonmyelomatous SCID-rab mice, suggesting that DKK1 is physiologically an important regulator of bone remodeling in adults. Anti-DKK1 agents, that is, BHQ880 (Norvatis), may therefore represent the next generation of therapeutic options for the enhancement of bone repair in some malignant and degenerative bone diseases.

Targeting Angiogenesis

VEGF is important for the formation of new blood vessels and plays a key role not only in solid tumors but also in hematologic malignancies, including MM.[150] A critical role for VEGF has been demonstrated in MM pathogenesis.[151] Previous studies showed that VEGF is expressed and secreted by MM cells and BMSCs and, in turn, stimulates IL-6 secretion by BMSCs , thereby augmenting paracrine MM cell growth. Moreover, IL-6 enhances the production and secretion of VEGF by MM cells. VEGF and VEGFR-1 (Flt-1) are coexpressed in both MM cell lines and patient MM cells, and VEGF-triggered effects in MM cells are mediated via Flt-1. Importantly, binding of VEGF increases MM cell growth, survival, and migration, thereby demonstrating the crucial role of VEGF in MM cell pathogenesis in the BM milieu.[152]

VEGF Inhibitor Becacizumab(Avastin)

Bevacizumab targets and blocks VEGF and its binding to its receptor on the vascular endothelium. Anti-VEGF Abs were active alone and in combination with radiation in earlier preclinical studies.[153,154] It is currently being studied clinically in many other solid and blood tumors including primary systemic amyloidosis and MM.[155,156] National Cancer Institute (NCI's) Cancer Therapy Evaluation Program is sponsoring a phase II study of bevacizumab and Thalomid (thalidomide, Celgene) in MM.[155]

Targeting BAFF/ARPIL Growth and Survival Pathway

BAFF/APRIL Promotes MM Cell Growth and Survival

Most recently, B-cell-activating factor of the TNF family (BAFF: also known as B lymphocyte stimulator, BLyS) and a proliferation-inducing ligand

(APRIL) were identified as new survival factors for MM.[157–159] In addition to BMSCs, osteoclasts produce these factors to support MM cells in the BM microenvironment.[157,159,160] BAFF (or APRIL) protects MM cells against apoptosis induced by serum deprivation or dexamethasone via AKT/nuclear factor-κB (NF-κB) activation, as well as upregulation of Bcl-2 and Mcl-1.158 Their cognate receptors are BAFF-R, TACI, and BCMA with heterogeneous expression among patient MM cells. Specifically, RNA expression of BCMA and TACI is approximately more than 30-fold and more than 10-fold higher, respectively, than that of BAFF-R.[157] These studies provide clinical rationale to target the BAFF/APRIL survival pathway in MM.

Atacicept/TACI-Ig

Atacicept (ZymoGenetics; Serono) acts as a decoy receptor (TACI-Ig) by binding to and neutralizing soluble BLyS and APRIL, and preventing these CD40L-related ligands from binding to their cognate receptors (TACI, BCMA, and BAFF-R) on B-cell tumors, thereby enhancing cytotoxicity. First, the safety, pharmacokinetics, and pharmacodynamics of atacicept was evaluated in healthy male volunteers in phase I study.[161] These results showed that single subcutaneous doses of Atacicept were well tolerated in healthy volunteers and demonstrated nonlinear pharmacokinetics and were biologically active, according to IgM levels. An open-label, dose-escalation phase I/II study enrolled 16 patients with refractory or relapsed MM or active, progressive Waldenstrom's macroglobulinemia (WM).[162] Sequential cohorts received one cycle of five weekly subcutaneous injections of atacicept at 2, 4, 7, or 10 mg/kg. Treatment with atacicept was well tolerated. No dose-limiting toxicity was observed. A biological response was observed in this heavily treated refractory population. Disease stabilization was seen in several patients and one patient with WM achieved a minimal response.

AMG523/BAFF Inhibitor

Because of the complexity of this pathway, drugs or mAbs could be developed against other components involving such ligand-receptor binding. The BAFF inhibitor, AMG523 (Amgen), specifically blocks BAFF but not APRIL binding to three receptors. The potential therapeutic utility of AMG523 was preclinically evaluated in MM lines, either sensitive or resistant to conventional chemotherapy, as well as freshly isolated patient MM cells, in the presence or absence of BMSCs[163] AMG523 induced modest cytotoxicity in MM cell lines and patient MM cells, suggesting a minor role of autocrine mechanism of BAFF for MM growth and survival. Pretreatment of AMG523 blocks BAFF-induced activation of AKT, nuclear factor kB, and ERK in MM cells, confirming its inhibitory effect on BAFF-mediated adhesion and survival. These data demonstrate that the novel therapeutic AMG523 blocks the interaction between BAFF and its receptors in human MM.

In addition, since the majority of MM cell lines and patient MM cells express BCMA, but not BAFF-R or TACI, BCMA might be a promising target for mAb development against MM.

Other Potential Targets

Other potential targets in MM include HLA-DR by 1D09C3,[164] HLA-class I by 2D7-DB,[165] KMA expression (on kappa MM),[166] kininogen by C11C1,[167] and polyclonal rabbit antithymocyte globulin (rATG).[168]

Conclusion

Therapeutic antibodies have made the transition from concept to clinical reality over the past two decades. The success of tumor-specific mAbs (i.e., anti-CD20 rituximab in NHL and anti-HER-2/c-erbB-2 Herceptin/trastuzumab in breast cancer) has fueled the optimism for this attractive approach to treat MM. Many are now being tested as single agent or as conjugate targets to assess their efficacy in improving response. However, mAbs targeting myeloma cells have not yet been included as part of standard myeloma therapy. Rituximab-based clinical trials in MM demonstrated very limited utility of this antibody to treat MM. Nevertheless, recent studies in gene expression profiling and oncogenomics have allowed the identification of new therapeutic MM targets. In the meantime, the ability to create essentially human antibody structures has reduced the likelihood of host-protective immune responses that otherwise limit the utility of therapy. Antibody structures now can be readily manipulated to facilitate selective interaction with host immune effectors. A better understanding of the immune defects that prevent patients with MM from mounting a strong response against their tumor cells should also improve establishment of effective mAb-based immunotherapy strategies. Several novel mAb targeting various receptors are already in clinical trials and number of others more are in clinical development. We expect that the use of potentially targeted therapies by mAbs, such as naked or immunoconjugate or bispecific, would soon claim defined therapeutic roles in patients with MM. The favorable toxicity profile of tumor-targeted therapy by mAbs, unlike other forms of therapy, would allow the maintenance of quality of life, while efficiently attacking the tumors.

References

1. Houghton AN, Scheinberg DA. Monoclonal antibody therapies—a 'constant' threat to cancer. Nat Med 2000;6(4):373–4.
2. Reichert JM, Valge-Archer VE. Development trends for monoclonal antibody cancer therapeutics. Nat Rev Drug Discov 2007;6(5):349–56.
3. Korte W, Jost C, Cogliatti S, Hess U, Cerny T. Accelerated progression of multiple myeloma during anti-CD20 (Rituximab) therapy. Ann Oncol 1999;10(10):1249–50.
4. Treon SP, Shima Y, Preffer FI, et al. Treatment of plasma cell dyscrasias by antibody-mediated immunotherapy. Semin Oncol 1999;26(5 Suppl 14):97–106.
5. Treon SP, Shima Y, Grossbard ML, et al. Treatment of multiple myeloma by antibody mediated immunotherapy and induction of myeloma selective antigens. Ann Oncol 2000;11 Suppl 1:107–11.
6. Treon SP, Raje N, Anderson KC. Immunotherapeutic strategies for the treatment of plasma cell malignancies. Semin Oncol 2000;27(5):598–613.
7. Stevenson FK, Bell AJ, Cusack R, et al. Preliminary studies for an immunotherapeutic approach to the treatment of human myeloma using chimeric anti-CD38 antibody. Blood 1991;77(5):1071–9.
8. Goldmacher VS, Bourret LA, Levine BA, . Anti-CD38-blocked ricin: an immunotoxin for the treatment of multiple myeloma. Blood 1994;84(9):3017–25.
9. Ellis JH, Barber KA, Tutt A, et al. Engineered anti-CD38 monoclonal antibodies for immunotherapy of multiple myeloma. J Immunol 1995;155(2):925–37.
10. Chan HT, Hughes D, French RR, . CD20-induced lymphoma cell death is independent of both caspases and its redistribution into triton X-100 insoluble membrane rafts. Cancer Res 2003;63(17):5480–9.

11. Jazirehi AR, Bonavida B. Cellular and molecular signal transduction pathways modulated by rituximab (rituxan, anti-CD20 mAb) in non-Hodgkin's lymphoma: implications in chemosensitization and therapeutic intervention. Oncogene 2005;24(13):2121–43.

12. Zhang N, Khawli LA, Hu P, Epstein AL. Generation of rituximab polymer may cause hyper-cross-linking-induced apoptosis in non-Hodgkin's lymphomas. Clin Cancer Res 2005;11(16):5971–80.

13. Zahalka MA, Okon E, Naor D. Blocking lymphoma invasiveness with a monoclonal antibody directed against the beta-chain of the leukocyte adhesion molecule (CD18). J Immunol 1993;150(10):4466–77.

14. Ruan HH, Scott KR, Bautista E, Ammons WS. ING-1(heMAb), a monoclonal antibody to epithelial cell adhesion molecule, inhibits tumor metastases in a murine cancer model. Neoplasia 2003;5(6):489–94.

15. Bautista DS, Xuan JW, Hota C, Chambers AF, Harris JF. Inhibition of Arg-Gly-Asp (RGD)-mediated cell adhesion to osteopontin by a monoclonal antibody against osteopontin. J Biol Chem 1994;269(37):23280–5.

16. Lutterbuese P, Brischwein K, Hofmeister R, et al. Exchanging human Fcgamma1 with murine Fcgamma2a highly potentiates anti-tumor activity of anti-EpCAM antibody adecatumumab in a syngeneic mouse lung metastasis model. Cancer Immunol Immunother 2007;56(4):459–68.

17. Holmberg LA, Maloney D, Bensinger W. Immunotherapy with rituximab/interleukin-2 after autologous stem cell transplantation as treatment for CD20[+] non-Hodgkin's lymphoma. Clin Lymphoma Myeloma 2006;7(2):135–9.

18. Khan KD, Emmanouilides C, Benson DM, Jr., et al. A phase 2 study of rituximab in combination with recombinant interleukin-2 for rituximab-refractory indolent non-Hodgkin's lymphoma. Clin Cancer Res 2006;12(23):7046–53.

19. Gluck WL, Hurst D, Yuen A, et al. Phase I studies of interleukin (IL)-2 and rituximab in B-cell non-hodgkin's lymphoma: IL-2 mediated natural killer cell expansion correlations with clinical response. Clin Cancer Res 2004;10(7):2253–64.

20. Parihar R, Dierksheide J, Hu Y, Carson WE. IL-12 enhances the natural killer cell cytokine response to Ab-coated tumor cells. J Clin Invest 2002;110(7):983–92.

21. Ansell SM, Geyer SM, Maurer MJ, et al. Randomized phase II study of interleukin-12 in combination with rituximab in previously treated non-Hodgkin's lymphoma patients. Clin Cancer Res 2006;12(20 Pt 1):6056–63.

22. Ansell SM, Witzig TE, Kurtin PJ, et al. Phase 1 study of interleukin-12 in combination with rituximab in patients with B-cell non-Hodgkin lymphoma. Blood 2002;99(1):67–74.

23. Hernandez-Ilizaliturri FJ, Reddy N, Holkova B, Ottman E, Czuczman MS. Immunomodulatory drug CC-5013 or CC-4047 and rituximab enhance antitumor activity in a severe combined immunodeficient mouse lymphoma model. Clin Cancer Res 2005;11(16):5984–92.

24. Tai YT, Li XF, Catley L, et al. Immunomodulatory drug lenalidomide (CC-5013, IMiD3) augments anti-CD40 SGN-40-induced cytotoxicity in human multiple myeloma: clinical implications. Cancer Res 2005;65(24):11712–20.

25. Xagoraris I, Paterakis G, Zolota B, Zikos P, Maniatis A, Mouzaki A. Expression of granzyme B and perforin in multiple myeloma. Acta Haematol 2001;105(3):125–9.

26. Dong M, Blobe GC. Role of transforming growth factor-beta in hematologic malignancies. Blood 2006;107(12):4589–96.

27. Robillard N, Avet-Loiseau H, Garand R, et al. CD20 is associated with a small mature plasma cell morphology and t(11;14) in multiple myeloma. Blood 2003;102(3):1070–1.

28. Treon SP, Pilarski LM, Belch AR, et al. CD20-directed serotherapy in patients with multiple myeloma: biologic considerations and therapeutic applications. J Immunother 2002;25(1):72–81.

29. Zojer N, Kirchbacher K, Vesely M, Hubl W, Ludwig H. Rituximab treatment provides no clinical benefit in patients with pretreated advanced multiple myeloma. Leuk Lymphoma 2006;47(6):1103–9.

30. Hofer S, Hunziker S, Dirnhofer S, Ludwig C. Rituximab effective in a patient with refractory autoimmune haemolytic anaemia and CD20-negative multiple myeloma. Br J Haematol 2003;122(4):690–1.

31. Moreau P, Voillat L, Benboukher L, et al. Rituximab in CD20 positive multiple myeloma. Leukemia 2007;21(4):835–6.

32. Gozzetti A, Fabbri A, Lazzi S, Bocchia M, Lauria F. Reply to Rituximab activity in CD20 positive multiple myeloma. Leukemia 2007;21(8):1842–3.

33. Musto P, Carella AM, Jr., Greco MM, et al. Short progression-free survival in myeloma patients receiving rituximab as maintenance therapy after autologous transplantation. Br J Haematol 2003;123(4):746–7.

34. Frassanito MA, Cusmai A, Iodice G, Dammacco F. Autocrine interleukin-6 production and highly malignant multiple myeloma: relation with resistance to drug-induced apoptosis. Blood 2001;97(2):483–9.

35. Bataille R, Klein B. Role of interleukin-6 in multiple myeloma. Ann Med Interne (Paris) 1992;143 Suppl 1:77–9.

36. Hideshima T, Mitsiades C, Tonon G, Richardson PG, Anderson KC. Understanding multiple myeloma pathogenesis in the bone marrow to identify new therapeutic targets. Nat Rev Cancer 2007;7(8):585–98.

37. Klein B, Zhang XG, Jourdan M, Portier M, Bataille R. Interleukin-6 is a major myeloma cell growth factor in vitro and in vivo especially in patients with terminal disease. Curr Top Microbiol Immunol 1990;166:23–31.

38. Lauta VM. A review of the cytokine network in multiple myeloma: diagnostic, prognostic, and therapeutic implications. Cancer 2003;97(10):2440–52.

39. Hargreaves PG, Wang F, Antcliff J, et al. Human myeloma cells shed the interleukin-6 receptor: inhibition by tissue inhibitor of metalloproteinase-3 and a hydroxamate-based metalloproteinase inhibitor. Br J Haematol 1998;101(4): 694–702.

40. Gaillard JP, Bataille R, Brailly H, et al. Increased and highly stable levels of functional soluble interleukin-6 receptor in sera of patients with monoclonal gammopathy. Eur J Immunol 1993;23(4):820–4.

41. Van Zaanen HC, Lokhorst HM, Aarden LA, Rensink HJ, Warnaar SO, Van Oers MH. Blocking interleukin-6 activity with chimeric anti-IL6 monoclonal antibodies in multiple myeloma: effects on soluble IL6 receptor and soluble gp130. Leuk Lymphoma 1998;31(5–6):551–8.

42. Hideshima T, Nakamura N, Chauhan D, Anderson KC. Biologic sequelae of interleukin-6 induced PI3-K/Akt signaling in multiple myeloma. Oncogene 2001;20(42):5991–6000.

43. Hideshima T, Chauhan D, Hayashi T, et al. Proteasome inhibitor PS-341 abrogates IL-6 triggered signaling cascades via caspase-dependent downregulation of gp130 in multiple myeloma. Oncogene 2003;22(52):8386–93.

44. Tai YT, Fulciniti M, Hideshima T, et al. Targeting MEK induces myeloma-cell cytotoxicity and inhibits osteoclastogenesis. Blood 2007;110(5):1656–63.

45. Tupitsyn N, Kadagidze Z, Gaillard JP, et al. Functional interaction of the gp80 and gp130 IL-6 receptors in human B cell malignancies. Clin Lab Haematol 1998;20(6):345–52.

46. Rebouissou C, Wijdenes J, Autissier P, et al. A gp130 interleukin-6 transducer-dependent SCID model of human multiple myeloma. Blood 1998;91(12):4727–37.

47. Chauhan D, Pandey P, Hideshima T, et al. SHP2 mediates the protective effect of interleukin-6 against dexamethasone-induced apoptosis in multiple myeloma cells. J Biol Chem 2000;275(36):27845–50.

48. Hideshima T, Chauhan D, Teoh G, et al. Characterization of signaling cascades triggered by human interleukin-6 versus Kaposi's sarcoma-associated herpes virus-encoded viral interleukin 6. Clin Cancer Res 2000;6(3):1180–9.

49. Podar K, Gouill SL, Zhang J, et al. A pivotal role for Mcl-1 in Bortezomib-induced apoptosis. Oncogene 2007 July 23; [Epub ahead of print].

50. Brocke-Heidrich K, Kretzschmar AK, Pfeifer G, et al. Interleukin-6-dependent gene expression profiles in multiple myeloma INA-6 cells reveal a Bcl-2 family-independent survival pathway closely associated with Stat3 activation. Blood 2004;103(1):242–51.

51. Jourdan M, De Vos J, Mechti N, Klein B. Regulation of Bcl-2-family proteins in myeloma cells by three myeloma survival factors: interleukin-6, interferon-alpha and insulin-like growth factor 1. Cell Death Differ 2000;7(12):1244–52.

52. Derenne S, Monia B, Dean NM, et al. Antisense strategy shows that Mcl-1 rather than Bcl-2 or Bcl-x(L) is an essential survival protein of human myeloma cells. Blood 2002;100(1):194–9.

53. Jourdan M, Veyrune JL, De Vos J, Redal N, Couderc G, Klein B. A major role for Mcl-1 antiapoptotic protein in the IL-6-induced survival of human myeloma cells. Oncogene 2003;22(19):2950–9.

54. Klein B, Wijdenes J, Zhang XG, et al. Murine anti-interleukin-6 monoclonal antibody therapy for a patient with plasma cell leukemia. Blood 1991;78(5):1198–204.

55. Bataille R, Barlogie B, Lu ZY, et al. Biologic effects of anti-interleukin-6 murine monoclonal antibody in advanced multiple myeloma. Blood 1995;86(2):685–91.

56. Moreau P, Harousseau JL, Wijdenes J, Morineau N, Milpied N, Bataille R. A combination of anti-interleukin 6 murine monoclonal antibody with dexamethasone and high-dose melphalan induces high complete response rates in advanced multiple myeloma. Br J Haematol 2000;109(3):661–4.

57. Rossi JF, Fegueux N, Lu ZY, et al. Optimizing the use of anti-interleukin-6 monoclonal antibody with dexamethasone and 140 mg/m^2 of melphalan in multiple myeloma: results of a pilot study including biological aspects. Bone Marrow Transplant 2005;36(9):771–9.

58. Lu ZY, Brailly H, Wijdenes J, Bataille R, Rossi JF, Klein B. Measurement of whole body interleukin-6 (IL-6) production: prediction of the efficacy of anti-IL-6 treatments. Blood 1995;86(8):3123–31.

59. Moreau P, Hullin C, Garban F, et al. Tandem autologous stem cell transplantation in high-risk de novo multiple myeloma: final results of the prospective and randomized IFM 99–04 protocol. Blood 2006;107(1):397–403.

60. van Zaanen HC, Koopmans RP, Aarden LA, et al. Endogenous interleukin 6 production in multiple myeloma patients treated with chimeric monoclonal anti-IL6 antibodies indicates the existence of a positive feed-back loop. J Clin Invest 1996;98(6):1441–8.

61. van Zaanen HC, Lokhorst HM, Aarden LA, et al. Chimaeric anti-interleukin 6 monoclonal antibodies in the treatment of advanced multiple myeloma: a phase I dose-escalating study. Br J Haematol 1998;102(3):783–90.

62. Trikha M, Corringham R, Klein B, Rossi JF. Targeted anti-interleukin-6 monoclonal antibody therapy for cancer: a review of the rationale and clinical evidence. Clin Cancer Res 2003;9(13):4653–65.

63. Nishimoto N, Sasai M, Shima Y, et al. Improvement in Castleman's disease by humanized anti-interleukin-6 receptor antibody therapy. Blood 2000;95(1):56–61.

64. Brochier J, Liautard J, Jacquet C, Gaillard JP, Klein B. Optimizing therapeutic strategies to inhibit circulating soluble target molecules with monoclonal antibodies: example of the soluble IL-6 receptors. Eur J Immunol 2001;31(1):259–64.

65. Honemann D, Chatterjee M, Savino R, et al. The IL-6 receptor antagonist SANT-7 overcomes bone marrow stromal cell-mediated drug resistance of multiple myeloma cells. Int J Cancer 2001;93(5):674–80.

66. Tassone P, Galea E, Forciniti S, Tagliaferri P, Venuta S. The IL-6 receptor super-antagonist Sant7 enhances antiproliferative and apoptotic effects induced by dexamethasone and zoledronic acid on multiple myeloma cells. Int J Oncol 2002;21(4): 867–73.

67. Tassone P, Neri P, Burger R, et al. Combination therapy with interleukin-6 receptor superantagonist Sant7 and dexamethasone induces antitumor effects in a novel SCID-hu in vivo model of human multiple myeloma. Clin Cancer Res 2005;11(11):4251–8.

68. Tassone P, Forciniti S, Galea E, et al. Synergistic induction of growth arrest and apoptosis of human myeloma cells by the IL-6 super-antagonist Sant7 and Dexamethasone. Cell Death Differ 2000;7(3):327–8.

69. Nishimoto N. [Humanized anti-human IL-6 receptor antibody, tocilizumab]. Nippon Rinsho 2007;65(7):1218–25.

70. Nishimoto N, Hashimoto J, Miyasaka N, et al. Study of active controlled monotherapy used for rheumatoid arthritis, an IL-6 inhibitor (SAMURAI): evidence of clinical and radiographic benefit from an x ray reader-blinded randomised controlled trial of tocilizumab. Ann Rheum Dis 2007;66(9):1162–7.

71. Yoshio-Hoshino N, Adachi Y, Aoki C, Pereboev A, Curiel DT, Nishimoto N. Establishment of a new interleukin-6 (IL-6) receptor inhibitor applicable to the gene therapy for IL-6-dependent tumor. Cancer Res 2007;67(3):871–5.

72. Nishimoto N, Kishimoto T. Inhibition of IL-6 for the treatment of inflammatory diseases. Curr Opin Pharmacol 2004;4(4):386–91.

73. Mitsiades CS, Mitsiades NS, McMullan CJ, et al. Inhibition of the insulin-like growth factor receptor-1 tyrosine kinase activity as a therapeutic strategy for multiple myeloma, other hematologic malignancies, and solid tumors. Cancer Cell 2004;5(3):221–30.

74. Stromberg T, Ekman S, Girnita L, et al. IGF-1 receptor tyrosine kinase inhibition by the cyclolignan PPP induces G2/M-phase accumulation and apoptosis in multiple myeloma cells. Blood 2006;107(2):669–78.

75. Menu E, Kooijman R, Van Valckenborgh E, et al. Specific roles for the PI3K and the MEK-ERK pathway in IGF-1-stimulated chemotaxis, VEGF secretion and proliferation of multiple myeloma cells: study in the 5T33MM model. Br J Cancer 2004;90(5):1076–83.

76. Tai YT, Podar K, Catley L, et al. Insulin-like growth factor-1 induces adhesion and migration in human multiple myeloma cells via activation of beta1-integrin and phosphatidylinositol 3'-kinase/AKT signaling. Cancer Res 2003;63(18):5850–8.

77. Menu E, Jernberg-Wiklund H, Stromberg T, . Inhibiting the IGF-1 receptor tyrosine kinase with the cyclolignan PPP: an in vitro and in vivo study in the 5T33MM mouse model. Blood 2006;107(2):655–60.

78. Cohen BD, Baker DA, Soderstrom C, et al. Combination therapy enhances the inhibition of tumor growth with the fully human anti-type 1 insulin-like growth factor receptor monoclonal antibody CP-751,871. Clin Cancer Res 2005;11(5):2063–73.

79. Chauhan D, Uchiyama H, Urashima M, Yamamoto K, Anderson KC. Regulation of interleukin 6 in multiple myeloma and bone marrow stromal cells. Stem Cells 1995;13 Suppl 2:35–9.

80. Westendorf JJ, Ahmann GJ, Lust JA, et al. Molecular and biological role of CD40 in multiple myeloma. Curr Top Microbiol Immunol 1995;194:63–72.

81. Tai YT, Catley LP, Mitsiades CS, . Mechanisms by which SGN-40, a humanized anti-CD40 antibody, induces cytotoxicity in human multiple myeloma cells: clinical implications. Cancer Res 2004;64(8):2846–52.

82. Hock BD, McKenzie JL, Patton NW, et al. Circulating levels and clinical significance of soluble CD40 in patients with hematologic malignancies. Cancer 2006;106(10):2148–57.

83. Urashima M, Chauhan D, Uchiyama H, Freeman GJ, Anderson KC. CD40 ligand triggered interleukin-6 secretion in multiple myeloma. Blood 1995;85(7):1903–12.

84. Teoh G, Urashima M, Greenfield EA, et al. The 86-kD subunit of Ku autoantigen mediates homotypic and heterotypic adhesion of multiple myeloma cells. J Clin Invest 1998;101(6):1379–88.

85. Tai YT, Podar K, Kraeft SK, et al. Translocation of Ku86/Ku70 to the multiple myeloma cell membrane: functional implications. Exp Hematol 2002;30(3):212–20.

86. Urashima M, Ogata A, Chauhan D, . Transforming growth factor-beta1: differential effects on multiple myeloma versus normal B cells. Blood 1996;87(5):1928–38.

87. Tai YT, Podar K, Gupta D, et al. CD40 activation induces p53-dependent vascular endothelial growth factor secretion in human multiple myeloma cells. Blood 2002;99(4):1419–27.

88. Tai YT, Podar K, Mitsiades N, et al. CD40 induces human multiple myeloma cell migration via phosphatidylinositol 3-kinase/AKT/NF-kappa B signaling. Blood 2003;101(7):2762–9.

89. Tai YT, Li X, Tong X, et al. Human anti-CD40 antagonist antibody triggers significant antitumor activity against human multiple myeloma. Cancer Res 2005;65(13):5898–906.

90. Law CL, Gordon KA, Collier J, et al. Preclinical antilymphoma activity of a humanized anti-CD40 monoclonal antibody, SGN-40. Cancer Res 2005;65(18):8331–8.

91. Mohamad A, Hussein JRB, Niesvizky R, Munshi NC, Matous J, Harrop K, Drachman JG. Results of a phase I trial of SGN-40 (Anti-huCD40 mAb) in patients with relapsed multiple myeloma. Blood 2006;108:3576.

92. Bensinger W, Jagannath S, Becker PS, Anderson KC, Stadtmauer EA, Aukerman L, Fox J, Girish S, Bilic S, Guzy S, Solinger A, Dort S, Wang Y, Hurst D. A phase 1 dose escalation study of a fully human, antagonist anti-CD40 antibody, HCD122 (formerly CHIR-12.12) in patients with relapsed and refractory multiple myeloma. Blood (ASH Annual Meeting Abstracts) 2006;108(11):3575–3575.

93. Davies FE, Raje N, Hideshima T, et al. Thalidomide and immunomodulatory derivatives augment natural killer cell cytotoxicity in multiple myeloma. Blood 2001;98(1):210–6.

94. Hsi ED, Steinle R, Balasa B, Draksharapu A, Shum B, Huseni M, Powers D, Nanisetti A, Williams M, Vexler V, Hussein M, Afar D. CS1: A potential new therapeutic target for the treatment of multiple myeloma. Blood (ASH Annual Meeting Abstracts) 2006;108:3457.

95. Szmania S, Balasa B, Malaviarachchi P, Zhan F, Huang Y, Draksharapu A, Vexler V, Shaughnessy, Jr., Barlogie B, Tricot G, Afar D, van Rhee F. CS1 is expressed on myeloma cells from early stage, late stage, and drug-treated multiple myeloma patients, and is selectively targeted by the HuLuc63 antibody. Blood 2006;108:660.

96. Tai YT, Dillon M, Song W, Leiba M, Li XF, Burger P, Lee AI, Podar K, Hideshima T, Rice AG, van Abbema A, Jesaitis L, Caras I, Law D, Weller E, Xie W, Richardson P, Munshi NC, Mathiot C, Avet-Loiseau H, Afar DE, Anderson KC. Anti-CS1 humanized monoclonal antibody HuLuc63 inhibits myeloma cell adhesion and induces antibody-dependent cellular cytotoxicity in the bone marrow milieu. Blood 2008 Aug 15;112(4):1329–1337. Epub 2007 Sep 28.

97. Rice A, Dillon M, van Abbema A, Jesaitis L, Wong M, Lawson S, Liu G, Zhang Y, Powers D, Rhodes S, Caras I, Law D, Afar D. Eradication of tumors in pre-clinical models of multiple myeloma by anti-CS1 monoclonal antibody HuLuc63: mechanism of action studies. Blood (ASH Annual Meeting Abstracts) 2006;108:3503.

98. Stevenson GT. CD38 as a therapeutic target. Mol Med 2006;12(11–12):345–6.

99. Rodig SJ, Abramson JS, Pinkus GS, . Heterogeneous CD52 expression among hematologic neoplasms: implications for the use of alemtuzumab (CAMPATH-1H). Clin Cancer Res 2006;12(23):7174–9.

100. Stanglmaier M, Reis S, Hallek M. Rituximab and alemtuzumab induce a non-classic, caspase-independent apoptotic pathway in B-lymphoid cell lines and in chronic lymphocytic leukemia cells. Ann Hematol 2004;83(10):634–45.

101. Villamor N, Montserrat E, Colomer D. Mechanism of action and resistance to monoclonal antibody therapy. Semin Oncol 2003;30(4):424–33.

102. Golay J, Gramigna R, Facchinetti V, Capello D, Gaidano G, Introna M. Acquired immunodeficiency syndrome-associated lymphomas are efficiently lysed through complement-dependent cytotoxicity and antibody-dependent cellular cytotoxicity by rituximab. Br J Haematol 2002;119(4):923–9.

103. Keating MJ, Cazin B, Coutre S, et al. Campath-1H treatment of T-cell prolymphocytic leukemia in patients for whom at least one prior chemotherapy regimen has failed. J Clin Oncol 2002;20(1):205–13.

104. Lundin J, Osterborg A, Brittinger G, CAMPATH-1H monoclonal antibody in therapy for previously treated low-grade non-Hodgkin's lymphomas: a phase II multicenter study. European Study Group of CAMPATH-1H Treatment in Low-Grade Non-Hodgkin's Lymphoma. J Clin Oncol 1998;16(10):3257–63.

105. Osterborg A, Dyer MJ, Bunjes D, Phase II multicenter study of human CD52 antibody in previously treated chronic lymphocytic leukemia. European Study Group of CAMPATH-1H Treatment in Chronic Lymphocytic Leukemia. J Clin Oncol 1997;15(4):1567–74.

106. Kumar S, Kimlinger TK, Lust JA, Donovan K, Witzig TE. Expression of CD52 on plasma cells in plasma cell proliferative disorders. Blood 2003;102(3):1075–7.

107. Carlo-Stella C, Guidetti A, Di Nicola M, et al. CD52 antigen expressed by malignant plasma cells can be targeted by alemtuzumab in vivo in NOD/SCID mice. Exp Hematol 2006;34(6):721–7.

108. Westermann J, Maschmeyer G, van Lessen A, Dorken B, Pezzutto A. CD52 is not a promising immunotherapy target for most patients with multiple myeloma. Int J Hematol 2005;82(3):248–50.

109. Rawstron AC, Laycock-Brown G, Hale G, et al. CD52 expression patterns in myeloma and the applicability of alemtuzumab therapy. Haematologica 2006;91(11):1577–8.

110. Kottaridis PD, Milligan DW, Chopra R, et al. In vivo CAMPATH-1H prevents GvHD following nonmyeloablative stem-cell transplantation. Cytotherapy 2001;3(3):197–201.

111. Piccaluga PP, Martinelli G, Malagola M, et al. Anti-leukemic and anti-GVHD effects of campath-1H in acute lymphoblastic leukemia relapsed after stem-cell transplantation. Leuk Lymphoma 2004;45(4):731–3.

112. Wandroo F, Auguston B, Cook M, Craddock C, Mahendra P. Successful use of Campath-1H in the treatment of steroid refractory liver GvHD. Bone Marrow Transplant 2004;34(3):285–7.

113. Harada H, Kawano MM, Huang N, et al. Phenotypic difference of normal plasma cells from mature myeloma cells. Blood 1993;81(10):2658–63.

114. Tassone P, Gozzini A, Goldmacher V, et al. In vitro and in vivo activity of the maytansinoid immunoconjugate huN901-N2'-deacetyl-N2'-(3-mercapto-1-oxopropyl)-maytansine against CD56+ multiple myeloma cells. Cancer Res 2004;64(13):4629–36.

115. Chanan-Khan AA, Jagannath S, Schlossman RL, Fram RJ, Falzone RM, Ruberti MF, Welch SK, DePaolo D, Anderson KC, Munshi NC. Phase I study of BB-10901 (huN901-DM1) in patients with relapsed and relapsed/refractory CD56-positive multiple myeloma. Blood 2006;108:3574.

116. Derksen PW, Keehnen RM, Evers LM, van Oers MH, Spaargaren M, Pals ST. Cell surface proteoglycan syndecan-1 mediates hepatocyte growth factor binding and promotes Met signaling in multiple myeloma. Blood 2002;99(4):1405–10.

117. Borset M, Hjertner O, Yaccoby S, Epstein J, Sanderson RD. Syndecan-1 is targeted to the uropods of polarized myeloma cells where it promotes adhesion and sequesters heparin-binding proteins. Blood 2000;96(7):2528–36.

118. Dhodapkar MV, Abe E, Theus A, et al. Syndecan-1 is a multifunctional regulator of myeloma pathobiology: control of tumor cell survival, growth, and bone cell differentiation. Blood 1998;91(8):2679–88.

119. Seidel C, Borset M, Hjertner O, et al. High levels of soluble syndecan-1 in myeloma-derived bone marrow: modulation of hepatocyte growth factor activity. Blood 2000;96(9):3139–46.

120. Yang Y, Yaccoby S, Liu W, et al. Soluble syndecan-1 promotes growth of myeloma tumors in vivo. Blood 2002;100(2):610–7.

121. Langford JK, Yang Y, Kieber-Emmons T, Sanderson RD. Identification of an invasion regulatory domain within the core protein of syndecan-1. J Biol Chem 2005;280(5):3467–73.

122. Seidel C, Sundan A, Hjorth M, et al. Serum syndecan-1: a new independent prognostic marker in multiple myeloma. Blood 2000;95(2):388–92.

123. Mahtouk K, Hose D, Raynaud P, et al. Heparanase influences expression and shedding of syndecan-1, and its expression by the bone marrow environment is a bad prognostic factor in multiple myeloma. Blood 2007;109(11):4914–23.

124. Tassone P, Goldmacher VS, Neri P, et al. Cytotoxic activity of the maytansinoid immunoconjugate B-B4-DM1 against CD138+ multiple myeloma cells. Blood 2004;104(12):3688–96.

125. Ozaki S, Kosaka M, Wakatsuki S, Abe M, Koishihara Y, Matsumoto T. Immunotherapy of multiple myeloma with a monoclonal antibody directed against a plasma cell-specific antigen, HM1.24. Blood 1997;90(8):3179–86.

126. Matsuda A, Suzuki Y, Honda G, et al. Large-scale identification and characterization of human genes that activate NF-kappaB and MAPK signaling pathways. Oncogene 2003;22(21):3307–18.

127. Ono K, Ohtomo T, Yoshida K, et al. The humanized anti-HM1.24 antibody effectively kills multiple myeloma cells by human effector cell-mediated cytotoxicity. Mol Immunol 1999;36(6):387–95.

128. Ozaki S, Kosaka M, Wakahara Y, et al. Humanized anti-HM1.24 antibody mediates myeloma cell cytotoxicity that is enhanced by cytokine stimulation of effector cells. Blood 1999;93(11):3922–30.

129. Kawai S, Yoshimura Y, Iida S, et al. Antitumor activity of humanized monoclonal antibody against HM1.24 antigen in human myeloma xenograft models. Oncol Rep 2006;15(2):361–7.

130. Jalili A, Ozaki S, Hara T, et al. Induction of HM1.24 peptide-specific cytotoxic T lymphocytes by using peripheral-blood stem-cell harvests in patients with multiple myeloma. Blood 2005;106(10):3538–45.

131. Rew SB, Peggs K, Sanjuan I, et al. Generation of potent antitumor CTL from patients with multiple myeloma directed against HM1.24. Clin Cancer Res 2005;11(9):3377–84.

132. Chiriva-Internati M, Liu Y, Weidanz JA, et al. Testing recombinant adeno-associated virus-gene loading of dendritic cells for generating potent cytotoxic T lymphocytes against a prototype self-antigen, multiple myeloma HM1.24. Blood 2003;102(9):3100–7.

133. Mitsiades CS, Treon SP, Mitsiades N, et al. TRAIL/Apo2L ligand selectively induces apoptosis and overcomes drug resistance in multiple myeloma: therapeutic applications. Blood 2001;98(3):795–804.

134. Spencer A, Yeh SL, Koutrevelis K, Baulch-Brown C. TRAIL-induced apoptosis of authentic myeloma cells does not correlate with the procaspase-8/cFLIP ratio. Blood 2002;100(8):3049; author reply 50–1.

135. Menoret E, Gomez-Bougie P, Geffroy-Luseau A, et al. Mcl-1L cleavage is involved in TRAIL-R1- and TRAIL-R2-mediated apoptosis induced by HGS-ETR1 and HGS-ETR2 human mAbs in myeloma cells. Blood 2006;108(4):1346–52.

136. Trudel S, Ely S, Farooqi Y, et al. Inhibition of fibroblast growth factor receptor 3 induces differentiation and apoptosis in t(4;14) myeloma. Blood 2004;103(9):3521–8.

137. Pollett JB, Trudel S, Stern D, Li ZH, Stewart AK. Overexpression of the myeloma-associated oncogene fibroblast growth factor receptor 3 confers dexamethasone resistance. Blood 2002;100(10):3819–21.

138. Xin X, Abrams TJ, Hollenbach PW, et al. CHIR-258 is efficacious in a newly developed fibroblast growth factor receptor 3-expressing orthotopic multiple myeloma model in mice. Clin Cancer Res 2006;12(16):4908–15.

139. Trudel S, Stewart AK, Rom E, et al. The inhibitory anti-FGFR3 antibody, PRO-001, is cytotoxic to t(4;14) multiple myeloma cells. Blood 2006;107(10):4039–46.

140. Lewiecki EM. RANK ligand inhibition with denosumab for the management of osteoporosis. Expert Opin Biol Ther 2006;6(10):1041–50.

141. Simonet WS, Lacey DL, Dunstan CR, et al. Osteoprotegerin: a novel secreted protein involved in the regulation of bone density. Cell 1997;89(2):309–19.

142. Giuliani N, Bataille R, Mancini C, Lazzaretti M, Barille S. Myeloma cells induce imbalance in the osteoprotegerin/osteoprotegerin ligand system in the human bone marrow environment. Blood 2001;98(13):3527–33.

143. Terpos E, Szydlo R, Apperley JF, et al. Soluble receptor activator of nuclear factor kappaB ligand-osteoprotegerin ratio predicts survival in multiple myeloma: proposal for a novel prognostic index. Blood 2003;102(3):1064–9.

144. Schwarz EM, Ritchlin CT. Clinical development of anti-RANKL therapy. Arthritis Res Ther 2007;9 Suppl 1:S7.

145. Bekker PJ, Holloway DL, Rasmussen AS, et al. A single-dose placebo-controlled study of AMG 162, a fully human monoclonal antibody to RANKL, in postmenopausal women. J Bone Miner Res 2004;19(7):1059–66.

146. McClung MR, Lewiecki EM, Cohen SB, et al. Denosumab in postmenopausal women with low bone mineral density. N Engl J Med 2006;354(8):821–31.

147. Body JJ, Facon T, Coleman RE, et al. A study of the biological receptor activator of nuclear factor-kappaB ligand inhibitor, denosumab, in patients with multiple myeloma or bone metastases from breast cancer. Clin Cancer Res 2006;12(4):1221–8.

148. Tian E, Zhan F, Walker R, et al. The role of the Wnt-signaling antagonist DKK1 in the development of osteolytic lesions in multiple myeloma. N Engl J Med 2003;349(26):2483–94.

149. Yaccoby S, Ling W, Zhan F, Walker R, Barlogie B, Shaughnessy JD, Jr. Antibody-based inhibition of DKK1 suppresses tumor-induced bone resorption and multiple myeloma growth in vivo. Blood 2007;109(5):2106–11.

150. Podar K, Anderson KC. Inhibition of VEGF signaling pathways in multiple myeloma and other malignancies. Cell Cycle 2007;6(5):538–42.

151. Kumar S, Witzig TE, Timm M, et al. Expression of VEGF and its receptors by myeloma cells. Leukemia 2003;17(10):2025–31.

152. Podar K, Tonon G, Sattler M, et al. The small-molecule VEGF receptor inhibitor pazopanib (GW786034B) targets both tumor and endothelial cells in multiple myeloma. Proc Natl Acad Sci U S A 2006;103(51):19478–83.

153. Ferrara N, Hillan KJ, Novotny W. Bevacizumab (Avastin), a humanized anti-VEGF monoclonal antibody for cancer therapy. Biochem Biophys Res Commun 2005;333(2):328–35.

154. Gorski DH, Beckett MA, Jaskowiak NT, et al. Blockage of the vascular endothelial growth factor stress response increases the antitumor effects of ionizing radiation. Cancer Res 1999;59(14):3374–8.

155. Goldman B. For investigational targeted drugs, combination trials pose challenges. J Natl Cancer Inst 2003;95(23):1744–6.

156. Hoyer RJ, Leung N, Witzig TE, Lacy MQ. Treatment of diuretic refractory pleural effusions with bevacizumab in four patients with primary systemic amyloidosis. Am J Hematol 2007;82(5):409–13.

157. Tai YT, Li XF, Breitkreutz I, et al. Role of B-cell-activating factor in adhesion and growth of human multiple myeloma cells in the bone marrow microenvironment. Cancer Res 2006;66(13):6675–82.

158. Moreaux J, Legouffe E, Jourdan E, et al. BAFF and APRIL protect myeloma cells from apoptosis induced by interleukin 6 deprivation and dexamethasone. Blood 2004;103(8):3148–57.

159. Abe M, Kido S, Hiasa M, et al. BAFF and APRIL as osteoclast-derived survival factors for myeloma cells: a rationale for TACI-Fc treatment in patients with multiple myeloma. Leukemia 2006;20(7):1313–5.

160. Moreaux J, Cremer FW, Reme T, et al. The level of TACI gene expression in myeloma cells is associated with a signature of microenvironment dependence versus a plasmablastic signature. Blood 2005;106(3):1021–30.

161. Munafo A, Priestley A, Nestorov I, Visich J, Rogge M. Safety, pharmacokinetics and pharmacodynamics of atacicept in healthy volunteers. Eur J Clin Pharmacol 2007;63(7):647–56.

162. Rossi JF, Moreaux J, Rose M, Picard M, Ythier A, Rossier C, Sievers E, Klein B. A Phase I/II study of atacicept (TACI-Ig) to neutralize APRIL and BLyS in

patients with refractory or relapsed multiple myeloma (MM) or active previously treated Waldenstrom's Macroglobulinemia (WM). Blood 2006;108:3578.

163. Tai Y-T, Xu J, Li X-F, Breitkreutz I, Podar K, Hideshima T, Schlossman R, Richardson P, Munshi NC, Anderson KC. The BAFF inhibitor AMG523 blocks adhesion and survival of human multiple myeloma cells in the bone marrow microenvironment: clinical implication. Blood 2006;108:3452.

164. Carlo-Stella C, Guidetti A, Di Nicola M, et al. IFN-gamma enhances the antimyeloma activity of the fully human anti-human leukocyte antigen-DR monoclonal antibody 1D09C3. Cancer Res 2007;67(7):3269–75.

165. Sekimoto E, Ozaki S, Ohshima T, et al. A single-chain Fv diabody against human leukocyte antigen-A molecules specifically induces myeloma cell death in the bone marrow environment. Cancer Res 2007;67(3):1184–92.

166. Asvadi P, Jones DR, Dunn RD, Choo ABH, Raison MJ, Raison RL. A monoclonal antibody specific for free human kappa light chains induces apoptosis of multiple myeloma cells and exhibits anti-tumor activity in vivo. Blood (ASH Annual Meeting Abstracts) 2004;104:2416.

167. Sainz IM, Isordia-Salas I, Espinola RG, Long WK, Pixley RA, Colman RW. Multiple myeloma in a murine syngeneic model: modulation of growth and angiogenesis by a monoclonal antibody to kininogen. Cancer Immunol Immunother 2006;55(7):797–807.

168. Zand MS, Vo T, Pellegrin T, et al. Apoptosis and complement-mediated lysis of myeloma cells by polyclonal rabbit antithymocyte globulin. Blood 2006;107(7):2895–903.

169. Kroger N, Shaw B, Iacobelli S, Comparison between antithymocyte globulin and alemtuzumab and the possible impact of KIR-ligand mismatch after dose-reduced conditioning and unrelated stem cell transplantation in patients with multiple myeloma. Br J Haematol 2005;129:631–643.

170. Rha S, Tolcher A, Stephenson J, et al. A phase I study of brevarex, a murine monoclonal antibody directed at the MUC1 antigen, in patients with advanced solid tumors. Proc Am Soc Clin Oncol 2000;19:abstr 1868

171. Somlo G, Bellamy W, Zimmerman TM, et al. Phase II randomized trial of bevacizumab versus bevacizumab and thalidomide for relapsed/refractory multiple myeloma. Blood 2005;106:abstract 2571.

172. Sapra P, Stein R, Pickett J, Qu Z, Govindan SV, Cardillo TM, Hansen HJ, Horak ID, Griffiths GL, Goldenberg DM.Anti-CD74 antibody-doxorubicin conjugate, IMMU-110, in a human multiple myeloma xenograft and in monkeys.Clin Cancer Res. 2005 Jul 15;11(14):5257–5264.

173. Rankin CT, Veri MC, Gorlatov S, Tuaillon N, Burke S, Huang L, Inzunza HD, Li H, Thomas S, Johnson S, Stavenhagen J, Koenig S, Bonvini E.CD32B, the human inhibitory Fc-gamma receptor IIB, as a target for monoclonal antibody therapy of B-cell lymphoma.Blood. 2006 Oct 1;108(7):2384–2391.

174. Yang J, Qian J, Wezeman M, Wang S, Lin P, Wang M, Yaccoby S, Kwak LW, Barlogie B, Yi Q.Targeting beta2-microglobulin for induction of tumor apoptosis in human hematological malignancies.Cancer Cell. 2006 Oct;10(4):295–307.

175. Coleman EJ, Brooks KJ, Smallshaw JE, Vitetta ES.The Fc portion of UV3, an anti-CD54 monoclonal antibody, is critical for its antitumor activity in SCID mice with human multiple myeloma or lymphoma cell lines.J Immunother. 2006 Sep-Oct;29(5):489–498.

176. Nimmanapalli R, Lyu MA, Du M, Keating MJ, Rosenblum MG, Gandhi V.The growth factor fusion construct containing B-lymphocyte stimulator (BLyS) and the toxin rGel induces apoptosis specifically in BAFF-R-positive CLL cells. Blood. 2007 Mar 15;109(6):2557–2564. Epub 2006 Nov 21.

177. Glennie MJ, van de Winkel JG.Renaissance of cancer therapeutic antibodies.Drug Discov Today. 2003 Jun 1;8(11):503–510. Review

Section 4

Existing Novel Agents

Chapter 13

Thalidomide in Patients with Relapsed Multiple Myeloma

Ashraf Badros

The Dark Remedy "History of Thalidomide"

More than half a century ago, thalidomide began an astonishing journey of endurance where fate rather than science transformed a dreadful drug to a great remedy.[1,2] In 1953, a chemist at a German pharmaceutical company, Chemie Grünenthal, first synthesized thalidomide after heating a commercially available chemical phthaloylisoglutamine; the new molecule was called thalidomide. The company patented the molecule and began searching for diseases thalidomide could treat. In absence of any scientific rationale, human clinical trials began. However, after extensive testing, they failed to establish pharmacological activity as an antibiotic, an anticonvulsant, or an antihistaminic. It is worth mentioning that thalidomide was evaluated in two clinical trials including 92 patients with advanced cancer, including two patients with multiple myeloma (MM). Many patients reported palliation of symptoms. However, with the lack of clinical responses, the drug was deemed ineffective and was abandoned as an anticancer drug.[3–5] These early trials showed that thalidomide was a hypnotic that directly induced sleep. Eventually, by 1957, thalidomide was marketed over the counter in over 50 countries as a sleeping pill and quickly became the drug of choice for pregnant women to treat morning sickness; the drug was never approved in the United States because of Food and Drug Administration (FDA) concerns about peripheral neuropathy (PN). In 1961, after 4 years on the market, thalidomide was withdrawn after its teratogenic effects were recognized; these malformations included deafness, blindness, cleft palate, malformed internal organs, and phocomelia, the devastating abnormalities of fetal limb development. There is no accurate census of the number of affected children, but there were ~5,000 thalidomide survivors and thousands of stillborns.[6,7] In 1964, a physician, Jacob Sheskin, gave two tablets of the banned drug "thalidomide" to a critically ill bedridden patient with erythema nodosum leprosum (ENL) to help him sleep. The patient slept for almost a day, and on waking up, he was able to walk and his condition markedly improved. This led to a revolution in the care of patients with leprosy. In 1998, the FDA approved thalidomide for therapy of ENL.[8] After recognition of its biological activities, thalidomide was tested in many clinical trials and on compassionate

From: *Contemporary Hematology Myeloma Therapy*
Edited by: S. Lonial © Humana Press, Totowa, NJ

use programs for therapy of inflammatory diseases, graft versus host disease, and various cancers with no real benefit.[9]

Fate, again, chartered the big breakthrough for thalidomide in another serendipitous discovery that grew out of the pleas and persistence of Beth Wolmer, who was desperate to find a treatment for her 35-year-old husband who was dying from MM after exhausting all available therapies. She called Judah Folkman, whose work on angiogenesis was publicized as a potential cure for cancer, to ask if thalidomide would help her husband; later, she contacted Bart Barlogie at the University of Arkansas who obtained thalidomide for few patients on compassionate-use basis. By the fall of 1997, Ira Wolmer received thalidomide; he did not respond. However, thalidomide was given to a second patient who achieved a near complete remission that lasted for 2 years. Thus, the first clinical trial for thalidomide began, starting a new era of novel agents for the treatment of MM.[10] This chapter presents a brief review of thalidomide pharmacokinetics and activity in patents with relapsed MM as well as possible mechanisms of actions and side effects.

Chemical Structure

Thalidomide is an alpha-phthalimidoglutarimide derived from glutamic acid. It has two-ring systems: a left-sided phthalimide and a right-sided glutarimide, existing in L- and R-isomer forms, with an asymmetric carbon atom at position 3' of the glutarimide ring (Fig. 1).[11,12] Early reports suggested that the L-isomer was linked to teratogenicity and the R-isomer was responsible for sedative purposes; however, under physiological conditions, both isomers are rapidly interconvertible in solution. The imide bonds in the two-ring system of both enantiomers are susceptible to hydrolytic cleavage in vitro at pH values greater than 6.[13]

Pharmacokinetics

The pharmacokinetics of thalidomide has been studied in healthy adult volunteers, in patients with prostate cancer, and in HIV-infected individuals.[14–16] Thalidomide is slowly absorbed from the gastrointestinal tract in a dose-dependent fashion from 200 mg to 1,200 mg. In healthy men, peak plasma levels of 0.8–1.4 µg/ml were reached in 4.4 h (range, 1.9–6.2 h) following a

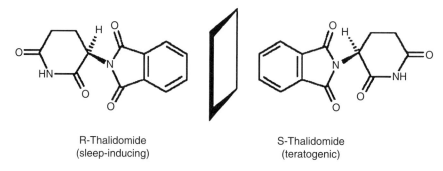

R-Thalidomide
(sleep-inducing)

S-Thalidomide
(teratogenic)

Fig. 1 The chemical structure of thalidomide.

single 200-mg oral dose with very little variability. Peak plasma levels could be maintained at steady state with thalidomide administration every 6 h. Volume of distribution for thalidomide was 120.69 ± 45.36 L. Plasma concentration versus time curves fit a one-compartment model with first-order absorption and elimination; absorption half-life was 1.7 ± 1.05 h, and elimination half-life of parent compound was 8.7 ± 4.11 h, about 3 times longer than that observed in animals. Total body clearance rate was relatively slow: 10.41 ± 2.04 L/h.[17] No information is available on the distribution of thalidomide in humans. Administration of radio-labeled drug into animals results in an even distribution of radioactivity with slight enhancement in kidneys, liver, biliary tissue, white matter, and peripheral nerves. Less than $0.6 \pm 0.22\%$ of thalidomide is excreted in urine as parent drug in the first 24 h, suggesting a nonrenal elimination. Thus, thalidomide can be used safely in patients with renal insufficiency.[18] Less than 15% of thalidomide is present in plasma 24 h after an oral dose, mostly protein bound; the rest is metabolized to over 100 compounds through two processes. The first is enzyme-mediated hepatic degradation involving the cytochrome P450 family: both phthalimide and glutaramide are isolated from the urine after oral administration as 3-hydroxyphthalimic acid and 4-phthalimidoglutarimic acid.[19] The second route of thalidomide metabolism is rapid spontaneous hydrolysis in aqueous solutions at pH 6.0 or greater to form three primary products: 4-phthalimidoglutarimic acid, 2-phthalimidoglutarimic acid, and *o*-carboxylbenzamido-glutarimide. Whether the parent compound or one or more of its metabolites are biologically active remains speculative. Antiangiogenic activity of thalidomide was not observed in vitro without the addition of fetal liver microsomes, suggesting that the parent compound does not possess this activity. In addition, the hydroxylation process is species specific; this explains the variability in side effects of thalidomide, such as teratogenicity, which was not seen in any animal models before the human tragedy.[18,20] Thalidomide does not induce or inhibit its own metabolism; in healthy women, thalidomide administrated at 200 mg/day for 18 days yielded similar pharmacokinetics on the first and last days.[21] There are emerging data that gender as well as race affect the metabolism of the drug.[22,23]

Thalidomide Antimyeloma Activity in the Relapsed Patients

Thalidomide Monotherapy

The efficacy of thalidomide in patients with relapsed MM has not been formally established in a randomized trial, but rather from several small phase I/II trials. The initial study of thalidomide in MM by Singhal et al. included 84 patients with relapsed/refractory MM; many had extensive prior therapy including stem cell transplantation. Thalidomide was started at 200 mg daily and the dose was escalated every 2 weeks as tolerated to 800 mg/day. Overall response rate (ORR) was 32%, mostly partial responses (PR); only two patients achieved complete responses (CR). Responses were apparent within 2 months with a trend for better responses with higher doses.[10] An update of the study with 169 patients confirmed the initial results: overall survival (OS) at 18 months was 55%, and event-free survival (EFS) was 30%; longer follow-up showed that 10% of the patients remain progression free at 6 years (Fig. 2).[24,25] A recent review of thalidomide monotherapy identified 42 studies

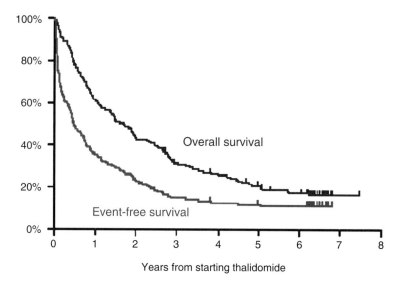

Fig. 2 Overall and event-free survival of 169 patients who had end-stage myeloma and were treated with thalidomide. Singhal, S. et al. Clin J Am Soc Nephrol 2006;1: 1322–1330. Lippincott Williams & Wilkins (permission pending).

published in peer-reviewed journals and abstracts reporting on 1674 patients with relapsed MM.[26,27] Thirty two trials used an escalating dosing regimen and four a fixed-dose regimen (one used 50 mg/day, three trials used 200 mg/day). The target dose in the dose-escalating trials was 800 mg/day in 17 trials, 400–600 mg/day in 10 trials, and 200 mg/day in 1 trial. The PR rate was ~30% (95% confidence interval [CI] 27–32%). The CR rate was 1% and the median OS from all these trials was 14 months.

There is no data to establish dose–response relationship for single-agent thalidomide, as randomization to different dose levels has not been done. Rather thalidomide is usually administered on as tolerated bases starting at 50–100 mg per day and the dose escalated in increments of 50 mg every 2 weeks; the target dose varied by study between 200 mg and 800 mg.[28]

Dexamethasone Plus Thalidomide

Dexamethasone was added to thalidomide mostly because of the traditional role of steroids in MM; however, after many patients who were refractory to single-agent thalidomide responded to the combination, dexamethasone plus thalidomide (DT) became the main salvage therapy for patients with MM. So far, no study had compared thalidomide single agent with DT and it is unlikely that such study will be done due to the higher ORR for the combination (45–60%); the additional impact of dexamethasone on EFS and OS has not been defined.[29] The combination DT was assessed in 44 patients with MM who were refractory to chemotherapy, 77% were resistant to dexamethasone-based regimens and 32% had previously received high-dose therapy. Thalidomide was administered at 200–400 mg orally daily and dexamethasone at 20 mg/m2 orally on days 1–4, 9–12, 17–20 of the 28-day cycle. Twenty-four patients (55%) achieved a PR with a median time to response of 1.3 months. The median time of progression-free survival (PFS) for responding patients was 10 months and the median OS for all patients was 12.6 months.[30] Lower doses of thalidomide (100 mg/day) and dexamethasone (40 mg, days 1–4) were assessed in 77 patients with MM. After 3 months of treatment, 41% of the patients had a PR and 25% had a minor response (25–50% reduction in paraprotein). Median PFS was 12 months.[31] This regimen was retrospectively compared to salvage conventional and high-dose chemotherapy for patients relapsing after autologous stem cell transplantation ($n = 90$). DT response rate (nCR 19% and PR 28%) was similar to high-dose chemotherapy (CR 11% and PR 71%) and was significantly higher than conventional therapy (CR 0% and PR 16%); however, time to progression (20 months) favored DT compared with 9 months for autologous transplant and 4–5 months for conventional chemotherapy. DT was also significantly superior to conventional chemotherapy in terms of OS (55 months vs 27 months, $p = 0.008$).[32] The addition of clarithromycin to DT seems to improve response in patients with MM, with ORR of 93% in 50 patients with refractory MM, including 13% CR, 40% nCR.[33] The mechanism by which clarithromycin enhances the activity of DT is unclear but is probably related to altered dexamethasone metabolism. Theoretically, downregulation of Bcl-2 and the apoptotic mitochondrial pathway could overcome resistance and enhance responses to DT. Bcl-2 antisense oligonucleotide, G3139, was combined with low-dose thalidomide (100–200 mg) and dexamethasone (20 mg daily for 4 days) every 28 days[34] in a phase I/II trial; ORR was 55% in 33 patients with relapsed MM including 15 patients who failed prior DT. However, myeloma cells isolated from the patients before and after G3139 infusion failed to document significant changes in Bc-2 levels and the level did not correlate with clinical response. The observed enhanced activity was independent of Bcl-2; all responding patients had significantly higher levels of IgM, suggesting that response is related to activation of the innate immune system by the CpG motif of the antisense molecule. From a practical prospect, the addition of dexamethasone allowed the use of lower doses of thalidomide without loss of activity, if anything improved responses. Whether dexamethasone should be added early or later if patients had no or minimal response to single-agent thalidomide is unclear. Finally, the upfront use of DT as induction may lead to diminished use of this regimen in the relapsed setting.[35,36]

Thalidomide Plus Chemotherapy

The lack of immune suppression and in vitro evidence of synergism make thalidomide an attractive drug to combine with traditional chemotherapeutic agents. Several combinations have been published with small number of patients and significant variability in patient selection making it difficult to compare the results. In the following section, a brief description of selected regimen will be reviewed (Table 1).

Thalidomide Plus Cyclophosphamide-Based Regimens

Kropff et al. treated 60 patients with advanced MM with hyperfractionated cyclophosphamide in combination with pulsed dexamethasone and thalidomide (HyperCDT): hyperfractionated cyclophosphamide (300 mg/m2 intravenously over 3 h twice daily × 6 doses) with pulsed dexamethasone (20 mg/m^2 on days 1–4, 9–12, 17–20) and thalidomide (100–400 mg daily as tolerated). CR and PR rates were 4% and 68%, respectively. Median EFS and OS were

Table 1 Summary of thalidomide therapy in relapsed multiple myeloma.

Regimen	No. of trialsa	No. of patients	Response rate[b]			OS	EFS
			ORR	CR	PR		
Thal monotherapy	42	1629	30	2	28	More than 14 months	
Thal + Dex	2	214	40–60	5–10	50	More than 12 months	10 months
DTPACE	1	235		16	32		
Thal + CTX	5	252	70–90	5–20	30–60	More than 16–19 months	11–13 months
Thal + Doxil + Dex	1	47	92				
MPT	3	72	60–70			10–12 months	9–11 months
Thal + Bortezomib + Dex	1	77	55				
MPT + Bortezomib	1	30	76	10	66	1 year 61%	1 year 83%

OS overall survival *EFS* event-free survival, *ORR* overall response rate, *CR* complete responses, *PR* partial responses, *Thal* thalidomide, *dex* dexamethasone, *CTX* cyclophosphamide, *MPT* melphalan, thalidomide, and prednisone, *DTPACE* 4 days of continuous-infusion cisplatin, doxorubicin, cyclophosphamide, and etoposide
aSee text for details of the studies.
bThese are approximate responses to various regimens; they cannot be compared with each other as the studies varied significantly in the patient selections dose and duration of therapy.

11 and 19 months, respectively. Side effects included neutropenia (67%) and infections (26%). Four patients developed myelodysplastic syndrome or secondary acute myeloid leukemia 2–4 months after study entry.[37] In a similar trial, 53 patients with relapsed/refractory MM received cyclophosphamide 150 mg/m^2 orally every 12 h before meals on days 1–5, thalidomide 400 mg *per os* (by mouth) in the evening on days 1–5 and 14–18, and dexamethasone 20 mg/m^2 in the morning after breakfast on days 1–5 and 14–18, repeated every 28 days. Thirty-two patients (60%) achieved a PR with a median time to response of 1.5 months. The median time to progression for responding patients was 12 months and the median OS was 17.5 months.[38] The Hoosier Oncology Group conducted a phase II trial of oral cyclophosphamide (50 mg twice daily for 21 days), thalidomide (200 mg daily) and prednisone (50 mg every other day), cycles repeated every 28 days, in patients with relapsed MM. Of the 37 patients enrolled, 16 had prior stem cell transplantation. The median follow-up time was 25.3 months. Twenty-two out of thirty-five patients (63%) responded: 7 (20%) achieved CR, 2 (6%) nCR, and 13 (37%) PR. The median time to response and PFS were 3.6 months (95% CI 2.8–10.9) and 13.2 months (95% CI 9.4–21.0), respectively.[39] The addition of etoposide to thalidomide, cyclophosphamide, and dexamethasone was studied in 56 patients with poor-prognosis MM. Of 50 patients evaluable for response, 4% achieved CR, 64% PR, and 18% minimal response (MR), and 6% had SD with an ORR of 77%. Subsequent to successful remission induction, 18 patients received autologous or allogeneic stem cell transplantation. The median PFS was 16 months. At a median follow-up of 14 months, OS was estimated at 55%.[40] A more intensive regimen using 4 days of oral dexamethasone, daily thalidomide, and 4 days of continuous-infusion cisplatin, doxorubicin, cyclophosphamide, and etoposide (DTPACE) was evaluated in patients with poor-risk MM who had received prior chemotherapy ($n = 236$), with documented progressive disease in 148 patients (63%). PR rate after two cycles of DTPACE was 32%, with 16% CR. Interestingly, patients with high lactate dehydrogenase (LDH; $n = 98$)

showed a better response than those with normal LDH ($n = 138$) and those with chromosome 13 abnormalities ($n = 55$) responded equally well as other patients ($n = 181$). No data has been presented on whether such induction can replace tandem autotransplantation.[41] This regimen has been moved to the upfront therapy for newly diagnosed patients with MM in combination with bortezomib with high response rate and no adverse effect on stem cell collection.[42] The data suggest that thalidomide improves antitumor activity of salvage cycolphosphamide-containing regimens in patients with poor-prognosis MM. In vivo coadministration of thalidomide with cyclophosphamide is not only synergistic but also increased thalidomide $t_{1/2}$ by 3.9-fold, in plasma and tumor tissue, with a corresponding increase in the area under the concentration curve (AUC).[43] Thalidomide can be administered at lower doses when combined with chemotherapy, thus allowing prolonged administration of the drug. Additional adverse events including infectious complications, cardiovascular events, and thrombosis are higher with chemotherapy combinations and may need additional supportive measures.

Thalidomide Plus Melphalan-Containing Regimens

Melphalan, the old gold standard therapy for MM, has been combined with thalidomide and dexamethasone or prednisone with impressive results, both in the newly diagnosed and in the relapsed setting.[44,45] The first report of this combination included 21 patients with relapsed MM who received up to four cycles of melphalan 50 mg intravenously, thalidomide titrated to target of 400 mg orally daily, and dexamethasone 40 mg orally on days 1–4; cycles were repeated every 4–6 weeks. Serum monoclonal protein reductions greater than 25% occurred in 14 (70%) out of 20 evaluable patients. Median EFS was 11 months and median OS was over 1 year.[46] In another study, patients were randomized to thalidomide starting at 100 mg/day and escalated weekly up to 600 mg alone ($n = 23$) or with melphalan ($n = 27$) given orally at 0.20 mg/kg/day for 4 days every month. PR was observed in 59% of the thalidomide and melphalan cohort compared with 26% of thalidomide-alone patients ($P = 0.009$). After a median follow-up of 13 months (range, 6–32), PFS at 2 years was significantly longer in the thalidomide/melphalan cohort (61 vs 45%; $P = 0.0376$), whereas OS did not differ significantly.[47,48] A recent trial evaluated intravenous melphalan 20 mg/m^2 every 4 months, thalidomide 50–100 mg and prednisone 50 mg daily in patients with advanced MM ($n = 24$). Fifteen patients (66%) had previously been treated with thalidomide. Overall, on an intent-to-treat basis, 14 patients responded: nCR ($n = 3$), PR ($n = 7$), and 4 had an MR. After a median follow-up of 14 months, median PFS was 9 months.[49] The use of melphalan increases the risk of myelodysplastic syndrome (MDS) and secondary acute myeloid leukemia in patients with MM, especially if used for prolonged periods.[50] Limiting the treatment duration to less than 1 year may decrease this risk; the addition of thalidomide is unlikely to have an impact on the development of MDS.[51]

Thalidomide Plus Pegylated Liposomal Doxorubicin, Doxil®-Containing Regimens

Thalidomide 100 mg daily was added to pegylated liposomal doxorubicin (PLD) in combination with dexamethasone and vincrestine (DVD), a highly effective regimen in patients with newly diagnosed and relapsed MM, in 49 relapsed patients. CR rate was 20%, 45% achieved a PR with an ORR of 90%. Median PFS was 15.5 months. After 50 months of follow-up, median OS was 39.9 months.[52,53] Case-matched study for age, beta2-microglobulin, and number of previous therapy showed significantly higher ORR when PDL was combined with DT (92% vs 63.5%; $P < 0.0001$); no data is provided for EFS or OS.[54]

Thalidomide Plus Bortezomib-Containing Regimens

Bortezomib has impressive results in patients with MM relapsing after chemotherapy (conventional and high-dose) as well as those refractory/intolerable to thalidomide and dexamethasone. The preclinical evidence of synergistic effect for bortezomib and thalidomide and the anecdotal responses for the combination in patients who progressed on either drug prompted the use of both drugs in patients with MM. In relapsed MM, Zangari et al. reported a phase I trial of bortezomib (0.7, 1, 1.3 mg/m^2) and thalidomide (50–150 mg daily) with dexamethasone added for nonresponders. Of 77 patients on the study, overall RR was 55% with 17% CR/nCR rate. Surprisingly, no grade 3 or 4 PN was reported and no thrombotic events.[55,56] This regimen has been used up to 3 years with impressive results in many refractory patients.[42] A smaller study of 18 patients with relapsed MM evaluated low-dose bortezomib 1.0 mg/m^2 intravenously on days 1, 4, 8, and 11 of a 28-day cycle for up to six cycles, dexamethasone 24 mg on the day of and the day after bortezomib, and daily thalidomide 100 mg. Nine out of seventeen (53%) patients responded: CR ($n = 2$) and PR ($n = 6$). Median time to best response was 2 months. No thrombotic events were reported. After a median follow-up of 11 months, 12 patients were alive.[57] In a phase I/II trial, bortezomib and thalidomide were added to melphalan and prednisone (VMPT). Bortezomib was administered at three dose levels, 1.0, 1.3, or 1.6 mg/m^2, on days 1, 4, 15, and 22; melphalan at 6 mg/m^2 on days 1–5, and prednisone at 60 mg/m^2 on days 1–5. Thalidomide was delivered at 50 mg on days 1–35. Cycles were repeated every 35 days. The maximum tolerated dose of bortezomib was 1.3 mg/m^2. Thirty patients with relapsed or refractory MM were enrolled: 20 patients (67%) achieved PR. Among 14 patients who received VMPT as second-line treatment, the PR rate was 79% and the CR rate was 36%. The 1-year PFS was 61%, and the 1-year OS was 84%. The incidence of neurotoxicities was unexpectedly low.[58] Higher doses of the same drugs were evaluated in the salvage setting in 26 patients with relapsed MM with hematopoietic stem cell support. The regimen included melphalan 50 mg/m^2, bortezomib 1.3 mg/m^2 on days -6 and -3 plus thalidomide 200 mg and dexamethasone 20 mg on days -6 through -3. ORR was 65%, including CR (4%), nCR (12%), and VGPR (8%).[59] The results of thalidomide and bortezomib in combination with chemotherapy are impressive efficacy with unexpected lower rates of neuropathy and thrombosis.

Predictors of Thalidomide Response

Early data from Arkansas suggested that cumulative thalidomide dose administrated during the first 3 months of treatment correlated with clinical outcome;

patients receiving 42 g of thalidomide had a higher rate of ORR (54 vs 21%) and a 2-year OS (63 vs 45%).[24] The cumulative 3 months thalidomide dose was also a prognostic factor for survival in other trials, supporting dose-dependent effect of single-agent thalidomide in patients with MM.[60] However, it is clear from the clinical experience that lower doses of thalidomide are effective in the majority of patients.[61,62] Lower doses allow tolerance to some adverse effects such as sedation. Clinically, if the response is less than a PR, with no improvement with the addition of dexamethasone, the dose should be titrated upward to 400–600 as tolerated or combined with chemotherapy before the drug is considered ineffective. Early response to thalidomide, defined as 25% reduction in M-spike within 3 weeks, predicated long-term response. The response duration was longer in those achieving PR versus minimal response (12.4 vs 9.7 months).[63] This can easily be used for early termination of therapy or addition of other agents such as dexamethasone or chemotherapy. Deletion of chromosome 13, high B2M, and elevation of LDH were independent unfavorable prognostic factors for response to thalidomide and predicted poor EFS and OS. Patients with low serum albumin, IgA isotype, and a platelet count less than 80 g/L had poor EFS and OS. High plasma cell-labeling index and elevated serum level of C-reactive protein were predictive of short EFS.[24] Since antiangiogenic effects were postulated as major mediator of thalidomide activity in MM pretreatment, angiogenesis was evaluated as a predictor of response. High pretreatment microvessel density (MVD) predicted a poor response to thalidomide therapy; however, there was no correlation between response and decreased MVD after therapy.[64] Two studies reported that high plasma basic fibroblast growth factor (bFGF) and vascular endothelial growth factor (VEGF) concentrations were associated with a better response to thalidomide.[65,66] Soluble interleukin-2 receptor (IL-2R) increased significantly after 3 weeks of therapy with thalidomide, probably indicating lymphocyte activation with thalidomide that correlated with improved EFS and OS in patients with relapsed MM.[67]

Relapse on Thalidomide

There are many reports suggesting lack of effect for thalidomide on extramedullary plasmacytomas even in patients who achieve a serological response (i.e., decrease in the M component).[68-70] Furthermore, it has been recently recognized that relapses that may occur in thalidomide maintenance can occur with an increase in bone marrow plasmacytosis and no increase in the monoclonal protein.[71] These data should alert physicians to consider therapy for patients with extramedullary MM carefully; combination chemotherapy is particularly effective in these cases. Also, patients should be screened carefully for extramedullary disease, which is more recognized now with the use of positron emission topography (PET) scans. Bone marrow evaluations yearly are recommended in patients on thalidomide maintenance, even in patients with no change in monoclonal protein. However, it is unclear if change of therapy is indicated for asymptomatic patients based on radiological or pathological relapse. Barlogie et al. randomized newly diagnosed patients with MM to receive thalidomide in combination with tandem autologous stem cell transplantation. Patients receiving thalidomide had a higher CR rate (62% vs

43%; $P < 0.001$) and longer 5-year EFS (56% vs 44%; $P = 0.01$); however, no statistically significant difference was observed for OS. Thalidomide-treated patients had a higher incidence of thromboembolic events (24% vs 12%) and PN (19% vs 12%), and shorter postrelapse survival (median 1.1 vs 2.7 years).[72] Although this study does not clearly address if drug holiday will be beneficial as patients remained on thalidomide until they relapsed. So far, no other investigator has reported a lower survival for patients after thalidomide.

Mechanisms of Actions

Thalidomide has been given to thousands of patients with more than 150 various medical conditions spanning half-a-century; however, thalidomide is still shrouded in mystery with limited data on its mechanisms of action. Several hypotheses have been described regarding the details of thalidomide effect on myeloma cell and bone marrow microenvironment. The following paragraph provides a brief summary of possible mechanism of action. Thalidomide has direct antitumor effect on proliferation and viability of drug-resistant myeloma cells, although such effect is at best modest in vitro. Thalidomide affects the adhesion molecules between MM and stromal cells, thus inhibiting the secretion of various cytokines such as interleukin-6 (IL-6), an essential antiapoptotic and proliferate cytokine for MM cells. Thalidomide antiangiogenesis and immune-modulating properties are crucial for its antimyeloma activity.[73–75] Angiogenic cytokines such as VEGF and bFGF are expressed by myeloma cells and play a role in the increased bone marrow angiogenesis in MM.[76] Orally administered thalidomide inhibits many angiogenic cytokines and suppresses tumor necrosis factor-alpha (TNF-alpha) and interferon alpha secretion, leading to inhibition of angiogenesis.[77,78] Although the first trial of thalidomide in MM had failed to show any correlation between response and bone marrow MVD,[10] others observed that thalidomide responses were linked to decrease in MVD as well as decrease in bFGF and VEGF production.[64] Thalidomide inhibits VEGF, bFGF, FGF-2, hepatocyte growth factor (HGF), IL-6, and TNF-alpha. Serum specimens were obtained from 38 patients with relapsed MM before thalidomide was started and at the time of maximum response in responding patients or at thalidomide discontinuation in nonresponders. VEGF serum levels were significantly higher in responding patients. In contrast, baseline serum levels of HGF and TNF were significantly lower in responders. The serum levels of FGF-2 and IL-6 did not correlate with response to thalidomide.[79] In patients receiving thalidomide, high pretreatment TNF-alpha levels (>11 pg/ml) and increased IL-6 of greater than 2 pg/ml predicted for poorer response (TNF-alpha, 48% vs 74% at 2 years, $P = 0.01$; IL-6, 24% vs 70% at 2 years, $P = 0.01$).[80] In a study of 30 patients with MM, cytokine secretion (VEGF, HGF, bFGF, TNF, IL-6, and sIL-6R) and Bcl-2 expression in PB and BM cell cultures significantly decreased after thalidomide but with no clinical correlations.[66] The changes in cytokine level are variable and overall does not correlate with response or survival in MM. Thalidomide has a broad range of inhibitory and stimulatory effects on the immune system.[81,82] Thalidomide triggers proliferation of stimulated T cells and natural killer (NK) "IL-2-primed" from patients with MM, accompanied by an increase in interferon-γ and IL-2 secretion.[83] The lysis of MM cells was mediated by NK cells rather than T-cells.[66] It seems probable that all the aforementioned mechanisms are relevant to the efficacy of thalidomide in MM.

Table 2 Adverse effects of thalidomide in multiple myeloma.

System affected	Side effect	Frequency (%)
Cardiovascular	Edema	57
	Bradycardia	50
	Hypotension	16
CNS	Fatigue	79
	Sensory PN	55
	Muscle weakness	40
	Motor PN	22
	Somnolence	36
	Confusion	28
	Tremors	15
Hematological	Leukopenia	15–30
	Neutropenia	30
	Thrombocytopenia	<5
Endocrine	Hypocalcemia	30
	Hyperlipemia	5–10
	Hypothyroidism	5
	Impotence	3–8
Respiratory	Dyspnea	42
Dermatological	Rash	20–30
Gastrointestinal	Constipation	55
	Weight change	20–40
	Nausea	4–25
Thrombosis	DVT	2–30

PN peripheral neuropathy, *CNS* central nervous system, *DVT* deep vein thrombosis.

Side Effects

Thalidomide side effects can be divided into selective that affect a specific patient population and general that affect all patients receiving the drug. The most common side effects are birth defects, sensorimotor PN, somnolence, rash, fatigue, and constipation. Less common side effects include deep venous thrombosis, Stevens-Johnson syndrome, elevated liver enzymes, malaise, and peripheral edema. The incidence and severity of adverse events are related to dose and duration of therapy (Table 2). Toxicity and intolerability lead to discontinuation of thalidomide in 15% of the patients. The description of side effects in the following section is derived from published clinical studies and relevant case reports. The recommendations for management are to a large extent observational as few studies implemented systematic interventions to provide firm conclusions.

Teratogenicity

Teratogenicity is the most feared toxicity of thalidomide.[84] Dispensation of thalidomide is controlled in the United States by the STEP (System for Thalidomide Education and Prescription Safety) Program. The main purpose of the program is restricting access of the drug to women of childbearing potential who must have a negative pregnancy test before starting thalidomide, and must use two effective methods of contraception; all must have monthly monitoring of pregnancy test while on therapy. Men receiving thalidomide must practice abstinence or use a latex condom during sexual intercourse. After almost a decade of thalidomide use in patients with MM , there are no reported cases of birth defects. There is no data that thalidomide is carcinogenic or genotoxic.

Neurological Effects

All patients receiving thalidomide will complain of sleepiness and drowsiness, especially in the first few weeks on therapy. Tolerance usually occurs as therapy continues. Fatigue, depression, visual disturbances, headache, and, rarely, seizures have been reported with thalidomide use. The most serious neurological complication of thalidomide is PN, which develops in majority of patients with MM receiving thalidomide.[85,86] PN incidence is independent of age, race, or sex, but is higher in patients with preexisting symptoms of PN secondary to diabetes and/or neurotoxic chemotherapy (e.g., vincristine, cisplatin, and paclitaxel) and correlate with the total cumulative dose of thalidomide. Genetic predisposition has been proposed to explain the variability in thalidomide-induced neurotoxicity that may be more common in patients with slower metabolism of the drug. Thalidomide induces an axonal length-dependent PN with electrophysiological evidence of a sensory more than motor damage.[87] Clinically, patients present with painful paresthesias or numbness and tingling that extends from the toes and digits proximally. Later, position sense is affected, leading to ataxia and progressive gait disturbance.[88] To a lesser degree, pyramidal tract damage can occur, leading to motor symptoms (weakness and atrophy) and autonomic dysfunction (incontinence and erectile dysfunction). Nerve biopsies showed evidence of Wallerian degeneration and loss of large myelinated fibers.

To minimize the risk of PN, the lowest dose of the thalidomide that controls the disease should be used. Electrophysiologic monitoring provides no clear benefit versus careful questioning and evaluation for signs and symptoms of PN. If PN grade II and higher develops, immediate discontinuation of thalidomide increases the probability of recovery. Improvement of symptoms occurs within 1–3 weeks in the majority of patients. At that point, restarting therapy at a lower dose can be considered against permanent discontinuation of thalidomide depending on the patient clinical scenario.[89] Patients with more severe symptoms benefit from the use of analgesics, antidepressant drugs such as amitriptylline, serotonin/norepinephrine reuptake inhibitors such as duloxetine, and anticonvulsant drugs such as gabapentin. The routine use of pyridoxine (vitamin B6) should be discouraged; it is well established that large doses of B6 worsen the PN symptoms.[90,91] Patients with painful cramps may benefit from vitamin E and L-carnitine supplement.[92] It is worth noting that patients receiving thalidomide in combination with bortezomib, both neurotoxic drugs, had no grade 4 PN; whether that represents a protective effect or selection bias will need to be further evaluated in a prospective trial.[58,93]

Thrombosis

Thalidomide increases the risk of developing venous thrombotic events (VTEs) probably through induction of prothrombotic factors and activation of platelets as well as vascular endothelial cells.[94] The incidence of VTE in patients with

Table 3 Incidence and risk of thrombo-embolic complications with thalidomide.

Regimen	Prophylaxis			Comments
	None	**Aspirin**	**LMWH**	
Thalidomide alone	2%	–	–	
Thal + dexamethasone	10–15%	5–7%	–	
Thal + chemotherapy	20–35%		10%	Data from total therapy II
Risk factors for VTE	Newly diagnosed with MM			
	Acquired protein C deficiency			
	Erythropoietin			

Thal thalidomide, *VTE* venous thrombotic events, *MM* multiple myeloma, *LMWH* low molecular weight heparin.

MM receiving thalidomide as a single agent is 2.7% (95% CI 1.1–4.3%); the incidence of VTE increases significantly if corticosteroids are used (15–20%) and may be as high as 30% with chemotherapy combinations (Table 3).[95,96] The Research on Adverse Drug Events and Reports (RADAR) project reported VTE in 1076 thalidomide-treated patients with cancer and confirmed higher incidence for thalidomide/dexamethasone-treated patients.[97] On multivariate analysis, the combination of thalidomide with doxorubicin was associated with the highest odds ratio (OR) for VTE (4.3; $P \leq 0.001$).[98] The risk is higher in newly diagnosed patients with MM (OR, 2.5; $P = 0.001$), which is possibly related to temporary resistance to activated protein C and central venous catheters.[99] The use of erythropoiesis-stimulating agents appears to increase the VTE risk in myelodysplastic syndrome but not in.[100] There is no consensus on the indications or the choice of agent for VTE prophylaxis. Most authorities do not recommend prophylaxis when thalidomide is used as a single agent. Aspirin was the preferred form of VTE prophylaxis for most thalidomide-containing regimens.[101] Von Willebrand levels and platelet aggregation increase significantly after thalidomide, suggesting that VTE involve platelet–endothelial interaction, thus making low-dose aspirin (81 mg) an attractive choice for prophylaxis. A randomized trial showed that aspirin decreases the incidence of VTE (58% vs 17.8%) in patients receiving the DVD regimen with thalidomide.[102,103] Doxorubicin-containing regimens have a high incidence of VTE for which low molecular weight heparin (LMWH) decreases the risk of VTE to 10%; however, it must be used carefully in the setting of renal insufficiency and in thrombocytopenic patients.[45,72,104] A survival benefit associated with anticoagulation therapy in MM has been suggested.[105] Patients who develop VTE can safely resume thalidomide after appropriate anticoagulation therapy with warfarin or LMWH. Recently, lower doses of dexamethasone in combination with lenalidomide were associated with a decreased risk of VTE compared to higher doses [18% vs 6%, Eastern Cooperative Oncology Group (ECOG) trial]; whether that is true for thalidomide is unclear.[106]

Dermatological Effects

The most common dermatological adverse effect is a pruritic maculopapular rash, starting on the trunk and extending to the back and proximal limbs.[107] The rash does not appear to be dose related, and is usually reported within

2 weeks after initiating treatment. Discontinuation of thalidomide leads to resolution of the rash; readministration at a lower dose can be done safely in many patients with no recurrence of the rash. Stevens-Johnson syndrome is a life-threatening condition that occurs in less than 1% of thalidomide-treated patients. The use of dexamethasone with thalidomide increases susceptibility to more severe dermatological adverse effects, such as toxic epidermic necrolysis, a serious hypersensitivity reaction with mortality rate over 30%.[108]

Cardiovascular Effects

Cardiac side effects of thalidomide include bradycardia, hypotension, and, rarely, syncope. Up to 50% of the patients on thalidomide are reported to have heart rate less than 60 beats per minute and 19% have symptoms related to bradycardia.[109] The cause of bradycardia is unclear; it occurs at lower doses and is reversible, suggesting no permanent autonomic dysfunction.[110] Pacemaker placement has been advocated to continue thalidomide therapy; however, such as extreme measure in newly diagnosed patients could not be justified with the availability of other effective therapies.[72] Hypotension is dose dependent in thalidomide-treated patients that is usually not accompanied by reflex tachycardia. To avoid orthostatic hypotension, patients should increase fluid intake and stand up slowly from sitting position. The concurrent administration of antidepressants and beta-blockers may induce or worsen hypotension and bradycardia.[111] Peripheral edema has been reported in up to 10% of patients, mostly when thalidomide is combined with corticosteroids.[112] Mild-to-moderate cases respond to diuretics, or, dose reduction, and in severe cases discontinuation of thalidomide.

Gastrointestinal Effects

The most common gastrointestinal adverse effect is constipation. Constipation is probably the most common side effect affecting 70% of the patients. It occurs early after initiation of therapy (2–4 days).[113] It can be severe in elderly patients and in those receiving narcotics. Thalidomide-induced hypothyroidism should be considered in patients with persistent constipation, or when the constipation occurs months after the initiation of thalidomide. Stool softeners and laxatives, maintaining a high fluid intake, and sufficient exercise can alleviate constipation. A temporary interruption of thalidomide may be necessary until bowel motility returns to normal. Nausea and emesis are not common side effects and usually resolve with continued treatment.[114]

Hematologic, Endocrine, and Respiratory Effects

Thalidomide induces a dose-dependent neutropenia that is mild in 3–14% of patients.[115,116] Thrombocytopenia can occur mostly when thalidomide is used as maintenance early after stem cell transplant and is reversible on stopping thalidomide. Subclinical hypothyroidism with elevated thyroid-stimulating hormone (TSH) levels and normal triiodothyronine and thyroxine levels was seen in 20% of thalidomide-treated patients within 3–4 months of therapy.[117] Measurements of TSH levels at baseline and at regular intervals is indicated, although supplementation should be limited to symptomatic cases. Thalidomide may result in erectile dysfunction in men; the incidence is unknown; most resolve with interruption of therapy.

Pulmonary hypertension has been reported with prolonged use of thalidomide; it is unclear if this is a direct effect on the blood vessel or secondary to pulmonary emboli.[118,119] Other thalidomide pulmonary toxicity includes symptomatic effusions, interstitial lung disease, and dyspnea on exertion without any objective pathologic injury.[120,121]

Conclusion

Thalidomide is a relatively safe drug which can be administered over a long period of time, offering many patients with MM longer EFS and OS. In relapsed patients, single-agent thalidomide has ORR of 30% that is further increased to 50% with the addition of dexamethasone. Lower doses of thalidomide (50–200 mg daily) are effective; higher doses (400–800 mg daily) should be carefully limited to nonresponders. Various chemotherapy combinations have response rates between 50% and 70% depending on the patient population and the extent of prior therapy; combinations with novel agents such as bortezomib are particularly interesting. Mechanism of antimyeloma activity of thalidomide remains speculative. The main side effects of thalidomide are drowsiness and constipation, which requires prophylactic use of stool softeners. Risk of thrombosis is low (2%) when thalidomide is used as a single agent. Prophylaxis is indicated in patients receiving combination therapy. There is no data about the best prophylaxis, although aspirin was safe and effective in one randomized trial. PN is the most serious complication of thalidomide treatment; it was reported in 70% of patients after prolonged use of thalidomide. Most patients recover after withdrawal of thalidomide. The role of thalidomide as salvage for patients who received thalidomide as upfront induction and as maintenance after transplant remains to be determined.

References

1. Stephens, T. & Brynner, R. (2001). *Dark Remedy*. First edn, Perseus Publishing Cambridge, Massachusetts.
2. Hales, B. F. (1999). Thalidomide on the comeback trail. *Nat Med* 5, 489–90.
3. Grabstald, H. & Golbey, R. (1965). Clinical experience with thaliomide in patients with cancer. *Clin Pharmacol Ther* 40, 298–302.
4. Alson, K., Hall, T., Horton, J. et al. (1965). Thalidomide in treatment of advanced cancer. *Clin Pharmaco Ther* 40, 292–7.
5. Pagnini, G. & Dicarlo, R. (1963). [Treatment of experimental tumors with thalidomide]. *Boll Soc Ital Biol Sper* 39, 1360–3.
6. Goldman, D. A. (2001). Thalidomide use: past history and current implications for practice. *Oncol Nurs Forum* 28, 471–7; quiz 478–9.
7. von Moos, R., Stolz, R., Cerny, T. & Gillessen, S. (2003). Thalidomide: from tragedy to promise. *Swiss Med Wkly* 133, 77–87.
8. Okafor, M. C. (2003). Thalidomide for erythema nodosum leprosum and other applications. *Pharmacotherapy* 23, 481–93.
9. Matthews, S. J. & McCoy, C. (2003). Thalidomide: a review of approved and investigational uses. *Clin Ther* 25, 342–95.
10. Singhal, S., Mehta, J., Desikan, R., Ayers, D., Roberson, P., Eddlemon, P., Munshi, N., Anaissie, E., Wilson, C., Dhodapkar, M., Zeddis, J. & Barlogie, B.

(1999). Antitumor activity of thalidomide in refractory multiple myeloma. *N Engl J Med* 341, 1565–71.

11. Jonsson, N. A. (1972). Chemical structure and teratogenic properties. IV. An outline of a chemical hypothesis for the teratogenic action of thalidomide. *Acta Pharm Suec* 9, 543–62.

12. Izumi, H., Futamura, S., Tokita, N. & Hamada, Y. (2007). Flip like motion in the thalidomide dimer: conformational analysis of (R)-thalidomide using vibrational circular dichroism spectroscopy. *J Org Chem* 72, 277–9.

13. Goosen, C., Laing, T. J., du Plessis, J., Goosen, T. C., Rao, T. B. & Flynn, G. L. (2002). Chemical stabilities and biological activities of thalidomide and its N-alkyl analogs. *Pharm Res* 19, 1232–5.

14. Figg, W. D., Raje, S., Bauer, K. S., Tompkins, A., Venzon, D., Bergan, R., Chen, A., Hamilton, M., Pluda, J. & Reed, E. (1999). Pharmacokinetics of thalidomide in an elderly prostate cancer population. *J Pharm Sci* 88, 121–5.

15. Chen, T. L., Vogelsang, G. B., Petty, B. G., Brundrett, R. B., Noe, D. A., Santos, G. W. & Colvin, O. M. (1989). Plasma pharmacokinetics and urinary excretion of thalidomide after oral dosing in healthy male volunteers. *Drug Metab Dispos* 17, 402–5.

16. Teo, S. K., Colburn, W. A., Tracewell, W. G., Kook, K. A., Stirling, D. I., Jaworsky, M. S., Scheffler, M. A., Thomas, S. D. & Laskin, O. L. (2004). Clinical pharmacokinetics of thalidomide. *Clin Pharmacokinet* 43, 311–27.

17. Eriksson, T., Bjorkman, S. & Hoglund, P. (2001). Clinical pharmacology of thalidomide. *Eur J Clin Pharmacol* 57, 365–76.

18. Chung, F., Lu, J., Palmer, B. D., Kestell, P., Browett, P., Baguley, B. C., Tingle, M. & Ching, L. M. (2004). Thalidomide pharmacokinetics and metabolite formation in mice, rabbits, and multiple myeloma patients. *Clin Cancer Res* 10, 5949–56.

19. Ando, Y., Fuse, E. & Figg, W. D. (2002). Thalidomide metabolism by the CYP2C subfamily. *Clin Cancer Res* 8, 1964–73.

20. Lu, J., Helsby, N., Palmer, B. D., Tingle, M., Baguley, B. C., Kestell, P. & Ching, L. M. (2004). Metabolism of thalidomide in liver microsomes of mice, rabbits, and humans. *J Pharmacol Exp Ther* 310, 571–7.

21. Lepper, E. R., Smith, N. F., Cox, M. C., Scripture, C. D. & Figg, W. D. (2006). Thalidomide metabolism and hydrolysis: mechanisms and implications. *Curr Drug Metab* 7, 677–85.

22. Thurmann, P. A. (2005). [Gender-related differences in pharmacokinetics and pharmacodynamics]. *Bundesgesundheitsblatt Gesundheitsforschung Gesundheitsschutz* 48, 536–40.

23. Kamikawa, R., Ikawa, K., Morikawa, N., Asaoku, H., Iwato, K. & Sasaki, A. (2006). The pharmacokinetics of low-dose thalidomide in Japanese patients with refractory multiple myeloma. *Biol Pharm Bull* 29, 2331–4.

24. Barlogie, B., Desikan, R., Eddlemon, P., Spencer, T., Zeldis, J., Munshi, N., Badros, A., Zangari, M., Anaissie, E., Epstein, J., Shaughnessy, J., Ayers, D., Spoon, D. & Tricot, G. (2001). Extended survival in advanced and refractory multiple myeloma after single-agent thalidomide: identification of prognostic factors in a phase 2 study of 169 patients. *Blood* 98, 492–4.

25. Barlogie, B. (2003). Thalidomide and CC-5013 in multiple myeloma: the University of Arkansas experience. *Semin Hematol* 40, 33–8.

26. Glasmacher, A., Hahn, C., Hoffmann, F., Naumann, R., Goldschmidt, H., von Lilienfeld-Toal, M., Orlopp, K., Schmidt-Wolf, I. & Gorschluter, M. (2006). A systematic review of phase-II trials of thalidomide monotherapy in patients with relapsed or refractory multiple myeloma. *Br J Haematol* 132, 584–93.

27. Prince, H. M., Schenkel, B. & Mileshkin, L. (2007). An analysis of clinical trials assessing the efficacy and safety of single-agent thalidomide in patients with relapsed or refractory multiple myeloma. *Leuk Lymphoma* 48, 46–55.

28. Thompson, J. L. & Hansen, L. A. (2003). Thalidomide dosing in patients with relapsed or refractory multiple myeloma. *Ann Pharmacother* 37, 571–6.

29. Weber, D. (2003). Thalidomide and its derivatives: new promise for multiple myeloma. *Cancer Control* 10, 375–83.

30. Dimopoulos, M. A., Zervas, K., Kouvatseas, G., Galani, E., Grigoraki, V., Kiamouris, C., Vervessou, E., Samantas, E., Papadimitriou, C., Economou, O., Gika, D., Panayiotidis, P., Christakis, I. & Anagnostopoulos, N. (2001). Thalidomide and dexamethasone combination for refractory multiple myeloma. *Ann Oncol* 12, 991–5.

31. Palumbo, A., Giaccone, L., Bertola, A., Pregno, P., Bringhen, S., Rus, C., Triolo, S., Gallo, E., Pileri, A. & Boccadoro, M. (2001). Low-dose thalidomide plus dexamethasone is an effective salvage therapy for advanced myeloma. *Haematologica* 86, 399–403.

32. Palumbo, A., Falco, P., Ambrosini, M. T., Petrucci, M. T., Musto, P., Caravita, T., Pregno, P., Bertola, A., Cavallo, F., Ciccone, G. & Boccadoro, M. (2005). Thalidomide plus dexamethasone is an effective salvage regimen for myeloma patients relapsing after autologous transplant. *Eur J Haematol* 75, 391–5.

33. Coleman, M., Leonard, J., Lyons, L., Pekle, K., Nahum, K., Pearse, R., Niesvizky, R. & Michaeli, J. (2002). BLT-D (clarithromycin [Biaxin], low-dose thalidomide, and dexamethasone) for the treatment of myeloma and Waldenstrom's macroglobulinemia. *Leuk Lymphoma* 43, 1777–82.

34. Badros, A. Z., Goloubeva, O., Rapoport, A. P., Ratterree, B., Gahres, N., Meisenberg, B., Takebe, N., Heyman, M., Zwiebel, J., Streicher, H., Gocke, C. D., Tomic, D., Flaws, J. A., Zhang, B. & Fenton, R. G. (2005). Phase II study of G3139, a Bcl-2 antisense oligonucleotide, in combination with dexamethasone and thalidomide in relapsed multiple myeloma patients. *J Clin Oncol* 23, 4089–99.

35. Rajkumar, S. V., Blood, E., Vesole, D., Fonseca, R. & Greipp, P. R. (2006). Phase III clinical trial of thalidomide plus dexamethasone compared with dexamethasone alone in newly diagnosed multiple myeloma: a clinical trial coordinated by the Eastern Cooperative Oncology Group. *J Clin Oncol* 24, 431–6.

36. Richardson, P. & Anderson, K. (2006). Thalidomide and dexamethasone: a new standard of care for initial therapy in multiple myeloma. *J Clin Oncol* 24, 334–6.

37. Kropff, M. H., Lang, N., Bisping, G., Domine, N., Innig, G., Hentrich, M., Mitterer, M., Sudhoff, T., Fenk, R., Straka, C., Heinecke, A., Koch, O. M., Ostermann, H., Berdel, W. E. & Kienast, J. (2003). Hyperfractionated cyclophosphamide in combination with pulsed dexamethasone and thalidomide (HyperCDT) in primary refractory or relapsed multiple myeloma. *Br J Haematol* 122, 607–16.

38. Dimopoulos, M. A., Hamilos, G., Zomas, A., Gika, D., Efstathiou, E., Grigoraki, V., Poziopoulos, C., Xilouri, I., Zorzou, M. P., Anagnostopoulos, N. & Anagnostopoulos, A. (2004). Pulsed cyclophosphamide, thalidomide and dexamethasone: an oral regimen for previously treated patients with multiple myeloma. *Hematol J* 5, 112–7.

39. Suvannasankha, A., Fausel, C., Juliar, B. E., Yiannoutsos, C. T., Fisher, W. B., Ansari, R. H., Wood, L. L., Smith, G. G., Cripe, L. D. & Abonour, R. (2007). Final report of toxicity and efficacy of a phase II study of oral cyclophosphamide, thalidomide, and prednisone for patients with relapsed or refractory multiple myeloma: a Hoosier Oncology Group Trial, HEM01–21. *Oncologist* 12, 99–106.

40. Moehler, T. M., Neben, K., Benner, A., Egerer, G., Krasniqi, F., Ho, A. D. & Goldschmidt, H. (2001). Salvage therapy for multiple myeloma with thalidomide and CED chemotherapy. *Blood* 98, 3846–8.

41. Lee, C. K., Barlogie, B., Munshi, N., Zangari, M., Fassas, A., Jacobson, J., van Rhee, F., Cottler-Fox, M., Muwalla, F. & Tricot, G. (2003). DTPACE: an effective, novel combination chemotherapy with thalidomide for previously treated patients with myeloma. *J Clin Oncol* 21, 2732–9.

42. Badros, A. & Gahres, N. (2005). Bortezomib, thalidomide, and dexamethasone for relapsed multiple myeloma: add it up and wait. *Clin Adv Hematol Oncol* 3, 916–7; discussion 918.

43. Chung, F., Wang, L. C., Kestell, P., Baguley, B. C. & Ching, L. M. (2004). Modulation of thalidomide pharmacokinetics by cyclophosphamide or 5,6-dimethylxanthenone-4-acetic acid (DMXAA) in mice: the role of tumour necrosis factor. *Cancer Chemother Pharmacol* 53, 377–83.

44. Dimopoulos, M. A., Anagnostopoulos, A., Terpos, E., Repoussis, P., Zomas, A., Katodritou, E., Kyrtsonis, M. C., Delibasi, S., Vassou, A., Pouli, A., Zervas, K., Anagnostopoulos, N. & Maniatis, A. (2006). Primary treatment with pulsed melphalan, dexamethasone and thalidomide for elderly symptomatic patients with multiple myeloma. *Haematologica* 91, 252–4.

45. Palumbo, A., Bringhen, S., Caravita, T., Merla, E., Capparella, V., Callea, V., Cangialosi, C., Grasso, M., Rossini, F., Galli, M., Catalano, L., Zamagni, E., Petrucci, M. T., De Stefano, V., Ceccarelli, M., Ambrosini, M. T., Avonto, I., Falco, P., Ciccone, G., Liberati, A. M., Musto, P. & Boccadoro, M. (2006). Oral melphalan and prednisone chemotherapy plus thalidomide compared with melphalan and prednisone alone in elderly patients with multiple myeloma: randomised controlled trial. *Lancet* 367, 825–31.

46. Srkalovic, G., Elson, P., Trebisky, B., Karam, M. A. & Hussein, M. A. (2002). Use of melphalan, thalidomide, and dexamethasone in treatment of refractory and relapsed multiple myeloma. *Med Oncol* 19, 219–26.

47. Offidani, M., Marconi, M., Corvatta, L., Olivieri, A., Catarini, M. & Leoni, P. (2003). Thalidomide plus oral melphalan for advanced multiple myeloma: a phase II study. *Haematologica* 88, 1432–3.

48. Offidani, M., Corvatta, L., Marconi, M., Olivieri, A., Catarini, M., Mele, A., Brunori, M., Candela, M., Malerba, L., Capelli, D., Montanari, M. & Leoni, P. (2004). Thalidomide plus oral melphalan compared with thalidomide alone for advanced multiple myeloma. *Hematol J* 5, 312–7.

49. Palumbo, A., Avonto, I., Bruno, B., Ambrosini, M. T., Bringhen, S., Cavallo, F., Falco, P. & Boccadoro, M. (2006). Intravenous melphalan, thalidomide and prednisone in refractory and relapsed multiple myeloma. *Eur J Haematol* 76, 273–7.

50. Economopoulos, T., Pappa, V., Panani, A., Stathakis, N., Dervenoulas, J., Papageorgiou, E., Asprou, N. & Raptis, S. (1991). Myelopathies during the course of multiple myeloma. *Haematologica* 76, 289–92.

51. Badros, A., Morris, C., Zangari, M., Barlogie, B. & Tricot, G. (2002). Thalidomide paradoxical effect on concomitant multiple myeloma and myelodysplasia. *Leuk Lymphoma* 43, 1267–71.

52. Hussein, M. A. (2003). Modifications to therapy for multiple myeloma: pegylated liposomal Doxorubicin in combination with vincristine, reduced-dose dexamethasone, and thalidomide. *Oncologist* 8 Suppl 3, 39–45.

53. Hussein, M. A., Baz, R., Srkalovic, G., Agrawal, N., Suppiah, R., Hsi, E., Andresen, S., Karam, M. A., Reed, J., Faiman, B., Kelly, M. & Walker, E. (2006). Phase 2 study of pegylated liposomal doxorubicin, vincristine, decreased-frequency dexamethasone, and thalidomide in newly diagnosed and relapsed-refractory multiple myeloma. *Mayo Clin Proc* 81, 889–95.

54. Offidani, M., Bringhen, S., Corvatta, L., Falco, P., Marconi, M., Avonto, I., Piersantelli, M. N., Polloni, C., Boccadoro, M., Leoni, P. & Palumbo, A. (2007). Thalidomide-dexamethasone plus pegylated liposomal doxorubicin vs. thalidomide-dexamethasone: a case-matched study in advanced multiple myeloma. *Eur J Haematol* 78(4), 297–302.

55. Zangari, M., Barlogie, B., Hollmig, K., Fassas, A., Rasmussen, E., Thertulien, R., Talamo, G., Lee, C. K. & Tricot, G. (2004). Marked activity of velcade plus thalidomide (V plus T) in advanced and refractory multiple myeloma (MM). *Blood* 104, 413A–414A.

56. Zangari, M., Barlogie, B., Jacobson, J., Rasmussen, E., Burns, M., Kordsmeier, B., Shaughnessy, J. D., Anaissie, E. J., Thertulien, R., Fassas, A., Lee, C. K., Schenkein, D., Zeldis, J. B. & Tricot, G. (2003). VTD regimen comprising velcade (V) plus thalidomide (T) and added DEX (D) for non-responders to V + T effects a 57% PR rate among 56 patients with myeloma (M) relapsing after autologous transplant. *Blood* 102, 236A–236A.

57. Ciolli, S., Leoni, F., Gigli, F., Rigacci, L. & Bosi, A. (2006). Low dose Velcade, thalidomide and dexamethasone (LD-VTD): an effective regimen for relapsed and refractory multiple myeloma patients. *Leuk Lymphoma* 47, 171–3.

58. Palumbo, A., Ambrosini, M. T., Benevolo, G., Pregno, P., Pescosta, N., Callea, V., Cangialosi, C., Caravita, T., Morabito, F., Musto, P., Bringhen, S., Falco, P., Avonto, I., Cavallo, F. & Boccadoro, M. (2007). Bortezomib, melphalan, prednisone and thalidomide for relapsed multiple myeloma. *Blood* 109, 2767–2772.

59. Palumbo, A., Avonto, I., Bruno, B., Falcone, A., Scalzulli, P. R., Ambrosini, M. T., Bringhen, S., Gay, F., Rus, C., Cavallo, F., Falco, P., Massaia, M., Musto, P. & Boccadoro, M. (2006). Intermediate-dose melphalan (100 mg/m2)/bortezomib/thalidomide/dexamethasone and stem cell support in patients with refractory or relapsed myeloma. *Clin Lymphoma Myeloma* 6, 475–7.

60. Neben, K., Moehler, T., Benner, A., Kraemer, A., Egerer, G., Ho, A. D. & Goldschmidt, H. (2002). Dose-dependent effect of thalidomide on overall survival in relapsed multiple myeloma. *Clin Cancer Res* 8, 3377–82.

61. Johnston, R. E. & Abdalla, S. H. (2002). Thalidomide in low doses is effective for the treatment of resistant or relapsed multiple myeloma and for plasma cell leukaemia. *Leuk Lymphoma* 43, 351–4.

62. Durie, B. G. (2002). Low-dose thalidomide in myeloma: efficacy and biologic significance. *Semin Oncol* 29, 34–8.

63. Cibeira, M. T., Rosinol, L., Ramiro, L., Esteve, J., Torrebadell, M. & Blade, J. (2006). Long-term results of thalidomide in refractory and relapsed multiple myeloma with emphasis on response duration. *Eur J Haematol* 77, 486–92.

64. Kumar, S., Witzig, T. E., Dispenzieri, A., Lacy, M. Q., Wellik, L. E., Fonseca, R., Lust, J. A., Gertz, M. A., Kyle, R. A., Greipp, P. R. & Rajkumar, S. V. (2004). Effect of thalidomide therapy on bone marrow angiogenesis in multiple myeloma. *Leukemia* 18, 624–7.

65. Neben, K., Moehler, T., Egerer, G., Kraemer, A., Hillengass, J., Benner, A., Ho, A. D. & Goldschmidt, H. (2001). High plasma basic fibroblast growth factor concentration is associated with response to thalidomide in progressive multiple myeloma. *Clin Cancer Res* 7, 2675–81.

66. Dmoszynska, A., Podhorecka, M., Manko, J., Bojarska-Junak, A., Rolinski, J. & Skomra, D. (2005). The influence of thalidomide therapy on cytokine secretion, immunophenotype, BCL-2 expression and microvessel density in patients with resistant or relapsed multiple myeloma. *Neoplasma* 52, 175–81.

67. Schutt, P., Ebeling, P., Buttkereit, U., Brandhorst, D., Opalka, B., Poser, M., Muller, S., Flasshove, M., Moritz, T., Seeber, S. & Nowrousian, M. R. (2005). Thalidomide in combination with dexamethasone for pretreated patients with multiple myeloma: serum level of soluble interleukin-2 receptor as a predictive factor for response rate and for survival. *Ann Hematol* 84, 594–600.

68. Blade, J., Perales, M., Rosinol, L., Tuset, M., Montoto, S., Esteve, J., Cobo, F., Villela, L., Rafel, M., Nomdedeu, B. & Montserrat, E. (2001). Thalidomide in multiple myeloma: lack of response of soft-tissue plasmacytomas. *Br J Haematol* 113, 422–4.

69. Juliusson, G., Celsing, F., Turesson, I., Lenhoff, S., Adriansson, M. & Malm, C. (2000). Frequent good partial remissions from thalidomide including best response ever in patients with advanced refractory and relapsed myeloma. *Br J Haematol* 109, 89–96.

70. Avigdor, A., Raanani, P., Levi, I., Hardan, I. & Ben-Bassat, I. (2001). Extramedullary progression despite a good response in the bone marrow in patients treated with thalidomide for multiple myeloma. *Leuk Lymphoma* 42, 683–7.

71. Rosinol, L., Cibeira, M. T., Blade, J., Esteve, J., Aymerich, M., Rozman, M., Segarra, M., Cid, M. C., Filella, X. & Montserrat, E. (2004). Extramedullary multiple myeloma escapes the effect of thalidomide. *Haematologica* 89, 832–6.

72. Barlogie, B., Tricot, G., Anaissie, E., Shaughnessy, J., Rasmussen, E., van Rhee, F., Fassas, A., Zangari, M., Hollmig, K., Pineda-Roman, M., Lee, C., Talamo, G., Thertulien, R., Kiwan, E., Krishna, S., Fox, M. & Crowley, J. (2006). Thalidomide and hematopoietic-cell transplantation for multiple myeloma. *N Engl J Med* 354, 1021–30.

73. Stirling, D. (2001). Thalidomide: a novel template for anticancer drugs. *Semin Oncol* 28, 602–6.

74. D'Amato, R. J., Lentzsch, S., Anderson, K. C. & Rogers, M. S. (2001). Mechanism of action of thalidomide and 3-aminothalidomide in multiple myeloma. *Semin Oncol* 28, 597–601.

75. Anderson, K. C. & Prince, H. M. (2005). Lenalidomide and thalidomide: an evolving paradigm for the management of multiple myeloma. *Semin Hematol* 42, S1–2.

76. Rajkumar, S. V. & Witzig, T. E. (2000). A review of angiogenesis and antiangiogenic therapy with thalidomide in multiple myeloma. *Cancer Treat Rev* 26, 351–62.

77. Du, W., Hattori, Y., Hashiguchi, A., Kondoh, K., Hozumi, N., Ikeda, Y., Sakamoto, M., Hata, J. & Yamada, T. (2004). Tumor angiogenesis in the bone marrow of multiple myeloma patients and its alteration by thalidomide treatment. *Pathol Int* 54, 285–94.

78. Jurczyszyn, A., Wolska-Smolen, T. & Skotnicki, A. B. (2003). [Multiple myeloma: the role of angiogenesis and therapeutic application of thalidomide]. *Przegl Lek* 60, 542–7.

79. Rosinol, L., Cibeira, M. T., Segarra, M., Cid, M. C., Filella, X., Aymerich, M., Rozman, M., Arenillas, L., Esteve, J., Blade, J. & Montserrat, E. (2004). Response to thalidomide in multiple myeloma: impact of angiogenic factors. *Cytokine* 26, 145–8.

80. Thompson, M. A., Witzig, T. E., Kumar, S., Timm, M. M., Haug, J., Fonseca, R., Greipp, P. R., Lust, J. A. & Rajkumar, S. V. (2003). Plasma levels of tumour necrosis factor alpha and interleukin-6 predict progression-free survival following thalidomide therapy in patients with previously untreated multiple myeloma. *Br J Haematol* 123, 305–8.

81. Dredge, K., Marriott, J. B. & Dalgleish, A. G. (2002). Immunological effects of thalidomide and its chemical and functional analogs. *Crit Rev Immunol* 22, 425–37.

82. Schutt, P., Buttkereit, U., Brandhorst, D., Lindemann, M., Schmiedl, S., Grosse-Wilde, H., Seeber, S., Nowrousian, M. R., Opalka, B. & Moritz, T. (2005). In vitro dendritic cell generation and lymphocyte subsets in myeloma patients: influence of thalidomide and high-dose chemotherapy treatment. *Cancer Immunol Immunother* 54, 506–12.

83. Davies, F. E., Raje, N., Hideshima, T., Lentzsch, S., Young, G., Tai, Y. T., Lin, B., Podar, K., Gupta, D., Chauhan, D., Treon, S. P., Richardson, P. G., Schlossman, R. L., Morgan, G. J., Muller, G. W., Stirling, D. I. & Anderson, K. C. (2001). Thalidomide and immunomodulatory derivatives augment natural killer cell cytotoxicity in multiple myeloma. *Blood* 98, 210–6.

84. Neiger, B. L. (2000). The re-emergence of thalidomide: results of a scientific conference. *Teratology* 62, 432–5.

85. Chaudhry, V., Cornblath, D. R., Corse, A., Freimer, M., Simmons-O'Brien, E. & Vogelsang, G. (2002). Thalidomide-induced neuropathy. *Neurology* 59, 1872–5.

86. Crawford, C. L. (2002). Thalidomide-induced neuropathy. Author's reply *Mayo Clin Proc* 77, 1395.

87. Isoardo, G., Bergui, M., Durelli, L., Barbero, P., Boccadoro, M., Bertola, A., Ciaramitaro, P., Palumbo, A., Bergamasco, B. & Cocito, D. (2004). Thalidomide neuropathy: clinical, electrophysiological and neuroradiological features. *Acta Neurol Scand* 109, 188–93.

88. Laaksonen, S., Remes, K., Koskela, K., Voipio-Pulkki, L. M. & Falck, B. (2005). Thalidomide therapy and polyneuropathy in myeloma patients. *Electromyogr Clin Neurophysiol* 45, 75–86.

89. Mileshkin, L., Stark, R., Day, B., Seymour, J. F., Zeldis, J. B. & Prince, H. M. (2006). Development of neuropathy in patients with myeloma treated with thalidomide: patterns of occurrence and the role of electrophysiologic monitoring. *J Clin Oncol* 24, 4507–14.

90. Katan, M. B. (2005). [How much vitamin B6 is toxic?]. *Ned Tijdschr Geneeskd* 149, 2545–6.

91. Levine, S. & Saltzman, A. (2004). Pyridoxine (vitamin B6) neurotoxicity: enhancement by protein-deficient diet. *J Appl Toxicol* 24, 497–500.

92. Offidani, M., Corvatta, L., Marconi, M., Malerba, L., Mele, A., Olivieri, A., Brunori, M., Catarini, M., Candela, M., Capelli, D., Montanari, M., Rupoli, S. & Leoni, P. (2004). Common and rare side-effects of low-dose thalidomide in multiple myeloma: focus on the dose-minimizing peripheral neuropathy. *Eur J Haematol* 72, 403–9.

93. van de Donk, N. W., Kroger, N., Hegenbart, U., Corradini, P., San Miguel, J. F., Goldschmidt, H., Perez-Simon, J. A., Zijlmans, M., Raymakers, R. A., Montefusco, V., Ayuk, F. A., van Oers, M. H., Nagler, A., Verdonck, L. F. & Lokhorst, H. M. (2006). Remarkable activity of novel agents bortezomib and thalidomide in patients not responding to donor lymphocyte infusions following nonmyeloablative allogeneic stem cell transplantation in multiple myeloma. *Blood* 107, 3415–6.

94. Zangari, M., Saghafifar, F., Mehta, P., Barlogie, B., Fink, L. & Tricot, G. (2003). The blood coagulation mechanism in multiple myeloma. *Semin Thromb Hemost* 29, 275–82.

95. Zangari, M., Anaissie, E., Barlogie, B., Badros, A., Desikan, R., Gopal, A. V., Morris, C., Toor, A., Siegel, E., Fink, L. & Tricot, G. (2001). Increased risk of deep-vein thrombosis in patients with multiple myeloma receiving thalidomide and chemotherapy. *Blood* 98, 1614–5.

96. Zangari, M., Siegel, E., Barlogie, B., Anaissie, E., Saghafifar, F., Fassas, A., Morris, C., Fink, L. & Tricot, G. (2002). Thrombogenic activity of doxorubicin in myeloma patients receiving thalidomide: implications for therapy. *Blood* 100, 1168–71.

97. Bennett, C. L., Hussain, Z., Courtney, M., Yarnold, P., Raisch, D. & McKoy, J. M. (2006). RADAR update on thalidomide (Thal)- and lenalidomide (Len)-associated venous thromboembolism (VTE): safety concerns persist for multiple myeloma (MM) despite FDA approvals in this setting. *ASH Annual Meeting Abstracts* 108, 3310A.

98. Zangari, M., Barlogie, B., Thertulien, R., Jacobson, J., Eddleman, P., Fink, L., Fassas, A., Van Rhee, F., Talamo, G., Lee, C. K. & Tricot, G. (2003). Thalidomide and deep vein thrombosis in multiple myeloma: risk factors and effect on survival. *Clin Lymphoma* 4, 32–5.

99. Zangari, M., Saghafifar, F., Anaissie, E., Badros, A., Desikan, R., Fassas, A., Mehta, P., Morris, C., Toor, A., Whitfield, D., Siegel, E., Barlogie, B., Fink, L. & Tricot, G. (2002). Activated protein C resistance in the absence of factor V Leiden mutation is a common finding in multiple myeloma and is associated with an increased risk of thrombotic complications. *Blood Coagul Fibrinolysis* 13, 187–92.

100. Zangari, M., Cavallo, F., Prasad, K., Fink, L., Coon, S., Barlogie, B. & Tricot, G. (2006). Erythropoietin therapy and venous thromboembolic events in patients with multiple myeloma receiving chemotherapy with or without thalidomide. *ASH Annual Meeting Abstracts* 108, 3572A.

101. Durie, B. G. M., Richardson, P., Palumbo, A., Dimopoulos, M. A., Cavo, M., Hajek, R., Joshua, D. E., Shimizu, K., Tricot, G. J., Gertz, M., Tosi, P., Vesole, D. H., Hussein, M. A., Ludwig, H., Goldschmidt, H., Miguel, J. F. S., Sonneveld, P. & Rajkumar, S. V. (2006). Deep vein thrombosis in myeloma: estimate of

prevelance and recommendations for therapy based upon a survey of members of the International Myeloma Working Group (IMWG). *ASH Annual Meeting Abstracts* 108, 3571–.

102. Baz, R., Li, L., Kottke-Marchant, K., Srkalovic, G., McGowan, B., Yiannaki, E., Karam, M. A., Faiman, B., Jawde, R. A., Andresen, S., Zeldis, J. & Hussein, M. A. (2005). The role of aspirin in the prevention of thrombotic complications of thalidomide and anthracycline-based chemotherapy for multiple myeloma. *Mayo Clin Proc* 80, 1568–74.

103. Jimenez, V. H., Dominguez, V., Reynoso, E. & Lopez, I. (2006). Thromboprophylaxis with aspirin for newly diagnosed multiple myeloma treated with thalidomide plus dexamethasone: a preliminary report. *ASH Annual Meeting Abstracts* 108, 5091A.

104. Zangari, M., Barlogie, B., Anaissie, E., Saghafifar, F., Eddlemon, P., Jacobson, J., Lee, C. K., Thertulien, R., Talamo, G., Thomas, T., Van Rhee, F., Fassas, A., Fink, L. & Tricot, G. (2004). Deep vein thrombosis in patients with multiple myeloma treated with thalidomide and chemotherapy: effects of prophylactic and therapeutic anticoagulation. *Br J Haematol* 126, 715–21.

105. Zangari, M., Cavallo, F., Fink, L. M., Barlogie, B., Bolejack, V., Burns, M. J., Anaissie, E., Hollmig, K. A., Mohiuddin, A., Pineda-Roman, M. & Tricot, G. J. (2006). Treatment associated venous thromboembolism (VTE) and survival in multiple myeloma patients. *ASH Annual Meeting Abstracts* 108, 3573–.

106. Rajkumar, S. V., Jacobus, S., Callander, N., Fonseca, R., Vesole, D. & Greipp, P. (2006). A randomized phase III trial of lenalidomide plus high-dose dexamethasone versus lenalidomide plus low-dose dexamethasone in newly diagnosed multiple myeloma (E4A03): a trial coordinated by the Eastern Cooperative Oncology Group. *ASH Annual Meeting Abstracts* 108, 799A.

107. Hall, V. C., El-Azhary, R. A., Bouwhuis, S. & Rajkumar, S. V. (2003). Dermatologic side effects of thalidomide in patients with multiple myeloma. *J Am Acad Dermatol* 48, 548–52.

108. Rajkumar, S. V., Gertz, M. A. & Witzig, T. E. (2000). Life-threatening toxic epidermal necrolysis with thalidomide therapy for myeloma. *N Engl J Med* 343, 972–3.

109. Fahdi, I. E., Gaddam, V., Saucedo, J. F., Kishan, C. V., Vyas, K., Deneke, M. G., Razek, H., Thorn, B., Bissett, J. K., Anaissie, E. J., Barlogie, B. & Mehta, J. L. (2004). Bradycardia during therapy for multiple myeloma with thalidomide. *Am J Cardiol* 93, 1052–5.

110. Coutsouvelis, J. & Corallo, C. E. (2004). Thalidomide-induced bradycardia and its management. *Med J Aust* 180, 366–7.

111. Haslett, P., Tramontana, J., Burroughs, M., Hempstead, M. & Kaplan, G. (1997). Adverse reactions to thalidomide in patients infected with human immunodeficiency virus. *Clin Infect Dis* 24, 1223–7.

112. Dispenzieri, A., Lacy, M. Q., Rajkumar, S. V., Geyer, S. M., Witzig, T. E., Fonseca, R., Lust, J. A., Greipp, P. R., Kyle, R. A. & Gertz, M. A. (2003). Poor tolerance to high doses of thalidomide in patients with primary systemic amyloidosis. *Amyloid* 10, 257–61.

113. Dimopoulos, M. A. & Eleutherakis-Papaiakovou, V. (2004). Adverse effects of thalidomide administration in patients with neoplastic diseases. *Am J Med* 117, 508–15.

114. Ghobrial, I. M. & Rajkumar, S. V. (2003). Management of thalidomide toxicity. *J Support Oncol* 1, 194–205.

115. Hattori, Y., Kakimoto, T., Okamoto, S., Sato, N. & Ikeda, Y. (2004). Thalidomide-induced severe neutropenia during treatment of multiple myeloma. *Int J Hematol* 79, 283–8.

116. McCarthy, D. A., Macey, M. G., Streetly, M., Schey, S. A. & Brown, K. A. (2006). The neutropenia induced by the thalidomide analogue CC-4047 in patients with

multiple myeloma is associated with an increased percentage of neutrophils bearing CD64. *Int Immunopharmacol* 6, 1194–203.

117. Badros, A. Z., Siegel, E., Bodenner, D., Zangari, M., Zeldis, J., Barlogie, B. & Tricot, G. (2002). Hypothyroidism in patients with multiple myeloma following treatment with thalidomide. *Am J Med* 112, 412–3.

118. Hattori, Y., Shimoda, M., Okamoto, S., Satoh, T., Kakimoto, T. & Ikeda, Y. (2005). Pulmonary hypertension and thalidomide therapy in multiple myeloma. *Br J Haematol* 128, 885–7; author reply 887–8.

119. Younis, T. H., Alam, A., Paplham, P., Spangenthal, E. & McCarthy, P. (2003). Reversible pulmonary hypertension and thalidomide therapy for multiple myeloma. *Br J Haematol* 121, 191–2.

120. Behrens, R. J., Gulley, J. L. & Dahut, W. L. (2003). Pulmonary toxicity during prostate cancer treatment with docetaxel and thalidomide. *Am J Ther* 10, 228–32.

121. Carrion Valero, F. & Bertomeu Gonzalez, V. (2002). [Lung toxicity due to thalidomide]. *Arch Bronconeumol* 38, 492–4.

Chapter 14

Thalidomide: Induction Therapy

Francis K. Buadi and S. Vincent Rajkumar

Introduction

Multiple myeloma (MM) is a clonal stem cell disorder characterized by the presence of a monoclonal protein in the serum or urine, osteolytic bone lesions, increased plasma cells in the bone marrow, anemia, renal insufficiency, and hypercalcemia.[1,2] The initial treatment of patients with MM has gone through changes over the years. The current management concept is to increase remission rates, progression-free survival (PFS), overall survival, and quality of life since MM is still incurable.[3,4] However, with the current availability of multiple targeted therapies with comparable and sometimes superior efficacy and improved survival, the side-effect profile and long-term toxicity has become a major factor.

High-dose therapy with autologous stem cell transplant as part of initial therapy is currently considered the standard of care for patients who are eligible for transplant.[5,6] It is therefore important to avoid stem cell toxic drugs as part of induction therapy in patients eligible for peripheral blood stem cell transplant so as to not compromise stem cell mobilization. The quality of remission before transplant may also have a significant effect on long-term outcome after transplant.[7] The search for the best or optimum induction therapy has gained momentum with the discovery of new drugs with significant antitumor activity either as single agent or in combination with well-known drugs.

Thalidomide is the first drug in several years to show significant single-agent activity in MM.[8] Thalidomide plus dexamethasone has recently been approved by the United States Food and Drug Administration for the treatment of newly diagnosed myeloma based on the results of an Eastern Cooperative Oncology Group (ECOG) trial.[9] Further, the addition of thalidomide to melphalan plus prednisone (MP) has emerged as the new standard of care for elderly patients with newly diagnosed myeloma. This chapter reviews the current role of thalidomide as initial therapy for myeloma.

From: *Contemporary Hematology Myeloma Therapy*
Edited by: S. Lonial © Humana Press, Totowa, NJ

Brief History and Pharmacology

Thalidomide (α-N-[phthalimido]glutarimide) is an oral formulation of a racemic mixture of its optically active dextrorotatory (R)- and levorotatory (S) isomers.[10] Under physiological conditions, both enantiomers undergo rapid interconversion making a total separation impossible. It is well absorbed, and upon absorption, undergoes spontaneous nonenzymatic cleavage to over 20 metabolites.[10] The role and fate of these metabolites are not well known. Most appear to be excreted in the urine. Although hepatic metabolites are felt to be involved in its antiangiogenic effect, most of the drug is not metabolized by the hepatic cytochrome P450 system.

The drug was first introduced in the 1950s as a sedative and later as treatment of morning sickness associated with pregnancy. However, because of the teratogenic effect of the levorotatory (S) isomer it was removed from the market in 1962. The discovery that it had antiangiogenic and immune modulation effect and that MM was associated with increased angiogenesis led to initial studies in MM.[11] The precise mechanism by which it induces remission in MM is, however, not well known. Multiple hypotheses have been proposed, including inhibition of angiogenesis through blockage of basic fibroblast growth factor (bFGF) and vascular endothelial growth factor (VEGF),[12] interfering with stromal cells, and altering production and activity of cytokines involved in plasma cell growth such as tumor necrosis factor alpha (TNF-α), interleukin (IL)-6, IL-10, IL-4, IL-5, IL-12, IL-8, and cyclooxygenase 2.

Early Clinical Studies

The efficacy of thalidomide in MM was initially confirmed in heavily pretreated patients with refractory and relapsed disease.[8,13–15] In a study of 84 patients who had received previous conventional chemotherapy and high-dose chemotherapy, single-agent thalidomide produced responses in 32% of the patients.[8] In responding patients, a partial response was typically seen after 2 months of therapy. With a median follow-up of 14.5 months (12–16) median response duration had not been reached, suggesting a median response duration of more than 1 year in responders.[8] A Mayo study in 16 patients showed partial response rates of 25%, and responses were durable.[13]

In the initial studies, dose escalation was performed often up to 800 mg/day, but all showed that lower doses of 100–200 mg daily were effective with acceptable toxicity.

Thalidomide Plus Dexamethasone

Phase II Studies in Newly Diagnosed Myeloma

In order to improve on the response rates, dexamethasone was combined with thalidomide, based on in vitro data suggesting synergy between thalidomide and dexamethasone.[16,17] In a phase II trial at the Mayo Clinic, 50 patients with newly diagnosed myeloma were treated on a schedule of thalidomide 200 mg daily combined with dexamethasone given at a dose of 40 mg/day on days 1–4, 9–12, and 17–20 (odd numbered cycles) and days 1–4 (even numbered cycles), with the cycle repeated every 28 days.[18] Patients were treated for a median of 5 months (range 1–42 months) and the median duration of follow-up was 21 months (1–52). Thirty-two (64%) of the patients had a response to therapy using ECOG criteria. This included two (8%) patients with a complete response (CR). Tumor response was accompanied by improvement in symptoms and cytopenias in anemia in most patients. There were three deaths on therapy, one each due to pancreatitis, pulmonary embolism, and infection. The most common grade 3 or higher toxicity seen was deep vein thrombosis (DVT) occurring in 12% of patients, followed by constipation and skin rash. Other common toxicities included constipation, neuropathy, fatigue, sedation, skin rash, tremor, and edema.

A study by Weber et al. at the MD Anderson Cancer Center obtained similar results.[19] Forty patients with newly diagnosed symptomatic MM were treated with thalidomide plus dexamethasone. Seventy-two percent of patients responded to therapy, including 16% with a CR. The median time to response was less than 1 month. With therapeutic doses of anticoagulation, only rare thrombotic events were noted among patients treated toward the latter part of the study. Cavo and colleagues confirmed similar results in a separate phase II trial (Table 1).[20] In this study, 71 patients were treated, and the partial response rate was 66%, with 17% achieving a CR or a very good partial response.

Thus, in phase II trials, thalidomide combined with dexamethasone in newly diagnosed myeloma produced response rates of 64–76% with CR rates of about 10–15%, which is comparable or better than those seen with infusional vincristine, doxorubicin, and dexamethasone (VAD).[21] In a case-control study, 100 patients who were treated with oral thalidomide plus dexamethasone as initial therapy before stem cell transplant were compared to a matched group of patients receiving infusional VAD.[22] The response rate was significantly higher with thalidomide plus dexamethasone (76%) compared to VAD (52%). There was also no difference in the proportion of patients proceeding to stem cell transplantation or in the ability to collect adequate stem cells. Based on these results, the use of VAD, one of the most commonly used induction regimens before thalidomide plus dexamethasone, has markedly declined.[23]

Phase III Trials in Newly Diagnosed Myeloma

Two hundred seven patients were studied in an ECOG randomized trial comparing thalidomide and dexamethasone (103 patients) versus dexamethasone alone (104 patients).[9] Thalidomide was administered at 200 mg daily for 4 weeks, and dexamethasone 40 mg orally on days 1–4, 9–12, and 17–21.

Table 1 Selected phase II studies of thalidomide plus dexamethasone in newly diagnosed multiple myeloma.

Study	No. of patients	Overall response rate (%)	Deep vein thrombosis rate (%)	Reference
Rajkumar et al.	50	64	12	18
Weber et al.	40	72	15	19
Cavo et al.	71	66	16	20

Each cycle was repeated every 4 weeks. The best response within four cycles of therapy was significantly higher with thalidomide plus dexamethasone compared to dexamethasone alone; 63% versus 41%, $P = 0.0017$. Adjusted response rates allowing for the use of serum M protein values alone in patients in whom a measurable urine protein at baseline was unavailable at follow-up were 72% with thalidomide plus dexamethasone versus 50% with dexamethasone alone. Stem cell harvest was successful in 90% of patients in each arm. Toxicity was minimal. DVT was more frequent with thalidomide plus dexamethasone (17% vs 3%). Overall, grade 3 or higher nonhematologic toxicities were seen in 67% of patients within four cycles with thalidomide plus dexamethasone and 43% with dexamethasone alone ($P < 0.001$). Early mortality (first 4 months) was 7% with thalidomide plus dexamethasone and 11% with dexamethasone alone.

In a separate randomized, double-blind, placebo-controlled study, thalidomide plus dexamethasone was compared to dexamethasone alone as primary therapy in 470 patients with newly diagnosed myeloma.[24] The response rate was significantly higher with thalidomide plus dexamethasone (59%) compared to placebo plus dexamethasone (42%), $P < 0.001$. The time to progression (TTP) was also significantly superior, $P < 0.001$. As in the ECOG trial, DVT and other grade 3–4 events were more frequent with thalidomide plus dexamethasone (Table 2).

Effect on Stem Cell Mobilization

As discussed above, in phase II and III trials, there was no significant adverse effect on stem cell mobilization with thalidomide-based initial therapy. Stem cell mobilization and engraftment is not impaired with thalidomide, although most studies usually discontinue thalidomide during stem cell mobilization.[18,20,25] The German Myeloma-Multicenter Group (GMMG) and the Dutch-Belgian Hemato-Oncology Cooperative Group (HOVON) investigated the influence of thalidomide on the outcome of peripheral blood stem cell collection using a mobilization regimen of cyclophosphamide, doxorubicin, dexamethasone (CAD) and GCSF compared to standard VAD chemotherapy.[26] Although patients receiving thalidomide had a significantly lower yield of stem cells, they were able to mobilize adequate stem cells and engraftment was not significantly impaired.

Table 2 Results of selected comparative studies of thalidomide plus dexamethasone.

| Study | Type of study | Comparison regimen | No. of patients | Response rate (%) | | Reference |
				With thalidomide plus dexamethasone	In control arm	
Cavo et al.	Case-control	VAD	200	76	52	22
Rajkumar et al. (ECOG)	Phase III	Dexamethasone	207	63	41	9
Rajkumar et al. (MM 003)	Phase III	Dexamethasone	470	63	46	24

VAD vincristine, doxorubicin, and dexamethasone, *ECOG* Eastern Cooperative Oncology Group, *MM* multiple myeloma.

Melphalan, Prednisone, Thalidomide

For elderly patients, MP has long been the standard of care. Numerous randomized trials with various chemotherapy regimens failed to improve on overall survival compared to MP. In these studies, combination chemotherapy with regimens such as VBMCP (vincristine, BCNU, melphalan, cyclophosphamide, prednisone) led to superior response rates (60–70%), but no survival benefit.[27–29] Recently, three randomized trials have compared MP to melphalan, prednisone, thalidomide (MPT).[30–32] Based on the results of these three trials discussed below, MPT has now emerged as the standard of care for elderly patients with newly diagnosed myeloma who are not candidates for stem cell transplantation (Table 3).

Palumbo et al. randomized patients to either standard dose MP for 6 months or to MPT for 6 months followed by maintenance thalidomide.[30] Overall response rates were significantly higher with the MPT compared to MP (76% vs 48%) as was the CR plus near-CR rate (28% vs 7%). MPT also resulted in superior 2-year event-free survival (EFS) rates (54% vs 27%, $P = 0.0006$), and a trend toward an improved 3-year overall survival.

Facon et al. recently reported results of the IFM 99-06 trial in which 436 patients between the ages of 65 and 75 were randomized to MP versus MPT versus tandem autologous stem cell transplantation (ASCT) with reduced dose melphalan (Mel 100 mg/m^{2}).[31] As in the study by Palumbo et al., significantly higher response and PFS rates were observed with MPT compared to either MP or tandem MEL100; median PFS was 29, 17, and 19 months, respectively. More importantly, the trial demonstrated a significant survival advantage with MPT, median overall survival not reached at 56, 30, and 39 months, respectively. Early (first 3 months) mortality rate was 3% with MPT compared to 8% with MP, indicating that the result was not just due to patients in the MP arm not having access to thalidomide. Hulin and colleagues tested MPT versus MP in patients over the age of 75 in a separate IFM trial. Preliminary results suggest superior event-free and overall survival with MPT compared to MP.[32] In contrast to MPT, thalidomide plus dexamethasone is not superior to MP in patients with newly diagnosed myeloma.[33]

Some caveats need to be considered with MPT. Access to thalidomide may be an issue based on availability and cost considerations. Moreover, MPT is

Table 3 Results of selected phase III studies of melphalan, prednisone, thalidomide in newly diagnosed myeloma.

Study	Age group	Comparison regimen (s)	Total no. of patients	Median progression-free survival (months)	Median overall survival	Reference
Palumbo et al.	65–85	MP	255	14	NR	30
		MPT		24+	NR	
Facon et al.	65–75	MP Mel 100 × 2	436	17 19	30 39	31
		MPT		30	56	
Hulin et al.	>75	MP MPT	232	19 24	28 45	32

MP melphalan plus prednisone, *MPT* melphalan, prednisone, thalidomide, *Mel* melphalan, *NR* not reached.

associated with greater toxicity than is MP. Therefore, not all elderly patients may be able to receive the regimen. Grade 3–4 adverse events occur in ~50% of patients treated with MPT, compared to 25% with MP. [30] As with Thal/Dex, there is a significant (20%) risk of DVT with MPT in the absence of thromboprophylaxis. However, this rate drops to ~3% with the use of thromboprophylaxis (e.g., daily subcutaneous enoxaparin).

Other Thalidomide-Based Combinations

Thalidomide has been combined with a variety of chemotherapy regimens with the hope of improving response rates.[34] To date, none of these regimens has shown significant superiority over MPT or thalidomide plus dexamethasone. The risk of DVT increases when thalidomide is combined with certain drugs such as doxorubicin, liposomal doxorubicin, and melphalan.

Thalidomide has also been tested in concert with high-dose therapy in the frontline setting. High-dose therapy followed by autologous stem cell transplantation is known to improve response rates and survival in myeloma.[35–37] Response rates with stem cell transplantation exceeds 75–90%[28,38] and CR rates range from 20% to 40%.[5,36] However, transplantation is not curative and there is a need to improve outcomes with the procedure.

Barlogie and colleagues studied the effect of thalidomide induction, consolidation, and maintenance on outcome in patients undergoing tandem autologous transplant.[39] They randomized 345 patients to standard induction, tandem transplant, and maintenance without thalidomide and 323 patients to the same treatment plus thalidomide. Thalidomide was administered in the latter group throughout the treatment duration from induction through maintenance. Patients in the "no thalidomide" arm (control group) could receive the drug at the time of relapse. The CR rate after transplant was 62% with thalidomide compared to 43% in the control group ($P < 0.001$). Five-year EFS was also better, 56% compared to 44%, respectively, $P = 0.01$. However, the 5-year overall survival was similar (65%) in both groups. There was a shorter median survival of 1.1 years after relapse in the thalidomide group compared to 2.7 years in the control group ($P = 0.001$). This study showed that in the context of patients undergoing intense therapy with induction, tandem transplantation, consolidation, and maintenance, there was no benefit to thalidomide therapy administered concurrently compared to delaying treatment with the drug until the time of relapse.

Adverse Effects

Thalidomide is generally well tolerated at lower doses (50–100 mg/day). At doses of 200 mg/day, the side effects increase significantly. Doses greater than 200 mg/day are not recommended. The extent and frequency of side effects depend on the combinations used. The most common side effects include sedation, fatigue, constipation, skin rash, and DVT.[8,10,40]

The incidence of DVT is 1–3% in patients receiving thalidomide alone. It increases to 15–20% with thalidomide plus dexamethasone, and over 25% in patients receiving the agent in combination with other cytotoxic chemotherapeutic agents, particularly doxorubicin.[41] Patients receiving thalidomide in combination with high-dose steroids or chemotherapy need routine thromboprophylaxis with coumadin (target INR 2–3) or low molecular weight heparin (equivalent of enoxaparin 40 mg once daily). Aspirin alone can be used instead in patients receiving only low doses of dexamethasone (40 mg once a week or lower) or prednisone in combination with thalidomide, provided no concomitant erythropoietic agents are used.[42]

Dryness of the skin, pruritus, and rash occurs in 25% of patients receiving thalidomide. If a skin rash occurs, the drug should be discontinued, and restarted at a lower dose after the rash has resolved. If severe exfoliation, Steven-Johnson syndrome, or toxic epidermal necrolysis occurs, the drug should be stopped and not used again.[43]

Thalidomide can cause peripheral neuropathy, generally following chronic use. Patients require close monitoring for symptoms such as numbness, tingling, or pain in the hands and feet. The neuropathy is axonal, and presents as asymmetric painful paresthesias and sensory loss. The toes and feet are affected first. Usually, the neuropathy is reversible upon prompt cessation of thalidomide, but permanent irreversible sensory loss has been reported.

Future Directions

The past decade has seen a significant increase in therapeutic options for MM. Several other newly diagnosed regimens are being tested and need to be compared prospectively with thalidomide plus dexamethasone.[29–32] For example, nonhematologic side effects of thalidomide could be reduced by using lenalidomide instead. In a phase II trial, lenalidomide in combination with dexamethasone has already shown higher response rates than those reported with thalidomide plus dexamethasone.[33,34] Similarly, melphalan, prednisone, lenalidomide (MPR)[44] and melphalan, prednisone, bortezomib (MPV)[45] are also proving to be very active and need to be compared with MPT in elderly patients.

Many of the advances in myeloma started with thalidomide. Future studies should be focused on testing the short- and long-term efficacy of other combinations compared to thalidomide-based regimens in patients with newly diagnosed myeloma .

References

1. Kyle RA, Rajkumar SV. Multiple myeloma. N Engl J Med 2004;351:1860–73.
2. Bataille R, Harousseau JL. Multiple myeloma (100 Refs) [Review]. N Engl J Med 1997 ;336 (23):1657–64.
3. Rajkumar SV, Kyle RA. Multiple myeloma: Diagnosis and treatment. Mayo Clin Proc 2005 ;80 : 1371–82.
4. Dispenzieri A, Rajkumar SV, Gertz MA, et al. Treatment of newly diagnosed multiple myeloma based on Mayo stratification of myeloma and risk-adapted therapy (mSMART): Consensus statement. Mayo Clin Proc 2007;82:323–41.
5. Attal M, Harousseau JL, Stoppa AM, et al. A prospective, randomized trial of autologous bone marrow transplantation and chemotherapy in multiple myeloma. Intergroupe Francais du Myelome. N Engl J Med 1996;335 (2):91–7.
6. Attal M, Harousseau JL, Facon T, et al. Single versus double autologous stem-cell transplantation for multiple myeloma [see comment] N Engl J Med 2003;349 (26):2495–502.

7. Harousseau J-L, Marit G, Caillot D, et al. VELCADE/Dexamethasone (Vel/Dex) versus VAD as induction treatment prior to autologous stem cell transplantation (ASCT) in newly diagnosed multiple myeloma (MM): An interim analysis of the IFM 2005–01 randomized multicenter phase III trial. Blood 2006;108(11):56.

8. Singhal S, Mehta J, Desikan R, et al. Antitumor activity of thalidomide in refractory multiple myeloma [see comments]. N Engl J Med 1999;341(21):1565–71.

9. Rajkumar SV, Blood E, Vesole DH, Fonseca R, Greipp PR. Phase III clinical trial of thalidomide plus dexamethasone compared with dexamethasone alone in newly diagnosed multiple myeloma: A clinical trial coordinated by the Eastern Cooperative Oncology Group. J Clin Oncol 2006;24:431–6.

10. Stirling DI. Pharmacology of thalidomide. Semin Hematol 2000;37:5–14.

11. D'Amato RJ, Loughnan MS, Flynn E, Folkman J. Thalidomide is an inhibitor of angiogenesis. Proc Natl Acad Sci USA 1994;91(9):4082–5.

12. Olson KB, Hall TC, Horton J, Khung CL, Hosley HF. Thalidomide (N-phthaloylglutamimide) in the treatment of advanced cancer. Clin Pharmacol Ther 1965;6(3):292–7.

13. Rajkumar SV, Fonseca R, Dispenzieri A, et al. Thalidomide in the treatment of relapsed multiple myeloma. Mayo Clin Proc 2000;75:897–902.

14. Kneller A, Raanani P, Hardan I, et al. Therapy with thalidomide in refractory multiple myeloma—The revival of an old drug. Br J Haematol 2000;108:391–3.

15. Juliusson G, Celsing F, Turesson I, Lenhoff S, Adriansson M, Malm C. Frequent good partial remissions from thalidomide including best response ever in patients with advanced refractory and relapsed myeloma. Br J Haematol 2000;109:89–96.

16. Hideshima T, Chauhan D, Shima Y, et al. Thalidomide and its analogs overcome drug resistance of multiple myeloma cells to conventional therapy . Blood 2000 ;96: 2943–50.

17. Weber DM, Gavino M, Delasalle K, Rankin K, Giralt S, Alexanian R. Thalidomide alone or with dexamethasone for multiple myeloma. Blood 1999;94 (Suppl 1):604a (A 2686).

18. Rajkumar SV, Hayman S, Gertz MA, et al. Combination therapy with thalidomide plus dexamethasone for newly diagnosed myeloma. J Clin Oncol 2002;20:4319–23.

19. Weber D, Rankin K, Gavino M, Delasalle K, Alexanian R. Thalidomide alone or with dexamethasone for previously untreated multiple myeloma. J Clin Oncol 2003;21(1):16–9.

20. Cavo M, Zamagni E, Tosi P, et al. First-line therapy with thalidomide and dexamethasone in preparation for autologous stem cell transplantation for multiple myeloma. Haematologica 2004;89:826–31.

21. Alexanian R, Barlogie B, Tucker S. VAD-based regimens as primary treatment for multiple myeloma. Am J Hematol 1990;33(2):86–9.

22. Cavo M, Zamagni E, Tosi P, et al. Superiority of thalidomide and dexamethasone over vincristine-doxorubicindexamethasone (VAD) as primary therapy in preparation for autologous transplantation for multiple myeloma. Blood 2005;106(1):35–9.

23. Rajkumar SV. The death of VAD as initial therapy for multiple myeloma. Blood 2005;106:2–3.

24. Rajkumar SV, Hussein M, Catalano J, et al. A randomized, double-blind, placebo-controlled trial of thalidomide plus dexamethasone versus dexamethasone alone as primary therapy for newly diagnosed multiple myeloma. Blood 2006;108(11):238a. Abstract 795.

25. Abdelkefi A, Torjman L, Ben Romdhane N, et al. First-line thalidomide-dexamethasone therapy in preparation for autologous stem cell transplantation in young patients (<61 years) with symptomatic multiple myeloma. Bone Marrow Transplant 2005;36(3):193–8.

26. Breitkreutz I, Lokhorst HM, Raab MS, et.al Thalidomide in newly diagnosed multiple myeloma: Influence of thalidomide treatment on peripheral blood stem cell collection yield. Leukemia 2007.

27. Myeloma Trialists' Collaborative Group. Combination chemotherapy versus melphalan plus prednisone as treatment for multiple myeloma: An overview of 6,633 patients from 27 randomized trials. J Clin Oncol 1998;16(12):3832–42.

28. Alexanian R, Dimopoulos M. The treatment of multiple myeloma. (54 Refs). N Engl J Med 1994;330(7):484–9.

29. Oken MM, Harrington DP, Abramson N, Kyle RA, Knospe W, Glick JH. Comparison of melphalan and prednisone with vincristine, carmustine, melphalan, cyclophosphamide, and prednisone in the treatment of multiple myeloma: Results of Eastern Cooperative Oncology Group Study E2479. Cancer 1997;79(8):1561–7.

30. Palumbo A, Bringhen S, Caravita T, et al. Oral melphalan and prednisone chemotherapy plus thalidomide compared with melphalan and prednisone alone in elderly patients with multiple myeloma: Randomised controlled trial. Lancet 2006;367:825–31.

31. Facon T, Mary JY, Hulin C, et al. Major superiority of melphalan-prednisone (MP) + thalidomide (THAL) over MP and autologous stem cell transplantation in the treatment of newly diagnosed elderly patients with multiple myeloma. Blood 2005;106(11):230a (A780).

32. Hulin C, Virion J, Leleu X, et al. Comparison of melphalan-prednisone-thalidomide (MP-T) to melphalan-prednisone (MP) in patients 75 years of age or older with untreated multiple myeloma (MM). Preliminary results of the randomized, double-blind, placebo controlled IFM 01–01 trial. J Clin Oncol (Meeting Abstracts) 2007;25(18_suppl):8001.

33. Ludwig H, Drach J, Tóthová E, et al. Thalidomide-dexamethasone versus melphalan-prednisolone as first line treatment in elderly patients with multiple myeloma: An interim analysis. J Clin Oncol 2005;23(16S):6537.

34. Offidani M, Corvatta L, Piersantelli M-N, et al. Thalidomide, dexamethasone, and pegylated liposomal doxorubicin (ThaDD) for patients older than 65 years with newly diagnosed multiple myeloma 10.1182/blood-2006-03-013086. Blood 2006;108(7):2159–64.

35. Harousseau JL, Attal M. The role of autologous hematopoietic stem cell transplantation in multiple myeloma [Review]. Semin Hematol 1997;34(1 Suppl 1):61–6.

36. Barlogie B, Jagannath S, Epstein J, et al. Biology and therapy of multiple myeloma in 1996 . Semin Hematol 1997;34:67–72.

37. Gertz MA, Pineda AA, Chen MG, et al. Refractory and relapsing multiple myeloma treated by blood stem cell transplantation. Am J Med Sci 1995;309(3):152–61.

38. Kovacsovics T, Delaly A. Intensive treatment strategies in myeloma. Semin Hematol 1997;34:49–60.

39. Barlogie B, Tricot G, Anaissie E, et al. Thalidomide and hematopoietic-cell transplantation for multiple myeloma [see comment]. N Engl J Med 2006;354(10):1021–30.

40. Fine HA, Figg WD, Jaeckle K, et al. A phase II trial of the anti-angiogenic agent thalidomide in patients with recurrent high-grade gliomas. J Clin Oncol 2000;18(4):708–15.

41. Barlogie B, Desikan R, Eddlemon P, et al. Extended survival in advanced and refractory multiple myeloma after single-agent thalidomide: Identification of prognostic factors in a phase 2 study of 169 patients. Blood 2001;98(2):492–4.

42. Rajkumar SV. Thalidomide therapy and deep venous thrombosis in multiple myeloma [comment]. Mayo Clin Proc 2005;80(12):1549–51.

43. Rajkumar SV, Gertz MA, Witzig TE. Life-threatening toxic epidermal necrolysis with thalidomide therapy for myeloma. N Engl J Med 2000;343:972–3.

44. Palumbo A, Falco P, Corradini P, et al. Melphalan, Prednisone and lenalidomide treatment for newly diagnosed myeloma. A report from the GIMEMA Italian Multiple Myeloma Network. J. Clin Oncol 2007;25:4459–4465.

45. Mateos M-V, Hernandez J-M, Hernandez M-T, et al. Bortezomib plus melphalan and prednisone in elderly untreated patients with multiple myeloma: Results of a multicenter phase 1/2 study 10.1182/blood-2006-04-019778. Blood 2006;108(7):2165–72.

Chapter 15

The Role of Bortezomib in the Treatment of Relapsed and Refractory Multiple Myeloma

Paul G. Richardson, Constantine S. Mitsiades, Robert Schlossman, Teru Hideshima, Irene Ghobrial, Nikhil C. Munshi, and Kenneth C. Anderson

Introduction

Relapsed and refractory multiple myeloma (MM) represents an unmet medical need in the management of this disease. Relapsed and refractory MM is defined as patients who achieve minor response or better followed by progression or relapse and then progress on salvage therapy, or experience progression within 60 days of their last therapy.[1–4] Historically, in the prethalidomide/prebortezomib era, median overall survival (OS) of relapsed and refractory MM has been short at 6–9 months, while responses to salvage regimens were of the order of few weeks to several months.[4] While comprehensive prognostic systems have been proposed for newly diagnosed MM, the identification and prospective validation of similar prognostic systems in the setting of relapsed and refractory MM are not as well developed. Nonetheless, patients with MM with chromosomal translocations t(4;14) or t(14;16), deletion of chromosomes 17 or 13, high β2 microglobulin, thrombocytopenia, and low serum albumin are considered to represent patients with higher-risk disease in the context of relapsed and refractory MM, particularly if accompanied by challenging clinical features such as light-chain disease or IgA isotype, renal failure, extramedullary disease, hyposecretory myeloma, and extensive bone disease.[5]

The emergence of novel anti-MM therapies which comprehensively target the MM tumor cells and their complex interactions with the bone marrow (BM) microenvironment have significantly improved the prognosis for patients with relapsed/refractory MM. The first-in-class proteasome inhibitor bortezomib (formerly known as PS-341) and the immunomodulatory agents, thalidomide (Thal) and lenalidomide, constitute Food and Drug Adminisration (FDA)-approved agents for the clinical management of relapsed/refractory MM. These three drugs now constitute "backbone" therapies in MM, with bortezomib in particular representing an example of accelerated FDA approval based on studies in relapsed/refractory MM, followed by full approval in the relapsed setting.[1–3] Moreover, there has now been extensive evaluation of bortezomib as a key partner for combination regimens with other anti-MM agents, both in advanced and in newly diagnosed MM.[5]

From: *Contemporary Hematology Myeloma Therapy*
Edited by: S. Lonial © Humana Press, Totowa, NJ

Preclinical Studies in Support of the Clinical Development of Bortezomib

The proteasome, the principal controller of intracellular protein degradation, is a multi-sub-unit complex that cleaves ubiquitin-tagged proteins via the coordinated action of three distinct proteolytic sites, with chymotryptic, tryptic, and postglutamyl peptide hydrolytic-like activities (as reviewed in Ciechanover[6]). Bortezomib is a boronic dipeptide that selectively binds to and reversibly inhibits the chymotryptic-like activity of the 20S proteasome core,[7–10] inhibiting the degradation of a set of protein substrates enriched in proteins with key regulatory roles in cell proliferation and survival. The accumulation of these proteins leads to cell cycle arrest; upregulation of stress response proteins; disruption of adhesion between MM and stromal cells; inhibition of cytokine signaling; antiangiogenic effects; and ultimately apoptosis of MM tumor cells.[7–9,11,12–16] The original rationale for the testing of proteasome inhibitors in MM was that the proliferation and survival of MM cells are dependent on constitutive activation of the heterodimeric transcription factor NF-κB and upregulation of the cytokine interleukin-6 (IL-6), both of which are indirectly triggered by proteasomal degradation of IκBα, a negative regulator of NF-κ;B activity, which binds to NF-κB and sequesters it in the cytoplasm, preventing its nuclear translocation. When proteasomal degradation of IκBα is inhibited by bortezomib, NF-κB remains in the cytoplasm, thereby blocking the production of IL-6 as well as other transcriptional targets of NF-κB, including caspase inhibitors.[17] However, the inhibition of NF-κB itself is not the only molecular event that accounts for the anti-MM activity of bortezomib. Indeed, proteasome inhibition by bortezomib also leads to accumulation of AP-1 and myc, which leads to upregulation of death receptors and their congnate ligands (e.g., Fas and FasL, respectively), triggering caspase-8-mediated apoptotic signaling. Furthermore, accumulation of bax and release of cytochrome-c from the mitochondria lead to activation of caspase-9-dependent apoptotic pathways. The fact that bortezomib both triggers activation of a dual caspase-8 and -9 apoptotic cascade and suppresses the expression of caspase inhibitors that can attenuate the activation of these two caspases explains in part why the proapoptotic effect of bortezomib is so potent and rapid, and why this agent can lead to enhanced anti-MM effect when combined with other agents that predominantly activate only caspase-8 (e.g., Thal and lenalidomide), or only caspase-9, for example, dexamethasone (Dex).[18,19] In addition, the known role of NF-κB in conferring chemoresistance to MM cells and other tumor types, combined with preclinical studies showing that bortezomib suppresses the expression of diverse DNA repair enzymes, suggests that proteasome inhibition can sensitize MM cells to conventional chemotherapeutic agents and so reverse chemoresistance.[20,21]

Clinical Studies of Bortezomib in Relapsed and/or Relapsed, Refractory MM

Following the encouraging results observed in patients with MM enrolled in a phase I trial of bortezomib for advanced hematologic malignancies[22], and the promising parallel preclinical studies of bortezomib, either alone or combined with Dex, was tested in a large multicenter phase II clinical program for relapsed/refractory MM, namely, the Study of Uncontrolled Multiple Myeloma Managed with Proteasome Inhibition Therapy (SUMMIT)[23] and Clinical Response and Efficacy Study of Bortezomib in the Treatment of Relapsing Multiple Myeloma (CREST)[24] studies. These trials showed that bortezomib, administered twice weekly .intravenously for the first 2 weeks of each 3-week cycle, was active in relapsed/refractory MM. In fact, the rate, depth, and durability of responses were sufficiently favorable to lead to accelerated FDA approval of bortezomib for the treatment of patients with MM who had received two lines of prior therapy.

Specifically, in the multicenter, open-label, nonrandomized, phase II trial SUMMIT, 202 patients with relapsed and refractory MM were enrolled. Patients received 1.3 mg/m^2 of bortezomib twice weekly for 2 weeks, followed by 1 week without treatment, for up to eight cycles. In patients with a suboptimal response, oral Dex (20 mg daily, on the day of and the day after bortezomib administration) was added to the regimen. Ninety-two percent of evaluable patients in this trial had previously received at least three of the major classes of anti-MM agents for myeloma, and 91% were confirmed at audit as being refractory to their most recently received therapy. According to modified European Group for Blood and Marrow Transplantation (EBMT) criteria, and based on an independent review committee evaluation, the response rate to bortezomib was 35%, including 7% complete response (CR) and 12% of near-CR (nCR, defined as CR with trace immunofixation positivity only). The median OS was significantly better than expected at 16 months, with a median duration of response (DOR) of 12 months.

In the CREST trial, 54 patients with MM who had relapsed after or were refractory to frontline therapy were randomized to receive intravenously. 1.0 or 1.3 mg/m^2 of bortezomib according to the same schedule (twice weekly for 2 weeks, every 3 weeks for a maximum of eight cycles), while Dex was permitted in patients with progressive disease (PD) or stable disease (SD) after two or four cycles, respectively. Responses were again determined using modified EBMT criteria. The complete response CR + partial response (PR) rate for bortezomib alone was 30% in the 1.0 mg/m^2 (8 out of 27 patients) group and 38% in the 1.3 mg/m^2 (10 out of 26 patients) group, and the CR + PR rate for patients who received bortezomib alone or in combination with Dex was 37% and 50% for the 1.0 and 1.3 mg/m^2 cohorts, respectively.

Based on the encouraging results of the phase II program of bortezomib, the international, randomized phase III Assessment of Proteasome Inhibition for Extending Remissions (APEX) trial enrolled patients with relapsed MM who had received one to three prior lines of therapy. In that trial, the single-agent bortezomib arm had significantly longer time to progression (TTP), higher response rate, and improved survival compared to the high-dose Dex arm[25]. Based on the results of that study, bortezomib is, at the moment, the only agent which has been shown, as single agent, to provide survival benefit in the setting of relapsed MM. An updated analysis of APEX after extended follow-up (median 22 months) revealed a median OS of 29.8 months with bortezomib versus 23.7 months with Dex. This 6-month benefit was seen despite the fact that 62% of the patients on the high-dose Dex arm crossed over to receive bortezomib.[26] The overall response rate (ORR) (43%) and CR/nCR rate (15%) with bortezomib monotherapy were also higher in the updated analysis than at initial analysis.[26] Results from the APEX trial also indicate that bortezomib is more active when used earlier in the relapsed setting, with TTP, DOR, and OS appearing longer and response rate higher among patients with only one prior therapy compared with those with two or three prior lines of therapy.[25]

The most common side effects associated with bortezomib therapy include fatigue, gastrointestinal events, and peripheral neuropathy. The most commonly reported grade 3 or higher adverse events are peripheral neuropathy, thrombocytopenia, neutropenia, and anemia. Bortezomib-emergent peripheral neuropathy is a key side effect because it can limit dose and duration of treatment with this agent, and thus curtail the clinical benefit that patients with bortezomib-responsive MM might otherwise achieve. Based on the experience from the SUMMIT and CREST trials, specific management guidelines were proposed[27] and prospectively tested in the APEX trial, where bortezomib-related neuropathy was shown to occur in about 30% of patients, be mainly mild to moderate, and be reversible in the majority of cases.[28] Consistent with this, bortezomib-related neuropathy resolved or improved in 71% of patients in the SUMMIT and CREST trials who had grade 3 or higher peripheral neuropathy and/or neuropathy requiring discontinuation.[27] Similar results have been observed in the frontline setting.[29–31] The hematologic side effects associated with bortezomib are also predictable and manageable. Bortezomib-emergent thrombocytopenia and neutropenia are transient and cyclical. For instance, bortezomib is associated with platelet count decrease and subsequent recovery which occur in a predictable pattern during each treatment cycle, without any evidence of cumulative toxicity.[28,32] Low baseline platelet count ($<70 \times 10^9$/L) is associated with increased risk of grade 3 or higher thrombocytopenia.[32] In the APEX trial, higher incidence of grade 3 or higher thrombocytopenia was observed in the bortezomib arm versus the Dex arm. However, the incidence of clinically significant bleeding events (including grade ≥ 3 bleeding events, serious bleeding, and cerebral haemorrhage) did not differ significantly between the two treatments.[33] It is also notable that in an extension study of the SUMMIT and CREST trials, no new or cumulative toxicities were reported.[34]

Combinations of Bortezomib with Conventional Anti-MM Agents

Bortezomib-Based Combinations Containing Anthracyclines

Preclinical studies had shown that combinations of bortezomib with anthracyclines can achieve significant anti-MM response in vitro, even against MM cells resistant to monotherapy with either of these two drug classes.[21] These studies provided the framework for clinical trials of combination regimens including bortezomib and doxorubicin or liposomal doxorubicin. In these trials, high OR and CR/nCR rates, as well as promising OS and time-to-event data, were observed.[35–41] For instance, bortezomib plus liposomal doxorubicin were administered in a phase I trial in patients with advanced hematologic malignancies, leading to a 73% response rate among 22 evaluable patients (including 36% CR/nCR).[40] Updated analysis of extended follow-up data showed that, compared with each patients' last prior regimen, the bortezomib plus liposomal doxorubicin had longer median TTP (9.3 vs 3.8 months) and median time between onset of therapy and start of a subsequent therapy (24.2 vs 5.9 months), while the median OS with the bortezomib plus liposomal doxorubicin was 38.3 months.[35] Importantly, among patients who had previously received an anthracycline-based regimen and had PD, SD, or initially responded but then had PD or SD, 8 out of 13 of these patients responded to the combination of bortezomib plus anthracycline.[40] These observations were consistent with the previous preclinical data which had suggested that bortezomib can sensitize MM cells to conventional chemotherapeutics, even in cases of patients with resistance to these agents.[20,21] A phase III trial comparing bortezomib and pegylated liposomal doxorubicin versus bortezomib monotherapy[42] showed a median TTP of 9.3 months with the combination versus 6.5 months with bortezomib monotherapy, as well as higher response rate and OS advantage with the combination. Based on these results, the FDA recently approved this combination for treatment of patients with MM who have not previously received bortezomib and who have received at least one prior line of anti-MM therapy.[42]

In further support of the concept of bortezomib-induced chemosensitization, the combination of bortezomib, Thal, and liposomal doxorubicin was tested in patients resistant to regimens containing bortezomib, doxorubicin, or Thal: the ORR was 65%, including 23% CR/nCR (according to Southwest Oncology Group [SWOG] criteria).[41] Similarly, a 63% response rate (including 25% CR/nCR) was reported with the combination of bortezomib, doxorubicin, Thal, and Dex, administered in patients who had previously received these agents in their course of MM.[37] Liposomal doxorubicin combined with bortezomib, Thal, and Dex (VTD) also leads to higher response rates compared with the triplet regimen (81% vs 55%; CR/nCR: 33% vs 17%), while the median TTP and OS were also longer with the liposomal doxorubicin-containing quartet versus the triplet regimen[39], despite the fact that patients had previously received bortezomib, doxorubicin, Thal, and Dex.[39]

Bortezomib-Based Combinations Containing Alkylating Agents

The chemosensitizing properties of bortezomib in preclinical models had been also observed with combinations of the proteasome inhibitor with alkylators.[21] Consistent with these results, combinations of bortezomib with alkylating agents have been shown to be active in advanced MM.[43–46] A dose-escalation trial of bortezomib plus oral melphalan reported response rate of 47%, with 15% CR/nCR rate and clinical responses observed in 5 out of 6 (83%) patients treated at the maximum tolerated dose of the combination.[43] In a dose-escalation trial of bortezomib with low-dose intravenous melphalan, the response rate was 43%, and was increased to 52% upon Dex addition for patients with suboptimal clinical response.[45] The clinical activity of the combination appeared more pronounced in patients who received the highest melphalan dose.[45] Addition of Thal, along with prednisone or Dex, seems to increase the activity of the combination, with response rates of 66% (37% CR/nCR) [46] and 67% (17% CR/nCR) [44] for the Dex- and prednisone-containing regimens, respectively.

Combination Regimens Based on a Bortezomib–Thalidomide "backbone"

Bortezomib monotherapy is active in relapsed/refractory MM, even in Thal-refractory patients.[23,25] The different molecular mechanism(s) of action of bortezomib, compared to conventional chemotherapy, glucocorticoids, Thal, or immunomodulatory drugs (IMiDs), allow it to act synergistically with either of them in preclinical models (Fig. 1).[47,48] The possibility of cumulative neurotoxocity is a particular concern about combinations of bortezomib with Thal. However, several clinical trials have shown that the neuropathy associated with bortezomib–Thal combination is usually manageable. Specifically, in a phase I/II trial, 85 patients with refractory MM who were bortezomib-naïve received a VTD regimen, at starting doses of 1.0 mg/m^2 (which could be increased up to 1.3) for bortezomib and 50 mg (which could be escalated up to 200 mg) daily for Thal, while Dex was added if PR or better was not achieved.[49] Based on the observed toxicities, including peripheral neuropathy, a final dose of bortezomib 1.0 mg/m^2, Thal 200 mg/day, and Dex 40 mg was proposed for further investigation. Most patients enrolled in that trial had abnormal cytogenetics (including chromosome 13 deletion in ~50% of them), one or two prior autotransplants, and the majority had previously received Thal. This VTD regimen achieved 55% PR or better (including 16% CR/nCR rate) and an additional 15% had minimal response (MR). The median event-free survival (EFS) and OS were 9 months and 22 months, respectively, and were shorter in patients with cytogenetic abnormalities, while prior Thal treatment was also associated with inferior EFS. However, EFS and OS were not

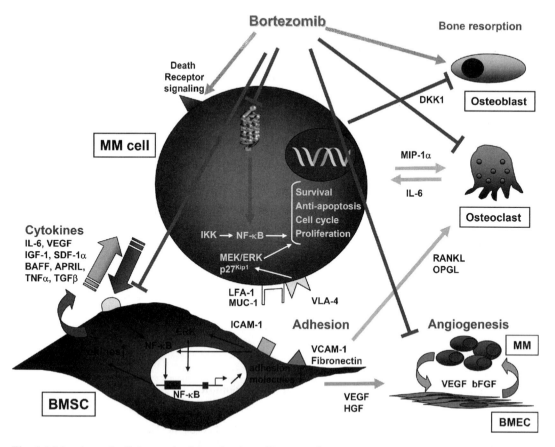

Fig. 1 Molecular and cellular mechanisms of action of bortezomib (*see* Plate 4).

influenced by the maximum daily dose of Thal administered (>100 mg/day vs <100 mg/day).

Extending even further the concept of multiagent combination regimens based on bortezomib–Thal "backbone," two clinical trials have evaluated the activity of quartet combinations containing bortezomib, Thal, alkylator, and glucocorticoids. Palumbo et al. treated 30 patients with relapsed or refractory MM with the VMPT combination (bortezomib, melphalan, Thal at 50 mg daily, and prednisone) and observed a 67% PR rate (including 43% rate of very good partial response [VGPR] or better), with 1-year progression-free survival (PFS) and 1-year survival rates of 61%, and 84%, respectively.[44] Neuropathy in particular was less in this study, likely due to the lower doses of Thal.[44] Terpos et al. evaluated a combination (for up to eight cycles) of bortezomib, oral melphalan, intermittent Thal (100 mg/day for 4 days), and pulsed Dex (12 mg/m^2) in 31 pretreated patients with MM (including 20 patients with relapsed refractory) and observed a 56% CR/PR rate (CR 8% and PR 48%) and another 8% of MR with a median time to response of 30 days, again with manageable toxicity.[50]

Combinations of Lenalidomide and Bortezomi*b*

Mechanistically, bortezomib triggers apoptosis of MM cells in a dual caspase-8 and -9-mediated manner,[51] while the direct anti-MM activity of lenalidomide and other IMiDs is mediated by caspase-8 activation. Although both bortezomib and Thal/IMIDs can suppress NF-κB transcriptional activity in MM cells, each of these drug classes achieves this effect by likely acting at different regulatory levels of the NF-κB pathway. These considerations suggested that perhaps combinations of proteasome inhibitors and IMiDs may have synergistic anti-MM activity and provided the rationale for preclinical in vitro studies, which confirmed enhanced anti-MM effect with combinations of immunomodulatory Thal derivatives, such as lenalidomide, with bortezomib. Since lenalidomide is not associated with peripheral neuropathy, its combination with bortezomib was expected to have more favorable safety profile than the bortezomib-Thal combinations. However, both lenalidomide and bortezomib can lead to hematologic adverse effects, indicating the need for careful clinical development of this combination to avoid pronounced myelosuppression. In a phase I study, combining lenalidomide and bortezomib in patients with refractory MM with prior exposure to lenalidomide, bortezomib, Thal, or transplant, the maximum tolerated doses were identified as 15 mg/day of lenalidomide for 14 days and 1.0 mg/m^2 of bortezomib on days 1, 4, 8, and 11 of each 21-day cycle. Consistent with the initial clinical rationale behind this trial, no significant peripheral neuropathy was reported. Furthermore, no anticoagulant prophylaxis was required and only one patient had deep-veinous thrombosis (DVT) while on lenalidomide alone at the time of this report.[30] After a median of six cycles (range: 4–17) in 36 evaluable patients, a 58% ORR (CR + PR + MR) (90% CI: 46–75%) was observed, including 6% CR/nCR rate. Responses were durable (median 6 months, range: 1–26), and 11 out of 36 evaluable patients remain on therapy beyond 1 year. Dex was subsequently added in 14 patients who had PD, resulting in PR/MR/SD in 10 (71%).[30] The combination of lenalidomide at 15 mg and bortezomib at 1.0 mg/m^2 has been selected for ongoing phase II studies in relapsed/refractory MM, while dose escalation in the upfront setting is also underway.

Clinical Trials of Bortezomib-Based Combinations with Investigational Agents

Bortezomib has been utilized in combination regimens with diverse investigational agents in clinical development for MM. One conceptual framework behind the design of some of these combination regimens involves the pairing of bortezomib with drug classes which may neutralize molecular pathway(s) that can confer resistance to proteasome inhibition. An example is the combination of bortezomib with hsp90 inhibitors: exposure of MM cells to bortezomib triggers upregulation of heat shock proteins, including hsp90.[52] This is likely a stress response, mounted by tumor cells in their effort to counteract the intracellular accumulation of misfolded proteins. This response may be insufficient, at least in vitro, to prevent the induction of cell death by bortezomib; however, it led to the hypothesis that small-molecule hsp90 inhibitors, such as 17-allylamino-17-demethoxy-geldanamcyin (17-AAG), may be able to precipitate more potent and/or more accelerated proapoptotic effects of bortezomib on MM cells. This hypothesis was confirmed in preclinical MM models [51,52] and provided the basis for ongoing clinical trials of tanespimycin (17-AAG in the KOS-953 cremophor-based formulation) as a single agent[53] or combined with bortezomib[54] in patients with relapsed or refractory MM. So far tanespimycin has exhibited a manageable profile of adverse events, without significant cardiotoxicity, peripheral neuropathy, or DVT. Furthermore, tanespimycin has been associated with durable disease stabilization and minimal responses with single-agent treatment in patients with relapsed and refractory MM, as well as showing encouraging anti-MM activity when combined with bortezomib both in patients who had prior received bortezomib and in patients who were refractory to bortezomib.[54] These results, together with the lack of major additive toxicity or pharmacokinetic interactions with bortezomib as well as a possible neuroprotective effect, have provided a platform for future phase III trials of tanespimycin in combination with bortezomib.

The Role of Bortezomib-Based Treatment in the Management of Advanced MM in the Context of Renal Dysfunction, Elderly Patients, or Higher-Risk Patients with Relapsed/Refractory MM

Bortezomib alone and in combination with Dex is active and well tolerated in patients 65 years or older with advanced MM.[55–57] A subgroup analysis on patients 65 years or older from the APEX trial showed longer TTP and higher response rate with bortezomib compared to high-dose Dex.[57] Furthermore, multivariate analyses from SUMMIT trial data indicated that age did not adversely affect TTP, DOR, or OS.[58] Bortezomib is also well tolerated and active in patients with adverse prognostic features. In subgroup analyses from the APEX trial, bortezomib offered longer TTP and higher response rate versus Dex in patients with more than one line of prior therapy, β^2-microglobulin (β^2-M) greater than 2.5 mg/L, or patients refractory to prior treatment.[57] Age, serum β^2-M level, and the number/type of previous therapies did not affect TTP, DOR, or OS in a multivariate analysis.[58] Interestingly, chromosome 13 deletion or translocation t(4;14) was not observed to have adverse prognostic impact on survival and response rates to bortezomib treatment in the SUMMIT and APEX trials.[59–63] However, the role of 1q21 amplification as putative marker of adverse prognosis remains to be further explored. Bortezomib has comparable ORRs in both light- and heavy-chain disease, it is notable though that most responders with light-chain disease achieved CR compared to ~25% of CRs in responders with heavy-chain MM.[58] The significant increase in bone-specific alkaline phosphatase (ALP) triggered by bortezomib treatment suggests that bortezomib stimulates osteoblast activity, providing additional rationale for the use of bortezomib for treatment of MM in the context of pronounced osteolytic disease.[64]

At least 30% of patients with MM at diagnosis have underlying renal dysfunction (serum creatinine levels ≥1.5 mg/dL)[65,66] and conceivably this frequency is higher in patients with relapsed and refractory MM. It was therefore important to evaluate the profile of safety and efficacy of bortezomib in patients with renal dysfunction. To this end, a subset analysis from the SUMMIT and CREST trials focused on patients with renal dysfunction and showed that renal function had little impact on the response rate to bortezomib.[67] Just like in entire patient population of these trials, adverse events to bortezomib were manageable in the subgroup of patients with renal impairment.[67] A prospective National Cancer Institute (NCI) trial in adult patients with cancer showed that bortezomib clearance is independent of renal function and that the standard bortezomib dose of 1.3 mg/m^2 is well tolerated in the context of mild-to-moderate renal dysfunction.[68] However, further studies are ongoing to address these questions for patients with more severe renal dysfunction or those who require dialysis.[68] A retrospective multicenter evaluation of 24 patients with MM with severe renal dysfunction, with the majority requiring dialysis, showed high response rates (including CR) and durable responses with bortezomib and bortezomib-based combinations.[69] Two clinical trials have provided data to support the notion that bortezomib-based treatment can reverse renal dysfunction in some patients and eliminate the need for dialysis or spare patients from imminent dialysis (Table 1).[69,70] These observations may reflect, at least in part, the potent antitumor effect of bortezomib and the corresponding decrease in the levels of M-protein (or fragments thereof) and/or the suppression of other nephrotoxic products (such as cytokines) released from the MM clone. It has not yet been formally studied whether bortezomib has any direct nephroprotective effect that would contribute to improvement of renal function in MM, but this remains an intriguing possibility.

Conclusions

Bortezomib alone and in combination with other agents for the treatment of relapsed/refractory MM is associated with high response rates, consistently high rates of CR, as well as a predictable and manageable side-effect profile. Accumulating data from ongoing clinical trials of bortezomib, lenalidomide (or Thal), and Dex combinations in relapsed/refractory MM are expected to offer important insights for these key components as part of combination regimens in the management of MM, not only for relapsed and refractory disease but also in earlier-stage MM. Such combination approaches are being further evaluated to incorporate cytotoxic drugs, other novel agents, and a large number of investigational approaches, including monoclonal antibodies. The outlook for patients with relapsed and refractory MM has thus been

Table 1 Clinical challenges in MM management that can be addressed with/overcome by bortezomib-based treatment.

Clinical challenges in MM management	Bortezomib treatment
• MM refractory to prior treatments (relapsed and refractory) has a short median OS and poor response to conventional salvage regimens	• Bortezomib is active in relapsed and refractory MM[57,58]
• Age > 65 years: majority of patients with MM are older (median age at diagnosis ~70 years)	• Favorable safety profile of bortezomib in patients older than 65 years, without adverse effect on TTP, DOR, or OS[58]
• Increased β2M, decreased serum albumin, and low platelet count are associated with inferior clinical outcome to standard salvage regimens	• Serum β_2-M level, albumin, and platelet count do not affect TTP, DOR, or OS after bortezomib treatment[58]
• Cytogenetic abnormalities, e.g., Chrom 13 deletion, t(4;14)	• Chromosome 13 deletion or t(4;14) was not observed to have adverse prognostic impact on survival and response rates to bortezomib treatment[59–63]
• Renal dysfunction	• Bortezomib is safe and active in patients with MM with renal dysfunction
– up to 50% of patients with MM have renal dysfunction – between 20% and 30% of patients have concomitant renal failure	– No significant impact of renal dysfunction on safety profile and response rate to bortezomib[67] – Bortezomib clearance is independent of renal function and the standard bortezomib dose of 1.3 mg/m^2 is well tolerated in mild-to-moderate renal dysfunction[68] – Patients with MM with severe renal dysfunction requiring dialysis showed high response rates (including CR rates) and durable responses with bortezomib and bortezomib-based combinations[69] – Two clinical trials suggest that bortezomib-based treatment can reverse renal dysfunction in some patients and eliminate the need for dialysis or spare patients from imminent dialysis[69,70]
• Extensive bone disease	• Bortezomib triggers significant increase in bone-specific ALP, suggesting stimulation of osteoblast activity[64]
• Extramedullary MM	• Bortezomib is a key "backbone" agent in combination regimens utilized for salvage of patients with plasma cell leukemia/extramedullary MM

MM multiple myeloma, *OS* overall survival, *DOR* duration of response, *TTP* time to progression, *CR* complete response, *ALP* alkaline phosphatase.

improved, and research in this vital patient population promises to be busier than ever.

References

1. Kane RC, Farrell AT, Sridhara R, Pazdur R. United States Food and Drug Administration approval summary: bortezomib for the treatment of progressive multiple myeloma after one prior therapy. Clin Cancer Res 2006; 12(10):2955–60.
2. Kane RC, Bross PF, Farrell AT, Pazdur R. Velcade: USFDA approval for the treatment of multiple myeloma progressing on prior therapy. Oncologist 2003; 8(6): 508–13.
3. Bross PF, Kane R, Farrell AT, et al. Approval summary for bortezomib for injection in the treatment of multiple myeloma. Clin Cancer Res 2004; 10(12 Pt 1): 3954–64.
4. Kumar SK, Therneau TM, Gertz MA, et al. Clinical course of patients with relapsed multiple myeloma. Mayo Clin Proc 2004; 79(7): 867–74.

5. Richardson PG, Mitsiades C, Schlossman R, Munshi N, Anderson K. New drugs for myeloma. Oncologist 2007; 12(6): 664–89.

6. Ciechanover A. The ubiquitin-proteasome proteolytic pathway. Cell 1994; 79(1): 13–21.

7. Adams J, Behnke M, Chen S, et al. Potent and selective inhibitors of the proteasome: dipeptidyl boronic acids. Bioorg Med Chem Lett 1998; 8(4): 333–8.

8. Adams J, Palombella VJ, Elliott PJ. Proteasome inhibition: a new strategy in cancer treatment. Invest New Drugs 2000; 18(2): 109–21.

9. Adams J, Palombella VJ, Sausville EA, et al. Proteasome inhibitors: a novel class of potent and effective antitumor agents. Cancer Res 1999; 59(11): 2615–22.

10. Teicher BA, Ara G, Herbst R, Palombella VJ, Adams J. The proteasome inhibitor PS-341 in cancer therapy. Clin Cancer Res 1999; 5(9): 2638–45.

11. Hideshima T, Richardson P, Chauhan D, et al. The proteasome inhibitor PS-341 inhibits growth, induces apoptosis, and overcomes drug resistance in human multiple myeloma cells. Cancer Res 2001; 61(7): 3071–6.

12. Mitsiades N, Mitsiades CS, Poulaki V, et al. Biologic sequelae of nuclear factor-kappaB blockade in multiple myeloma: therapeutic applications. Blood 2002; 99(11): 4079–86.

13. Adams J. The proteasome: a suitable antineoplastic target. Nat Rev Cancer 2004; 4(5): 349–60.

14. Adams J. Development of the proteasome inhibitor PS-341. Oncologist 2002; 7(1): 9–16.

15. Adams J. The development of proteasome inhibitors as anticancer drugs. Cancer Cell 2004; 5(5): 417–21.

16. Voorhees PM, Dees EC, O'Neil B, Orlowski RZ. The proteasome as a target for cancer therapy. Clin Cancer Res 2003; 9(17): 6316–25.

17. Hideshima T, Chauhan D, Hayashi T, et al. Proteasome inhibitor PS-341 abrogates IL-6 triggered signaling cascades via caspase-dependent downregulation of gp130 in multiple myeloma. Oncogene 2003; 22(52): 8386–93.

18. Hideshima T, Mitsiades C, Akiyama M, et al. Molecular mechanisms mediating antimyeloma activity of proteasome inhibitor PS-341. Blood 2003; 101(4): 1530–4.

19. Mitsiades CS, Treon SP, Mitsiades N, et al. TRAIL/Apo2L ligand selectively induces apoptosis and overcomes drug resistance in multiple myeloma: therapeutic applications. Blood 2001; 98(3): 795–804.

20. Ma MH, Yang HH, Parker K, et al. The proteasome inhibitor PS-341 markedly enhances sensitivity of multiple myeloma tumor cells to chemotherapeutic agents. Clin Cancer Res 2003; 9(3): 1136–44.

21. Mitsiades N, Mitsiades CS, Richardson PG, et al. The proteasome inhibitor PS-341 potentiates sensitivity of multiple myeloma cells to conventional chemotherapeutic agents: therapeutic applications. Blood 2003; 101(6): 2377–80.

22. Orlowski RZ, Stinchcombe TE, Mitchell BS, et al. Phase I trial of the proteasome inhibitor PS-341 in patients with refractory hematologic malignancies. J Clin Oncol 2002; 20(22): 4420–7.

23. Richardson PG, Barlogie B, Berenson J, et al. A phase 2 study of bortezomib in relapsed, refractory myeloma. N Engl J Med 2003; 348(26): 2609–17.

24. Jagannath S, Barlogie B, Berenson J, et al. A phase 2 study of two doses of bortezomib in relapsed or refractory myeloma. Br J Haematol 2004; 127(2): 165–72.

25. Richardson PG, Sonneveld P, Schuster MW, et al. Bortezomib or high-dose dexamethasone for relapsed multiple myeloma. N Engl J Med 2005; 352(24): 2487–98.

26. Richardson P, Sonneveld P, Schuster M, et al. Bortezomib continues to demonstrate superior efficacy compared with high-dose dexamethasone in relapsed multiple myeloma: updated results of the APEX trial. Blood 2005; 106(11): 715A–6A.

27. Richardson PG, Briemberg H, Jagannath S, et al. Frequency, characteristics, and reversibility of peripheral neuropathy during treatment of advanced multiple myeloma with bortezomib. J Clin Oncol 2006; 24(19): 3113–20.

28. San Miguel JF, Richardson P, Sonneveld P, et al. Frequency, characteristics, and reversibility of peripheral neuropathy (PN) in the APEX trial. Blood 2005; 106(11): 111A.

29. Richardson P, Schlossman R, Munshi N, et al. A phase 1 trial of lenalidomide (REVLIMID (R)) with bortezomib (VELCADE (R)) in relapsed and refractory multiple myeloma. Blood 2005; 106(11): 110A–1A.

30. Richardson P. Jagannath S. Avigan DE, et al. Lenalidomide plus bortezomib (Rev-Vel) in relapsed and/or refractory multiple myeloma (MM): final results of a multicenter phase 1 trial Annual Meeting of the American Society of Hematology, Blood 2006; 108: 405.

31. Oakervee HE, Popat R, Curry N, et al. PAD combination therapy (PS-341/bortezomib, doxorubicin and dexamethasone) for previously untreated patients with multiple myeloma. Br J Haematol 2005; 129(6): 755–62.

32. Lonial S, Waller EK, Richardson PG, et al. Risk factors and kinetics of thrombocytopenia associated with bortezomib for relapsed, refractory multiple myeloma. Blood 2005; 106(12): 3777–84.

33. Lonial S, Richardson P, Sonneveld P, et al. Hematologic profiles in the phase 3 APEX trial. Blood 2005; 106(11): 970A.

34. Berenson JR, Jagannath S, Barlogie B, et al. Safety of prolonged therapy with bortezomib in relapsed or refractory multiple myeloma. Cancer 2005; 104(10): 2141–8.

35. Biehn SE, Moore DT, Voorhees PM, et al. Extended follow-up of outcome measures in multiple myeloma patients treated on a phase I study with bortezomib and pegylated liposomal doxorubicin. Ann Hematol 2007; 86(3): 211–6.

36. Friedman J, Al-Zoubi A, Kaminski M, Kendall T, Jakubowiak A. A new model predicting at least a very good partial response in patients with multiple myeloma after 2 cycles of velcade-based therapy. Haematologica 2006; 91: 273. Abstract P.0741

37. Hollmig K, Stover J, Talamo G, et al. Bortezomib (VelcadeTM) plus AdriamycinTM plus thalidomide plus dexamethasone (VATD) as an effective regimen in patients with refractory or relapsed multiple myeloma (MM). Blood 2004; 104(11): 659A.

38. Jakubowiak AJ, Brackett L, Kendall T, Friedman J, Kaminski MS. Combination therapy with velcade, doxil, and dexamethasone (VDD) for patients with relapsed/refractory multiple myeloma (MM). Blood 2005; 106(11): 378B.

39. Leoni F, Casini C, Breschi C, et al. Low dose bortezomib, dexamethasone, thalidomide plus liposomal doxorubicin in relapsed and refractory myeloma. Haematologica 2006; 9(s1): 281.

40. Orlowski RZ, Voorhees PM, Garcia RA, et al. Phase 1 trial of the proteasome inhibitor bortezomib and pegylated liposomal doxorubicin in patients with advanced hematologic malignancies. Blood 2005; 105(8): 3058–65.

41. Padmanabhan S, Miller K, Musiel L, et al. Bortezomib (Velcade) in combination with liposomal doxorubicin (Doxil) and thalidomide is an active salvage regimen in patients with relapsed or refractory multiple myeloma: final results of a phase II trial. Haematologica 2006; 91(s1): 277.

42. Orlowski RZ, Zhuang SH, Parekh T, Xiu L, Harousseau JL. The combination of pegylated liposomal doxorubicin and bortezomib significantly improves time to progression of patients with relapsed/refractory multiple myeloma compared with bortezomib alone: results from a planned interim analysis of a randomized phase III study. Blood 2006; 108(11): 124A.

43. Berenson JR, Yang HH, Sadler K, et al. Phase I/II trial assessing bortezomib and melphalan combination therapy for the treatment of patients with relapsed or refractory multiple myeloma. J Clin Oncol 2006; 24(6): 937–44.

44. Palumbo A, Ambrosini MT, Benevolo G, et al. Bortezomib, melphalan, prednisone and thalidomide for relapsed multiple myeloma. Blood 2006; 108: 3560.

45. Popat R, Oakervee HE, Foot N, et al. A phase I/II study of bortezomib and low dose intravenous melphalan (BM) for relapsed multiple myeloma. Blood 2005; 106(11): 718A.

46. Terpos E, Anagnostopoulos A, Heath D, et al. The combination of bortezomib, melphalan, dexamethasone and intermittent thalidomide (VMDT) is an effective regimen for relapsed/refractory myeloma and reduces serum levels of Dickkopf-1, RANKL, MIP-1 alpha and angiogenic cytokines. Blood 2006; 108(11): 1010A–1A.

47. Hideshima T, Chauhan D, Shima Y, et al. Thalidomide and its analogs overcome drug resistance of human multiple myeloma cells to conventional therapy. Blood 2000; 96(9): 2943–50.

48. Mitsiades N, Mitsiades CS, Poulaki V, et al. Apoptotic signaling induced by immunomodulatory thalidomide analogs in human multiple myeloma cells: therapeutic implications. Blood 2002; 99(12): 4525–30.

49. Zangari M, Barlogie B, Burns MJ, et al. Velcade (V)-thalidomide (T)-dexamethasone (D) for advanced and refractory multiple myeloma (MM): long-term follow-up of phase I-II trial UARK 2001–37: superior outcome in patients with normal cytogenetics and no prior T. Blood 2005; 106(11): 717A.

50. Terpos E, Anagnostopoulos A, Kastritis E, et al. The combination of bortezomib, melphalan, dexamethasone and intermittent thalidomide (VMDT) is an effective treatment for relapsed/refractory myeloma: results of a phase II clinical trial. Blood 2005; 106(11): 110A.

51. Mitsiades N, Mitsiades CS, Poulaki V, et al. Molecular sequelae of proteasome inhibition in human multiple myeloma cells. Proc Natl Acad Sci USA 2002; 99(22): 14374–9.

52. Mitsiades CS, Mitsiades NS, McMullan CJ, et al. Antimyeloma activity of heat shock protein-90 inhibition. Blood 2006; 107(3): 1092–100.

53. Richardson PG, Chanan-Khan AA, Alsina M, et al. Safety and activity of KOS-953 in patients with relapsed refractory multiple myeloma (MM): interim results of a phase 1 trial. Blood 2005; 106(11): 109a.

54. Richardson P, Chanan-Khan A, Lonial S, et-al. A multicenter phase 1 clinical trial of tanespimycin (KOS-953) + bortezomib (BZ): encouraging activity and manageable toxicity in heavily pre-treated patients with relapsed refractory multiple myeloma (MM). In: Annual Meeting of the American Society of Hematology; 2006; Orlando FL.

55. Mateos MV, Hernandez JM, Hernandez MT, et al. Bortezomib plus melphalan and prednisone in elderly untreated patients with multiple myeloma: results of a multicenter phase 1/2 study. Blood 2006; 108(7): 2165–72.

56. Hrusovsky I, Heidtmann HH. Combination therapy of bortezomib with low-dose bendamustine in elderly patients with advanced multiple myeloma. Blood 2005; 106(11): 363B–B.

57. Richardson PG, Sonneveld P, Schuster MW, et al. Safety and efficacy of bortezomib in high-risk and elderly patients with relapsed myeloma. J Clin Oncology 2005; 23(16): 568S.

58. Richardson PG, Barlogie B, Berenson J, et al. Clinical factors predictive of outcome with bortezomib in patients with relapsed, refractory multiple myeloma. Blood 2005; 106(9): 2977–81.

59. Jagannath S, Richardson PG, Sonneveld P, et al. Bortezomib appears to overcome the poor prognosis conferred by chromosome 13 deletion in phase 2 and 3 trials. Leukemia 2007; 21(1): 151–7.

60. Drach J, Kuenburg E, Sagaster V, et al. Short survival, despite promising response rates, after bortezomib treatment of multiple myeloma patients with a 13q-deletion. Blood 2005; 106(11): 152A.

61. Drach J, Sagaster V, Odelga V, et al. Amplification of 1q21 is associated with poor outcome after treatment with bortezomib in relapsed/refractory multiple myeloma. Blood 2006; 108(11): 970A–1A.

62. Kropff MH, Bisping G, Wenning D, et al. Bortezomib in combination with dexamethasone for relapsed multiple myeloma. Leuk Res 2005; 29(5): 587–90.

63. Chang H, Trieu Y, Qi X, Xu W, Stewart KA, Reece D. Bortezomib therapy response is independent of cytogenetic abnormalities in relapsed/refractory multiple myeloma. Leuk Res 2007; 31(6): 779–82.

64. Zangari M, Yaccoby S, Cavallo F, Esseltine D, Tricot G. Response to bortezomib and activation of osteoblasts in multiple myeloma. Clin Lymphoma Myeloma 2006; 7(2): 109–14.

65. Knudsen LM, Hippe E, Hjorth M, Holmberg E, Westin J. Renal function in newly diagnosed multiple myeloma—a demographic study of 1353 patients. The Nordic Myeloma Study Group. Eur J Haematol 1994; 53(4): 207–12.

66. Knudsen LM, Hjorth M, Hippe E. Renal failure in multiple myeloma: reversibility and impact on the prognosis. Nordic Myeloma Study Group. Eur J Haematol 2000; 65(3): 175–81.

67. Jagannath S, Barlogie B, Berenson JR, et al. Bortezomib in recurrent and/or refractory multiple myeloma. Cancer 2005; 103(6): 1195–200.

68. Mulkerin D, Remick S, Ramanathan R, et al. A dose-escalating and pharmacologic study of bortezomib in adult cancer patients with impaired renal function. J Clin Oncol 2006; 24(18): 87S.

69. Chanan-Khan A, Kaufman J, Mehta J et al. Activity and safety of bortezomib in multiple myeloma patients with advanced renal failure: a multicenter retrospective study. Blood 2007; 109(6): 2604–6.

70. Mohrbacher A, Levine AM. Reversal of advanced renal dysfunction on bortezomib treatment in multiple myeloma patients. J Clin Oncol 2005; 23(16): 612S.

Chapter 16

Bortezomib as Induction Therapy in Patients with Multiple Myeloma

San Miguel J.F. and Mateos M.V.

Introduction

In 2006, ~16,570 individuals (9,250 men and 7,320 women) developed multiple myeloma (MM) in the United States, while another 11,310 individuals (5,680 men and 5,630 women) died from the disease. Although deaths from MM accounted for only 2% of all cancer deaths in the United States in 2006, this disease remains as an incurable disease with the worst ratio of deaths to newly diagnosed cases at 4:3.[1] Therefore, new treatment approaches are needed to improve patients' outcome. The increased knowledge in MM biology is already contributing to a more specific drug design, and we have recently learned that in the pathogenesis of MM, as important as the malignant plasma cells themselves, is their interaction with the microenvironment.[2] One novel therapeutic strategy focuses on the proteasome, a large complex of proteolytic enzymes responsible for degradation of ubiquitinated proteins. Bortezomib (Velcade®, Millennium Pharmaceuticals, Inc., and Johnson & Johnson Pharmaceutical Research & Development, L.L.C., CA) is the first proteasome inhibitor used in clinical practice that targets the malignant plasma cells, as well as their interaction with the bone marrow microenvironment.

Based on the results obtained with bortezomib-based regimens in patients with relapsed and refractory MM, bortezomib was approved by the US Food and Drug Administration (FDA) and the European Agency for the Evaluation of Medicinal Products (EMEA) for patients with relapsed and refractory MM who have received at least two prior lines of therapy and progressed on their last therapy. One year later, both the FDA and the EMEA also granted approval for the use of bortezomib after only one prior line of therapy. Once the role of bortezomib has been established in relapsed and refractory MM, attention was turned to activity in patients with newly diagnosed symptomatic MM and numerous clinical trials have been designed to assess the activity and toxicity of this agent as frontline therapy for young and elderly patients with newly diagnosed MM. In these studies, the role of bortezomib has been explored as monotherapy or, more frequently, in combination with other agents.

From: *Contemporary Hematology Myeloma Therapy*
Edited by: S. Lonial © Humana Press, Totowa, NJ

First, we will review the trials in which bortezomib has been used in young patients with newly diagnosed MM as induction therapy and, afterward, the use of bortezomib in the setting of elderly untreated patients not candidates for autologous stem cell transplant (ASCT).

Bortezomib as Induction Therapy in Young Patients with Untreated MM

Bortezomib as Monotherapy

Several clinical trials have been designed for young patients with untreated MM using bortezomib as monotherapy and, more frequently, in combination with other drugs. In particular, in the setting of young patients, an important aim of these trials has been to explore the rate, rapidity, and magnitude of responses to consolidate them with ASCT. In addition, all these trials also included as an important endpoint the effect of bortezomib in stem cell collection and engraftment.

Bortezomib as single agent in patients with newly diagnosed MM has been explored in a phase II trial conducted by Richardson and colleagues.[3] Bortezomib was given at dose of 1.3 mg/m^2 on days 1, 4, 8, and 11 of a 21-day treatment cycle; this represents a conventional cycle of bortezomib at standard dose. Response rate was assessed after every two cycles. Eligible patients could then receive ASCT, whereas those who did not qualify for transplantation could continue on bortezomib for up to eight cycles if a clear treatment benefit and acceptable tolerability were observed. The addition of dexamethasone was not permitted in this trial. Among the 60 patients included in the trial, the median age was 60 years (range, 33–77 years) and 47% had stage III MM. Among 60 patients who completed at least two cycles of therapy, the overall response rate (ORR) was 38%, including 10% of complete remission (CR); in addition, 25% of patients had a minimal response, while another 32% exhibited stable disease. This figure is similar to that previously reported in refractory patients, which could suggest that the sensitivity to bortezomib is not very different between patients with refractory and "de novo" MM. One additional aim of this trial was to evaluate the frequency of peripheral neuropathy (PN) at baseline and during treatment. Half of all patients assessed by clinical examination at baseline showed evidence of PN, and an even higher incidence of PN (75%) was observed by neurophysiologic testing. In fact, PN was the commonest adverse event reported, with an incidence of 55%. During treatment, 23 patients developed grade 1 PN, 12 patients grade 2 PN, and 1 patient developed grade 3 PN. Despite the emergence of PN on bortezomib, the majority experienced an improvement in or resolution of PN symptoms when the dosage was reduced. The frequency of other adverse events was similar to that reported in patients with relapsed and refractory MM, including fatigue (21%), rash (17%), nausea (10%), constipation (10%), varicella zoster virus (10%), and infections (7%); all of these events were mild to moderate (grade 1/2). Dispenzieri et al. have conducted a similar trial using bortezomib as monotherapy but in patients with newly diagnosed high-risk MM (43 cases).[4] High-risk MM was defined by the presence of β2 microglobulin levels of at least 5.5 mg/dL, a plasma cell labeling index of at least 1, or deletion of chromosome 13 (del 13q). Patients received induction treatment with bortezomib at standard dose on days 1, 4, 8, and 11 every 21 days for eight cycles. After induction, patients were scheduled to receive bortezomib at the same dose every other week indefinitely. Alternatively, eligible patients could receive peripheral stem cell mobilization after four cycles of bortezomib. Those patients who relapsed while on maintenance bortezomib were candidates to receive the full bort-ezomib induction schedule again. Responses were determined after each cycle and required reconfirmation after at least 6 weeks. Among the 43 eligible patients, median age was 63 (range, 41–81 years) and 88% had stage II/III MM. Response data are available for 37 out of 43 patients. The ORR was 49%, including very good partial response (VGPR) in 2%, partial response (PR) in 36%, and minor response (MR) in 2% of patients. The median progression-free survival was 9.9 months. Thirty-three percent of patients completed the eight cycles of planned induction therapy and moved to maintenance therapy. Among the 15 patients who received maintenance therapy, 3 progressed. Of these 3, 2 received reinduction, and none of them responded. Median time to progression for those entering maintenance was 20.5 months from the time of starting therapy. The commonest grade 3 or higher adverse events included neutropenia (33%), diarrhea (31%), hyponatremia (21%), anemia (19%), thrombocytopenia (16%), and fatigue (14%). Grade 1–2 PN occurred in 53% of patients, with only 5% having grade 3 PN. In summary, these data suggest that upfront bortezomib may be an effective strategy in patients with high-risk MM, although either consolidation therapy or combination with other agents will be required since, at 10 months, 50% of these patients have shown progressive disease.

Bortezomib Plus Dexamethasone

Both in vitro studies and the experience accumulated with patients with relapsed and refractory MM indicate that there is a synergistic effect when bortezomib is combined with dexamethasone, and accordingly this combination has been explored as induction therapy in newly diagnosed patients in several clinical trials. Jagannath and colleagues conducted a phase II trial in which patients with newly diagnosed MM received bortezomib at standard dose in the conventional schedule for a maximum of six cycles.[5] Patients received bortezomib alone for the first two treatment cycles. Dexamethasone at dose of 40 mg on the day of and the day after each bortezomib dose was added for patients who failed to achieve at least a PR after two bortezomib treatment cycles and for those who failed to achieved a complete response (CR) after four bortezomib treatment cycles. ASCT was not specified by protocol, but the decision to proceed with it was guided by patient eligibility and investigator criteria. Interim results were reported with the first 32 patients and updated at the 2006 American Society of Hematology (ASH) annual meeting with 49 patients and longer-term follow-up, including analysis of patients by stem cell transplantation status.[6] The median time to first response was 1.9 months. Response rate improved with time: after only two treatment cycles, the ORR was 49%, including 10% of CRs/nCRs. However, by the end of the study, 18% of patients were in CRs/nCRs and other 69% in PR who represent an ORR of 87%. Thirty-six out of 49 patients included in the trial received dexamethasone due to suboptimal response. The addition of dexamethasone to bortezomib improves the response in 69% of patients, the majority being improvements from either stable disease or MR to PR. The estimated survival rate at 2 years for all patients was 85%. ASCT was performed in 25 patients; median number of harvested CD34+ cells, after granulocyte colony-stimulating factor (G-CSF) alone, was 12.6×10^6/kg during 2 days (median number of collection days). All patients showed complete hematologic recovery following ASCT, with a median time to neutrophil recovery (>1,000 cells/μL) of 17 days (range, 8–13 days) and a median time to platelet recovery (>100,000 cells/μL) of 17 days (range, 10–98 days). The estimated survival at 2 years for transplanted patients was 91%, while the estimated 2-year overall survival for patients not candidates for ASCT was 81%. The commonest adverse events (grade 2 or higher) included PN in 36% (24% grade 2 and 12% grade 3), fatigue (20%), constipation (16%), neutropenia (12%), and nausea (12%). Only two patients experienced grade 4 adverse events (one with neutropenia and the other with thrombocytopenia). These results show that bortezomib in combination with dexamethasone provides an added benefit over bortezomib single agent in terms of response rate and this response improves after ASCT; in addition, all observed toxicities were predictable and manageable.

Bortezomib in combination with dexamethasone as induction therapy for ASCT has been also explored by the Intergroupe Francais du Myélome.[7] In a phase II trial, 48 patients with untreated MM received four cycles consisting of standard-dose bortezomib in the conventional schedule plus dexamethasone, 40 mg on days 1–4 and 9–12 for the first two cycles and on days 1–4 only for the following two cycles. ORR after induction therapy was 66%, including 21% CRs, 10% VGPR (>90% reduction in the M-component), and 35% PRs. Five patients progressed while receiving therapy. Response to treatment improved along the therapy: the CR rate increased from 6% after two cycles to 21% after four cycles. Likewise, the VGPR rate increased from 2% after two cycles to 10% after four cycles. The CR plus VGPR rate did not appear to be related to initial prognostic characteristics, such as International Staging System (ISS) stage, or β2 microglobulin serum value. On the same line, the CR plus VGPR and the ORRs were identical in patients with or without del 13q; one patient with both t(4;14) and del 17p progressed on therapy, while out of the six patients with either abnormality, four had a PR, one had a VGPR, and one achieved CR. Forty patients could proceed to ASCT, after priming with G-CSF alone and a median number of cytapheresis procedures of 2 days (range, 1–4). The median number of CD34+ cells collected was 6.7×10^6/kg and all patients had enough CD34+ cells to perform one ASCT. Following ASCT, the response rates improved: the CRs plus VGPR rate increased from 31% to 54%. No significant side effects were observed with this combination, and these were usually mild (grade 1/2), with gastrointestinal toxicity being the most frequently reported. PN was observed in the 30% of patients but was grade 2–3 in only seven cases (14%). In all three patients with grade 3 PN, the neuropathic symptoms improved to grade 1 after drug withdrawal or dose reduction. Based on these results, this same group has activated a phase III trial in which standard dose of bortezomib plus dexamethasone in the schedule previously reported is compared with a conventional VAD induction regimen (vincristine, adriamicyn, and dexamethasone) in young patients with untreated MM who were candidates for ASCT. The primary objective is to determine the CR rate (CR + nCR) with bortezomib-dexamethasone versus VAD, and secondary objectives include the contribution of a consolidation cycle DCEP (Dexamethasone plus cyclophosphamide, etoposide, and cisplatinum as continuous infusion) after induction therapy in half of patients receiving either bortezomib plus dexamethasone or VAD; posttransplant outcome and the toxicity profile will also be evaluated as secondary objectives. Preliminary result on first 165 patients included has been presented at the 2006 ASH annual meeting,[8] and bortezomib–dexamethasone resulted in a higher response rate as compared to VAD: PR (82% vs 67%) and CR/nCR (20% vs 9%). The improvement in CR/nCR rate with bortezomib–dexamethasone treatment was also observed in poor prognosis patients (high B2M and 13q). The addition of a consolidation schedule with DCEP resulted in an increase in response rate as compared to that of patients not receiving this consolidation: CR/nCR of 28% versus 11% in patients not receiving DCEP without consolidation, respectively. Preliminary safety data show no significant differences in side effects between bortezomib plus dexamethasone and VAD treatments: similar incidences of serious adverse events (17% in VAD vs 15% in bortezomib plus dexamethasone), infections, thromboembolic events, and mucositis; only a slight higher incidence of grade 3–4 neutropenia was observed in patients receiving VAD (7% vs 4%) and by contrast, 4% of patients receiving bortezomib plus dexamethasone developed grade 3–4 PN while none of the patients treated with VAD developed this grade 3–4 adverse event.

Bortezomib plus dexamethasone has been also explored by the PETHEMA/GEM group (Spanish Myeloma Group) as induction therapy, but instead of giving both drugs concomitantly, using alternating bortezomib and dexamethasone cycles (a total of six alternating cycles, three of each one) previous to ASCT.[9] Forty patients have been included receiving bortezomib at standard dose, in the conventional schedule, during cycles 1, 3, and 5 and dexamethasone at dose of 40 mg on days 1–4, 9–12, and 17–20 during cycles 2, 4, and 6, respectively. The ORR was 60% with 12.5% of patients achieving CR. The response was quick with 82% M-protein reduction achieved with the first two cycles. In addition, responses were not influenced by the presence of cytogenetic abnormalities and there were no differences in response rate among patients with or without Rb deletion (90% vs 78%, $p = NS$); similarly, the response rate in patients with or without IgH translocation was not significantly different (93% vs 75%, $p = NS$). Stem cell harvest was performed in 36 patients after priming with G-CSF (10 mcg/kg per day). The median number of CD34$^+$ cells was 5.2×10^6 CD34$^+$ cells/kg with a median of 1 (range, 1–3) collection procedure. There were no mobilization failures. Overall, 36 patients received high-dose melphalan followed by ASCT. Responses improved after the procedure and the ORR at 3 months was 90% with 40% CR, 20% VGPR, and 30% PR. This schedule was associated with very low toxicity, and mainly consisted of grade 1 or 2 neutropenia, fever, gastrointestinal symptoms, fatigue, PN, and thrombocytopenia. No patient developed grade 4 toxicity. One additional aim of this trial was to analyze the tumor response kinetics to bortezomib and dexamethasone: the total reduction in bortezomib-treated cycles was not significantly different from that in dexamethasone-treated cycles. Taking together all this information, we can conclude that the combination of bortezomib plus dexamethasone is more effective than bortezomib alone as induction therapy, this regimen does not adversely affect the collection of peripheral blood stem cells, the response rate is upgraded following ASCT, and the toxicity profile is very low.

Bortezomib in Combination with Other Drugs

Laboratory studies have demonstrated synergy between bortezomib and a number of conventional cytotoxic agents, showing that even chemoresistant

MM cell lines were sensitive to combinations of bortezomib with melphalan, doxorubicin, or mitoxantrone.[10] Similarly, bortezomib potently sensitizes primary patient tumor cells to doxorubicin and melphalan and overcomes drug resistance.[11] These in vitro studies have laid the rationale for several trials investigating bortezomib-based combinations in patients with relapsed and refractory MM with highly encouraging response rates, even in patients with prior resistance to conventional agents, such as melphalan and doxorubicin. This fact, together with the additional benefit of dexamethasone when combined with bortezomib, provided the rationale for combining bortezomib, doxorubicin, and dexamethasone (PAD) in patients with newly diagnosed MM as induction therapy, followed by peripheral blood stem cell collection and ASCT. This regimen consists of the administration of four 21-day cycles of bortezomib, at standard dose and conventional schedule, and dexamethasone at dose of 40 mg in three pulses during the first cycle and only one pulse during the cycles 2–4 and escalating doses of doxorubicin (0.4–5.9 mg/m^2) during the first 4 days of each cycle.[12] The primary endpoint of the trial was to determine whether stem cell mobilization was compromised after PAD, and as secondary objectives included response rates and safety, 21 patients, who were candidates for ASCT, were included in the trial. The ORR to PAD at all treatment levels was 95%, including CR in five patients (24%) and nCR in one patient (5%). Responses were very rapid, with 71% of patients achieving PR after only one cycle, and 95% after two cycles. High-quality responses were observed in all cohorts receiving different doses of doxorubicin, although the small number of patients treated precludes any meaningful comparison of response rates between the different dose levels. All patients underwent peripheral stem cell mobilization, and 20 of them mobilized (median of 3.75×10^6 CD34$^+$ cells/kg collected, with a median of two collection procedures). Finally, 18 out of 21 patients received ASCT and 10 of them improved response status following transplant; the rate of CR/nCR increased from 29% after PAD to 55% after ASCT. Regarding toxicity, no dose-limiting toxicity was observed in any of the treatment levels. Most of adverse events were grade 1–2, but PN was reported in 48% of the patients. Importantly, all patients who experienced PN improved over time, with complete resolution in a minority of them. In an attempt to decrease this toxicity, the same group included a subsequent cohort of 19 patients receiving four 21-day cycles in which the dose of bortezomib was reduced to 1.0 mg/m^2 in combination with doxorubicin at dose of 9 mg/m^2 during the first 4 days of each cycle and dexamethasone in three pulses on cycle 1 and one pulse during cycles 2–4. This schedule, with reduced dose of bortezomib, has maintained the high efficacy for this combination, with an ORR of 89%, including 16% of CR/nCR.[13] Fifteen patients completed all four cycles and all successfully mobilized with a median of 5×10^6 CD34$^+$ cells/kg collected. Eleven patients have received ASCT so far with adequate hematologic recovery. ORR improved also after ASCT, from 89% to 100% and the CR/nCR from 16% to 54%. Toxicities were modest, and importantly, grade 3–4 neuropathy was not seen, and the incidence of grade 1–2 neuropathy was 16%. Although because of the small number of patients, a meaningful comparison with the previous schedule PAD using bortezomib at dose of 1.3 mg/m^2 is not possible, this data support the continued use of dose-adjusted bortezomib in PAD, especially if patients develop PN. This reduced dose regimen may also be of use in patients with preexisting neuropathy or those with a poor performance status.

Based on the above-mentioned synergistic effect observed with bortezomib in combination with anthracyclines, bortezomib was also combined with pegylated liposomal doxorubicin (PegLD), in a phase I trial conducted by Orlowski et al., in relapsed and refractory patients with hematologic malignancies, demonstrating encouraging efficacy in patients with MM.[14] PegLD was used instead of conventional doxorubicin due to the lower cardiac toxicity of the former drug. In addition, the prolonged half-life of doxorubicin in the liposomal formulation would allow maximal overlap between the two agents. These facts were the rationale for a phase II trial in which 63 untreated symptomatic patients with MM received up to eight 21-day cycles consisting of bortezomib, at standard dose in the conventional schedule, plus PegLD, at dose of 30 mg/m^2 on day 4.[15] Fifty-seven patients have completed at least two cycles of therapy and results of efficacy show an ORR of 58% with 16% of CR/nCR; but if we consider the 29 patients who have completed the study, the ORR increased up to 79% with 28% of CR/nCR. Stem cell collection data is available for 6, in whom a median of 13.6×10^6 CD34$^+$ cells/kg were mobilized (range 11.2–48.6×10^6). Regarding toxicity, grade 3–4 nonhematologic adverse events were reported in 58% of patients, being grade 4 in only 9% of them; the most common side effects included fatigue (16%), PN (13%), hand-foot syndrome (9%), and syncope (9%). Grade 3–4 hematologic adverse events occurred in 35%, with neutropenia being the most frequently reported (18%). In conclusion, this trial suggests that the bortezomib/PegLD, a steroid-free regimen, is well tolerated, has promising activity, and does not seem to compromise stem cell collection for later transplantation. This same combination, using standard dose of bortezomib plus PegLD (30 mg/m^2 on day 4), but adding dexamethasone, 40 mg on day one and after each bortezomib dose in cycle 1, and 20 mg during cycles 2–6, is being explored by Jakubowiak and colleagues in a trial in which 36 patients have been included.[16] This combination has demostranted high efficacy as induction therapy, improving slightly the efficacy of bortezomib plus PegLD without dexamethasone; the ORR with this schedule was 89%, including 32% CR/nCR; in the same line of previous studies, these responses increased after ASCT (ORR of 96% with 54% CR/nCR). This regimen was well tolerated with a toxicity profile similar to those previously reported in other trials, and surprisingly, PN was limited to grade 1 or 2.

The therapeutic efficacy of thalidomide in patients with MM has been confirmed in numerous clinical trials and, on the contrary, the nonmyelosuppresive profile of thalidomide has favored its combination with other agents, including bortezomib. Moreover, thalidomide has been reported to restore the sensitivity of myeloma cells to other drugs and to enhance the antimyeloma activity of dexamethasone. These facts have been the support for the combination of bortezomib with thalidomide-based regimens in patients with untreated MM. Wang and colleagues have explored escalating dose of bortezomib (1.3–1.6 mg/m^2), thalidomide (100–200 mg), and dexamethasone at fixed dose of 20 mg/m^2 for 4 days in three pulses in a series of 38 untreated patients.[17] The ORR was 92% with 18% CR; this response rate was 30% higher than those observed previously among similar patients treated with thalidomide plus dexamethasone. Responses were not influenced by the dose of bortezomib, suggesting no added value with a dose higher than 1.3 mg/m^2. Time to response was less than 1.5 months, so that only two cycles of this regimen were necessary to prepare the patients for subsequent ASCT, avoiding the potential side effects and costs of additional therapy. Because of the short treatment duration, adverse events were generally mild and reversible; in fact, only three patients developed short-term PN of grade 3, despite the potential additive neurologic toxicity of thalidomide and bortezomib. A more complicated schedule has been investigated by Badros and colleagues to determine the maximum tolerated dose (MTD) of bortezomib (dose escalation from 0.7 to 1.3 mg/m^2) in combination with DT-PACE (cisplatin, doxorubicin, cyclophosphamide, etoposide, dexamethasone, and thalidomide).[18] Twelve patients completed the study, and all received ASCT. After two cycles of therapy, the ORR was 80% with 16% CR/nCR. After ASCT, this ORR improved up to 90%, including a 66% of CR/nCR. This schedule did not appear to have any untoward effects on the quality of the collected stem cells and did not adversely affect engraftment. The overall toxicity of this regimen was predictable, although 25% of the patients required hospitalization and intravenous antibiotics for neutropenic fever despite the use of prophylactic antibiotics, probably due to the myeloablative effect of the DT-PACE regimen. PN affected 25% of patients in this trial, an incidence no higher than what is observed with bortezomib as a single agent despite the combined use of thalidomide, cisplatin, and bortezomib.

Bortezomib as Induction Therapy in Elderly Patients with Untreated MM

Upon considering the value of novel treatment strategies, it is important to keep in mind that half of the patients with MM are 65 years or older and therefore not transplant candidates. In this setting, melphalan–prednisone (MP) remains the "unsatisfactory" gold standard: response rate of 45–60%, with rare CR and a progression-free survival of 18 months. Thus, new treatment strategies are urgently needed for these patients. Based on the efficacy of bortezomib in patients with relapsed and refractory MM as well as the synergistic effect observed in in vitro studies when bortezomib was combined with melphalan and corticosteroids, the Spanish Myeloma Group/PETHEMA decided to explore the value of adding bortezomib to the standard MP in elderly patients with untreated MM.[19] The schedule of therapy included an induction therapy with 4–6-week cycles consisting of bortezomib administered on days 1, 4, 8, and 11, followed by a 10-day rest period (this represents a conventional 3-week cycle of bortezomib), and the same cycle was repeated during the following 3 weeks, which makes one 6-week cycle; melphalan and prednisone were given at dose of 9and 60 mg/m^2 during the first 4 days of each 6-week cycle. Afterward, patients received a maintenance therapy consisting of five 5-week cycles, but bortezomib was administered once a week, instead of twice a week, in combination with the same doses of MP. Dose of bortezomib was not initially defined since the first step of this trial was to define the appropriate dose of bortezomib in combination with MP. Accordingly, during the phase I trial, we investigated the appropriate dose of bortezomib for this combination, which was eventually defined to be 1.3 mg/m^2 and it was used during the phase II trial. A total of 60 patients were recruited (half of them ≥75 years). After a median of eight cycles, the ORR was 88% with 32% CR by immunofixation plus 13% nCR. Moreover, half of these patients achieved CR by immunophenotyping (undetectable malignant PC with a detection limit ranging between 10^{-4} and 10^{-5}). Interestingly, responses were not influenced by the presence of cytogenetic abnormalities (Rb deletions or IgH translocations). Regarding the toxicity profile, a higher incidence of PN (18% grade 3) was observed as compared to that previously reported in other trials, which is probably due to the physical conditions of the patients included. The hematologic toxicity, particularly neutropenia, was also higher (neutropenia grade 3 in 43%) which is probably due to the myeloablative effect of melphalan. Nevertheless, the overall toxicity is not significantly higher than that observed in Assessment of Proteasome Inhibition for Extending Remissions (APEX) or Study of Uncontrolled Multiple Myeloma Managed with Proteasome Inhibition Therapy (SUMMIT) trials and significantly decreased after the third cycle of therapy. These results have been the rationale for the randomized trial in which bortezomib in combination with MP has been compared with the standard MP, Velcade as initial standard therapy in Multiple Myeloma: Assessment with melphalan and prednisone (VISTA trial). No results are yet available for this trial, but it will evaluate the efficacy and toxicity of these regimens and also whether bortezomib-MP is superior to MP to change the gold standard for elderly patients with MM.

Conclusion

The results of all trials in which bortezomib-based schedules have been used as induction therapy before ASCT confirm a high efficacy with encouraging CR rates which significantly improve after ASCT. In addition, stem cell mobilization does not appear to be affected with adequate hematologic recovery. These data speak in favor of the complementary value of this sequential strategy: novel drugs combinations upfront, followed by ASCT.

In addition, the high preliminary efficacy observed with the combination of bortezomib plus MP suggests that this regimen may replace the conventional MP as the standard of care for elderly patients with myeloma (Table 1 and 2).

Table 1 Results of the trials of bortezomib as upfront therapy in patients with multiple myeloma.

References	No. of patients	Regimen	Dose of bortezomib (mg/m^2)	Response rate (CR + PR) (%)
Young patient				
Richardson et al.[3]	60	Bz as monotherapy	1.3	28 (10 CR)
Dispenzieri et al.[4]	42	Bz as monotherapy	1.3	43
Jagannath et al.[6]	49	Bz/Bz + Dex	1.3	4488 (18 CR)
Harousseau et al.[7]	48	Bz + Dex	1.3	66 (21 CR)
Harousseau et al.[8]	165	Bz + Dex vs VAD	1.3	82 vs 67(20 vs 9CR)
Rosiñol et al.[9]	40	Alternating Bz-Dex cycles	1.3	60 (13 CR)
Oarkowee et al.[12]	21	Bz + doxorubicin + Dex	1.3	95 (29 CR)
Popat et al.[13]	19	Bz + doxorubicin + Dex	1.0	89 (16 CR)
Orlowski et al.[15]		Bz + PegLD	1.3	58 (16 CR)
Jakubowiak et al.[16]	28	Bz + PegLD + Dex	1.3	89 (32 CR)
Wang et al.[17]	38	Bz + thalidomide + Dex	Escalating doses	92 (18 CR)
Badros et al.[18]	12	Bz-DT-PACE	Escalating doses	80 (16 CR)
Elderly patient				
Mateos et al.[19]	53	Bz-melphalan-prednisone	Escalating doses	88 (32 CR)

Bz bortezomib, *Dex* dexamethasone, *VAD* vincristine, adriamicine, Dex, *PegLD* pegylated liposomal doxorubicin, *DT-PACE* cisplatin, doxorubicin, cyclophosphamide, etoposide, dexamethasone, and thalidomide, *PR* partial response, *CR* complete response.

Table 2 Improvement in ORR and CR rates when bortezomib-based induction schedules are followed by ASCT.

References	No. of patients	Regimen	Response rate (CR + PR) (%)	CR + nCR rate (%)
Young patient				
Harousseau et al.[7]	48	Bz + Dex	Pre-ASCT: 66	Pre-ASCT: 21
			Post-ASCT: 90	Post-ASCT: 33
Rosiñol et al.[9]	40	Alternating Bz-Dex cycles	Pre-ASCT: 60	Pre-ASCT: 12.5
			Post-ASCT: 90	Post-ASCT: 20
Oarkowee et al.[12]	21	Bz + doxorubicin + Dex	Pre-ASCT: 95	Pre-ASCT: 29
			Post-ASCT: 95	Post-ASCT: 57
Popat et al.[13]	19	Bz + doxorubicin + Dex	Pre-ASCT: 89	Pre-ASCT: 16
			Post-ASCT: 100	Post-ASCT: 54
Jakubowiak et al.[16]	28	Bz + PegLD + Dex	Pre-ASCT: 89	Pre-ASCT: 32
			Post-ASCT: 96	Post-ASCT: 54
Badros et al.[18]	12	Bz-DT-PACE	Pre-ASCT: 80	Pre-ASCT: 16
			Post-ASCT: 90	Post-ASCT: 66

Bz bortezomib, *Dex* dexamethasone, *PegLD* pegylated liposomal doxorubicin, *DT-PACE* cisplatin, doxorubicin, cyclophosphamide, etoposide, dexamethasone, and thalidomide, *Pre-ASCT* previous to autologous stem cell transplant, *Post-ASCT* posterior to autologous stem cell transplant, *PR* partial response, *CR* complete response, *ORR* overall response rate.

Acknowledgments: This work was partially supported by grants from the Scientific Foundation of Spanish Association against Cancer (AECC), FISS and Myeloma Network (Red de Mieloma G03-136), and SaCyL (Ref 51-05).

References

1. Jenal A, Murray T, Ward E, et al. Cancer statistics, 2005. CA Cancer J Clin 2005; 55: 10–30.
2. San Miguel JF, Gutiérrez N, García-Sanz R, et al. Thalidomide and new drugs for treatment of multiple myeloma. Hematol J 2003; 4: 201–7.
3. Richardson P, Chanan-Khan A, Schlossman R, et al. Phase II trial of single agent bortezomib (VELCADE®) in patients with previously untreated multiple myeloma (MM). Blood 2004; 104(11): Abstract 336.
4. Dispenzieri A, Zhang L, Fonseca R, et al. Single agent bortezomib is associated with a high response rate in patients with high risk myeloma. A phase II study from the Eastern Cooperative Oncology Group (E2A02). Blood 2006; 108(11): Abstract 3527.
5. Jagannath S, Wolf H, Camacho E, et al. Bortezomib therapy alone and in combination with dexamethasone for previously untreated symptomatic multiple myeloma. Br J Haematol 2005; 129: 776–83.
6. Jagannath S, Durie B, Wolf H, et al. Long-term follow-up of patients treated with bortezomib alone and in combination with dexamethasone as frontline therapy for multiple myeloma. Blood 2006; 108(11): Abstract 796.
7. Harousseau JL, Attal M, Leleu X, et al. Bortezomib (VELCADE®) plus dexamethasone as induction treatment prior to autologous stem cell transplantation (ASCT) in patients with newly diagnosed multiple myeloma: preliminary results of an IFM phase II study. Hematologica 2006; 91(11): 1498–505.
8. Harousseau JL, Marit G, Caillot D, et al. VELCADE/dexamethasone (Vel/Dex) versus VAD as induction treatment prior to autologous stem cell transplantation (ASCT) in newly diagnosed multiple myeloma (MM): an interim analysis of the IFM 2005–01 randomized multicenter phase III trial. Blood 2006; 108(11): Abstract 56

9. Rosiñol L, Oriol A, Mateos MV, et al. Alternating bortezomib and dexamethasone as induction regimen prior to autologous stem-cell transplantation in newly diagnosed younger patients with multiple myeloma: results of a PETHEMA phase II trial. Blood 2006; 108(11): Abstract 3086.

10. Ma MH, Yang HH, Parker K, et al. The proteasome inhibitor PS-341 markedly enhances sensitivity of multiple myeloma tumor cells to chemotherapeutic agents. Clin Cancer Res 2003; 9: 1136–44.

11. Mitsiades N, Mitsiades CS, Richardson PG, et al. The proteasome inhibitor PS-341 potentiates sensitivity of multiple myeloma cells to conventional chemotherapeutic agents; therapeutic applications. Blood 2003; 101: 2377–80.

12. Oarkowee HE, Popat R, Curry N, et al. PAD combination therapy (PS-341/bortezomib, Adriamycin and dexamethasone) for previously untreated patients with multiple myeloma. Br J Haematol 2005; 129:755–62.

13. Popat R, Oakervee HE, Curry N, et al. Reduced dose PAD combination therapy (PS-341/bortezomib, Adriamycin and dexamethasone) for previously untreated patients with multiple myeloma. Blood 2005; 106(11): Abstract 717.

14. Orlowski RZ, Stinchcombe TE, Mitchell BS, et al. Phase I trial of the proteasome inhibitor PS-341 in patients with refractory hematologic malignancies. J Clin Oncol 2002; 20: 4420–7.

15. Orlowski RZ, Peterson BL, Sanford B, et al. Bortezomib/PLD as induction therapy for symptomatic MM; CALGB Study 10301. Blood 2006; 108(11): Abstract 797

16. Jakubowiak AJ, Al-Zoubi A, Kendall T, et al. High rate of complete and near complete responses (CR/nCR) after initial therapy with bortezomib (Velcade®), Doxil®, and dexamethasone (VDD) is further increased after autologous stem cell transplantation (ASCT). Blood 2006; 108(11): Abstract 3096

17. Wang M, Delasalle K, Giralt S, and Alexanian R. Rapid control of previously untreated multiple myeloma with bortezomib-thalidomide-dexamethasone followed by early intensive therapy. Blood 2005; 106(11): Abstract 232.

18. Badros A, Goloubeva O, Fenton R, et al. Phase I trial of first-line bortezomib/thalidomide plus chemotherapy for induction and stem cell mobilization in patients with multiple myeloma. Clin Lymphoma Myeloma 2006; 7(3): 210–6.

19. Mateos MV, Hernández JM, Hernández MT, et al. Bortezomib plus melphalan and prednisone in elderly untreated patients with multiple myeloma: results of a multicenter phase I/II trial. Blood 2006; 108: 2165–72.

Chapter 17

Lenalidomide in Relapsed or Refractory Multiple Myeloma

Sheeba K. Thomas, Tiffany A. Richards, and Donna M. Weber

Introduction

Until the late-1990s, combinations of alkylating agents, steroids, and anthracyclines formed the basis of therapy for patients with multiple myeloma (MM), with regimens such as melphalan–prednisone, high-dose dexamethasone, and VAD (vincristine, Adriamycin®, dexamethasone) providing partial response (PR) rates of up to 55% and complete response (CR) rates of up to 10% in previously untreated patients.[1–3] Among patients with either primary refractory or relapsing myeloma, only 25–40% achieved PR with these regimens, and rates of CR were negligible.[4,5] The introduction of thalidomide in 1999 began a new era of agents effective for the treatment of MM, with single-agent response rates of 28–36% in relapsing/refractory patients.[6–9] When given together with dexamethasone, response rates approximated 47–55% in this population.[7,10–12] More recently, lenalidomide, an analogue of thalidomide, has emerged, and is associated with single-agent response rates of 25–35% in patients with relapsing or refractory myeloma.[13–15] When combined with dexamethasone, overall response rates (ORRs) of 68% have been achieved.[16–18] Among patients resistant to thalidomide, lenalidomide–dexamethasone has been associated with a response rate of 43%.[18] Most importantly, lenalidomide is able to achieve these response rates, while maintaining a lower incidence of neuropathy, somnolence, and constipation than its parent compound. In this chapter, we will review the role of lenalidomide and its combinations for treatment of patients with primary refractory or relapsed MM.

Mechanism of Action

In vitro and in vivo models suggest that lenalidomide's effects on cell adhesion, apoptosis, the marrow microenvironment, host immunity, and angiogenesis may all contribute to its cytotoxic effect on myeloma cells, but its precise mechanism of action remains unclear.

From: *Contemporary Hematology Myeloma Therapy*
Edited by: S. Lonial © Humana Press, Totowa, NJ

Cell Adhesion

Interleukin-6 (IL-6) is one of the most important factors promoting myeloma cell growth and survival; vascular endothelial growth factor (VEGF) is important to tumor angiogenesis, and tumor necrosis factor-α (TNF-α) promotes vascular endothelial cell migration.[19,20] Adhesion of myeloma cells to bone marrow stromal cells (BMSCs) leads BMSCs to secrete increased levels of IL-6, insulin-like growth factor-1 (IGF-1), VEGF, and TNF-α.[19] Lenalidomide modulates expression of cell surface adhesion molecules such as TNF-α, ICAM-1, VCAM-1, E-selectin, and L-selectin in both endothelial cells and leukocytes, downregulating secretion of IL-6, IGF-1, VEGF, and TNF-α.[19,21] It also reduces tumor growth factor-β(TGF-β)-induced IL-6 and VEGF secretion by myeloma cells contributing to growth inhibition of myeloma cells.[19]

Fas-Mediated Apoptosis

Caspase-8 is integral to Fas-mediated apoptosis. Lenalidomide promotes caspase-8 activity, and downregulates antiapoptotic signaling by such proteins as the cellular inhibitor of apoptosis protein 2 (cIAP2) and the FLICE inhibitory protein (FLIP).[19,22,23] It also inhibits nuclear factor-κB (NF-κB), which regulates transcription of cIAP2 and FLIP.[19] When used together with dexamethasone, an activator of caspase-9, lenalidomide augments myeloma cell kill.[19,22]

Modulation of Host Immunity

Costimulatory signaling by CD28 is integral to maximizing T cell proliferation. It also increases secretion of cytokines, such as IL-2, which promote T cell clonal expansion.[19,20] Lenalidomide stimulates T cell proliferation by activating the T cell receptor (TCR) with 50–20,000 times the potency of thalidomide. It also costimulates CD28 on T cells leading to nuclear translocation of nuclear factor of activated T cells 2 (NFAT2).[24] This promotes the transcriptional activity of T cells, thereby increasing expression of IL-2 and interferon-γ (IFN-γ) genes.[25] The resulting rise in IL-2 and IFN-γ, of 50–100 times that seen with thalidomide, increases T cell and natural killer (NK) cell-mediated lysis of myeloma cells.[19,20]

Anti-angiogenesis

In mouse models of myeloma, the use of lenalidomide has been associated with decreased microvessel density.[19,21,26] This is thought to occur because lenalidomide downregulates basic fibroblast growth factor (bFGF), VEGF, and TNF-α-induced migration of vascular endothelial cells.[19,26,27] It is as yet unclear how much the antiangiogenic properties of lenalidomide contribute to its effect on myeloma cells.

Pharmacokinetics

A single dose of lenalidomide was rapidly absorbed with maximum plasma concentrations at a median of 0.5–4 h after oral administration in healthy volunteers; food did not impair absorption of the drug.[14] The half-life of lenalidomide ranges from 3 to 9 h, with steady-state levels achieved after the fourth dose.[14] The drug appears to be renally metabolized, with two-thirds of each dose excreted unchanged in the urine.[14] In phase III trials, as well as in an expanded access program (EAP) of lenalidomide–dexamethasone, impaired kidney function was associated with a higher incidence of thrombocytopenia.[28,29] Accordingly, patients with a creatinine clearance greater than 2.5 mg/dl have been excluded from clinical trials; although phase I trials in myeloma patients with renal failure are planned. Pharmacokinetic studies in patients with hepatic insufficiency are unavailable. However, co-administration with warfarin or digoxin does not appear to affect prothrombin times or digoxin levels, and lenalidomide is *not* metabolized by, nor does it induce, the cytochrome P450 pathway.[30]

Toxicity Profile

Myelosuppression is the most frequent side effect associated with lenalidomide. In a phase II study of 102 patients with relapsed/refractory myeloma treated with 30 mg of lenalidomide daily in either single or divided doses, 69% of those who received once-daily dosing, and 61% of those who received twice-daily dosing, experienced grade 3 or higher neutropenia, with 43% and 31% experiencing grade 3 or 4 thrombocytopenia, respectively.[13] A significantly higher incidence of myelosuppression was noted among patients who had previously been treated with high-dose therapy followed by autologous stem cell transplant (82% vs 58%, $p < 0.01$), but there was no correlation with the number of prior therapies in patients who had not received prior myeloablative therapy.[13] Temporary cessation of therapy for myelosuppression and appropriate institution of G-CSF until recovery of lenalidomide neutropenia, followed by subsequent dose-reduction appears warranted for patients with significant neutropenia. By comparison, in two phase III studies of 705 patients with relapsed or refractory myeloma treated with lenalidomide–dexamethasone or dexamethasone alone, 16.5% and 24% of patients treated with lenalidomide–dexamethasone had grade 3 or higher neutropenia compared with 1.2% and 3.5% of patients receiving dexamethasone alone.[16,17] Impaired renal function was associated with a higher incidence of grade 3–4 thrombocytopenia (<50 ml/min, 13.8%; > 50 ml/min, 4.6%, $p = 0.01$) in these studies as well as in an expanded access program (EAP) of lenalidomide. Thus appropriate caution must be instituted when using lenalidomide in these patients until phase I studies are complete.[28,29]

Single-agent lenalidomide has not been associated with an increased risk of thromboembolism.[14] However, when combined with dexamethasone, thromboembolic rates of 15% and 8.5% were seen in each of the two phase III studies, compared with rates of 3.5% and 4.5% when dexamethasone alone was used.[16,17] Concomitant use of erythropoietic growth factors such as erythropoietin and darbepoietin may further increase the risk of thromboembolism among patients receiving lenalidomide–dexamethasone, although subsequent reports have not confirmed these findings.[16,17,32] In a phase III study of patients with relapsed myeloma, randomized to receive lenalidomide/dexamethasone or placebo/dexamethasone, 75% of the first 21 patients enrolled on the lenalidomide/dexamethasone arm developed thromboembolic events.[33,34] Upon the initiation of prophylactic aspirin, the incidence of thromboembolism fell to 19%.[34] Among previously untreated patients who received lenalidomide–dexamethasone and were given prophylactic aspirin, only 3% developed thrombosis.[35] Similarly, low rates of thrombosis were observed in previously untreated patients receiving lenalidomide, melphalan, and prednisone.[30] For patients receiving low-dose steroid schedules who are not otherwise at risk for thrombosis, aspirin prophylaxis maybe sufficient, however prophylactic anticoagulation with low molecular weight heparin or warfarin (target INR of 2–3) is warranted for patients receiving high-dose steroids, anthracyclines, or for those with other risk factors for thromboembolic disease.[37]

The teratogenic potential of lenalidomide in humans is not known, but as its parent compound, thalidomide, is associated with phocomelia, precautions must be taken to avoid pregnancy among patients taking lenalidomide as well as in their partners. Accordingly, all patients treated in the United States must be registered on the RevAssist program before lenalidomide can be prescribed and dispensed.[38] Women of childbearing potential (premenopausal and <2 years postmenopausal) must take a pregnancy test, use two effective forms of birth control, and have repeated pregnancy tests every 4 weeks for the duration of treatment with lenalidomide. Men receiving lenalidomide must either abstain from sex or use a latex condom.[38]

Treatment-emergent neuropathy has been a limiting factor to prolonged treatment with thalidomide. In comparison, lenalidomide is associated with a lower incidence of neuropathy.[13,14,16,17] Twice daily dosing of lenalidomide should be avoided since it has been associated with a higher incidence of grade 3 or higher neuropathy (23% vs 10%).[13]

Other side effects associated with lenalidomide include rash, constipation, and elevated liver function tests.[13,14,16,17] One case of cold agglutinin hemolytic anemia has also been recently reported. A rash (morbiliform, acneiform, or urticarial) is seen in ~30% of patients treated with lenalidomide.[39]

Lenalidomide as Single Agent

In a phase I dose-escalation study of lenalidomide, 27 patients were treated with 5 mg/day, 10 mg/day, 25 mg/day, or 50 mg/day.[14] Response to therapy was noted at all doses levels, with the highest response rate (38%) seen in patients treated with 50 mg/day.[14] However, since grade 3 myelosuppression developed in all 13 patients treated with 50 mg/day, and since dose reduction to 25 mg/day was well tolerated, 25 mg/day was defined as the maximum tolerated dose (MTD).[14] In a second phase I study of 15 patients conducted by Zangari et al., the MTD of 25 mg was confirmed, with an ORR of 29% for patients treated with either 25 mg/day or 50 mg/day.[40] The most frequently observed toxicities included myelosuppression, syncope, and thromboembolism.

A subsequent phase II study compared lenalidomide dosing schedules of 15 mg twice daily and 30 mg once daily, for 21 of every 28 days, in 102 patients with relapsing or refractory disease.[13] Patients with stable or progressive disease after two cycles were allowed to receive 40 mg/day of dexamethasone orally for 4 of every 14 days with subsequent cycles of therapy. After 70 patients were enrolled, the rate of grade 3–4 myelosuppression observed among patients treated twice daily was found to be significantly higher than among patients receiving once-daily dosing (41% vs 13%, $p = 0.03$), prompting all subsequent 32 patients to receive once-daily dosing. PR rates of patients treated with single-agent lenalidomide were 12% and 14% in the once- and twice-daily dosing arms, respectively. CR was seen in 6% of patients who received once-daily dosing. However, no patients who received twice-daily dosing achieved CR.[13] When dexamethasone was added, an additional 20% of patients achieved PR, and 1% achieved CR in the once-daily group; in the twice-daily group, an additional 2% achieved PR, but no CRs were observed. Because of the increased rate of cytopenias seen with twice-daily dosing, a study of 222 patients with relapsed or refractory myeloma was performed to further evaluate once-daily dosing with 30 mg of lenalidomide on 21 days out of a 28-day cycle.[41] The ORR with this regimen was 25%. Based on these studies, a dosing recommendation of 25 mg/day of lenalidomide for 21 days out of a 28-day cycle was established (Table 1)[41].

Combination Studies

When lenalidomide is combined with dexamethasone, both caspase-8 and caspase-9 are activated, resulting in enhanced in vitro apoptosis of myeloma cells.[19] This observation prompted initiation of two pivotal phase III trials, one in North America (MM-009) and the other in Australia, Europe, and Israel (MM-010).[16,17] These double-blind, placebo-controlled studies randomized 705 patients to receive 40 mg of dexamethasone on days 1–4, 9–12, and 17–20 of a 28-day cycle together with either 25 mg of lenalidomide on days 1–21 and identical placebo on days 22–28, or placebo on all 28 days. After four cycles, the frequency of dexamethasone, in both study arms, was reduced to days 1–4 only. Lenalidomide–dexamethasone was associated with significantly higher rates of response than placebo–dexamethasone (60.2–61.0% vs 19.9–24%) ($p < 0.001$) and time to progression (TTP) similarly favored the lenalidomide–dexamethasone arm (11.1–11.3 months vs 4.7 months) ($p < 0.001$).[16,17] These benefits in response and TTP translated into an improved overall survival (OS) as demonstrated by an approximately 9 month prolongation in median OS for patients who received lenalidomide–dexamethasone and were comparable in both patients younger than 65 years of age and in those older 65 years of age and older.[31,42] Among patients receiving lenalidomide–dexamethasone whose creatinine clearance was less than 30 ml/min, TTP and OS were shorter than in those whose creatinine clearance was greater than 30 ml/min. However, regardless of creatinine clearance, TTP and OS remained significantly longer than in patients treated with placebo–dexamethasone.[28]

Before FDA approval of lenalidomide, the drug was made available to patients with relapsed or refractory myeloma, through an EAP. At the University of Calgary, fluorescence in situ hybridization (FISH) was performed on interphase bone marrow aspirates of patients enrolling on the EAP to detect deletion 13q (del 13) and translocation (4;14), t(4;14).[43] Among 36 patients, del 13 and t(4;14) were detected by FISH in 16 (44.5%) and 7(19.4%) patients, respectively; 6 out of 16 (37.5%) patients with del 13 also had t(4;14) whereas only 1 patient (5%) without del 13 had t(4;14). The presence of these chromosomal abnormalities by FISH did not affect ORRs or the 6-month event-free survival of these patients. However, the prognostic weight of del 13 and t(4;14) detected by FISH requires further validation and comparison with conventional cytogenetic analysis before it is known if lenalidomide–dexamethasone is able to overcome the poor prognosis associated with detection of del 13.[43]

Combination therapy with thalidomide–cyclophosphamide–dexamethasone has been associated with an ORR of 57% in patients with relapsed or primary refractory myeloma.[44] On the basis of this finding, Morgan et al. investigated

Table 1 Single-agent lenalidomide for refractory/relapsing myeloma.

Reference	Regimen	Oral dose	No. of evaluable patients	PR (%)	CR (%)	EFS/PFS/TTP (median no. of months)	OS (median no. of months)	DVT (%)	DVT prophylaxis
Richardson et al.[14]	L	L 5 mg/d × 28 d	3	33		NI	NI	0**	None
		L 10 mg/d × 28 d	5	20					
		L 25 mg/d × 28 d	3	0					
		L 50 mg/d × 28 d	13	38					
Zangari et al.[15]	L	L 5 mg/d × 28 d	3	0	0	NI	NI	7**	None
		L 10 mg/d × 28 d	3	0	0				
		L 25 mg/d × 28 d	3	20*	0				
		L 50 mg/d × 28 d	6		0				
Richardson et al.[13]	L	L 15 mg bid × 21 d, q28 d vs	35	14	0	PFS 2.8	27	6	None
Richardson et al.[41]	L	L 30 mg/d × 21 d, q28 d	67	12	6	PFS 3	28	2	
	L	L 30 mg/d × 21 d, q28 d	212	25*		TTP 22.4 weeks	NI	0	None
Zangari et al.[40]	L	L 25 mg/d × 20 d ,q28 d	58	40		EFS 30%*	61	0	None
	L	L 50 mg/d × 10 d, q28 d		15					

DVT deep-vein thrombosis, PR partial response, CR complete response, EFS event-free survival, PFS progression-free survival, TTP time to progression, OS overall survival, d day, q every, L Lenalidomide, bid twice a day, NI no information.
*Response rate for both the 25 mg and 50 mg levels were combined
**Total for all dose cohorts

the combination of lenalidomide (25 mg/day p.o. days 1–21), cyclophosphamide (500 mg p.o. bid, days 1, 8, 15, and 21), and dexamethasone (40 mg
p.o. days 1–4 and 12–15) repeated on a 28-day cycle.[45,46] All patients were
given prophylaxis with acyclovir, trimethoprim–sulfamethoxazole, and a pro-
ton pump inhibitor. Among 17 evaluable patients, 65% achieved PR and 6%
achieved CR. The most notable toxicities were deep-vein thrombosis (11%)
and febrile neutropenia (22%).[45,46]

Since anthracyclines have shown in vitro synergy with lenalidomide, lenalidomide has also been combined with doxorubicin and dexamethasone.[47] In
a phase I/II dose-escalation study of 41 patients, PR rate of 45% and CR rate
of 3% were seen among 31 evaluable patients. Overall, this regimen was well
tolerated. However, febrile neutropenia was noted in two patients, prompting a
protocol amendment to institute support with pegylated filgrastim. Other adverse
events seen were catheter-related infection, pneumocystis pneumonitis, and acute
renal failure secondary to emesis and hypovolemia, in one patient each.[47]

A similar study evaluated pegylated liposomal doxorubicin (40 mg/m^2 intravenously on day 1), vincristine (2 mg intravenously on day 1), dexamethasone
(40 mg p.o. on days 1–4) and lenalidomide (10 mg p.o. on days 1–21) (DVd-R),
based on the previous high response rates achieved with DVd-thalidomide.[48]
Among 45 evaluable patients, 29% obtained CR and 46% obtained PR. Grade
3–4 toxicities of note included leukopenia (35%), infections (29%), thrombocytopenia (20%), venous thromboembolic events (9%), neuropathy (6.7%), and
tumor lysis syndrome (4.4%) (Table 2).[48]

In vitro, lenalidomide and bortezomib inhibit osteoclast growth and survival, and block the growth and survival of myeloma cells co-cultured with
osteoclasts. It is postulated that these effects occur via inhibition of B-cell
activating factor (BAFF) and may prevent development of osteolytic lesions
in MM, making the combination of bortezomib and lenalidomide worthy of
study.[49] In a phase I study of 38 patients with relapsed or refractory myeloma,
patients received 5–20 mg of lenalidomide on days 1–14 with 1–1.3 mg/m^2 of
bortezomib on days 1, 4, 8, and 11. Patients were enrolled in eight separate
cohorts of three, with an additional ten patients enrolled at the MTD.[50,51] In
patients having progressive disease, 20 mg of dexamethasone was added on
days 1, 2, 4, 5, 8, 9, 11, and 12. Patients enrolled on the first five cohorts had a
PR rate of 50%; however, upon completing enrollment of all eight cohorts, the
PR rate fell to 34% with a CR rate of 3%. Dose-limiting toxicities of one episode of grade 3 herpes zoster reactivation and one episode of grade 4 neutropenia occurred with lenalidomide 15 mg and bortezomib 1.3 mg/m^2. The MTD
was declared at doses of lenalidomide 15 mg on days 1–14 with bortezomib
1.0 mg/m^2 on days 1, 4, 8, and 11. No grade 3 or higher fatigue or peripheral
neuropathy was seen, and no anticoagulant prophylaxis was required.[50,51] This
regimen is of particular interest, for its steroid-sparing design, as many of the
side effects associated with the systemic therapy of myeloma relate to the use
of high-dose steroids (Table 3).

Conclusion

Lenalidomide is an effective agent for patients with relapsed or refractory
myeloma, particularly when combined with conventional chemotherapeutic
agents, as well as novel therapeutic agents, such as bortezomib. Even among

Table 2 Lenalidomide combinations for relapsing/refractory myeloma

Reference	Regimen	Dose[a]	No. of Evaluable Patients	PR (%)	CR (%)	PFS/TTP (median no. of months)	OS (median no. of months)	DVT (%)	DVT prophylaxis
Weber et al.[16]	L/D	L 25 mg/d × 21 d D 40 mg/d Cycles 1–4: d 1–4, 9–12, and 17–20 Cycles ≥ 5: d 1–4 only Repeat q28 d	354	46.9	14.1	TTP11.1	29.6	14.7	None
Dimopoulos et al.[17]	L/D	Same as above	351	44.3	15.9	TTP11.3	NR	8.5	None
Knop et al.[47]	RAd	L 15 mg/d × 21 d Do 9 mg/m²/d × 4 d CI D 40 mg/d d 1–4, and 17–20 Repeat q28 d	31	45	3	NA	NA	0	None
Baz et al.[48]	DVd-R	PLD 40 mg/m²IV d 1 V 2 mg IV d 1 D 40 mg/d × 4 d L 10 mg/d × 21 d Cycle 1:35 d, cycles 2–5: 28 d	52	46	29	NA	NA	9	ASA 81 mg/day
Morgan et al.[45,46]	CRd	Cy 500 mg/d d 1, 8, 15, and 21 L 25 mg/d × 21 d D 40 mg/d d 1–4, and 12–15 Repeat q28 d	17	65	6	NA	NA	11	One patient received prophylactic anticoagulation

PR partial response, *CR* complete response, *PFS* progression-free survival, *TTP* time to progression, *DVT* deep-vein thrombosis, *OS* overall survival, *L* lenalidomide, *D* dexamethasone, *RAd* lenalidomide, doxorubicin, dexamethasone, *DVd-R* doxorubicin, vincristine, dexamethasone, and lenalidomide, *Do* doxorubicin, *PLD* pegylated liposomal doxorubicin, *V* vincristine, *Cy* cyclophosphamide, *CRd* cyclophosphamide, lenalidomide, dexamethasone, *ASA* aspirin, *IV* intravenously, *d* day, *q* every, *CI* confidence interval.
[a]All drugs given orally unless otherwise specified.
[b]Represents overall response rate. Rate of CR not available.

Table 3 Steroid-sparing lenalidomide combinations in relapsed/refractory multiple myeloma.

Reference	Regimen	Dose[a]	No. of evaluable Patients	PR (%)	CR (%)	EFS/PFS/TTP (median no. of months)	OS (median no. of months)	DVT (%)	DVT prophylaxis
Richardson et al.[51]	L-B	L 5–15 mg/d × 14 d B 1–1.3 mg/m^2/d IV d 1, 4, 8, and 11 D 40 mg/d (added for PD) d 1, 2, 4, 5, 8, 9, 11, and 12 Repeat q21 d	38	34	3	NI	NI	4	None

PR partial response, *CR* complete response, *EFS* event-free survival, *PFS* progression-free survival, *TTP* time to progression, *L* lenalidomide, *D* dexamethasone, *B* bortezomib, *DVT* deep-vein thrombosis, *OS* overall survival, *IV* intravenously, *d* day, *q* every, *NI* no information.
[a]All drugs given orally unless otherwise specified.

those patients with prior thalidomide exposure, lenalidomide–dexamethasone has been associated with response rates of 43–63%, depending on thalidomide sensitivity. Importantly, such response rates can be achieved with a lower incidence of treatment-emergent neuropathy, sedation, and constipation than seen with thalidomide. Prospective, randomized studies of lenalidomide in combination with currently available therapies, as well as novel agents, including phase I compounds, are necessary to improve understanding of how to incorporate lenalidomide into the current and future therapy of myeloma. Other studies of lenalidomide combinations with or without high-dose chemotherapy and stem cell support need be done to understand the place of stem cell transplant in the era of novel agents. Finally, an improved understanding of how to synthesize FISH, cytogenetic analysis, molecular profiles, and clinical presentation of patients with myeloma is integral to developing optimal patient-tailored lenalidomide combinations.

References

1. Alexanian R, Barlogie B, Tucker S, et al. VAD-based regimens as primary treatment for multiple myeloma. American Journal of Hematology. 1990;33(2):86–9.
2. Alexanian R, Bergsagel DE, Migliore PJ, et al. Melphalan therapy for plasma cell myeloma. Blood. 1968;31(1):1–10.
3. Alexanian R, Dimopoulos MA, Delasalle K, et al. Primary dexamethasone treatment of multiple myeloma. Blood. 1992;80(4):887–90.
4. Alexanian R, Barlogie B, Dixon D, et al. High-dose glucocorticoid treatment of resistant myeloma. Annals of Internal Medicine. 1986;105(1):8–11.
5. Barlogie B, Smith L, Alexanian R. Effective treatment of advanced multiple myeloma refractory to alkylating agents. The New England Journal of Medicine. 1984;310(21):1353–6.
6. Singhal S, Mehta J, Desikan R, et al. Antitumor activity of thalidomide in refractory multiple myeloma. New Engl J Med. 1999; 341 (21): 1565–71.
7. Alexanian R, Weber D, Anagnostopoulos A, et al. Thalidomide with or without dexamethasone for refractory or relapsing multiple myeloma. Seminars in Hematology. 2003;40(4 Suppl 4):3–7.
8. Glasmacher A, Hahn C, Hoffmann F, et al. A systematic review of phase-II trials of thalidomide monotherapy in patients with relapsed or refractory multiple myeloma. British Journal of Haematology. 2006;132(5):584–93.
9. Barlogie B, Desikan R, Eddlemon P, et al. Extended survival in advanced and refractory multiple myeloma after single-agent thalidomide: Identification of prognostic factors in a phase 2 study of 169 patients. Blood. 2001;98(2):492–4.
10. Dimopoulos MA, Anagnostopoulos A, Weber D. Treatment of plasma cell dyscrasias with thalidomide and its derivatives. Journal of Clinical Oncology. 2003;21(23):4444–54.
11. Dimopoulos MA, Zervas K, Kouvatseas G, et al. Thalidomide and dexamethasone combination for refractory multiple myeloma. Annals of Oncology. 2001;12(7):991–5.
12. Weber DM, Gavino M, Delasalle K, et al. Thalidomide alone or with dexamethasone for multiple myeloma. Blood. 1999;94(604a).
13. Richardson PG, Blood E, Mitsiades CS, et al. A randomized phase 2 study of lenalidomide therapy for patients with relapsed or relapsed and refractory multiple myeloma. Blood. 2006;108(10):3458–64.
14. Richardson PG, Schlossman RL, Weller E, et al. Immunomodulatory drug CC-5013 overcomes drug resistance and is well tolerated in patients with relapsed multiple myeloma. Blood. 2002;100(9):3063–7.

15. Zangari M, Tricot G, Zeldis J, et al. Results of a phase I study of CC-5013 for the treatment of multiple myeloma (MM) patients who relapse after high dose chemotherapy (HDCT). Blood. 2001:98(775a).

16. Weber DM, Chen C, Niesvizky R, et al. Lenalidomide plus dexamethasone for relapsed multiple myeloma in North America. New England Journal of Medicine. 2007;357:2133–2142.

17. Dimopoulos MA, Spencer A, Attal M, et al. Lenalidomide plus dexamethasone for relapsed or refractory multiple myeloma. New England Journal of Medicine. 2007; 357:2123–2132.

18. Wang M, Knight R, Dimopoulos M, et al. Lenalidomide in combination with dexamethasone was more effective than dexamethasone in patients who have received prior thalidomide for relapsed or refractory multiple myeloma. ASH Annual Meeting Abstracts. 2006;108(11):3553.

19. Anderson KC. Lenalidomide and thalidomide: Mechanisms of action—similarities and differences. Seminars in Hematology. 2005;42(4 Suppl 4):S3–8.

20. De Raeve H, Vanderkerken K. Immunomodulatory drugs as a therapy for multiple myeloma. Current Pharmaceutical Biotechnology. 2006;7:415–21.

21. Gupta D, Treon SP, Shima Y, et al. Adherence of multiple myeloma cells to bone marrow stromal cells upregulates vascular endothelial growth factor secretion: therapeutic applications. Leukemia. 2001; 15(12): 1950–61.

22. Hideshima T, Chauhan D, Shima Y, et al. Thalidomide and its analogs overcome drug resistance of human multiple myeloma cells to conventional therapy. Blood. 2000;96(9):2943–50.

23. Mitsiades N, Mitsiades CS, Poulaki V, et al. Apoptotic signaling induced by immunomodulatory thalidomide analogs in human multiple myeloma cells: therapeutic implications. Blood. 2002;99(12):4525–30.

24. Davies FE, Raje N, Hideshima T, et al. Thalidomide and immunomodulatory derivatives augment natural killer cell cytotoxicity in multiple myeloma. Blood. 2001;98(1):210–6.

25. Chang DH, Liu N, Klimek V, et al. Enhancement of ligand-dependent activation of human natural killer T cells by lenalidomide: Therapeutic implications. Blood. 2006;108(2):618–21.

26. Dredge K, Marriott JB, MacDonald CD, et al. Novel thalidomide analgues display anti-angiogenic activity independently of immunomodulatory effects. British Journal of Cancer. 2002;87(10):1166–72.

27. Kumar S, Rajkumar SV. Thalidomide and lenalidomide in the treatment of multiple myeloma. European Journal of Cancer. 2006;42(11):1612–22.

28. Weber D, Wang M, Chen C, et al. Lenalidomide plus high-dose dexamethasone provides improved overall survival compared to high-dose dexamethasone alone for relapsed or refractory multiple myeloma (MM): Results of 2 phase III studies (MM-009, MM-010) and subgroup analysis of patients with impaired renal function. ASH Annual Meeting Abstracts. 2006;108(11):3547.

29. Reece DE, Masih-Khan E, Chen C, et al. Use of lenalidomide (Revlimid®) + / – Corticosteroids in relapsed/refractory multiple myeloma patients with elevated baseline serum creatinine levels. Blood (ASH Annual Meeting Abstracts). 2006;108:3548.

30. Kastritis E, Dimopoulos MA. The evolving role of lenalidomide in the treatment of hematologic malignancies. Expert Opinion on Pharmacotherapy. 2007;8(4):497–509.

31. Reece DE, Masih-Khan E, Chen C, et al. Lenalidomide (Revlimid®) + / – Corticosteroids in elderly patients with relapsed/refractory multiple myeloma. Blood (ASH Annual Meeting Abstracts). 2006;108:3550.

32. Knight R. Lenalidomide and venous thrombosis in multiple myeloma. The New England Journal of Medicine. 2006;354(19):2079.

33. Zonder JA, Durie BGM, McCoy J, Crowley J, Zeldis JB, Ghannam, et al. High incidence of thrombotic events observed in patients receiving lenalidomide

(L) + Dexamethasone (D) (LD) as first-line therapy for multiple myeloma (MM) without aspirin (ASA) prophylaxis. ASH Annual Meeting Abstracts. 2005;106(11):3455.

34. Zonder JA, Barlogie B, Durie BGM, et al. Thrombotic complications in patients with newly diagnosed multiple myeloma treated with lenalidomide and dexamethasone: Benefit of aspirin prophylaxis. Blood. 2006;108(1):403–4.

35. Rajkumar SV, Hayman SR, Lacy MQ, et al. Combination therapy with lenalidomide plus dexamethasone (Rev/Dex) for newly diagnosed myeloma [see comment]. Blood. 2005;106(13):4050–3.

36. Palumbo A, Falco P, Falcone A, et al. Oral Revlimid(R) plus melphalan and prednisone (R-MP) for newly diagnosed multiple myeloma: Results of a multicenter phase I/II study. ASH Annual Meeting Abstracts. 2006;108(11):800.

37. Palumbo A, Rajkumar SV, Dimopoulos MA, et al. Prevention of thalidomide- and lenalidomide-associated thrombosis in myeloma. Leukemia. 2008;22(2):414–23.

38. Zeldis JB, Williams BA, Thomas SD, et al. S.T.E.P.S.: A comprehensive program for controlling and monitoring access to thalidomide. Clinical Therapeutics. 1999;21(2):319–30.

39. Sviggum HP, Davis MDP, Rajkumar SV, et al. Dermatologic adverse effects of lenalidomide therapy for amyloidosis and multiple myeloma. Archives of Dermatology. 2006;142(10):1298–302.

40. Zangari M, Barlogie B, Jacobson J, et al. Revlimid 25 mg (REV 25) x 20 versus 50 mg (REV 50) x 10 q 28 days with bridging of 5 mg x 10 versus 10 mg x 5 as posttransplant salvage therapy for multiple myeloma (MM). Blood. 2003.102(11):1642.

41. Richardson P, Jagannath S, Hussein M, et al. A multicenter, single-arm, open-label study to evaluate the efficacy and safety of single-agent lenalidomide in patients with relapsed and refractory multiple myeloma: Preliminary results. ASH Annual Meeting Abstracts. 2005;106(11):1565.

42. Chanan-Khan AA, Weber D, Dimopoulos M, et al. Lenalidomide (L) in combination with dexamethasone (D) improves survival and time to progression in elderly patients (pts) with relapsed or refractory (rel/ref) multiple myeloma (MM). Blood (ASH Annual Meeting Abstracts). 2006;108:3551.

43. Bahlis NJ, Mansoor A, Lategan JC, et al. Lenalidomide overcomes poor prognosis conferred by deletion of chromosome 13 and t(4;14) in multiple myeloma: MM016 trial. Blood (ASH Annual Meeting Abstracts). 2006;108:3557.

44. Garcia-Sanz R, Gonzalez-Porras JR, Hernandez JM, et al. The oral combination of thalidomide, cyclophosphamide and dexamethasone (ThaCyDex) is effective in relapsed/refractory multiple myeloma. Leukemia. 2004;18(4):856–63.

45. Morgan GJ, Schey SA, Wu P, Srikanth M, et al. Lenalidomide (Revlimid), in combination with cyclophosphamide and dexamethasone (RCD), is an effective and tolerated regimen for myeloma patients. British Journal of Haematology. 2007;137(3):268–9.

46. Morgan GJ, Schey S, Wu P, et al. Lenolidamide (Revlimid), in combination with cyclophosphamide and dexamethasone (CRD) is an effective regimen for heavily pre-treated myeloma patients. ASH Annual Meeting Abstracts. 2006;108(11):3555.

47. Knop S, Gerecke C, Topp MS, et al. Lenalidomide (Revlimid™), Adriamycin and dexamethasone chemotherapy (RAD) is safe and effective in treatment of relapsed multiple myeloma—First results of a German multicenter phase I/II trial. Blood (ASH Annual Meeting Abstracts). 2006;108(11):408.

48. Baz R, Walker E, Karam MA, et al. Lenalidomide and pegylated liposomal doxorubicin-based chemotherapy for relapsed or refractory multiple myeloma: safety and efficacy. Annals of Oncology. 2006;17(12):1766–71.

49. Breitkreutz I, Tai Y, Li X, Coffey R, et al. Lenalidomide and bortezomib induce osteoclast cytotoxicity and decrease BAFF secretion in osteoclasts in human multiple myeloma: Clinical implications. Journal of Clinical Oncology. 2006;24(18S):7606.

50. Richardson P, Schlossman R, Munshi N, et al. A phase 1 trial of lenalidomide (REVLIMID(R)) with bortezomib (VELCADE(R)) in relapsed and refractory multiple myeloma. ASH Annual Meeting Abstracts. 2005;106(11):365.
51. Richardson PG, Jagannath S, Avigan DE, et al. Lenalidomide plus bortezomib (Rev-Vel) in relapsed and/or refractory multiple myeloma (MM): Final results of a multicenter phase 1 trial. ASH Annual Meeting Abstracts. 2006;108(11):405.

Chapter 18

Lenalidomide for Initial Therapy of Newly Diagnosed Multiple Myeloma

Shaji Kumar

Introduction

Multiple myeloma (MM) is the second most common hematologic malignancy after non-Hodgkin's lymphoma, and over 19,000 individuals were estimated to be diagnosed with this disease in 2007, with nearly 12,000 myeloma-related deaths during this time period.[1] It is characterized by accumulation of clonal plasma cells in the bone marrow that secrete a monoclonal protein in the majority and usually presents with destructive bone lesions, anemia, hypercalcemia, and/or renal insufficiency.[2] Conventional therapy with alkylating agents and steroids or other chemotherapy combinations result in a median survival of 3–4 years, which is prolonged by nearly a year with high-dose therapy and stem cell rescue.[2–4] Myeloma is believed to be incurable with the current approaches, but several new promising therapies have been introduced in the past few years that have vastly improved the treatment options for these patients. These include the immunomodulatory derivatives of thalidomide (IMiDs), of which lenalidomide (Revlimid®) is approved for use in myeloma.

Historical Background

Thalidomide was initially introduced as a sedative hypnotic in the late-1950s and was found to be particularly effective for morning sickness. Soon, there was a rash of birth defects including absence or hypoplasia of arms (phocomelia), absence of ears, deafness, defects of the femur and tibia as well as malformations of the heart and the bowel, which was traced back to the use of thalidomide during the early embryogenesis period. This led to its initial withdrawal from the market; however, given its effect on the proliferating fetal tissue, several small clinical trials were performed in the 1960s evaluating its antitumor properties, none of which appeared promising.[5–7] Subsequent work in the mid-1990s by D'Amato and colleagues led to the recognition of the antiangiogenic properties of thalidomide and together with the description of increased bone marrow angiogenesis and its prognostic value in myeloma laid the framework

From: *Contemporary Hematology Myeloma Therapy*
Edited by: S. Lonial © Humana Press, Totowa, NJ

for its evaluation in MM.[8–11] In the first large study from the University of Arkansas, remarkable antimyeloma activity was observed with nearly a third of patients with relapsed and refractory disease responding to thalidomide.[12,13] Thalidomide, when used in combination with dexamethasone led to high response rates and was eventually approved by Food and Drug Administration (FDA) for use in newly diagnosed myeloma. However, the concern for the teratogenic potential necessitating multiple safeguards for its prescription as well as the significant side-effect profile led to evaluation of its analogues in the setting of myeloma. Two of the immunomodulatory analogues of thalidomide (immunomodulatory drugs; IMiDs), CC4047 (IMiD1; Actimid™, Celgene Corporation) and lenalidomide (CC5013; IMiD3; CDC-501; Revlimid™, Celgene Corporation), were the first to reach clinical trials.[14,15]

Pharmacology

Lenalidomide is a second-generation analogue of thalidomide that shares a similar chemical structure (Fig. 1). The structural modifications introduced in lenalidomide enhanced its ability to inhibit tumor necrosis factor-α (TNF-α) in vitro several fold. Lenalidomide also possesses higher inhibitory effect on the HUVEC (human umbilical vein endothelial cells) proliferation and tube formation assays. Lenalidomide appears not to be teratogenic in the New Zealand rabbit preclinical model, which is sensitive to the teratogenic effect of thalidomide.[16]

In single-dose pharmacokinetic studies performed in healthy volunteers, lenalidomide when administered on empty stomach was rapidly absorbed with peak concentration achieved in 0.5–2.0 h (Investigator's Brochure, Celgene Corporation). Peak levels and area under curve (AUC) were proportional to the administered dose across the dose levels studied (5–400 mg). There was an initial rapid decline in plasma concentrations with a slower decline afterward with an elimination half-life of 3.2–8.7 h. Very little protein binding has been seen in these normal volunteer studies. When administered with a high fat meal, the rate of absorption was slowed though no decrease was seen in the AUC. In multiple dosing studies, a steady-state plasma level was achieved in 4 days. In a dose-escalation study of lenalidomide (5–50 mg/day) in patients with relapsed myeloma, drug absorption was rapid with maximum plasma concentrations at a median of 1 h or 1.5 h on day 1 and day 28 in patients treated at each dose level.[14] The mean terminal elimination half-lives were 3.1–4.2 h on both day 1 and day 28 and there was little or no accumulation of the drug. Patient to patient variability was generally low to moderate for AUC and maximum plasma levels.

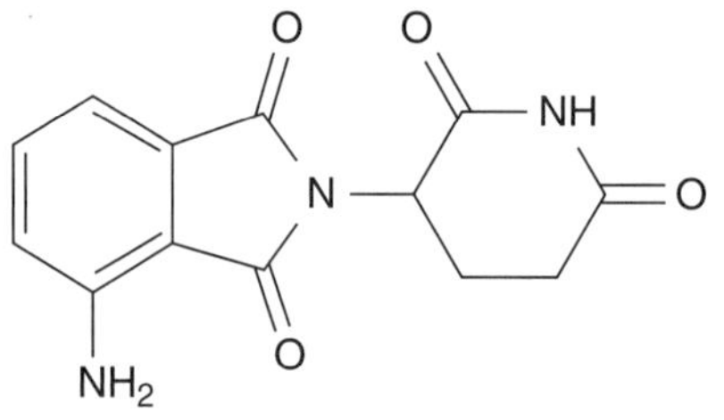

Fig. 1 Chemical structure of lenalidomide (CC-5013).

Limited information is available on the use of lenalidomide in patients with renal failure.

Preclinical Activity and Mechanism of Action

Studies so far have identified several potential mechanisms for the antimyeloma effect of lenalidomide, but it is likely that other yet unidentified mechanisms exist. It is likely that lenalidomide has activity against the myeloma cells directly as well as other cells in the bone marrow microenvironment, including the immune cells and endothelial cells. Lenalidomide possesses significant direct cytotoxic activity against the myeloma cells and induces apoptosis or growth arrest of myeloma cell lines in vitro as well as patient-derived primary myeloma cells.[17] In a mouse model of myeloma, lenalidomide led to significant regression of established tumors as well as complete disappearance in some.[18] The apoptotic signaling by the lenalidomide appear to be related at least in part to activation of related adhesion focal tyrosine kinase. IMiDs trigger activation of caspase-8 without any effect on caspase-9 activation, enhance MM cell sensitivity to Fas-induced apoptosis, and downregulate nuclear factor (NF)-κB activity as well as expression of cellular inhibitor of apoptosis protein-2 and FLICE inhibitory protein.[19] In vitro, lenalidomide was able to overcome the protective effect of the tumor microenvironment simulated by coculture with marrow stromal cells or coculture with various cytokines such as interleukin-6 (IL-6).[17]

As suggested by its classification as an immunomodulatory agent, its effects on the immune system likely contribute to its antimyeloma activity. In in vitro studies, lenalidomide inhibits the production of various proinflammatory mediators (IL-6, IL-1β, TNF-α, IL-12) by monocytes as well as inhibits the expression of cycloxygenase-2 (COX-2) and release of prostaglandin E_2.[20,21] Similar to thalidomide, lenalidomide is a potent inhibitor of TNF-α, being 400–2,000 times more effective than thalidomide in its ability to block lipopolysaccharide (LPS)-induced TNF-α production by peripheral blood mononuclear cells (PBMCs). Lenalidomide is 1,000 times more potent than thalidomide in stimulating T-cell proliferation following T-cell receptor activation. It is also 100–200 times more potent in terms of its ability to augment IL-2 and IFN-γ production by PBMCs following T-cell receptor activation. Lenalidomide induces an increased proliferation of CD3+ cells from healthy donors and patients with myeloma, when cultured in the presence of either anti-CD3 or dendritic cells, which is also accompanied by increased IFN-γ and IL-2 secretion.[22,23] Increased lysis of myeloma plasma cells is observed when PBMCs are treated with lenalidomide in the presence of IL-2, which is mediated by modulation of natural killer cell activity. When patient's PBMCs are treated with lenalidomide, there is enhanced lysis of autologous tumor cells highlighting the immunomodulatory role of the drug in patients with myeloma.[22] Lenalidomide can stimulate production of IL-2 from activated human CD4+ and CD8+ peripheral blood T cells, IL-2 and IFN-γ from T helper (Th)1-type cells, and IL-5 and IL-10 from Th2-type cells. Studies suggest that drug-induced costimulation is likely mediated via the B7-CD28 pathway and lenalidomide is able to trigger tyrosine phosphorylation of CD28 on T cells, followed by activation of NF-κB.[23]

Lenalidomide also exerts an indirect effect through its actions on the marrow microenvironment. These drugs can inhibit the upregulation of IL-6 and vascular endothelial growth factor (VEGF) that is usually seen when myeloma cells come in contact with marrow stromal cells.[24] Lenalidomide has been shown to have significant antiangiogenic activity in vitro and in vivo.[25] It significantly inhibits rat aortic microvessel sprouting and human endothelial cell tubule development, likely related to its ability to inhibit endothelial cell migration. It is able to inhibit TNF-α and basic fibroblast growth factor (bFGF)-induced HUVEC migration which may be related to its ability to downregulate phosphorylation of Akt in the endothelial cell.[25] In a mouse model of myeloma, lenalidomide was shown to have significant antiangiogenic activity as demonstrated by decreased microvessel density in the tumors.[26] The extent to which the antiangiogenic properties of lenalidomide play a role in its antimyeloma activity is not very well understood.

Clinical Activity

Lenalidomide was first evaluated in the setting of relapsed MM, where a phase I dose-escalation study enrolled 27 patients with relapsed and refractory MM at doses of 5–50 mg/day.[14] A reduction of at least 25% in paraprotein was seen in 71% in this group of heavily treated patients with —two to six prior therapies, including autologous stem cell transplantation and thalidomide. Most of the responses were seen at the 25 mg/day and 50 mg/day doses. The dose-limiting toxicity in this study was myelosuppression and a dose of 25 mg/day was determined to be the optimum dose for subsequent clinical trials. Richardson et al. in a phase II trial of two different doses of lenalidomide (30 mg daily either as a single dose or two equally divided doses) accrued 102 patients with relapsed myeloma. The study included a cohort of heavily pretreated patients, with patients having received a median of four different lines of therapy (range 1–13) at the time of enrollment. Most importantly, 61% of patients had previous stem cell transplantation and 76% had previous exposure to thalidomide. Thirty-five patients were treated on the twice daily schedule and 68 patients received their lenalidomide as a single daily dose. Nearly a quarter of these heavily pretreated patients had at least a minimal response to single-agent lenalidomide within the first 2 months of initiating therapy, and the remaining patients had dexamethasone added to their treatment protocol, 40 mg for 4 days every 2 weeks. Among these patients, 12 (18%) had a complete response (CR) or partial response (PR) among those receiving single daily dose and there were 5 (14%) PRs in the twice daily treatment group with none in CR. The median duration of response, with censoring at addition of dexamethasone, was remarkable given the disease characteristics of this population and was 19 months (range 2–22) for the once daily cohort and 23 months (range 2–25) in the twice daily cohort. The overall survival for this group of patients was 27 months from start of therapy, which is remarkable for a group of patients with a median of four previous failed therapies. Lenalidomide used alone or in combination with dexamethasone was well tolerated, with bone marrow suppression being the dominant side effect. Two phase III trials have evaluated the combination of lenalidomide plus dexamethasone (Rev-Dex) versus dexamethasone plus placebo. Preliminary results show significantly

Table 1 Adverse effects of lenalidomide.

Common side effects	Less common side effects
Neutropenia	Myocardial infarction, stroke, and sudden death
Thrombocytopenia	Cardiac arrhythmias
Deep-vein thrombosis and pulmonary embolism (when used in combination with corticosteroids or chemotherapy)	Warm autoantibody hemolytic anemia
	Pulmonary hypertension
	Diverticulitis, bowel perforation
	Skin rash, itching, and dry skin
	Fatigue
	Light headedness
	Leg cramps
	Diarrhea/constipation
	Nausea, vomiting
	Alteration of taste, loss of appetite
	Dry mouth
	Muscle cramps, muscle pains, and sore joints
	Anemia
	Tremors
	Neuropathy
	Hyperthyroidism
	Cardiac arrhythmias

better response rates with the lenalidomide plus dexamethasone regimen compared to dexamethasone plus placebo, 51% versus 30% (North American trial) and 48% versus 18% (Europe/Australian trial), respectively.[27] Time to progression was also significantly better with lenalidomide plus dexamethasone, over 14 months versus 5 months (North American trial) and 11 months versus 5 months (Europe/Australian trial), respectively. Lenalidomide is well tolerated and is associated with an acceptable side-effect profile (Table 1).

Treatment of Newly Diagnosed Myeloma

Treatment approach to newly diagnosed myeloma has traditionally been based on the eligibility of patients for autologous stem cell transplant (SCT), given the survival benefit seen with this modality in phase III trials compared to conventional therapies. Patients considered eligible for SCT are often treated with four to six cycles of a treatment regimen with the aim of initial control of the disease. The regimens employed in the past have typically been devoid of alkylating agents given the potential impact of drugs like melphalan on the stem cell pool and have included VAD, single-agent dexamethasone, and thalidomide plus dexamethasone. Along these lines, initial trials of lenalidomide and dexamethasone were designed to allow for pursuit of SCT in patients considered eligible for SCT, after a limited number of treatment cycles.

Lenalidomide Plus Dexamethasone

Based on the results from the trials in relapsed disease, lenalidomide and dexamethasone were studied in two phase II trials conducted in newly diagnosed patients as initial therapy. In a trial conducted at the Mayo Clinic, we reported significant activity in patients with newly diagnosed myeloma. Lenalidomide was given orally 25 mg daily on days 1–21 of a 28-day cycle along with dexamethasone given orally at 40 mg daily on days 1–4, 9–12, and 17–20 of each cycle. All patients received aspirin for prophylaxis against thrombotic events. Granulocyte-colony stimulating factors (G-CSFs) were utilized for isolated neutropenia before initiating dose reduction steps for lenalidomide. Thirty-one of 34 (91%) of the enrolled patients achieved an objective response, including 2 (6%) CRs, and 11 (32%) with near-CRs. Of the remaining three patients, two had a minor response and one had stable disease. Ten patients went on to stem cell transplantation following four cycles of therapy. Forty-seven percent of patients experienced grade 3 or higher nonhematologic toxicity, most commonly fatigue (15%), muscle weakness (6%), anxiety (6%), pneumonitis (6%), and rash (6%). Long-term follow-up of these patients identified six patients (18%) with a CR and thirteen patients (38%) with very good partial response (VGPR) for a CR + VGPR rate of 56%. The CR + VGPR rate among the 21 patients staying on lenalidomide plus dexamethasone as primary therapy without proceeding to a SCT was 67% (CR 24%, VGPR 43%).[28]

This was followed by two large phase III trials in patients with newly diagnosed myeloma, one conducted by the Southwest Oncology Group (SWOG) comparing dexamethasone (40 mg/day on days 1–4, 9–11, and 17–20 every 35 days for three induction cycles, then 40 mg/day on days 1–4 and 15–18 every 28 days as maintenance thereafter) plus placebo to dexamethasone (same schedule) plus lenalidomide (25 mg/day on days 1–28 every 35 days during induction, then 25 mg/day on days 1–21 every 28 days during maintenance) and a second trial by the Eastern Cooperative Oncology Group (ECOG) that compared the same dose of lenalidomide with two different doses of dexamethasone (standard-dose dexamethasone [LD]: 40 mg/day on days 1–4, 9–11, and 17–20 every 28 days for four induction cycles, then 40 mg/day on days 1, 8, 15, and 22 every 28 days thereafter or low-dose dexamethasone [Ld]: 40 mg/day on days 1, 8, 15, and 22 of every 28-day cycle). The planned interim analysis of the ECOG clinical trial demonstrated a survival benefit to using the lower dose of dexamethasone and led to early closure of the high-dose dexamethasone arm as well as the SWOG trial, the results of which are awaited.[29]

In the ECOG phase III trial, 445 patients (median age, 65 years.) were accrued; 223 were randomized to high-dose dexamethasone (LD), 222 to low-dose dexamethasone (Ld). Overall survival at interim analysis was significantly superior with Ld; 1-year survival 96.5% (Ld) versus 86% (LD) and the advantage was applicable to younger (<65 years; 98% vs 90%) as well as older patients (>65 years; 95% vs 83%). Major grade 3 or higher toxicities included thromboembolism (22.1% with LD vs 6.1% with Ld), infection (15.7% vs 7.5%), and hyperglycemia (9.7% vs 6.6%). Grade 3 or higher nonhematologic toxicities occurred in 65.9% with LD versus 54.9% with Ld; corresponding grade 4 or higher rates were 20.3% versus 13.1%, respectively.

The 1-year survival seen with the combination of lenalidomide and low-dose dexamethasone is remarkably higher than what has been historically observed with other approaches including those using SCT-based therapies. This dramatic decrease in the early mortality seen in this trial has led us and others to prefer this combination for initial therapy for patients with myeloma. Patients with newly diagnosed myeloma receiving this regimen will have the option to collect stem cells and proceed to SCT after a limited number of cycles of treatment if they so desire. Alternatively, patients can elect to defer SCT to a later date, potentially at the time of relapse after the initial therapy. The excellent tolerance that we have seen with extended follow-up in patients treated with lenalidomide and dexamethasone supports the continued use of the drug according to patient preferences.

The risk of thromboembolic complications need to be highlighted in the context of therapy with lenalidomide and dexamethasone. In the phase III trials of lenalidomide in relapsed myeloma, higher rates of thrombotic episodes were reported in the group receiving lenalidomide and dexamethasone and additional analysis from these studies suggested dramatic elevation of the risk with concurrent use of erythropoietic agent use. These studies also suggested benefit for routine antithrombotic prophylaxis with aspirin. In the ECOG phase III trial, at interim safety analysis, the rate of venous thromboembolic events was 18.2% in those receiving high-dose dexamethasone compared to 3.7% among those with lower-dose dexamethasone. These findings led to modification of the study mandating aspirin prophylaxis in all patients. Similar rates of thrombosis were also observed in the SWOG phase III trial, and the results there suggested lesser benefit with aspirin prophylaxis. Clearly the dose of dexamethasone employed as well as the use of erythropoietic agents enhanced the thrombogenicity of lenalidomide-based treatments.

Another aspect of lenalidomide-based therapies that deserves mention in the context of planned SCT is its potential effect on growth factor-based peripheral blood stem cell collection. In a study of patients undergoing stem cell collection at our institution, among those mobilized with G-CSF alone, there was a significant decrease in total CD34+ cells collected, average daily collection, day 1 collection, and increased number of aphereses in patients treated with lenalidomide compared to those receiving dexamethasone, thalidomide plus dexamethasone, or VAD. A similar trend was seen in those mobilized with chemotherapy and G-CSF. A trend was seen toward decreased PBSC yield with increasing duration of lenalidomide therapy as well as increasing age. However, there was no effect on quality of PBSC collected based on similar engraftment across all groups who proceeded to a SCT. This effect needs to be considered when transplant-eligible patients want to defer SCT as a primary therapy option and early collection and storage of stem cells should be addressed.

Lenalidomide has been studied in combination with other drugs in the setting of initial therapy for MM. Niesvizky et al. studied the combination of lenalidomide, dexamethasone, and clarithromycin (Biaxin®) (BIRD).[30] Patients with newly diagnosed myeloma were treated with lenalidomide (25 mg/day for 21 days), dexamethasone (40 mg weekly), and clarithromycin (500 mg twice daily continuously in four weekly cycles). Among the 22 evaluable patients, 21(95%) obtained at least a PR including six patients with CR and one patient with an nCR. Grade 3 or higher adverse events included anemia, neutropenia, thrombocytopenia, increased liver enzymes, anxiety, insomnia, tremors, hyperglycemia, syncope, Stevens-Johnson syndrome, thrombotic events, and colonic perforation. The contribution of clarithromycin to the lenalidomide plus dexamethasone combination needs further study, preferably in randomized trials. Ongoing clinical trials are examining the combination of lenalidomide and dexamethasone with cyclophosphamide or bortezomib.

Melphalan, Prednisone, Lenalidomide (MPR)

A different approach has been pursued in patients considered ineligible for SCT or those who decline SCT. The combination of melphalan and prednisone has been the mainstay of therapy for these patients. Addition of thalidomide to MP (MPT, melphalan, prednisone, thalidomide) has already been shown in separate phase III trials to confer survival advantage in patients with newly diagnosed myeloma.[31,32] Similarly, lenalidomide has been combined with melphalan and prednisone in patients not undergoing SCT. Palumbo et al. conducted a multicenter phase I/II clinical trial evaluating this combination in patients over 65 years of age with newly diagnosed symptomatic myeloma.[33] These patients were treated with nine cycles of lenalidomide (5–10 mg/day for 21 days every 4–6 weeks) with melphalan (0.18–.25 mg/kg for 4 days every 4–6 weeks) and prednisone (2 mg/kg for 4 days every 4–6 weeks). Six patients were studied at each dose level with 15 additional patients at levels 3 and 4 (melphalan 0.18 and.25 mg/kg, respectively, with 10 mg of lenalidomide). No dose-limiting toxicities were observed in levels 1 and 2 (melphalan 0.18 and 0.25 mg/kg, respectively, with 5 mg of lenalidomide). In level 3, 1 patient experienced a dose-limiting toxicity (grade 4 neutropenia > 7 days) and in level 4, 3 patients had a dose-limiting toxicity (neutropenic fever, skin rash, pulmonary embolism, and delayed cycle 2 due to neutropenia). After one cycle, 51% of patients showed a response of 50–99% (PR) and 49% a response less than 50% with no patients having progressive disease. After three cycles of therapy, a CR was seen in 10% and a PR in 60%. Significant toxicities included grade 3–4 hematologic toxicities (neutropenia and thrombocytopenia). Major grade 3–4 nonhematologic toxicities were skin rash, infections, and febrile neutropenia. Ongoing phase III studies are comparing the combination of MP with either thalidomide or lenalidomide.

Future Directions

Introduction of lenalidomide and other novel agents has clearly resulted in a paradigm shift in how we manage myeloma today. While these approaches have significantly diminished the early mortality in this disease, further improvements in therapy are needed to continue to maintain the advantage through the course of the disease. Success of this effort will depend on the ability to better understand the disease biology and developing therapies through introduction of new agents and skillful application of current therapies, alone or in rational combinations.

References

1. Jemal A, Murray T, Ward E, Samuels A, Tiwari RC, Ghafoor A, et al. Cancer statistics, 2005. CA Cancer J Clin 2005;55(1):10–30.
2. Kyle RA, Rajkumar SV. Multiple myeloma. N Engl J Med 2004;351(18):1860–73.

3. Kyle RA, Gertz MA, Witzig TE, Lust JA, Lacy MQ, Dispenzieri A, et al. Review of 1027 patients with newly diagnosed multiple myeloma. Mayo Clin Proc 2003;78(1):21–33.

4. Kumar SK, Therneau TM, Gertz MA, Lacy MQ, Dispenzieri A, Rajkumar SV, . Clinical course of patients with relapsed multiple myeloma. Mayo Clin Proc 2004;79(7):867–74.

5. Rogerson G. Thalidomide and congenital abnormalities. Lancet 1962;1:691.

6. Grabstad H, Golbey R. Clinical experience with thalidomide in patients with cancer. Clin Pharmacol Ther 1965;6:298–302.

7. Olson KB, Hall TC, Horton J, Khung CL, Hosley HF. Thalidomide (N-phthaloylglutamimide) in the treatment of advanced cancer. Clin Pharmacol Ther 1965;6(3):292–297.

8. D'Amato RJ, Loughnan MS, Flynn E, Folkman J. Thalidomide is an inhibitor of angiogenesis. Proc Natl Acad Sci USA 1994;91(9):4082–5.

9. Kenyon BM, Browne F, D'Amato RJ. Effects of thalidomide and related metabolites in a mouse corneal model of neovascularization. Exp Eye Res 1997;64(6):971–8.

10. Folkman J. Tumor angiogenesis: therapeutic implications. N Engl J Med 1971;285(21):1182–6.

11. Folkman J. Seminars in Medicine of the Beth Israel Hospital, Boston. Clinical applications of research on angiogenesis. N Engl J Med 1995;333(26):1757–63.

12. Singhal S, Mehta J, Desikan R, Ayers D, Roberson P, Eddlemon P, et al. Antitumor activity of thalidomide in refractory multiple myeloma. N Engl J Med 1999;341(21):1565–71.

13. Rajkumar SV. Thalidomide: tragic past and promising future. Mayo Clin Proc 2004;79(7):899–903.

14. Richardson PG, Schlossman RL, Weller E, Hideshima T, Mitsiades C, Davies F, . Immunomodulatory drug CC-5013 overcomes drug resistance and is well tolerated in patients with relapsed multiple myeloma. Blood 2002;100(9):3063–7.

15. Schey SA, Fields P, Bartlett JB, Clarke IA, Ashan G, Knight RD, . Phase I study of an immunomodulatory thalidomide analog, CC-4047, in relapsed or refractory multiple myeloma. J Clin Oncol 2004;22(16):3269–76.

16. Bartlett JB, Dredge K, Dalgleish AG. The evolution of thalidomide and its IMiD derivatives as anticancer agents. Nat Rev Cancer 2004;4(4):314–22.

17. Hideshima T, Chauhan D, Shima Y, Raje N, Davies FE, Tai YT, . Thalidomide and its analogs overcome drug resistance of human multiple myeloma cells to conventional therapy. Blood 2000;96(9):2943–50.

18. Davies FE, Raje N, Hideshima T, Lentzsch S, Young G, Tai Y-T, . Thalidomide and immunomodulatory derivatives augment natural killer cell cytotoxicity in multiple myeloma. Blood 2001;98(1):210–216.

19. Mitsiades N, Mitsiades CS, Poulaki V, Chauhan D, Richardson PG, Hideshima T, et al. Apoptotic signaling induced by immunomodulatory thalidomide analogs in human multiple myeloma cells: therapeutic implications. Blood 2002;99(12):4525–30.

20. Fujita J, Mestre JR, Zeldis JB, Subbaramaiah K, Dannenberg AJ. Thalidomide and its analogues inhibit lipopolysaccharide-mediated induction of cyclooxygenase-2. Clin Cancer Res 2001;7(11):3349–55.

21. Payvandi F, Wu L, Haley M, Schafer PH, Zhang LH, Chen RS, et al. Immunomodulatory drugs inhibit expression of cyclooxygenase-2 from TNF-alpha, IL-1beta, and LPS-stimulated human PBMC in a partially IL-10-dependent manner. Cell Immunol 2004;230(2):81–8.

22. Davies FE, Raje N, Hideshima T, Lentzsch S, Young G, Tai YT, et al. Thalidomide and immunomodulatory derivatives augment natural killer cell cytotoxicity in multiple myeloma. Blood 2001;98(1):210–6.

23. LeBlanc R, Hideshima T, Catley LP, Shringarpure R, Burger R, Mitsiades N, et al. Immunomodulatory drug costimulates T cells via the B7-CD28 pathway. Blood 2004;103(5):1787–90.

24. Gupta D, Treon SP, Shima Y, Hideshima T, Podar K, Tai YT, .et al Adherence of multiple myeloma cells to bone marrow stromal cells upregulates vascular endothelial growth factor secretion: therapeutic applications. Leukemia 2001;15(12):1950–61.

25. Dredge K, Horsfall R, Robinson SP, Zhang LH, Lu L, Tang Y, et al. Orally administered lenalidomide (CC-5013) is anti-angiogenic in vivo and inhibits endothelial cell migration and Akt phosphorylation in vitro. Microvasc Res 2005;69(1–2):56–63.

26. Lentzsch S, LeBlanc R, Podar K, Davies F, Lin B, Hideshima T, et al. Immunomodulatory analogs of thalidomide inhibit growth of Hs Sultan cells and angiogenesis in vivo. Leukemia 2003;17(1):41–4.

27. Dimopoulos MA, Weber D, Chen C, Spencer A, Niesvizky R, Attal M, et al. Evaluating oral lenalidomide (Revlimid-) and dexamethasone versus placebo and dexamethasone in patients with relapsed or refractory multiple myeloma. Haematologica 2005;90(S2):160.

28. Lacy M, Gertz M, Dispenzieri A, Hayman S, Geyer S, Zeldenrust S, . Lenalidomide plus dexamethasone (Rev/Dex) in newly diagnosed myeloma: response to therapy, time to progression, and survival. ASH Annual Meeting Abstracts 2006;108(11):798-.

29. Rajkumar SV, Jacobus S, Callander N, Fonseca R, Vesole D, Williams M, et al. Phase III trial of lenalidomide plus high-dose dexamethasone versus lenalidomide plus low-dose dexamethasone in newly diagnosed multiple myeloma (E4A03): a trial coordinated by the Eastern Cooperative Oncology Group. J Clin Oncol (Meeting Abstracts) 2007;25(18_suppl):LBA8025-.

30. Niesvizky R, Jayabalan DS, Furst JR, Cho HJ, Pearse RN, Zafar F, et al. Clarithromycin, lenalidomide and dexamethasone combination therapy as primary treatment of multiple myeloma. J Clin Oncol (Meeting Abstracts) 2006;24(18_suppl):7545-.

31. Palumbo A, Bringhen S, Caravita T, Merla E, Capparella V, Callea V, et al. Oral melphalan and prednisone chemotherapy plus thalidomide compared with melphalan and prednisone alone in elderly patients with multiple myeloma: randomised controlled trial. Lancet 2006;367(9513):825–31.

32. Facon T, Mary J, Harousseau J, Huguet F, Berthou C, Grosbois B, et al. Superiority of melphalan-prednisone (MP) + thalidomide (THAL) over MP and autologous stem cell transplantation in the treatment of newly diagnosed elderly patients with multiple myeloma. J Clin Oncol (Meeting Abstracts) 2006;24(18_suppl):1-.

33. Palumbo A, Falco P, Benevolo G, Canepa L, D'Ardia S, Gozzetti A, et al. Oral lenalidomide plus melphalan and prednisone (R-MP) for newly diagnosed multiple myeloma. J Clin Oncol (Meeting Abstracts) 2006;24(18_suppl):7518-.

Section 5

Current and Future Targets

Chapter 19

The Role of Heat Shock Protein 90 as a Therapeutic Target for Multiple Myeloma

Constantine S. Mitsiades, Teru Hideshima, Nikhil C. Munshi,
Paul G. Richardson, and Kenneth C. Anderson

Introduction

Heat shock protein 90 (hsp90) is a molecular chaperone ubiquitously present in eukaryotic cells (as reviewed in Neckers and Ivy,[1] Xu and Neckers,[2] and Workman et al.[3]). It interacts intracellularly with a broad range of client proteins and functions to preserve their 3-dimensional (3-D) conformation to a functionally competent state, as well as facilitate their intracellular trafficking.[4] The interaction of hsp90 with its client proteins involves formation of a multiprotein complex whereby binding of ATP to the ATP-binding domain of hsp90 allows it to facilitate the proper folding and conformational stabilization of a target protein. In the absence of this ATP–hsp90 interaction, client proteins are more likely to remain unfolded or misfolded and become ubiquitinated, thus leading to their proteasomal degradation. Compared to many other heat shock proteins, hsp90 has the intriguing feature that it interacts with a set of client proteins which include cell surface receptors for diverse cytokines and growth factors, intracellular kinases and kinase targets, as well as other effectors of signal transduction cascades.[1–4] Although many of these hsp90 client proteins share limited, if any, structural similarities, their respective functions tend to promote cell proliferation, survival, and resistance to proapoptotic stimuli. Neoplastic cells, in particular, typically require a high degree of hsp90 function, not only because many of these hsp90-depenent molecular cascades play critical roles in the biological behavior of tumor cells but also because the 3-D conformations of many mutated oncoproteins (including mutant versions of src, raf, or p53), as well as chimeric oncogenic kinases (including bcr/abl), which drive the malignant phenotype, are more dependent on hsp90 function compared to their respective wild-type counterparts.[1–3] Therefore, inhibition of hsp90 function would present the advantage of being directed against a singular molecular target, which, in turn, facilitates the biological activities of a multitude of pathways that contribute to the establishment and progression of neoplasias.

   Work from many centers, including our own, has shown that small molecule inhibitors which competitively inhibit the ATP-binding domain of hsp90, such as the ansamycin geldanamycin and its analogues, including

From: *Contemporary Hematology Myeloma Therapy*
Edited by: S. Lonial © Humana Press, Totowa, NJ

17-allylamino-17-demethoxygeldanamycin (17-AAG) or 17-dimethylami-noethylamino-17-demethoxygeldanamycin (DMAG), can suppress the function of hsp90 and therefore perturb its client proteins, leading to antiproliferative and proapoptotic effects in various solid tumor models and hematologic neoplasias. In particular, our studies in multiple myeloma (MM) models have shown that MM cells are responsive to hsp90 inhibitors in vitro (at pharmacologically achievable concentrations) and in clinically relevant orthotopic in vivo xenograft models.[5] They can also function to sensitize MM cells to other proapoptotic agents.[6] In this review, we summarize the current preclinical and clinical experience in MM with hsp90 inhibition and highlight some of the unanswered questions regarding the mechanism(s) of anti-MM actions of these agents, as well as the challenges that lie ahead in the clinical development and applications of this promising class of agents.

The Molecular Basis for Chaperoning Function of hsp90 and Its Inhibition by Pharmacological Modulators

The precise sequence of molecular events that are intertwined in the process of hsp90 function remains the focus of ongoing research efforts. The current view on the hsp90 functional cycle (as reviewed in Powers and Workman[4]) is that misfolded intracellular client proteins of hsp90 are initially engaged by the hsp70–hsp40 complex, which is subsequently transferred onto the ADP-bound dimer of hsp90 via the tetracopeptide repeat cochaperone HOP (also known as hsp70/hsp90-organizing protein). When ADP is exchanged for ATP at the N-terminal ATP-binding site of hsp90, the latter undergoes a conformational change which releases hsp70/hsp40 and HOP, allowing for ATP-dependent association with hsp90 of other cochaperones, including P23, p50CDC37, the immunophilins, or AHA1, a cochaperone which increases the ATPase activity of hsp90. This assortment of interacting proteins is collectively referred to as the "mature complex." It is presently believed that the precise compliment of cochaperones in this mature complex is dependent upon the specific type of client protein which is being chaperoned. The formation of the mature complex allows for the client protein to undergo changes in its 3-D conformation and eventually adopt the active conformation that is conducive to a functionally competent state. For this entire process, the exchange of ADP for ATP in the N-terminal-binding pocket of hsp90 is essential: small molecules of the ansamycin family (such as geldanamycin and its various analogues) bind to this pocket and block its ATPase activity, so preventing the formation of the mature complex. This results, in turn, in proteasome-dependent degradation of associated client proteins, possibly via the recruitment of the E3 ubiquitin ligase CHIP (Carboxyl terminus of the Hsc70-Interacting Protein), as reviewed in Powers and Workman[4] and pearl and Prodromou.[7]

The Rationale Behind the Preclinical Evaluation of hsp90 Inhibitors in MM

We initiated our studies of hsp90 inhibition in MM in the early part of this decade, at a time when hsp90 was not deemed to be a major therapeutic target for MM. We know now that several key proteins are regulated directly or indirectly by hsp90 (e.g., Akt, IGF-1R, and IKK).[8–13] However, at the beginning of our preclinical studies of hsp90 inhibitors in MM, there was little, if any, evidence that might directly and specifically implicate hsp90 in the pathophysiology of MM. For instance, hsp90 transcripts had not emerged from any major molecular profiling studies as being differentially expressed in MM cells compared to normal plasma cells,[14–17] a finding that was also later supported by subsequent studies.[5] Nevertheless, despite the apparent lack of differential expression of hsp90 transcripts between MM cells and normal plasma cells, we proceeded with preclinical studies of hsp90 inhibitors. This decision was influenced by a constellation of key factors, which included the molecular/genetic heterogeneity/complexity of MM cells, the functional redundancy that can exhibited by molecular lesions contributing to the pathophysiology of each MM subtype, as well as the relatively higher dependence of mutated/chimeric oncoproteins, compared to their wild-type counterparts, on hsp90 for their 3-D structure and oncogenic function.

High-resolution genomic and transcriptional analyses of MM cells have recently characterized in detail that MM encompasses a series of molecularly defined subtypes.[18,19] Even before those more recent advances, it was already recognized for several years now, that MM patients can vary considerably in terms of the molecular features of their tumor cells. Even within each of the molecularly defined subgroups of MM, the biological behavior of MM tumor cells is dictated not by any single molecular lesion but by multiple ones which coexist in the same MM cell. Indeed, while patients within each of subsets of MM may share certain similar molecular features (e.g., chromosomal translocations which juxtapose, in nonhyperdiploid MM cases, diverse proto-oncogenes to immunoglobulin promoter regions[18,19]), very few, if any, specific and well-credentialed therapeutic targets are present across all molecularly defined subtypes of MM. Furthermore, within each of these MM subgroups, substantial genetic complexity exists and the molecular lesions (e.g., chromosomal translocations and patterns of expression of D-type cyclins) which are now used to distinguish one subtype of MM from another are not the sole determinants of the biological behavior of MM cells (as reviewed in Mitsiades et al.[20]). For instance, nonhyperdiploid MM cases not only harbor the primary immunoglobulin translocations which are considered a key driving force for these cells but also have a broad constellation of other genetic events (e.g., chromosome 13 abnormalities, Ras mutations).[21] An example that supports this point comes from studies of newly diagnosed MM patients harboring the t(4;14) translocation.[22] Although collectively this subgroup of patients has inferior median overall survival and event-free survival with double autologous stem cell transplant in the IFM 99 trials compared to patients without t(4;14), patients who present at diagnosis with both low β(2)-microglobulin (β2M) (<4 mg/l) and high hemoglobin (Hb) (≥10g/l) have significantly better clinical outcome than do those patients with high β2M and/or low Hb, indicating a heterogeneous underlying biology for MM cases harboring the t(4;14) translocation.[22] Similarly, the biological behavior of hyperdiploid MM cases cannot be attributed to any single individual molecular target because these cells harbor by default a multitude of upregulation genes which are resident in supernumerary chromosomes. Further adding to this complexity, both hyperdiploid and nonhyperdiploid MM cases accumulate, as the disease progresses, a wide range of additional genetic lesions that contribute to increased proliferation, survival, and drug resistance. These secondary events can include secondary immunoglobulin gene translocations (e.g., secondary myc translocations), inactivation of components of the Rb pathway (e.g., p18[INK4c] or Rb itself), mutations and/or mono-allelic deletion of p53, PTEN mutations/deletions, etc. (as reviewed in Fonseca et al.[21,23]).

From the standpoint of developing new therapies for MM, the conclusion derived from the molecular heterogeneity and complexity of MM is that single-agent therapeutic which is exclusively directed against any individual molecular target is unlikely to offer curative treatment for MM, in general, or for any one of its molecularly defined subtypes. The multiplicity of cascades that contribute to MM cell proliferation, survival, and drug resistance, and, importantly, the fact that these cascades are not the same for patients in different molecular subgroups of MM, or even within the same one, highlight the importance of the concept of multitargeted treatment approaches. One strategy to simultaneously target multiple molecular cascades is to administer regimens which combine conventional and/or investigational anti-MM agents. Another approach is to utilize single chemical entities which can either simultaneously target multiple molecular targets (e.g., as the case is with broad-spectrum small molecule kinase inhibitors[24]) or which target a single molecular target which in turn regulates the activity of diverse molecular pathways at the same time. Hsp90 inhibitors fall into the latter category, and, as described previously, by virtue of its ability to chaperone a broad spectrum of client proteins involved in proliferation, survival, and drug resistance in solid tumor, we hypothesized that hsp90 would likely play a similar role in MM.

Some additional considerations made the study of hsp90 inhibitors particularly attractive for MM. Prior studies in other tumor types had shown that mutated or chimeric oncoproteins (such as bcr/abl, mutated p53, and B-Raf) are often more dependent on hsp90 function for their proper 3-D structure, compared to their wild-type counterparts.[1] Consequently, these mutated/chimeric oncoproteins are more sensitive to inhibition of hsp90. On the basis of this experience, we hypothesized that at least some cases of MM would harbor mutated or chimeric oncoproteins which would be sensitive to hsp90 inhibition and would drive the pathophysiology of these MM cells in a manner that would render them responsive to hsp90 inhibitors.

Another attractive feature of the multitargeted nature of hsp90 inhibition is that it may be applied even without specific pretreatment information on which molecular pathways might be activated in MM cells of a particular patient. In a hypothetical clinical scenario where a cocktail of highly selective targeted agents would have to be designed to specifically counteract the pro-liferative/drug resistance cascades of the tumor cells, a prescribing physician would also by default need to have access to detailed and specific information on which pathways must be targeted, in order for the patient to receive the right combination of selective inhibitors for each target of interest. Omitting from that cocktail an inhibitor for one or more of those critical pathways could comprise the activity of the entire regimen, due to unopposed activity of these pathway(s) in stimulating tumor cell proliferation/survival/drug resistance. Despite the progress in molecular profiling, such a level of clinically oriented molecular information is not routinely available for therapeutic decision-making in MM or most other cancers. However, such pieces of data, while probably useful, are not indispensable in the case of treatment with hsp90 inhibitors. Indeed, most critical nodal points in proliferative and antiapoptotic signaling cascades are regulated directly or indirectly by hsp90 (as reviewed in Neckers and Ivy[1]). Therefore, the probability that hsp90 can effectively target one or more pathways driving the biological behavior of a patient's MM cells is considerably higher than the probability of achieving the same molecular sequelae and antitumor effect through combining highly selective targeted monotherapies in random, without the benefit of validated insight on the molecular features of the MM cells of the individual patient. This pleiotropicity of hsp90 inhibitors could be a therapeutic advantage in terms of decreasing the probability of emergence of drug-resistant clones. The multitargeted nature of the action of an hsp90 inhibitor not only allows for increased probability that the multiple pathways responsible for MM cell proliferation and survival are inhibited but also leads to an increased probability that any collateral pathways that might emerge to confer drug resistance are also blocked. It is also conceivable that the molecular lesions that might lead to emergence of drug resistance involve mutated/chimeric oncoproteins, which again may have a high probability of being themselves quite sensitive to hsp90 inhibition, as previously mentioned.

Preclinical Results of In Vitro and In Vivo Studies of hsp90 Inhibitors in MM

The in vitro and in vivo anti-MM activity of hsp90 inhibitors was initially evaluated in the studies of Mitsiades et al.,[5,6] which utilized several members of the ansamycin family of hsp90 inhibitors, including the parent compound geldanamycin and its various analogues, such as 17-AAG. We observed that submicromolar and low micromolar concentrations of these hsp90 inhibitors, which are clinically achievable in trials of 17-AAG in solid tumors, led to in vitro induction of MM cell death. This effect was observed in a wide range of MM cell lines and primary MM tumor samples, including cells resistant to conventional (including dexamethasone, doxorubicin, and melphalan), novel (e.g., bortezomib, thalidomide, lenalidomide), or investigational (e.g., Apo2L/TRAIL) anti-MM agents.[5] Importantly, we observed significant in vivo anti-MM activity of 17-AAG in a model of diffuse MM bone lesions in SCID/NOD mice.[5] Our original preclinical observations have since been confirmed by multiple groups in diverse MM experimental settings, both in vitro[25–30] and in vivo,[25,27,31] using diverse members of the ansamycin class, as well as different drug formulations.[25,27,31] Of particular interest is the development of alternative formulations of ansamycin hsp90 inhibitors: geldanamycin and many of its analogues are poorly soluble in aqueous solutions and the originally clinical uses of 17-AAG have required formulations based on DMSO-egg phospholipid vehicles, which were difficult to prepare for clinical use and also were associated with substantial side effects that limited the ability to deliver maximal doses to the patients enrolled in those trials.[32] Subsequent improvements in formulations of hsp90 inhibitors have included the use of cremophor as vehicle for 17-AAG (as in the KOS-953 formulation)[33,34] as well as the development of the water-soluble isomers of 17-AAG, such as IPI-504.[35]

As expected by the pleiotropic molecular functions of hsp90, its inhibition in MM cells by small molecular weight inhibitors confers a pleiotropic constellation of molecular sequelae, which are considered to account, at least in part, for the mechanistic basis of their anti-MM effects.[5] The aggregate preclinical experience with hsp90 inhibitors indicates that hsp90 inhibitors abrogate cytokine (e.g., IGF-1R and IL-6)-induced signaling cascades at multiple molecular levels, including suppression of cell surface expression of IGF-1R and IL-6R and inhibition of downstream signaling (via PI-3K/Akt/mTOR, Ras/Raf/MAPK, IKK/NF-κB), via molecular events which include the suppression of expression and/or function of Akt, Raf, IKK-α, and p70S6K5. These events lead to multiple downstream proapoptotic sequelae, including increased nuclear translocation of proapoptotic members of the Forkhead family of transcription factors; suppressed expression of intracellular inhibitors of apoptosis (e.g., the caspase inhibitors FLIP, XIAP, cIAP-2); as well as decreased constitutive and IGF-induced activity of NF-κB, telomerase, HIF-1a, and 20S proteasome.[5] These molecular events not only contribute to decreased MM proliferation but can also increase their sensitivity to chemotherapy or dexamethasone (e.g., through NF-κB inhibition), suppress the long-term replicative potential of MM cells (e.g., through inhibition of telomerase function), or blunt proangiogenic effects (e.g., via suppression of HIF-1a transcriptional activity).[5] These pleiotropic antiproliferative/proapoptotic events allow hsp90 inhibitors to abrogate bone marrow stromal cell (BMSC)-derived protection on MM tumor cells, and sensitize them to other anticancer drugs, including cytotoxic chemotherapy.[5]

Specifically, many of the diverse cascades that are regulated by hsp90 and suppressed by its inhibition are known to contribute to resistance of MM cells to apoptosis induced by other anti-MM agents. For instance, IGF-1R signaling has been implicated to decreased response of MM cells to dexamethasone, doxorubicin, and the proteasome inhibitor bortezomib (PS-341).[6,11,36] Stimulation of MM cells with IL-6, either exogenously administered or produced by BMSCs cocultured with MM cells, also confers to MM cells attenuated response to dexamethasone.[37] The inhibitors of apoptosis (IAPs), FLIP, XIAP, cIAP-2, and survivin, are known to suppress the activity of caspase-8 (e.g., in the case of FLIP and cIAP-2), caspase-9 (in the case of XIAP), and caspase-3 (in the case of survivin). Given the role of these caspases for induction of MM cell death by various anti-MM agents (e.g., caspase-8 mediates the direct anti-MM effects of thalidomide, lenalidomide, and TRAIL; caspase-9 mediates through caspase-3 the effects of dexamethasone; while a dual caspase-8 and -9 apoptotic signaling mediates the effects of bortezomib), the effects of hsp90 in suppressing the expression/function of caspase inhibitors should enhance the ability of MM cells to respond to anti-MM therapies operating through these cascades. Indeed, we confirmed that hsp90 inhibition can enhance the response of MM cells to bortezomib, cytotoxic chemotherapy, immunomodulatory thalidomide derivatives, and TRAIL.[5] Another important reason why hsp90 inhibition may function to sensitize MM cells to diverse other therapies may be related to the role of heat shock proteins in general, and hsp90 more specifically, as master regulators for intracellular programs designed to protect cells, both normal and malignant.[32] For instance, when MM cells are exposed to the proteasome inhibitor bortezomib, they upregulate the expression of heat shock proteins, including hsp90.[6] This event is conceivably related to the intracellular accumulation of the transcription factor HSF-1 (heat shock factor-1) which results in concomitant upregulation in the transcription and eventually protein levels of multiple heat shock proteins.[32] The upregulation of heat shock proteins appears to be a stress response mounted by tumor cells in an effort to counteract the intracellular accumulation of misfolded proteins, given the role of heat shock proteins in facilitating correct protein folding and preventing protein aggregation.[6] Although this stress response is not sufficient per se to rescue MM cells from bortezomib treatment in vitro, we hypothesized that its inhibition could precipitate a more potent and/or rapid induction of MM cell death compared to proteasome inhibition alone. Indeed, we observed that hsp90 inhibitors can sensitize MM cells to the anti-MM effects of bortezomib.[6] This effect has not only been confirmed by several different groups in diverse in vitro MM models[5,26,27,38] but has also been validated in preclinical in vivo studies,[27] and has been translated clinically, where hsp90 inhibitors tested in combination with bortezomib have led to clinical responses in both bortezomib-pretreated and bortezomib refractory patients.[34]

Importantly, Hsp90 inhibition not only targets the MM cells directly but also targets the interaction of MM cells with their local microenvironment. Specifically, hsp90 inhibition suppresses, in MM cells, the expression and function of the growth factor receptors and downstream effectors utilized for signaling cascades (e.g., IGFs/IGF-1R, IL-6/IL-6R) that mediate protective effects of the bone marrow microenvironment on MM cells.[5] This explains why hsp90 inhibitors can overcome the protective effect conferred to MM cells by BMSCs.[5] In addition, hsp90 inhibition decreases the constitutive, IGF-1-induced, and stroma-induced production of proangiogenic cytokines (e.g., VEGF) by MM cells[5], and also decreases the ability of endothelial cells to respond to such proangiogenic cytokines with increased survival and proliferation.[5] These latter direct effects of hsp90 inhibition on endothelial cells in vitro are associated with, but not exclusively linked to, decreased expression and function of hsp90 client proteins such as IGF-1R.[5]

Why are Neoplastic Cells More Sensitive to hsp90 Inhibition Than Their Normal Counterparts?

At the moment, there is no definitive answer as to why neoplastic cells are generally more sensitive to hsp90 inhibition compared to their normal counterparts or why MM cells are among the most sensitive malignant cell types to hsp90 inhibition.[39] Although some studies have suggested that heat shock proteins such as hsp90 are expressed at higher levels in certain types of tumor cells compared to their normal counterparts, the hsp90 transcripts in MM cells (either MM cell lines or primary MM tumor cells) are expressed in levels comparable to those in normal plasma cells.[5] The levels of hsp90 expression may vary in normal tissues, but generally represent a high level of expression (~2% of the intracellular proteome) and are typically not significantly lower than those in MM cells.[32] Therefore, the therapeutic window associated with hsp90 inhibition cannot be attributed to differential expression of the target in tumor versus normal cells. Instead, it appears that the function of hsp90 is differentially required for tumor cell biology versus normal cell function[32]: tumor cells harbor mutated or chimeric oncoproteins which are absent from normal cells, but present and often indispensable for tumor cell proliferation and survival, as well as exquisitely sensitive to hsp90 inhibition compared to their wild-type counterparts present in nonmalignant cells. Because of these considerations, it is plausible that that the role of hsp90 in chaperoning of mutated and/or chimeric oncoproteins can account at least in part for its tumor-selective effects.[32] In the case of MM, it has not been feasible yet to identify specific mutated/chimeric oncoproteins that specifically drive the pathophysiology of MM cells. However, the broad spectrum of hsp90 client proteins encompasses several ones that are known to play critical roles in MM cell biology (e.g., Akt, Raf, p70S6K, and IKK). It is therefore plausible that even if these proteins are not mutationally activated in MM cells, they are constitutively activated in MM cells present in their BM microenvironment and that perhaps MM cells have become "addicted" to the survival signals mediated by these cascades and are thus more sensitive to their loss in the context of hsp90 inhibition than normal cells. It has also been reported that hsp90 derived from tumor cells has a 100-fold higher binding affinity for ansamycin hsp90 inhibitors such as 17-AAG compared to hsp90 from normal cells and that tumor hsp90 is present entirely in multichaperone complexes with high ATPase activity, whereas hsp90 from normal tissues is in a latent, uncomplexed state.[40] These data have provided the basis for the hypothesis that the tumor selectivity of hsp90 inhibitors such as 17-AAG is related to an activated, high-affinity conformation of hsp90 complexes in tumor cells, which not only facilitates malignant progression but also renders its function significantly more sensitive to 17-AAG than hsp90 function in normal tissues. More studies will be needed to confirm this hypothesis in a broader range of experimental conditions and in terms of its relevance to hsp90 inhibitors of other nonansamycin chemical families.

Post-Translational Regulation of hsp90 Function

Recent studies from various groups[41–44] have suggested that hsp90 acetylation attenuates its chaperoning activity and that inhibition of cytoplasmic deacetylases can lead to decreased hsp90 function, mimicking the effects of small molecule inhibitors of the ATP-binding pocket of hsp90. Treatment of MM cells with broad-spectrum deacetylase inhibitors, such as the nuclear (histone) and cytoplasmic deactylase inhibitor vorinostat (SAHA, suberolyanilide hydroxamic acid) or other deacetylase inhibitors (including LBH589 or LAQ824), can lead to molecular sequelae that exhibit substantial overlap with those of hsp90 inhibitors (e.g., suppression of expression of diverse oncogenic kinases).[45,46] However, it should be noted that hsp90 ATP-binding pocket inhibitors, despite their functional overlap with deacetylase inhibitors, have differences, which are probably related to the different kinetics and magnitude of hsp90 functional inhibition with these two strategies. It is plausible that the anti-hsp90 effect of deacetylase inhibitors requires concentrations higher than those necessary to achieve antitumor effects through effects on regulation of the histone code and gene transcription.[46] Nonetheless, combinations of hsp90 ATP-binding pocket inhibitors and deacetylase inhibitors could perhaps be used in the future to achieve more comprehensive suppression of hsp90 function.

Clinical Development of hsp90 Inhibitors

The preclinical studies of our Center and others[5] provided the rationale for clinical trials of tanespimycin (17-AAG in the KOS-953 cremophor-based formulation) either as a single agent[33] or in combination with bortezomib[34] in patients with relapsed or refractory MM. In these trials, tanespimycin has shown a manageable profile of side effects (without significant cardiotoxicity, peripheral neuropathy, or deep vein thrombosis), durable disease stabilization, and minor responses with single agent treatment in relapsed and refractory MM patients, as well as encouraging anti-MM activity with the combination of tanespimycin with bortezomib.[34] This experience, coupled with the lack of additive toxicity or pharmacokinetic interactions in the tanespimycin + borte-zomib combination, has now provided a platform for future phase III trials of this regimen. Clinical trials of the water-soluble ansamycin IPI-504 have also taken place in MM[47–49] and in other diseases.[50]

Barriers to Improvement of Clinical Responses to hsp90 Inhibitors

The clinical activity of the combination of hsp90 inhibitors with bortezomib has been promising in the ongoing clinical trials. Although historical comparisons of results from different trials should be interpreted with caution, the activity of single-agent 17-AAG has been more modest compared with the historical experience of clinical responses in MM patients enrolled in the original phase I and II trials of bortezomib[51,52] or lenalidomide[53,54] or the original phase II studies of thalidomide.[55] However, the patient population in the contemporary phase I trial of KOS-953 as single agent was enriched for patients with more aggressive MM, was all relapsed or relapsed refractory, and had been previously exposed to the major new classes of anti-MM agents that have recently become FDA approved, such as thalidomide, bortezomib, or lenalidomide.[33,34]

One of the key barriers toward improved clinical outcome with hsp90 inhibitors is related to the significant room that exists for improvement in not only the dosing and schedule of hsp90 inhibitors but also in the formulation utilized for their administration, at least for the family of ansamycin hsp90 inhibitors that have been tested clinically so far (i.e., 17-AAG and 17-DMAG). 17-AAG, in particular, is poorly soluble in aqueous solutions and the original clinical studies of this agent required its administration with a DMSO-based, egg phospholipid-containing formulation which not only required a laborious preparation procedure for clinical pharmacies in participating centers but also posed significant clinical challenges related to hypersensitivity reactions to the egg phospholipid component of the formulation, as well as adverse events related to the DMSO. These side effects limited the dose escalation of 17-AAG. Specifically, in the 17-AAG clinical trials that utilized the DMSO-based, egg phospholipid-containing formulation, the recommended phase II doses for further evaluation in adult cancer patients were, depending on the schedule of administration, as high as 450 mg/m^2 (with once weekly dosing)[56] but also as low as 40 mg/m^2 (with daily administration for five consecutive days, every 3 weeks).[57] As Table 1 indicates, the cremophor-based formulation of 17-AAG (KOS-953) utilized in the MM clinical trials allowed for the 420 mg/m2 dose level to be easily administered as a monotherapy while no MTD was determined in that trial,[33] suggesting that even higher doses of 17-AAG may be administered safely using improved formulation(s) of this compound. A comparison of the cumulative 17-AAG dose administered over a 3-week period (i.e., the equivalent of one cycle in the KOS-953 trials) for those trials where the DMSO/egg phospholipid formulation was used in adult[56–61]

Table 1 Summary data from clinical trials of 17-AAG using the egg phospholipid (EPL)/DMSO formulation (references 55–60 for clinical trials in adults and 61 and 62 in pediatric populations) versus trials of 17-AAG in the cremophor formulation (KOS-953) (references 32 and 33) for treatment of MM.

Study	No. of patients	Schedule of 17-AAG administration	Formulation	Recommended phase II1 dose (mg/m2)	Dose delivered (mg/m2)/3 weeks	Response
Banerji et al.[56]	30	Weekly (no rest period)	EPL/DMSO	450	1,350	2 SD (melanoma)
Ramanathan et al.[58]	45	Weekly × 3	EPL/DMSO	295	885	
Goetz et al.[59]	21	Weekly × 3	EPL/DMSO	308	924	
Grem et al.[57]	19	Daily × 5, every 3 weeks	EPL/DMSO	40	200	
Solit et al.[60]	40	Daily × 5, every 3 weeks	EPL/DMSO	56	280	
Solit et al.[60]		Daily × 3 every 2 weeks	EPL/DMSO	112	672	2 SD (renal & breast cancer)
		Weekly × 2, for 2 weeks, every 3 weeks	EPL/DMSO	220	880	2 SD (lung & thyroid)
Ramanathan et al.[61]	32	Weekly × 2 for 3 weeks, every 4 weeks	EPL/DMSO	175	1,050	1 SD
Ramanathan et al.[61]	12	Weekly × 2, for 2 weeks, every 3 weeks	EPL/DMSO	200	800	
Weigel BJ et al. (pediatric)[62]	12	Weekly × 2, for 2 weeks, every 3 weeks	EPL/DMSO	360	1,440	5 SD
Bagatell et al. (pediatric)[63]	13	Weekly × 2, for 2 weeks, every 3 weeks	EPL/DMSO	270	1,080	
Richardson et al.[33] (MM)	19	Weekly × 2, for 2 weeks, every 3 weeks	Cremophor	420 (MTD not yet reached)	1,680	12/19 SD or better
Richardson et al.[34] (MM)	23	Weekly × 2, for 2 weeks, every 3 weeks (plus bortezomib)	Cremophor		1,400	13/23 MR/PR/ CR (8/15 in relapsed or refractory MM)

SD stable disease, *MR* minor response, *PR* partial response, *CR* complete response, *MM* multiple myeloma.

or pediatric patients[62,63] versus the two trials so far utilizing the cremophor formulation[33,34] indicates that a higher cumulative dose was delivered in trials with the latter formulation. Interestingly, clinical responses were observed predominantly in the KOS-953 clinical trials and in those trials of the DMSO/egg phospholipid formulation where the highest cumulative doses were achieved (e.g., in the study of Banerji et al.[56]). These observations suggest that it may be feasible to further improve the clinical outcome of single-agent, as well as combination trials of 17-AAG, through the development of improved clinical formulations of this class of drug in order to deliver higher doses of the compounds to the tumor cells.

Because of the poor solubility in aqueous solutions for many hsp90 inhibitors of the ansamycin family, including 17-AAG, the development of improved formulations is not an easy task for this group of compounds. One of the efforts to address this issue involves the development of isomers of 17-AAG that are water-soluble, with the hope that this would allow for easier and safer administration of drug doses sufficient to induce antitumor activity. An example of that approach is the development of IPI-504, a highly soluble hydroquinone hydrochloride derivative of 17-AAG.[27,64,65] IPI-504 and 17-AAG interconvert in vitro and in vivo via an oxidation–reduction equilibrium and have comparable in vitro antitumor potencies. However, the hydroquinone hydrochloride salt of IPI-504 can be isolated in high purity as a solid; is less prone to air oxidation than the free base hydroquinone ring of 17-AAG[66]; and exhibits dramatically different physical–chemical properties compared with 17-AAG. For instance, IPI-504 is readily soluble in water (at concentrations > 250 mg/ml) compared with 17-AAG (50 µg/ml), which enables aqueous delivery formulations of IPI-504 which do not require organic solubilizing agents which have their own limitations.[27]

So far, clinical testing of IPI-504 has shown minimal adverse events, and some evidence of clinical responses in gastrointestinal stromal tumors[50] but not in MM,[48] even at IPI-504 dose levels comparable to KOS-953 doses that led to manageable side effects (e.g., asymptomatic elevation of liver function tests) and clinical responses in the MM trials.[33] The pharmacokinetic data from the clinical trials of IPI-504 (as well as from preclinical models) indicate that achievable serum levels of IPI-504 and 17-AAG (derived from the in vivo interconversion of IPI-504) are within the range of concentrations that lead to in vitro antitumor activity as well as in the same order of magnitude as serum 17-AAG levels reported to be achieved in clinical trials of 17-AAG in its different formulations.[27,48] One possible explanation for these observations is that the nature of the formulation that is utilized for clinical administration of hsp90 inhibitors influences their tissue-specific bioavailability (J. Adams, personal communication). For instance, it is possible that lipid-soluble formulations, such as the ones in the early clinical trials with the DMSO/egg phospholipid vehicle or in the cremophor-based trials of KOS-953, may allow better delivery of the drug into tissues with high content in fat, as the case is for liver (which might explain the asymptomatic liver function test increases with these formulations) or the bone marrow (which might explain the clinical responses observed in the KOS-953 trials for MM), while formulations that involve aqueous solutions, as is the case for IPI-504, are associated with lower drug levels in these aforementioned tissues. Although more data will be needed to provide definitive conclusions on this question, it is plausible, based on all the currently available information, that the choice of vehicle/ formulation for hsp90 inhibitors of the ansamycin family can affect the safety and efficacy of this drug class not only by changing the maximum dose level that can be administered but also by influencing the tissue-specifc bioavailability of these agents. It remains to be seen whether this same property applies for nonansamycin hsp90 inhibitors, which are currently in preclinical and/or clinical development (references [67–69] and as reviewed in references[70,71]).

The Role of hsp90 in Immune Function: Implications for Anti-MM Immunotherapy

Hsp90 plays critical roles in the pathophysiology of tumor cells and in the ability of normal cells to survive diverse conditions of stress. Although the activation of immune effector cells may not be per se a form of cellular stress, it has been known for years that hsp90, as well as other heat shock proteins, is upregulated when T-lymphocytes are stimulated by mitogens, such as phytohemagglutinin, and cytokines such as interleukin-2 (IL-2).[72] The stimulation of hsp90 expression during activation of lymphocyte mitogenesis was at the time viewed as reflection of genetic mechanisms evolved from primitive stress/adaptation responses.[72] Since then, a large body of data has supported the notion that heat shock proteins including hsp90 are implicated in various aspects of immune system function, including antigen presentation and tumor immunity. For instance, hsp90 has been proposed to function as potent activator of the innate immune system, inducing the proinflammatory cytokines by the monocyte-macrophage system, as well as activation and maturation of dendritic cells (DCs) via the Toll-like receptor 2 and 4 signal transduction pathways (as reviewed in Tsan and Gao[73]). Despite some controversy, fueled by evidence suggesting that the reported cytokine effects of heat shock proteins might have been affected, at least in part, by contaminating bacterial cell wall products in the corresponding experiments,[73] it is still widely accepted that heat shock proteins play important roles in immune responses not only by functioning to support intracellular signal transduction mediating survival and activation of immune effector cells but also in the form of extracellularly located or membrane-bound heat shock proteins, which contribute to or mediate the elicitation of immunological responses of the adaptive or innate immune system.[74]

As a direct consequence of these data, when hsp90 inhibitors became the focus of research efforts for their direct antitumor properties in preclinical models, questions were raised about their potential effects on the function of the immune system. In the MM field, two preclinical studies so far have addressed this question. Spisek et al. showed that human MM cells which have been killed by exposure to bortezomib are uptaken by DCs, leading to induction of antitumor immunity, including immunity against primary tumor cells, without the need for any additional adjuvants.[38] However, the delivery of activating signal from bortezomib-killed MM cells to DCs depends on cell–cell contact between DCs and dying MM cells and is mediated by bortezomib-induced exposure of hsp90 on the surface of dying cells.[38] So while the combination of bortezomib and the hsp90 inhibitor geldanamycin led to increased apoptosis of MM cells, this combination may abrogate the immunogenicity triggered by the exposure of MM cells to bortezomib.[38] A separate study,[75] which evaluated the role of hsp90 in human DC phenotype and function, showed that hsp90 inhibition by relatively higher concentrations of geldamaycin family members significantly decreased cell surface expression of costimulatory (CD40, CD80, CD86), maturation (CD83), and MHC (HLA-A, B, C and HLA-DP, DQ, DR) markers in immature DC and mature DC and was associated with downregulation of both RNA and intracellular protein expression.[75] Hsp90 inhibition also inhibited DC function: it decreased Ag uptake, processing, and presentation by immature DC, leading to reduced T cell proliferation in response to tetanus toxoid as a recall antigen; decreased the ability of mature DC to present Ag to T cells; and secrete IL-12 as well as induce IFN-γ secretion by allogeneic T cells.[75] These observations indicated that hsp90-mediated protein folding is important for DC function, which is disrupted by hsp90 inhibition.

So far, no significant clinical evidence of immunosuppression or any other evidence that might be deemed compatible with deficient DC function has been observed in the clinical trials of hsp90 inhibitors. However, these studies were not specifically designed to include corrolary studies evaluating the response of patients to antigen stimulation or how hsp90 inhibition may have affected other immune system parameters. Therefore, appropriate caution should be exercised in the timing of hsp90 inhibitor-containing therapies in relationship to patient vaccinations (if needed) or participation of patients in clinical trials of immune-based therapies, until more clinical and translational studies resolve these questions.

The Role of Heat Shock Proteins Other Than hsp90

Hsp90 is not the only heat shock protein. Even though it has emerged so far as the first one to become the target of clinical interventions for anticancer purposes, other heat shock proteins have also attracted interest, including hsp70 and hsp27. Expression of hsp70 is upregulated, just as hsp90, in the context of treatment of tumor cells with diverse antitumor agents, including bortezomib and hsp90 inhibitors, themselves.[5,6] Stable transfection of a small interfering RNA (siRNA) against hsp70 blocks 17-AAG-mediated hsp70 induction, resulting in sensitization of K562/siRNA-hsp70 leukemic cells to 17-AAG-induced apoptosis.[76] Furthermore, KNK437, a benzylidine lactam inhibitor of hsp70 induction, increased 17-AAG-induced apoptosis and loss of clonogenic survival of HL-60 leukemic cells.[76] Taken together, these data supported the notion that inhibition of hsp70 upregulation may increase the activity of other antitumor agents, including hsp90 inhibitors.[76] Other studies have shown that inhibition of hsp70 can enhance apoptosis induction by farnesyl transferase inhibitors.[77]

In regard to hsp27, antisense constructs against hsp27 restore the apoptotic response of DHL4 lymphoma cells to the proteasome inhibitor bortezomib (PS-341), while ectopic expression of wild-type hsp27 renders the bortezomib-sensitive DHL6 cells resistant to PS-341.[78] These data suggest that hsp27 is one of the heat shock proteins that can be targeted to regulate resistance of tumor cells to proteasome inhibitors.

Conclusions

Hsp90 inhibition with small molecules represents a promising therapeutic strategy that has already translated from the bench to the bedside, with encouraging results so far in clinical trials combining hsp90 and proteasome inhibitors in patients with advanced MM. Preclinical studies of hsp90 inhibition in MM started at a time when the rationale for evaluation of this pathway would not have been deemed as promising or exciting as perhaps other investigational avenues. However, with the generation of more preclinical data, hsp90 inhibition has proved an interesting and promising strategy that may at least enhance the activity of other antitumor agents. In terms of the potential of hsp90 inhibitor monotherapy, more work is needed to optimize their clinical activity. This may be accomplished through further optimization of the properties of the vehicles utilized for clinical administration of this class of drugs, in order to allow for safer administration of higher cumulative drug doses and with improved bioavailability at the sites of tumor involvement. Furthermore, the development of new hsp90 inhibitors from nonansamycin classes of chemical entities may perhaps lead to safer and clinically active orally bioavailable inhibitors, which can then be conveniently, in terms of schedule and sequence, incorporated into combination regimens with other agents.

References

1. Neckers L, Ivy SP. Heat shock protein 90. Curr Opin Oncol 2003;15(6):419–24.
2. Xu W, Neckers L. Targeting the molecular chaperone heat shock protein 90 provides a multifaceted effect on diverse cell signaling pathways of cancer cells. Clin Cancer Res 2007;13(6):1625–9.
3. Workman P, Burrows F, Neckers L, Rosen N. Drugging the cancer chaperone HSP90: combinatorial therapeutic exploitation of oncogene addiction and tumor stress. Ann N Y Acad Sci 2007.
4. Powers MV, Workman P. Inhibitors of the heat shock response: biology and pharmacology. FEBS Lett 2007.
5. Mitsiades CS, Mitsiades NS, McMullan CJ, et al. Antimyeloma activity of heat shock protein-90 inhibition. Blood 2006;107(3):1092–100.
6. Mitsiades N, Mitsiades CS, Poulaki V, et al. Molecular sequelae of proteasome inhibition in human multiple myeloma cells. Proc Natl Acad Sci USA 2002;99(22):14374–9.
7. Pearl LH, Prodromou C. Structure and mechanism of the Hsp90 molecular chaperone machinery. Annu Rev Biochem 2006;75:271–94.
8. Hideshima T, Nakamura N, Chauhan D, Anderson KC. Biologic sequelae of interleukin-6 induced PI3-K/Akt signaling in multiple myeloma. Oncogene 2001;20(42):5991–6000.
9. Hsu JH, Shi Y, Hu L, Fisher M, Franke TF, Lichtenstein A. Role of the AKT kinase in expansion of multiple myeloma clones: Effects on cytokine-dependent proliferative and survival responses. Oncogene 2002;21(9):1391–400.
10. Hsu J, Shi Y, Krajewski S, et al. The AKT kinase is activated in multiple myeloma tumor cells. Blood 2001;98(9):2853–5.
11. Mitsiades CS, Mitsiades NS, McMullan CJ, et al. Inhibition of the insulin-like growth factor receptor-1 tyrosine kinase activity as a therapeutic strategy for multiple myeloma, other hematologic malignancies, and solid tumors. Cancer Cell 2004;5(3):221–30.

12. Hideshima T, Neri P, Tassone P, et al. MLN120B, a novel IkappaB kinase beta inhibitor, blocks multiple myeloma cell growth in vitro and in vivo. Clin Cancer Res 2006;12(19):5887–94.

13. Hideshima T, Chauhan D, Richardson P, et al. NF-kappa B as a therapeutic target in multiple myeloma. J Biol Chem 2002;277(19):16639–47.

14. Davies FE, Dring AM, Li C, et al. Insights into the multistep transformation of MGUS to myeloma using microarray expression analysis. Blood 2003;102(13):4504–11.

15. Zhan F, Hardin J, Kordsmeier B, et al. Global gene expression profiling of multiple myeloma, monoclonal gammopathy of undetermined significance, and normal bone marrow plasma cells. Blood 2002;99(5):1745–57.

16. Tarte K, De Vos J, Thykjaer T, et al. Generation of polyclonal plasmablasts from peripheral blood B cells: A normal counterpart of malignant plasmablasts. Blood 2002;100(4):1113–22.

17. De Vos J, Thykjaer T, Tarte K, et al. Comparison of gene expression profiling between malignant and normal plasma cells with oligonucleotide arrays. Oncogene 2002;21(44):6848–57.

18. Bergsagel PL, Kuehl WM, Zhan F, Sawyer J, Barlogie B, Shaughnessy J, Jr. Cyclin D dysregulation: an early and unifying pathogenic event in multiple myeloma. Blood 2005;106(1):296–303.

19. Bergsagel PL, Kuehl WM. Molecular pathogenesis and a consequent classification of multiple myeloma. J Clin Oncol 2005;23(26):6333–8.

20. Mitsiades CS, Mitsiades N, Munshi NC, Anderson KC. Focus on multiple myeloma. Cancer Cell 2004;6(5):439–44.

21. Fonseca R, Blood E, Rue M, et al. Clinical and biologic implications of recurrent genomic aberrations in myeloma. Blood 2003;101(11):4569–75.

22. Moreau P, Attal M, Garban F, et al. Heterogeneity of t(4;14) in multiple myeloma. Long-term follow-up of 100 cases treated with tandem transplantation in IFM99 trials. Leukemia 2007;21(9):2020–4.

23. Fonseca R, Barlogie B, Bataille R, et al. Genetics and cytogenetics of multiple myeloma: A workshop report. Cancer Res 2004;64(4):1546–58.

24. Negri J, Mitsiades N, Deng QW, et al. PKC412 is a multi-targeting kinase inhibitor with activity against multiple myeloma in vitro and in vivo. Blood 2005;106(11):75a.

25. Mitsiades CS, Mitsiades N, Rooney M, et al. Anti-tumor activity of KOS-953, a cremophor-based formulation of the hsp90 inhibitor 17-AAG. Blood 2004;104(11):660A-1A.

26. Duus J, Bahar HI, Venkataraman G, et al. Analysis of expression of heat shock protein-90 (HSP90) and the effects of HSP90 inhibitor (17-AAG) in multiple myeloma. Leuk Lymphoma 2006;47(7):1369–78.

27. Sydor JR, Normant E, Pien CS, et al. Development of 17-allylamino-17-demethoxygeldanamycin hydroquinone hydrochloride (IPI-504), an anti-cancer agent directed against Hsp90. Proc Natl Acad Sci U S A 2006;103(46):17408–13.

28. Chatterjee M, Jain S, Stuhmer T, et al. STAT3 and MAPK signaling maintain overexpression of heat shock proteins 90 alpha and beta in multiple myeloma cells, which critically contribute to tumor-cell survival. Blood 2007;109(2):720–8.

29. Francis LK, Alsayed Y, Leleu X, et al. Combination mammalian target of rapamycin inhibitor rapamycin and HSP90 inhibitor 17-allylamino-17-demethoxygeldanamycin has synergistic activity in multiple myeloma. Clin Cancer Res 2006;12(22):6826–35.

30. Davenportel, Moore HE, Dunlop AS, et al. Heat shock protein inhibition is associated with activation of the unfolded protein response (UPR) pathway in myeloma plasma cells. Blood 2007.

31. Mitsiades CS, Mitsiades N, Rooney M, et al. IPI-504: A novel hsp90 inhibitor with in vitro and in vivo antitumor activity. Blood 2004;104(11):660A-A.

32. Mitsiades CS, Richardson PG, Munshi NC, Anderson KC. Inhibition of heat shock proteins: Therapeutic perspectives. Haematol Hematol J 2007;92(6):26–7.

33. Richardson PG, Chanan-Khan AA, Alsina M, et al. Safety and activity of KOS-953 in patients with relapsed refractory multiple myeloma (MM): Interim results of a phase 1 trial. Blood 2005;106(11):109a.

34. Richardson P, Chanan-Khan A, Lonial S, et al A multicenter phase 1 clinical trial of tanespimycin (KOS-953) + bortezomib (BZ): Encouraging activity and manageable toxicity in heavily pre-treated patients with relapsed refractory multiple myeloma (MM). In: Annual Meeting of the American Society of Hematology; 2006; , FL.

35. Ge J, Normant E, Porter JR, et al. Design, synthesis, and biological evaluation of hydroquinone derivatives of 17-amino-17-demethoxygeldanamycin as potent, water-soluble inhibitors of Hsp90. J Med Chem 2006;49(15):4606–15.

36. Mitsiades CS, Mitsiades N, Poulaki V, et al. Activation of NF-kappaB and upregulation of intracellular anti-apoptotic proteins via the IGF-1/Akt signaling in human multiple myeloma cells: Therapeutic implications. Oncogene 2002;21(37):5673–83.

37. Grigorieva I, Thomas X, Epstein J. The bone marrow stromal environment is a major factor in myeloma cell resistance to dexamethasone. Exp Hematol 1998;26(7):597–603.

38. Spisek R, Charalambous A, Mazumder A, Vesole DH, Jagannath S, Dhodapkar MV. Bortezomib enhances dendritic cell (DC)-mediated induction of immunity to human myeloma via exposure of cell surface heat shock protein 90 on dying tumor cells: Therapeutic implications. Blood 2007;109(11):4839–45.

39. Chiosis G, Neckers L. Tumor selectivity of Hsp90 inhibitors: The explanation remains elusive. ACS Chem Biol 2006;1(5):279–84.

40. Kamal A, Thao L, Sensintaffar J, et al. A high-affinity conformation of Hsp90 confers tumour selectivity on Hsp90 inhibitors. Nature 2003;425(6956):407–10.

41. Aoyagi S, Archer TK. Modulating molecular chaperone Hsp90 functions through reversible acetylation. Trends Cell Biol 2005;15(11):565–7.

42. Bali P, Pranpat M, Bradner J, et al. Inhibition of histone deacetylase 6 acetylates and disrupts the chaperone function of heat shock protein 90: A novel basis for antileukemia activity of histone deacetylase inhibitors. J Biol Chem 2005;280(29):26729–34.

43. Kovacs JJ, Murphy PJ, Gaillard S, et al. HDAC6 regulates Hsp90 acetylation and chaperone-dependent activation of glucocorticoid receptor. Mol Cell 2005;18(5):601–7.

44. Murphy PJ, Morishima Y, Kovacs JJ, Yao TP, Pratt WB. Regulation of the dynamics of hsp90 action on the glucocorticoid receptor by acetylation/deacetylation of the chaperone. J Biol Chem 2005;280(40):33792–9.

45. Mitsiades N, Mitsiades CS, Richardson PG, et al. Molecular sequelae of histone deacetylase inhibition in human malignant B cells. Blood 2003;101(10):4055–62.

46. Mitsiades CS, Mitsiades NS, McMullan CJ, et al. Transcriptional signature of histone deacetylase inhibition in multiple myeloma: biological and clinical implications. Proc Natl Acad Sci U S A 2004;101(2):540–5.

47. Phase I trial with IPI-504 in relapsed/refractory multiple myeloma. Clin Lymphoma Myeloma 2007;7(5):341–2.

48. Siegel D, Jagannath S, Mazumder A, et al. Update on phase I clinical trial of IPI-504, a novel, water-soluble Hsp90 inhibitor, in patients with relapsed/refractory multiple myeloma (MM). Blood 2006;108(11):1022A-A.

49. Jagannath S, Siegel D, Richardson P, et al. Phase I clinical trial of IPI-504, a novel, water-soluble Hsp90 inhibitor, in patients with Relapsed/Refractory multiple myeloma (MM). Blood 2005;106(11):719A-20A.

50. Demetri GD, George S, Morgan JA, et al. Overcoming resistance to tyrosine kinase inhibitors (TKIs) through inhibition of Heat Shock Protein 90 (Hsp90) chaperone function in patients with metastatic GIST: Results of a Phase I Trial of IPI-504, a water-soluble Hsp90 inhibitor. Ejc Suppl 2006;4(12):173.

51. Orlowski RZ, Stinchcombe TE, Mitchell BS, et al. Phase I trial of the proteasome inhibitor PS-341 in patients with refractory hematologic malignancies. J Clin Oncol 2002;20(22):4420–7.

52. Richardson PG, Barlogie B, Berenson J, et al. A phase 2 study of bortezomib in relapsed, refractory myeloma. N Engl J Med 2003;348(26):2609–17.

53. Richardson PG, Schlossman RL, Weller E, et al. Immunomodulatory drug CC-5013 overcomes drug resistance and is well tolerated in patients with relapsed multiple myeloma. Blood 2002;100(9):3063–7.

54. Richardson PG, Blood E, Mitsiades CS, et al. A randomized phase 2 study of lenalidomide therapy for patients with relapsed or relapsed and refractory multiple myeloma. Blood 2006;108(10):3458–64.

55. Singhal S, Mehta J, Desikan R, et al. Antitumor activity of thalidomide in refractory multiple myeloma. N Engl J Med 1999;341(21):1565–71.

56. Banerji U, O'Donnell A, Scurr M, et al. Phase I pharmacokinetic and pharmacodynamic study of 17-allylamino, 17-demethoxygeldanamycin in patients with advanced malignancies. J Clin Oncol 2005;23(18):4152–61.

57. Grem JL, Morrison G, Guo XD, et al. Phase I and pharmacologic study of 17-(allylamino)-17-demethoxygeldanamycin in adult patients with solid tumors. J Clin Oncol 2005;23(9):1885–93.

58. Ramanathan RK, Trump DL, Eiseman JL, et al . Phase I pharmacokinetic-pharmacodynamic study of 17-(allylamino)-17-demethoxygeldanamycin (17AAG, NSC 330507), a novel inhibitor of heat shock protein 90, in patients with refractory advanced cancers. Clin Cancer Res 2005;11(9):3385–91.

59. Goetz MP, Toft D, Reid J, et al. Phase I trial of 17-allylamino-17-demethoxygeldanamycin in patients with advanced cancer. J Clin Oncol 2005;23(6):1078–87.

60. Solit DB, Ivy SP, Kopil C, et al. Phase I trial of 17-allylamino-17-demethoxygeldanamycin in patients with advanced cancer. Clin Cancer Res 2007;13(6):1775–82.

61. Ramanathan RK, Egorin MJ, Eiseman JL, et al. Phase I and pharmacodynamic study of 17-(allylamino)-17-demethoxygeldanamycin in adult patients with refractory advanced cancers. Clin Cancer Res 2007;13(6):1769–74.

62. Weigel BJ, Blaney SM, Reid JM, et al. A phase I study of 17-allylaminogeldanamycin in relapsed/refractory pediatric patients with solid tumors: A Children's Oncology Group study. Clin Cancer Res 2007;13(6):1789–93.

63. Bagatell R, Gore L, Egorin MJ, et al. Phase I pharmacokinetic and pharmacodynamic study of 17-N-allylamino-17-demethoxygeldanamycin in pediatric patients with recurrent or refractory solid tumors: A pediatric oncology experimental therapeutics investigators consortium study. Clin Cancer Res 2007;13(6):1783–8.

64. Porter JR, Ge J, Normant E, et al Synthesis and biological evaluation of IPI-504, an aqueous soluble analog of 17-AAG and potent inhibitor of Hsp90. Abs Pap Am Chem Soc 2006;231.

65. Peng C, Brain J, Hu YG, et al. IPI-504, a Novel, orally active HSP90 inhibitor, prolongs survival of mice with BCR-ABL T315I CML and B-ALL. Blood 2006;108(11):619A-A.

66. Ge J, Normant E, Porter JR, et al. Design, synthesis, and biological evaluation of hydroquinone derivatives of 17-amino-17-demethoxygeldanamycin as potent, water-soluble inhibitors of Hsp90. J Med Chem 2006;49(15):4606–15.

67. Kasibhatla SR, Hong K, Biamonte MA, et al. Rationally designed high-affinity 2-amino-6-halopurine heat shock protein 90 inhibitors that exhibit potent antitumor activity. J Med Chem 2007;50(12):2767–78.

68. Zhang L, Fan J, Vu K, et al. 7'-substituted benzothiazolothio- and pyridinothiazolothio-purines as potent heat shock protein 90 inhibitors. J Med Chem 2006;49(17):5352–62.

69. Biamonte MA, Shi J, Hong K, et al. Orally active purine-based inhibitors of the heat shock protein 90. J Med Chem 2006;49(2):817–28.

70. Chiosis G. Discovery and development of purine-scaffold Hsp90 inhibitors. Curr Top Med Chem 2006;6(11):1183–91.

71. McDonald E, Jones K, Brough PA, Drysdale MJ, Workman P. Discovery and development of pyrazole-scaffold Hsp90 inhibitors. Curr Top Med Chem 2006;6(11):1193–203.

72. Ferris DK, Harel-Bellan A, Morimoto RI, Welch WJ, Farrar WL. Mitogen and lymphokine stimulation of heat shock proteins in T lymphocytes. Proc Natl Acad Sci U S A 1988;85(11):3850–4.

73. Tsan MF, Gao B. Heat shock protein and innate immunity. Cell Mol Immunol 2004;1(4):274–9.

74. Schmitt E, Gehrmann M, Brunet M, Multhoff G, Garrido C. Intracellular and extra-cellular functions of heat shock proteins: Repercussions in cancer therapy. J Leukoc Biol 2007;81(1):15–27.

75. Bae J, Mitsiades C, Tai YT, et al. Phenotypic and functional effects of heat shock protein 90 inhibition on dendritic cell. J Immunol 2007;178(12):7730–7.

76. Guo F, Rocha K, Bali P, et al. Abrogation of heat shock protein 70 induction as a strategy to increase antileukemia activity of heat shock protein 90 inhibitor 17-allylamino-demethoxy geldanamycin. Cancer Res 2005;65(22):10536–44.

77. Hu W, Wu W, Verschraegen CF, et al. Proteomic identification of heat shock protein 70 as a candidate target for enhancing apoptosis induced by farnesyl trans-ferase inhibitor. Proteomics 2003;3(10):1904–11.

78. Chauhan D, Li G, Shringarpure R, et al. Blockade of Hsp27 overcomes Bortezomib/proteasome inhibitor PS-341 resistance in lymphoma cells. Cancer Res 2003;63(19):6174–7.

Chapter 20

The PI3 Kinase/Akt Pathway as a Therapeutic Target in Multiple Myeloma

R. Donald Harvey, Jeannine Silberman, and Sagar Lonial

Introduction

The development of novel therapies for multiple myeloma (MM) depends on a comprehensive understanding of the events leading to cellular proliferation and survival. Controlling pathways that regulate growth signals is an emerging and complementary approach to myeloma treatment. Dysregulation of the phosphotidylinositol 3-kinase (PI3K)/Akt pathway has been implicated in malignant transformation and progression of a number of cancers, including MM.[1-10] When activated, the PI3K/Akt pathway leads to downstream activators of cellular proliferation, adhesion, migration, survival, angiogenesis, and drug resistance (Fig. 1).[11,12] The PI3K/Akt pathway is a central gatekeeper for these critical cellular functions. Established proteins and genes such as mTOR (mammalian target of rapamycin), p53, NF-κB (nuclear factor kappa B), and BAD (Bcl-2 antagonist of cell death) are all regulated through PI3K and Akt activation, making them attractive targets for broad downstream effects. Direct PI3K inhibition has demonstrated impressive tumor inhibition and regression in cell line and animal models, and multiple agents including SF1126 are currently in clinical trials. Drugs such as perifosine that are specific for Akt are also in development. Combinations of these agents with existing therapies are rational approaches on the path to improving myeloma treatment.

The PI3K/Akt Pathway as a Signaling Convergence Point

Cells integrate a variety of signals to determine survival, proliferation, and function. Rarely is there a single checkpoint for signaling convergence, but information to date suggests that the PI3K pathway is a gatekeeper for tumor growth. Because it is a central regulation point and can become constitutively activated due to direct and indirect PI3K/Akt mutations or loss of function of a tumor suppressor gene, it is an attractive therapeutic target for a variety of cancers, including MM.

From: *Contemporary Hematology Myeloma Therapy*
Edited by: S. Lonial © Humana Press, Totowa, NJ

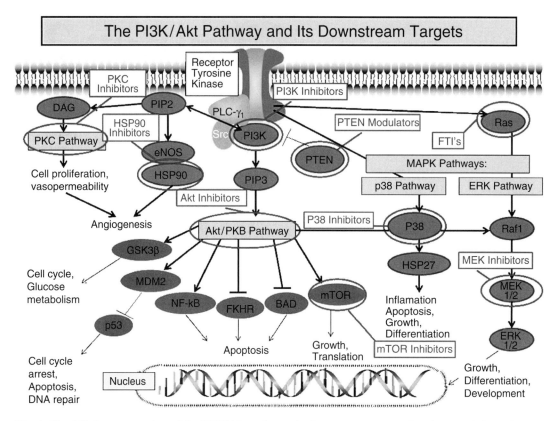

Fig. 1 Simplified representation of the PI3K/Akt pathway, its downstream targets, functions, and sites of therapeutic intervention.

Mechanisms of PI3K/Akt Dysregulation in Cancer

Several different mechanisms of deranged PI3K/Akt signaling have been identified in the development of malignant diseases (Table 1). The unifying theme, however, is that they all result in constitutive activation of the pathway due to pathologic membrane localization and activation of Akt. Currently three forms of Akt are known: Akt1/PKBa, Akt2/PKBb, and Akt3/PKBg[11] and of the three, the Akt2 gene and its RNA and/or protein products are the most frequently amplified in human cancers. Recently, though, an activating mutation in the pleckstrin homology domain of Akt1, which mediates its membrane translocation, was identified in breast, colorectal, and ovarian carcinomas in humans and leukemias in mice.[12] More often activation of Akt is the result of aberrant events upstream. Indirect activation of Akt can occur as the result of mutations in upstream enzymes regulating second messenger phospholipids, such as PtdIns (3,4,5)P3 and PtdIns (3,4)P2, dysregulated production of growth factors, activating mutations of PIK3CA, amplification of PI3K, inactivation of the PTEN (phosphatase and tensin homolog deleted on chromosome 10) tumor suppressor gene, and/or mutations of receptor tyrosine kinases, Ras, and Srcas. Studies have shown that pathologic activation of Akt induces drug resistance to both conventional chemotherapeutic agents and novel-targeted agents such as gefitinib, imatinib, trastuzumab, and retinoic acid.[13–17]

Table 1 Known mechanisms of PI3K/Akt dysregulation causing constitutive activation in cancer.

Location of activation/mutation	Function	Malignancy
Enzymes regulating phospholipids PtdIns(3,4,5)P3 PtdIns(3,4)P2	Second messengers	Breast, ovarian, small cell lung cancer
PIK3CA gene	Catalytic subunit of PI3K	Breast (18–40%), ovarian (4–12%), hepatocellular (36%), gastric (25%), and lung (4%)
Pleckstrin homology domain of Akt1	Mediates membrane translocation	Breast, colorectal, ovarian, and leukemia in mice
Akt1	Inhibits cell motility in breast cancer cell lines Cell proliferation survival Drug resistance	Ovarian, breast, colorectal, and gastric
Akt2- most frequently mutated of Akt isoforms	Motility, invasion in breast cancer cell lines Glucose metabolism	Ovarian, breast, pancreatic, colorectal, glioblastoma, gastric, and lung
Akt3	Role in cell motility unknown	Ovarian, breast, prostate, and murine thymoma
PTEN inactivation	Tumor suppressor	Somatic: gallbladder, prostate, and endometrial Germline: Cowden's disease (breast, thyroid, and endometrial)

Regulation by PTEN

Inactivation or mutation of tumor suppressor genes and amplification of oncogenes lead to initiation and progression of MM. The tumor suppressor gene PTEN is located on 10q23.3 and negatively regulates the function of the PI3K/Akt pathway. Loss of function may be an early and continuing event in carcinogenesis and has been associated with cell survival and resistance in MM and poor clinical outcome in breast, brain, endometrial, prostate, lung, and ovarian cancers, among others.[18–25] Germline mutations of PTEN are causative in Cowden's disease, a hereditary condition which predisposes patients to breast, thyroid, and endometrial cancer.[26] Normally, the protein encoded by the PTEN gene removes phosphate groups from key regulatory lipids, specifically, phophatidylinositol 3,4,5-triphosphate (PIP3). Loss of this phosphate group renders activation of PI3K impossible, turning the pathway off at an early stage in signaling. Inactivation of PTEN through somatic mutation or loss of heterozygosity allows PI3K activation and downstream signaling to proceed unchecked.

In addition to PI3K regulation, PTEN normally shares a feedback loop with another tumor suppressor gene, p53, such that PTEN expression upregulates p53 and vice versa.[27] In addition to increasing function, PTEN also appears to prolong p53 half-life.[28]

PI3K Activation and Effects

The family of phosphoinositide kinase enzymes is characterized by the ability to phosphorylate the inositol ring 3'-OH group in cellular phospholipids.[29] Class I PI3K enzymes catalyze phosphorylation of multiple phosphotidylinositols, and are divided further into A (activated by tyrosine kinase-linked receptors) and B (activated by G-protein coupled receptors) subtypes.[30] The class IA PI3K enzyme is a heterodimer with regulatory (p85) and catalytic (p110) subunits that are activated by extracellular receptor tyrosine kinases (RTK), including the insulin-like growth factor receptor 1 (IGFR1), HER2, and EGFR. Activation of RTKs leads to allosteric joining to the cellular membrane and subsequent tyrosine phosphorylation of the regulatory subunit of PI3K.[31] Following PI3K activation, PIP3 is generated from the substrate PIP2. PIP3 has the ability to recruit the serine-threonine kinase Akt (protein kinase B) and the phosphoinositide-dependent kinase 1 (PDK1) to the cellular membrane and catalyze their function.[32] Initial phosphorylation of Akt through PIP3 leads to increased PDK1 interaction and direct activation of Akt. Once Akt is activated, it is able to phosphorylate multiple downstream targets with various functions.

Akt Actions

Phosphorylation of mTOR, BAD, IKK (IκB kinase), p27, FOXO (forkhead box subgroup O), MDM2 (murine double minute 2), and GSK3β (glycogen synthase kinase-3 beta) occurs through direct activation by Akt (Fig. 1). Each of these substrate kinases has a vital role in cell cycle regulation, either directly or through an intermediary (Table 2). Activation of mTOR leads to protein synthesis and translation through its ability to sense glucose and amino acid availability.[33] mTOR also inhibits the translation repressor PHAS-1, another pathway to upregulate proteins that drive cell cycle progression from G1 to S phase.[34] Efficacy of mTOR inhibition can be seen in the activity of CCI-779 (temsirolimus), RAD001 (everolimus), and AP23573 in renal cell carcinoma and breast, nonsmall cell lung, and endometrial cancers.[35–37] Direct inhibition of PI3K leads to reduced mTOR signaling, effectively mimicking effects on cancer cell proliferation.[38] One drawback to mTOR blockade is upstream activation of Akt through a loss of feedback inhibition, potentially requiring combination PI3K/mTOR blockade to overcome attenuation.[39,40]

Phosphorylation of BAD via Akt prevents inactivation of the survival factor Bcl-XL, leading to uncontrolled proliferation via the Bcl-2 and 14-3-3 pathways.[41] Activation of NFκB occurs through an indirect mediator, IκB kinase (IKK), which negates an NFκB control mechanism.[42] The overall effect

Table 2 PI3K/Akt pathway downstream proteins.

Protein	Intermediary	Stimulatory effects on cancer growth
mTOR	S6K1, 4EBP1	Transcription, protein synthesis
BAD	Bcl-2, Bcl-XL	Proliferation, apoptosis escape
IKK	NFκB	Transcription, protein synthesis
FOXO	14-3-3, TRAIL	Uncontrolled cell cycle progression, drug resistance
p27	CDK2	Uncontrolled cell cycle progression
MDM2	p53	Apoptosis escape, uncontrolled cell cycle progression, DNA repair
GSK3β	β-catenin	Transcription of survival genes

mTOR mammalian target of rapamycin, *S6K1* p70-S6 Kinase 1, *4EBP1* eukaryotic initiation factor 4E (eIF4E) binding protein 1, *BAD* Bcl-2 antagonist of cell death, *Bcl-2* B cell lymphoma 2, *IKK* I kappa B kinase, *NFκB* nuclear factor kappa B, *FOXO* forkhead box subgroup O, *TRAIL* NF-related apoptosis-inducing ligand, *DK2* cyclin-dependent kinase 2, *MDM2* murine double minute 2, *GSK3β* glycogen synthase kinase-3 beta of Akt-induced IKK phosphorylation is promotion of cell survival through increased mRNA transcription and protein synthesis.

Antiproliferative signals are impaired due to Akt-induced phosphorylation of p27, primarily due to a loss of G1 arrest and due to reduced p27 transport to the nucleus and cytoplasmic accumulation. Breast cancers with increased p27 activation have been shown to have a poor prognosis compared to those without.[43]

The FOXO family of Forkhead transcription factors and their role in inhibiting tumor proliferation is not currently well defined; however, a loss of function due to Akt activation appears to play at least a supportive role in allowing lymphoma and prostate cancer cell lines to grow unchecked.[44,45]

MDM2 is a growth factor that, when phosphorylated by Akt, migrates to the nucleus and inhibits the tumor suppressor gene p53.[46] This effect may occur independently and in addition to PTEN loss-induced p53 downregulation at the cellular membrane. Restoration of PTEN function in glioblastoma and acute lymphocytic leukemia leads to increased p53 activity, cell cycle arrest, and chemotherapy sensitivity in the nucleus, demonstrating partial reliance on the MDM2 pathway for control.[47,48]

The serine kinase GSK3β normally phosphorylates β-catenin, a protein that stimulates proliferation and cell-to-cell adhesion, which leads to its clearance through ubiquitination-dependent proteosomal degradation.[49] Inhibition of GSK3β by Akt therefore allows β-catenin to migrate to the nucleus and aid transcription of cell survival genes. A second function of GSK3β is promotion of the storage of glucose as glycogen in the presence of high levels of insulin.[50] Inhibition of the PI3K/Akt pathway could therefore potentially lead to hyperglycemia that is nonresponsive to exogenous insulin administration.

Another regulator of Akt function is heat shock protein 90 (hsp90), a chaperone protein involved in an array of cellular functions that assist protein folding. Normally, hsp90 binds to Akt and stabilizes and promotes evasion of degradation pathways and apoptosis.[51] The precise mechanism is under investigation, but it is clear that the hsp90-specific inhibitor geldanamycin reduces phosphorylation of Akt and subsequent downstream signaling, although it does not inhibit the hsp90/Akt interaction directly.[52] Another analogue, 17-allylaminogeldanamycin (17-AAG), induces proteosome-mediated Akt degradation, suggesting that combination with agents that induce apoptosis could yield synergistic activity.[53]

The cellular survival processes regulated by Akt involve a number of substrates. Activation of antiapoptotic pathways, silencing of tumor suppressor genes, and disruption of negative feedback signals all contribute to the diversity of downstream effects controlled by the PI3K/Akt pathway.

The PI3K/Akt Pathway in Multiple Myeloma

Evidence that the PI3K/Akt pathway is important in MM has been demonstrated in cell line and xenograft models. Restoration of a functional PTEN/PI3K/Akt axis in PTEN null cell lines leads to apoptosis in dexamethasone-resistant cell lines.[25] Myeloma growth cytokines such as IL-6 and IGF1 have activating effects via the PI3K/Akt pathway.[54,55] Activation of mTOR has been shown to reduce apoptosis in myeloma cell lines, and the mTOR inhibitor CCI-779 (temsirolimus) sensitizes previously resistant cells to dexamethasone.[56,57]

Crosstalk between surface glycoproteins and extracellular receptors can lead to increased activity of the PI3K/Akt pathway in myeloma. Plasma cell migration is stimulated by CD40-induced activation of PI3K.[58] The growth of CD45 (−) myeloma cells is dependent on stimulation of the IGF1R, with subsequent phosphorylation of Akt.[59] Blocking the PI3K pathway with the selective inhibitor wortmannin (a fungal derivative that irreversibly binds to the p110 subunit) causes a 70–85% reduction in CD45 (−) myeloma cell growth compared to 20% for CD45 (+) cells, demonstrating the reliance on this pathway for proliferation.

Therapeutic Manipulation of Upstream Regulators of PI3/Akt

PTEN Restoration

If the primary genomic event that leads to uncontrolled proliferation and survival can be reversed through gene transfer, normal signaling and processes could be restored. Experience with this approach to date has been in glioma and endometrial, gastric, colorectal, prostate, and lung cancer using adenoviral vectors. Results have been encouraging, with suppression of the neoplastic phenotype occurring in most cases. Downregulation of VEGF expression, elimination of G2/M arrest, and a reduction in IGF signaling are all results of PTEN restoration.[60–62] In MM, restoration of PTEN function in human cell lines using a retroviral vector reduced IGF-mediated Akt activity by 50%.[63] The use of gene array techniques may help define the specific patient population that would benefit from these approaches.

Inhibitors of the MAPK Pathways

Ras Inhibitors (Inhibitors of Prenylation)

Farnesylation, a type of protein prenylation or posttranslational lipid modification, is necessary for oncogenesis to occur via the GTPase Ras. Ras represents an important target in MM as N and K-Ras activating mutations are frequently found in both MM plasma cell leukemia.[64] The clinical course when these mutations are present tend to be more aggressive and is associated with progressive disease and decreased survival.[65] The farnesyl transferase inhibitors (FTIs) R115777 (tipifarnib) and SCH66336 (lonafarnib) have shown marginal single-agent activity in both solid and hematologic malignancies, but significant activity in combination. The sequence of bortezomib followed by lonafarnib induces synergistic cell death in both MM cell lines and primary patient samples and is associated with downregulation of p-Akt.[66] The addition of tipifarnib to paclitaxel or docetaxel in MM cell lines, primary patient samples, and SCID-hu bone models of MM was more effective at inducing apoptosis than either agent alone, providing the basis for clinical trials in patients.[67]

MEK Inhibitors

Constitutive activation of the RAS/MEK/ERK signaling cascade has been implicated in the pathogenesis of MM. Mutations of NRAS and RAF have been identified and are sensitive to MEK inhibitors such as AZD6211, a novel specific MEK1/2 inhibitor. Recently, Tai et al.[68] published data showing that it inhibits constitutive and cytokine-stimulated ERK1/2 phosphorylation inducing MM cell cytotoxicity and inhibiting osteoclastogenesis in human MM cell lines in bone marrow milieau. Tumor growth in a plasmacytoma xenograft model is also inhibited, prolonging survival.

p38 Inhibitors

In 2003, Hideshima et al. published data indicating that the p38/MAPK inhibitor VX-745 inhibits IL-6 and VEGF secretion in bone marrow stromal cells, effectively inhibiting paracrine MM cell growth in bone marrow and overcoming cell adhesion-related drug resistance in MM cell lines.[69] Subsequently, Hideshima et al. reported that the p38 inhibitor SCIO-469 overcomes bortezomib resistance in MM cell lines by inhibiting HSP27, which is frequently overexpressed in bortezomib-resistant MM.[70]

More recently, Wang et al. found that p38 inhibitors were capable of restoring dysfunctional monocyte dendritic cell function in primary MM patient derived samples, which has implications for the development of immunotherapies.[71]

PI3K Inhibition

Direct inhibition of the PI3K enzyme complex will have a maximal effect on all downstream targets. While this is optimal for the impact on cellular proliferation and survival, it may lead to more toxicity. To date, animal data has not suggested excessive toxicity following PI3K inhibition, but clinical data is needed. Two inhibitors frequently used in laboratory evaluations are wortmannin and LY294002. Both inhibit all class I PI3K enzymes but are poorly soluble and have off target activity. More water-soluble forms of wortmannin with longer half-lives are in preclinical development. LY204002 is a reversible pan-PI3K inhibitor limited by poor solubility and a short half-life, which lead to the development of SF1126, a soluble covalent conjugate of LY294002 that localizes to tumor vasculature.[72] In myeloma, dexamethasone-resistant xenografts were inhibited 95% compared to controls following treatment with SF1126, with IC50 values of 2.8 µM for p-Akt inhibition.[73] Microvessel density analysis showed significant antiangiogenic activity.

Inhibition of PI3K also activates other proapoptotic events. The SAPK/JNK pathway is downregulated in tumorigenesis, and inhibition of PI3K with wortmannin leads to restoration of the signals lost during uncontrolled cellular proliferation.[74] In myeloma, downregulation of the antiapoptotic mitogen-activated protein kinase/extracellular signal-regulated kinase (MAPK/ERK) pathway has also been demonstrated following PI3K inhibition with wortmannin, with a resultant reduction in VEGF secretion from myeloma cells.[75]

Combinations Including PI3K Inhibition

Combination therapy with PI3K inhibitors and conventional antimyeloma therapies are intriguing since preclinical studies suggest more than additive activity.[76–78] It will be important to design clinical trials that take full advantage of the combination of agents based on laboratory evaluations that incorporate validated measurements of the timeline and extent of myeloma cell death following inhibition of the PI3K pathway.

Akt Inhibition

Inhibition of Akt holds promise for therapy since it serves as a second nodal point for cellular proliferation, survival signaling, angiogenesis, and resistance. The oral Akt inhibitor perifosine has shown promising activity in MM cell lines and xenografts.[79–81] Preliminary results of a phase II trial combining perifosine 150 mg daily in relapsed and refractory patients with add-on dexamethasone at progression have been presented.[82] In 25 evaluable patients who had a median of 4 previous lines of therapy, stable disease (SD) was seen in 24% prior to the addition of dexamethasone. Of nine patients on the combination, three achieved a minor response and two had SD. Common adverse events were nausea, vomiting, diarrhea, fatigue, and increased creatinine seen in 14 patients with progressive disease and light chain nephropathy.

The broad, nonselective Akt inhibitor 7-hydroxystaurosporine (UCN-01) is a staurosporine analogue that has been evaluated in phase I trials in solid tumors and leukemias alone and in combination. Initially, data suggested a 72-h infusion would provide optimal activity; however, more recent trials have shown the maximum tolerated dose to be 90 mg/m^2 infused over 3 h on cycle 1, followed by 47.5 mg/m^2 on subsequent cycles.[83] It has been associated with hypotension, nausea/vomiting, and hyperglycemia. Insulin-resistant hyperglycemia was observed in the initial 72-h infusion trials; however, the severity appears to be reduced with shorter infusion times.[84] Evidence of activity in myeloma is limited to cell line data, with the combination of UCN-01 and the HMG CoA reductase inhibitor lovastatin producing a fourfold increase in apoptosis as measured by annexin V compared to either agent alone.[85] Synergy was also observed in combination with interruption of the NFκB pathway in cell lines, suggesting dual-agent therapy with bortezomib may be effective.

Triciribine phosphate monohydrate (TCN-PM, VQD-002) is a tricyclic nucleoside that inhibits activated Akt. It has been evaluated as an antiviral and antineoplastic for over 20 years, but formulation challenges and toxicities prevented development. A novel oral formulation is currently in phase I trials in solid tumors and leukemias and is undergoing laboratory evaluation in myeloma (Table 3).

Combinations Including Akt Inhibition

Inhibition of Akt alone may be ineffective in myeloma cells not under cellular stress, leading to a potential for survival and reexpansion upon discontinuation of an Akt inhibitor. Combination therapies that place cells under apoptotic stress and inhibit Akt actions could provide more effective and less toxic results. The farnesyl transferase inhibitor tipifarnib has been shown to inhibit Akt phosphorylation in vivo and in vitro and is synergistic with bortezomib in inducing apoptosis in myeloma.[86,87] Clinical trials of this combination are underway.

Conclusion

Activation of the PI3K/Akt pathway is a critical event in malignant transformation and survival, and its importance in MM continues to emerge. The inciting event, PTEN loss, occurs early in many cancers, demonstrating the pivotal role

Table 3 Inhibitors of the PI3K/Akt pathway currently in development.

Agent	Route	Sponsor	Phase	Disease(s)
PI3K inhibitors				
SF1126	IV	Semafore	Phase I	Solid tumors, myeloma
XL147	PO	Exelixis	Phase I	Solid tumors
XL765 (PI3K/mTOR)	PO	Exelixis	Phase I	Solid tumors
BEZ235	PO	Novartis	Phase I /II	Solid tumors
Akt inhibitors				
Perifosine (KRX-0401)	PO	Keryx	Phase I/II	Solid tumors, myeloma, Leukemias, MDS, lymphoma
XL418	PO	Exelixis	Phase I	Solid tumors
GSK690693	IV	GlaxoSmithKline	Phase I	Solid tumors, lymphoma
Triciribine (TCN-PM, VQD-002)	IV (Prodrug PO)	VioQuest	Phase I/II	Solid tumors, leukemias
UCN-01	IV	National Cancer Institute	Phase I/II	Solid tumors, leukemias, MDS, lymphoma

this pathway plays in malignancy. It is also clear that multiple proteins along the pathway stimulate and contribute to cellular proliferation, migration, and resistance; however, because PI3K integrates many extracellular and intracellular signals, it functions as a central locus for signal transduction. Interventions that reverse PI3K/Akt activation, therefore, hold promise in rational approaches to myeloma therapy. Combinations of novel agents with existing treatment will likely be more effective than monotherapy, particularly in patients whose disease requires overcoming resistance and inducing sensitivity. The diversity of potential targets along the PI3K/Akt pathway will necessitate careful preclinical evaluation of combinations both internal and external to the pathway in order to ensure optimal activity, minimal toxicity, and lack of resistance. Current information on laboratory activity of these agents is encouraging, and clinical trial experience is accumulating. Further translational efforts to understand the activity and toxicity of these agents is likely to lead to successes in development and in the clinic.

Future Perspective

Comprehension of the PI3K/Akt pathway and its role in cancer development and progression is far from complete. Additionally, interventions to reverse constitutive activation of the pathway appear promising, but understanding the best target or combination of targets is currently minimal. The PI3K enzyme itself is probably the most attractive approach to inhibiting downstream proliferation due to its centrality in signaling. While this may prove to have the broadest effect on inhibiting survival and restoring apoptosis, toxicity concerns are real due to the diversity of function of many effector proteins. To date, animal models with PI3K inhibitors slated for clinical development have not shown marked toxicity; however, experience in humans is minimal. Both PI3K and Akt inhibition induce apoptosis in cancer cells, and combination therapy with existing antineoplastics will likely offer synergy above either class of agent alone. The most biologically elegant approach to the pathway is restoration of PTEN function; however, practical challenges of delivering the gene to cancer cells safely and effectively are daunting. Individualizing therapy through genomics and proteomics is possible through tissue typing for PTEN loss, and this should help personalize patients for response to agents that act through the PI3K/Akt pathway.

Summary

- Activation of the PI3K/Akt pathway is increasingly being recognized as a central event in both solid tumors and hematologic malignancies.
- Multiple attractive targets exist along the pathway, including the abnormal tumor suppressor gene (PTEN), PI3K, Akt, the chaperone protein HSP90, and end proteins and genes including mTOR, BAD, IKK, FOXO, p27, MDM2, and GSK3β.
- Many inhibitors of these targets are already in use, and more are in clinical trials and preclinical development. Specifically, the PI3K inhibitors and Akt inhibitors are in phase I testing.
- Preclinical studies of PI3K and Akt inhibitors show that turning off this pathway induces apoptosis, reduces angiogenesis, and reverses drug resistance.
- Based on preclinical data, combinations of agents with PI3K and Akt inhibitors will likely produce synergistic clinical response.

References

1. Lim, W.T., et al, PTEN and phosphorylated AKT expression and prognosis in early- and late-stage non-small cell lung cancer. Oncol Rep, 2007. **17**(4): 853–7.
2. Bahlis, N.J., et al, CD28-mediated regulation of multiple myeloma cell proliferation and survival. Blood, 2007. **109**(11): 5002–10.
3. Govindarajan, B., et al, Overexpression of Akt converts radial growth melanoma to vertical growth melanoma. J Clin Invest, 2007. **117**(3): 719–29.
4. Meng, Q., et al, Role of PI3K and AKT specific isoforms in ovarian cancer cell migration, invasion and proliferation through the p70S6K1 pathway. Cell Signal, 2006. **18**(12): 2262–71.
5. Opel, D., et al, Activation of Akt predicts poor outcome in neuroblastoma. Cancer Res, 2007. **67**(2): 735–45.
6. Tazzari, P.L., et al, Multidrug resistance-associated protein 1 expression is under the control of the phosphoinositide 3 kinase/Akt signal transduction network in human acute myelogenous leukemia blasts. Leukemia, 2007. **21**(3): 427–38.
7. Tokunaga, E., et al, Activation of PI3K/Akt signaling and hormone resistance in breast cancer. Breast Cancer, 2006. **13**(2): 137–44.
8. Uddin, S., et al, Role of phosphatidylinositol 3″-kinase/AKT pathway in diffuse large B-cell lymphoma survival. Blood, 2006. **108**(13): 4178–86.
9. Cantrell, D.A., Phosphoinositide 3-kinase signalling pathways. J Cell Sci, 2001. **114**(Pt 8): 1439–45.
10. Chang, F., et al, Involvement of PI3K/Akt pathway in cell cycle progression, apoptosis, and neoplastic transformation: a target for cancer chemotherapy. Leukemia, 2003. **17**(3): 590–603.
11. Testa, J.R., et al and Bellacosa, A., AKT plays a central role in tumorigenesis. Proc Natl Acad Sci USA, 2001. **98**(20): 10983–10985.
12. Carpten, J., et al, A transforming mutation in the pleckstrin homology domain of AKT1 in cancer. Nature, 2007. **448**: 439–444.
13. Cheng, J.Q., Activation of the PI3K/Akt pathway and chemotherapeutic resistance. Drug Resist Update, **5**: 131–146.

14. Arlt, A., et al, Role of NF- βB and Akt/PI3K in the resistance of pancreatic carcinoma cell lines against gemcitabine-induced cell death. Oncogene, 2003. **22**: 3242–3251.

15. Kneufermann, C., et al, HER2/PI-3K/Akt activation leads to a multidrug resistance in human breast adenocarcinoma cells. Oncogene, 2003. **22**: 3205–3512.

16. Yuan, Z.-Q., et al, AKT2 inhibition of cisplatin-induced JNK/p38 and Bax activation by phosphorylation of ASK1: Implication of AKT2 in chemoresistance. J Biol Chem, 2003. **19**: 2324–2330.

17. Nagata, Y., et al, PTEN activation contributes to tumor inhibition by trastuzumab, and loss of PTEN predicts trastuzumab resistance in patients. Cancer Cell, 2004. **6**: 117–127.

18. Athanassiadou, P., et al, The prognostic value of PTEN, p53, and beta-catenin in endometrial carcinoma: A prospective immunocytochemical study. Int J Gynecol Cancer, 2007. **17**(3): 697–704.

19. Bepler, G., et al, RRM1 and PTEN as prognostic parameters for overall and disease-free survival in patients with non-small-cell lung cancer. J Clin Oncol, 2004. **22**(10): 1878–1885.

20. Edwards, L.A., et al, Inhibition of ILK in PTEN-mutant human glioblastomas inhibits PKB/Akt activation, induces apoptosis, and delays tumor growth. Oncogene, 2005. **24**(22): 3596–3605.

21. Ferraro, B., et al, EGR1 predicts PTEN and survival in patients with non-small-cell lung cancer. J Clin Oncol, 2005. **23**(9): 1921–1926.

22. Schmitz, M., et al, Complete loss of PTEN expression as a possible early prognostic marker for prostate cancer metastasis. Int J Cancer, 2007. **120**(6): 1284–92.

23. Sui, L., et al, Alteration and clinical relevance of PTEN expression and its correlation with survivin expression in epithelial ovarian tumors. Oncol Rep, 2006. **15**(4): 773–8.

24. Tsutsui, S., et al, Reduced expression of PTEN protein and its prognostic implications in invasive ductal carcinoma of the breast. Oncology, 2005. **68**(4–6): 398–404.

25. Zhang, J., et al, Preferential killing of PTEN-null myelomas by PI3K inhibitors through Akt pathway. Oncogene, 2003. **22**(40): 6289–95.

26. Eng, C., PTEN: One gene, many syndromes. Hum Mutat, 2003. **22**(3): 183–98.

27. Feng, Z., et al, The regulation of AMPK beta1, TSC2, and PTEN expression by p53: stress, cell and tissue specificity, and the role of these gene products in modulating the IGF-1-AKT-mTOR pathways. Cancer Res, 2007. **67**(7): 3043–53.

28. Blanco-Aparicio, C., et al, PTEN, more than the AKT pathway. Carcinogenesis, 2007. **28**(7): 1379–86.

29. Fruman, D.A., Meyers, R.E., and Cantley, L.C., Phosphoinositide kinases. Annu Rev Biochem, 1998. **67**: 481–507.

30. Wymann, M.P., and Marone, R., Phosphoinositide 3-kinase in disease: Timing, location, and scaffolding. Current Opinion in Cell Biology, 2005. **17**(2): 141–149.

31. Hunter, T., Signaling—2000 and beyond. Cell, 2000. **100**(1): 113–27.

32. Datta, S.R., Brunet, A., and Greenberg, M.E., Cellular survival: a play in three Akts. Genes Dev, 1999. **13**(22): 2905–27.

33. Hay, N., and Sonenberg, N., Upstream and downstream of mTOR. Genes Dev, 2004. **18**(16): 1926–45.

34. Brunn, G.J., et al, Direct inhibition of the signaling functions of the mammalian target of rapamycin by the phosphoinositide 3-kinase inhibitors, wortmannin and LY294002. EMBO J, 1996. **15**(19): 5256–67.

35. Cho, D., et al, The role of mammalian target of rapamycin inhibitors in the treatment of advanced renal cancer. Clin Cancer Res, 2007. **13**(2 Pt 2): 758s–763s.

36. Smolewski, P., Recent developments in targeting the mammalian target of rapamycin (mTOR) kinase pathway. Anticancer Drugs, 2006. **17**(5): 487–94.

37. Sun, S.Y., Fu, H., and Khuri, F.R., Targeting mTOR signaling for lung cancer therapy. J Thorac Oncol, 2006. **1**(2): 109–11.

38. Sun, S.Y., et al, Activation of Akt and eIF4E survival pathways by rapamycin-mediated mammalian target of rapamycin inhibition. Cancer Res, 2005. **65**(16): 7052–8.

39. Hay, N., The Akt-mTOR tango and its relevance to cancer. Cancer Cell, 2005. **8**(3): 179–83.

40. Franke, T.F., et al, PI3K/Akt and apoptosis: Size matters. Oncogene, 2003. **22**(56): 8983–98.

41. Downward, J., PI 3-kinase, Akt and cell survival. Semin Cell Dev Biol, 2004. **15**(2): 177–82.

42. Liang, J., et al, PKB/Akt phosphorylates p27, impairs nuclear import of p27 and opposes p27-mediated G1 arrest. Nat Med, 2002. **8**(10): 1153–60.

43. Paik, J.H., et al, FoxOs are lineage-restricted redundant tumor suppressors and regulate endothelial cell homeostasis. Cell, 2007. **128**(2): 309–23.

44. Dong, X.Y., et al, FOXO1A is a candidate for the 13q14 tumor suppressor gene inhibiting androgen receptor signaling in prostate cancer. Cancer Res, 2006. **66**(14): 6998–7006.

45. Mayo, L.D., and Donner, D.B., A phosphatidylinositol 3-kinase/Akt pathway promotes translocation of Mdm2 from the cytoplasm to the nucleus. Proc Natl Acad Sci U S A, 2001. **98**(20): 11598–603.

46. Mayo, L.D., et al, PTEN protects p53 from Mdm2 and sensitizes cancer cells to chemotherapy. J Biol Chem, 2002. **277**(7): 5484–9.

47. Zhou, M., et al, PTEN reverses MDM2-mediated chemotherapy resistance by interacting with p53 in acute lymphoblastic leukemia cells. Cancer Res, 2003. **63**(19): 6357–62.

48. Hino, S., et al, Phosphorylation of beta-catenin by cyclic AMP-dependent protein kinase stabilizes beta-catenin through inhibition of its ubiquitination. Mol Cell Biol, 2005. **25**(20): 9063–72.

49. Cross, D.A., et al, Inhibition of glycogen synthase kinase-3 by insulin mediated by protein kinase B. Nature, 1995. **378**(6559): 785–9.

50. Workman, P., Combinatorial attack on multistep oncogenesis by inhibiting the Hsp90 molecular chaperone. Cancer Lett, 2004. **206**(2): 149–157.

51. Fujita, N., et al, Involvement of Hsp90 in signaling and stability of 3-phosphoinositide-dependent kinase-1. J Biol Chem, 2002. **277**(12): 10346–53.

52. Basso, A.D., et al, Ansamycin antibiotics inhibit Akt activation and cyclin D expression in breast cancer cells that overexpress HER2. Oncogene, 2002. **21**(8): 1159–66.

53. Hideshima, T., et al, Biologic sequelae of interleukin-6 induced PI3-K/Akt signaling in multiple myeloma. Oncogene, 2001. **20**(42): 5991–6000.

54. Tu, Y., Gardner, A., and Lichtenstein, A., The phosphatidylinositol 3-kinase/AKT kinase pathway in multiple myeloma plasma cells: Roles in cytokine-dependent survival and proliferative responses. Cancer Res, 2000. **60**(23): 6763–70.

55. Pene, F., et al, Role of the phosphatidylinositol 3-kinase/Akt and mTOR/P70S6-kinase pathways in the proliferation and apoptosis in multiple myeloma. Oncogene, 2002. **21**(43): 6587–97.

56. Yan, H., et al, Mechanism by which mammalian target of rapamycin inhibitors sensitize multiple myeloma cells to dexamethasone-induced apoptosis. Cancer Res, 2006. **66**(4): 2305–13.

57. Tai, Y.T., et al, CD40 induces human multiple myeloma cell migration via phosphatidylinositol 3-kinase/AKT/NF-kappa B signaling. Blood, 2003. **101**(7): 2762–9.

58. Descamps, G., et al, The magnitude of Akt/phosphatidylinositol 3″-kinase proliferating signaling is related to CD45 expression in human myeloma cells. J Immunol, 2004. **173**(8): 4953–9.

59. Gomez-Manzano, C., et al, Mechanisms underlying PTEN regulation of vascular endothelial growth factor and angiogenesis. Ann Neurol, 2003. **53**(1): 109–17.

60. Saito, Y., et al, Adenovirus-mediated PTEN treatment combined with caffeine produces a synergistic therapeutic effect in colorectal cancer cells. Cancer Gene Ther, 2003. **10**(11): 803–13.

61. Yi, H.-K., et al, Impact of PTEN on the expression of insulin-like growth factors (IGFs) and IGF-binding proteins in human gastric adenocarcinoma cells. Biochem Biophys Res Commun, 2005. **330**(3): 760–767.

62. Hyun, T., et al, Loss of PTEN expression leading to high Akt activation in human multiple myelomas. Blood, 2000. 96(10): 3560–8.

63. Garlich, J., Development of a vascular targeted pan-PI3K inhibitor for cancer therapy. 3rd Focused Meeting on P13K signalling and disease Bath, UK 6–8 November 2006.

64. Bezieau, S., et al, High incidence of N and K-Ras activating mutations in multiple myeloma and primary plasma cell leukemia at diagnosis. Hum Mutat, 2001. **18**: 212–242.

65. Liu, P., et al, Activating mutations of N and K-Ras in multiple myeloma show different clinical associations: Analysis of the Eastern Cooperative Oncology Group phase III trial. Blood, 1996. **88**: 2699–2706.

66. David, E., et al, The combination of farnesyl transferase inhibitor lonafarnib and the proteosome inhibitor bortezomib induces synergistic apoptosis in human myeloma cells that is associated with down-regulation of p-AKT. Blood, 2005. **106**: 4322–4329.

67. Zhu, K., Bloodet al, , 2005. **105**: 4759–4766.Farnesyl transferase inhibitor R115777 (Zarnestra, Tipifarnib) synergizes with paclitaxel to induce apoptosis and mitotic arrest and to inhibit tumor growth of multiple myeloma cells.

68. Tai, Y.T., et al, Targeting MEK induces myeloma-cell cytotoxicity and inhibits osteoclastogenesis. Blood, 2007. **110**: 1656–1663.

69. Hideshima, T., et al, Targeting p38 MAPK inhibits multiple myeloma cell growth in the bone marrow milieu. Blood, 2003. **101**: 703–705.

70. Hideshima, T., et al, p38 MAPK inhibition enhances PS-341 (bortezomib) induced cytotoxicity against multiple myeloma cells. Oncogene, 2004. **23**: 8766–8776.

71. Wang, S., et al, Optimizing immunotherapy in multiple myeloma: Restoring the function of patients' monocyte derived dentritic cells by inhibiting p38 or activating MEK/ERK/MAPK and neutralizing IL-6 in progenitor cells. Blood, 2006. **108**: 4071–4077.

72. Garlich, J.R., et al, A vascular targeted pan phosphoinositide 3-kinase inhibitor prodng, SF1126, with antitumor and antiangiogenic activity. Cancer Res, 2008. **68**(1): 206–15.

73. Ruiter, G.A., et al, Anti-cancer alkyl-lysophospholipids inhibit the phosphatidylinositol 3-kinase-Akt/PKB survival pathway. Anticancer Drugs, 2003. **14**(2): 167–73.

74. Giuliani, N., et al, Downmodulation of ERK protein kinase activity inhibits VEGF secretion by human myeloma cells and myeloma-induced angiogenesis. Leukemia, 2004. **18**(3): 628–35.

75. Ihle, N.T., et al, Molecular pharmacology and antitumor activity of PX-866, a novel inhibitor of phosphoinositide-3-kinase signaling. Mol Cancer Ther, 2004. **3**(7): 763–72.

76. Ohta, T., et al, Inhibition of phosphatidylinositol 3-kinase increases efficacy of cisplatin in in vivo ovarian cancer models. Endocrinology, 2006. **147**(4): 1761–9.

77. Fujiwara, Y., et al, Blockade of the phosphatidylinositol-3-kinase-Akt signaling pathway enhances the induction of apoptosis by microtubule-destabilizing agents in tumor cells in which the pathway is constitutively activated. Mol Cancer Ther, 2007. **6**(3): 1133–42.

78. Catley, L., et al, Alkyl phospholipid perifosine induces myeloid hyperplasia in a murine myeloma model. Exp Hematol, 2007. **35**(7): 1038–46.

79. Gajate, C., and Mollinedo, F., Edelfosine and perifosine induce selective apoptosis in multiple myeloma by recruitment of death receptors and downstream signaling molecules into lipid rafts. Blood, 2007. **109**(2): 711–9.

80. Hideshima, T., et al, Perifosine, an oral bioactive novel alkylphospholipid, inhibits Akt and induces in vitro and in vivo cytotoxicity in human multiple myeloma cells. Blood, 2006. **107**(10): 4053–62.

81. Richardson, P., et al, A Multicenter Phase II Study of perifosine (KRX-0401) alone and in combination with dexamethasone (Dex) for patients with relapsed or relapsed/refractory multiple myeloma (MM). ASH Annual Meeting Abstracts, 2006. **108**(11): Abstract 3582.

82. Dees, E.C., et al, A phase I and pharmacokinetic study of short infusions of UCN-01 in patients with refractory solid tumors. Clin Cancer Res, 2005. **11**(2 Pt 1): 664–71.

83. Sausville, E.A., et al, Phase I trial of 72-hour continuous infusion UCN-01 in patients with refractory neoplasms. J Clin Oncol, 2001. **19**(8): 2319–33.

84. Dai, Y., , Statins synergistically potentiate 7-hydroxystaurosporine (UCN-01) lethality in human leukemia and myeloma cells by disrupting Ras farnesylation and activation. Blood, 2007. **109**(10): 4415–23.

85. Jiang, K., et al, The phosphoinositide 3-OH kinase/AKT2 pathway as a critical target for farnesyltransferase inhibitor-induced apoptosis. Mol Cell Biol, 2000. **20**(1): 139–48.

86. Yanamandra, N., et al, Tipifarnib and bortezomib are synergistic and overcome cell adhesion-mediated drug resistance in multiple myeloma and acute myeloid leukemia. Clin Cancer Res, 2006. **12**(2): 591–9.

Chapter 21

The Mammalian Target of Rapamycin and Multiple Myeloma

Patrick Frost and Alan Lichtenstein

The Biochemistry and Molecular Biology of TOR

Eukaryotic cells have evolved a highly integrated regulatory process linking progrowth environmental stimuli (e.g., growth factors, nutrient, and energy levels) with the activation and regulation of the protein synthesis machinery, thereby ensuring that the proteins critical for cell growth and cell cycle progression are expressed only when conditions are appropriate. While multiple intracellular proteins and signaling pathways are involved in this process, the mammalian target of rapamycin (mTOR) is an especially important component and acts as a convergence point for these diverse regulatory and sensory pathways. The TOR protein (also known as FRAP, RAFT, RAPT, or SEP) is a −290 kD serine/threonine kinase that belongs to the phosphatidylinositol kinase-related kinase (PIKK) family and was initially identified by mutations that conferred resistance to the growth inhibitory effects of rapamycin in the budding yeast *Saccharomyces cereviseae*.[1] Subsequent studies have demonstrated that the gene for mTOR is highly conserved (40–60% homology) and present in all eukaryotic genomes.[2–4]

Structurally, mTOR is a complex protein that contains multiple subdomains; the N-terminus contains the HEAT domain whose putative function is a scaffold for protein–protein binding.[5] The C-terminus contains the catalytic kinase domain, a putative autoinhibitor or repressor domain, and the FKBPl2-rapamycin-binding domain, which mediates rapamycin's inhibitory effect.[6] Furthermore, the function and regulation of mTOR is dependent on interactions with a number of accessory and scaffold proteins, such as the regulatory-associated protein of mTOR (raptor),[7,8] mLST8 (also known as GpL), and rictor.[9]

When growth conditions are favorable, activated mTOR upregulates ribosome biogenesis and initiates protein translation.[10,11] However, in cells with inactivated mTOR, such as those exposed to rapamycin or depleted of energy, nutrients, or growth factors, general protein synthesis is depressed and cell cycle transit slows, while proteasome and autophagy activity increases and stress-responsive transcription factors become activated (reviewed

From: *Contemporary Hematology Myeloma Therapy*
Edited by: S. Lonial © Humana Press, Totowa, NJ

in Wullschleger et al.[12]) Thus, when the environment is favorable, mTOR signaling acts as a rheostat, promoting pathways responsible for induction of protein synthesis and cell growth, while unfavorable conditions result in mTOR-mediated triggering of survival pathways.

In yeast, two separate genes for TOR (TOR1 and TOR2) were identified that perform separate functions and that are differentially regulated.[1] TOR1, which is sensitive to inhibition by rapamycin, regulates growth of cells, while TOR2, which is insensitive to rapamycin, regulates the spatial and cytoskeletal aspects of growth.[9] In contrast to yeasts, only one TOR gene is present in the mammalian genome. However, differential sensitivity to rapamycin is conserved by the formation of two functionally distinct mTOR complexes, the rapamycin-sensitive mTORCl, which consists of mTOR, raptor, and GpL and the rapamycin-resistant mTORC2, which consists of mTOR, rictor, and GpL. Emerging evidence indicates that these two distinct complexes may also perform separate functions.[8,12]

Upstream Activating mTOR Signaling Components

The cascade that results in mTOR activation consists of the AKT kinase, the tuberous sclerosis (TSC) TSCl–TSC2 protein complex, and the GTP/GDP-bound Ras homolog enriched in brain (Rheb) protein (Fig. 1). The TSCl–TSC2 complex negatively curtails Rheb through its GTPase-activating protein (GAP) activity, which converts GTP to GDP.[13] AKT phosphorylates TSC2, inhibiting its GAP activity against Rheb.[14,15] This results in a concomitant increase in Rheb–GTP levels, which binds directly to the kinase domain of mTOR and activates it in a GTP-dependent manner.[16]

Conditions that regulate mTOR activity modulate afferent pathways that impact this main activating axis at different levels (Fig. 1). Growth factor positive input into this cascade occurs via stimulation of phosphoinositol 3-kinase (PI3-K) with subsequent AKT activation. The PTEN (phosphatase and tensin

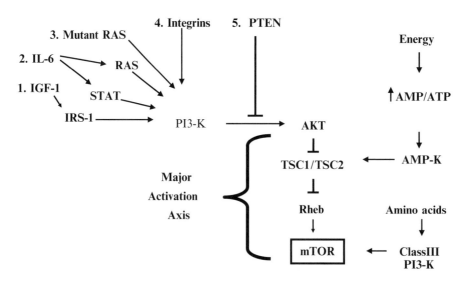

Fig. 1 Pathways that activate mTOR in multiple myeloma. Arrows represent activation pathways, whereas bars represent inhibitory pathways.

homolog deleted on chromosome 10) phosphatase is a brake that curtails AKT activation.[17] In contrast, the cellular energy-sensing pathway occurs through the AMP-activated protein kinase (AMP-K)[18] that enters the main signaling axis at the level of TSC l/TSC2 (Fig. 1). Low cellular energy (i.e., a high AMP/ATP ratio) activates AMP-K, which then enhances the Rheb-GAP activity of TSCl/TSC2, resulting in lower levels of Rheb-GTP and decreased mTOR activity. An increase in cellular ATP and decrease in AMP prevents AMP-K activation, depresses the Rheb-GAP activity ofTSC1/TSC2, and thus activates mTOR. In contrast to the primary AKT-TSC1/TSC2 Rheb axis, early evidence suggests that a sensory mechanism for intracellular amino acids uses the class III PI3-K for activation directly at the level of mTOR.[19]

Activation of mTOR in Multiple Myeloma

Immunohistochemical studies of bone marrow demonstrate frequent tumor cell AKT activation in myeloma patients.[20] As AKT is a major inducer of the TSCl/TSC2/Rheb axis, it is anticipated that concurrent mTOR activation is also present in situ in these marrow tumor cells. The following are potential mechanisms by which mTOR is activated in myeloma: In myeloma cell lines and selected primary specimens, the myeloma growth factors IL-6 and IGF-1 have been shown to activate mTOR and this activation is an important player in cell growth stimulated by these cytokines.[21] After IGF-1 binds to IGF receptors, the IRS-1 adapter induces PI3-K and AKT activation with subsequent signals transferred through TSCl/TCS2 and Rheb to mTOR (pathway 1, Fig. 1). IL-6 induces PI3-K activation in myeloma cells by two separate pathways: through its activation of RAS and, possibly, STAT-3 (pathway 2 Fig.1).[22] GTP-bound Ras activates PI3-K by directly binding to its p110 kinase subunit, while activated STAT-3 can function as an adapter binding the p85 regulatory subunit of PI3-K with ensuing activation. In most multiple myeloma cell line studies,[23] IGF-I is usually more effective than IL-6 in activation of AKT and mTOR. Activating mutations of N-Ras or K-Ras, occurring in up to 40% of patients,[24,25] also directly activate PI3-K by binding to p110 with subsequent downstream stimulation of mTOR (pathway 3, Fig. 1).

Several other potential molecular stimuli in myeloma could result in enhanced downstream signaling through AKT to mTOR. Stimulation of the integrin-linked kinase occurs via binding of myeloma cells to supporting cells or extracellular matrix in the marrow, and it may activate PI3-K (pathway 4, Fig. 1).[26] In addition, the finding of loss-of-function PTEN mutations in some multiple myeloma cell lines suggests a possible pathogenic role (pathway 5, Fig. 1).[27] This would theoretically amplify downstream signaling through AKT to mTOR. However, although such mutations have been found in some primary multiple myeloma specimens, the frequency is low (−5%).[28] Another potential mechanism of PTEN inactivation in myeloma is via a PKC-dependent pathway. Enhanced myeloma cell PKC activity results in PTEN phosphorylation and loss-of-function.[29]

Downstream Targets of mTOR

The activation of mTOR results in phosphorylation of P70S6 kinase and the 4E-BPI translational repressor, factors that are responsible for ribosome biogenesis and cap-dependent protein translation of critical proliferation-dependent proteins such as D-type cyclins and c-myc (pathway 1, Fig. 2).[30,31] Specifically, activated P70S6 kinase induces phosphorylation of the S6 ribosomal component which results in translational upregulation of mRNA transcripts containing a polypyrimidine tract at their 5' transcriptional start sites, such as those encoding ribosomal proteins and elongation factors.[32] These proteins are important components of the translation machinery that would be needed for a theoretical stimulation of protein expression. The 4E-BPl translational repressor is normally bound to the translational initiation factor, eIF4E. When mTOR induces phosphorylation of 4E-BPl, it is inactivated and releases eIF4E. Liberated elF4E then participates in assembly of the translation initiation complex that mediates the so-called "cap-dependent" translation, thus named because the mechanism utilizes the cap structure that is found on mRNAs.[33–35] Thus, both mTOR-dependent phosphorylation events on p70S6K and 4E-BP1 result in an upregulation of translation via effects on the translational machinery and on translation initiation factors. Thus, it is not surprising that mTOR activity is critical for cell cycle transit in myeloma cells stimulated with growth factors[22,36] or containing activating mutations of Ras.[37]

In addition to its role in regulating protein expression, recent studies have demonstrated that mTOR is involved in regulation of additional intracellular pathways, such as autophagy and apoptosis. Autophagy is a nonselective vacuolar-mediated protein degradation pathway involved in the turnover of long-lived proteins and organelles.[38] Autophagy occurs in all cells, providing critical housekeeping and homeostatic regulation of the cytoplasmic protein and organelle milieu. It recycles critical amino acids and metabolites that are needed for survival when exogenous supplies are deficient.[39] Autophagy is also induced under conditions of cellular stress, such as in response to starvation, changes in cell volume, oxidative stress, irradiation, and accumulation of

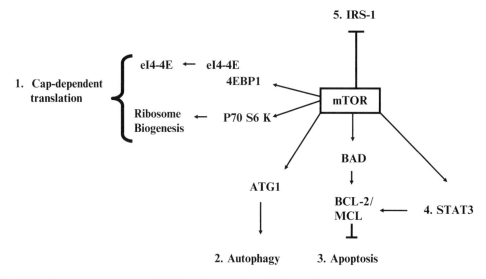

Fig. 2 The downstream targets of mTOR activation in multiple myeloma cells. Arrows represent activation pathways, whereas bars represent inhibitory pathways.

misfolded proteins.[40] mTOR inhibits autophagy by downregulating the function of protein kinase ATG1,[41] which is an early initiator of the autophagic process (pathway 2, Fig. 2). Although not yet investigated in myeloma cells, the theoretic activation of autophagy by mTOR inhibitors, potential therapeutic agents in the disease, and by an unfolded protein response suggests this is a ripe area of study.

Another cell function regulated by mTOR is apoptosis (pathway 3, Fig. 2). mTOR may protect myeloma cells from apoptotic death by several potential mechanisms: mTOR-induced activation of P70 results in a P70-mediated phosphorylation BAD (ser136),[42] causing its sequestration in the cytoplasm. Sequestered BAD cannot heterodimerize with BCL-2/BCL-XL and, thus, cannot prevent their antiapoptotic function (pathway 3,Fig. 2). P70 activity also phosphorylates STAT-3 on serine 727 (pathway 4, Fig. 2),[43] which enhances STAT-3 gene expression of antiapoptotic proteins such as BCL-2 and MCL-1.[44] In contrast to mTOR's potential to protect multiple myeloma cell viability, its phosphorylation of IRS-1 (pathway 5, Fig. 2) with resulting downregulation of IRS-1 function could diminish IGF-1-induced AKT activity, rendering cells more sensitive to apoptosis. This is a real concern with the use of mTOR inhibitors in myeloma cells as it has been shown that they can prevent IRS-l phosphorylation and induce activity of AKT, resulting in theoretical protection against drugs such as bortezomib.[45]

Use of mTOR Inhibitors in Myeloma: Preclinical and Clinical Studies

Several mTOR inhibitors, including rapamycin,[46,47] CCI-779,[48–51] and RAD001,[52] have shown potential in preclinical studies. The antimyeloma effect in vitro is associated with dephosphorylation of p70S6 kinase and 4E-BP1 and induction of G liS cell cycle arrest,[23,27] whereas in vivo, mTOR inhibitors inhibit tumor proliferation and angiogenesis and induce apoptosis.[48,51] In attempts to enhance a cytoreductive effect, mTOR inhibitors have been combined with other agents and a strong apoptotic effect on myeloma cells has been observed when they are combined with dexamethasone,[49,50] heat shock protein (HSP)-90 inhibitor,[53] sunitinib,[52] farnesyl transferase inhibitors,[47] or revlimid.[46] However, the above-described potential for mTOR inhibitors to induce activation of AKT via effects on IRS-l suggests caution in combination therapy. This feedback about unwanted activation of AKT has been noted in several other tumor models as well[54] and could potentially prevent tumor cell apoptosis when mTOR inhibitors are combined with specific agents against which the IGF/IRS-I/PI3K/AKT pathway provides protection. This suggests a rationale for combining mTOR inhibitors with agents that could interrupt this pathway.

The mTOR inhibitor CCI-779 has shown significant efficacy in early phase I–II trials of patients with renal cell carcinoma and mantle cell lymphoma. Latter studies[55] which demonstrate clear responses in up to 38% of refractory/resistant lymphoma are notable, as mantle cell lymphoma displays some similar molecular characteristics to myeloma, namely, Ig-D-type cyclin translocations and a proliferative drive probably dependant on D-cyclin expression.[56] As noted above, D-cyclin expression is a particularly susceptible protein to downregulation by mTOR inhibition.[57] To date, one phase II study with CCI-779 has been reported in myeloma. An initial report described 14 patients with resistant/refractory disease who were treated with CCI -779 at 25 mg every week. Overall, six patients (43%) demonstrated response (at least 26% decrease in M-protein), and response was associated with maximal reduction in phosphorylation of P70 and 4E-BPl in peripheral blood mononuclear cells.[58] Thus, mTOR inhibitors have demonstrated potential as therapeutic agents against myeloma, and further studies will be needed to decide how best to use them and what molecular markers predict for responsiveness.

References

1. Heitman J, Movva NR, Hall MN. Targets for cell cycle arrest by the immunosuppressant rapamycin in yeast. Science 1991; 253:905–9.
2. Sabatini DM, Erdjument-Bromage H, Lui M, Tempst P, Snyder SH. RAFT 1: A mammalian protein that binds to FKBP 12 in a rapamycin-dependent fashion and ishomologous to yeast TORs. Cell 1994; 78:35–43.
3. Brown EJ, Albers MW, Shin TB, et al. A mammalian protein targeted by Gl-arresting rapamycin-receptor complex. Nature 1994; 369:756–8.
4. Chiu MI, Katz H, Berlin V. RAPTl, a mammalian homolog of yeast Tor, interacts with the FKBPl2/rapamycin complex. Proc Natl Acad Sci USA 1994; 91:12574–8.
5. Groves MR, Hanlon N, Turowski P, Hemmings BA, Barford D. The structure of the protein phosphatase 2A PR65/ A subunit reveals the conformation of its 15 tandemly repeated HEAT motifs. Cell 1999; 96:99–110.
6. Choi J, Chen J, Schreiber SL, Clardy J. Structure of the FKBPl2-rapamycin complex interacting with the binding domain of human FRAP. Science 1996; 273:239–42.
7. Hara K, Maruki Y, Long X, et al. Raptor, a binding partner of target of rapamycin (TOR), mediates TOR action. Cell 2002; 110:177–89.
8. Kim DH, Sarbassov DD, Ali SM, et al. mTOR interacts with raptor to form a nutrient-sensitive complex that signals to the cell growth machinery. Cell 2002; 110:163–75.
9. Jacinto E, Loewith R, Schmidt A, et al. Mammalian TOR complex 2 controls the actin cytoskeleton and is rapamycin insensitive. Nat Cell Biol 2004; 6:1122–8.
10. Gingras AC, Raught B, Sonenberg N. Regulation of translation initiation by FRAP/mTOR. Genes Dev 2001; 15:807–26.
11. Abraham RT. Identification of TOR signaling complexes: More TORC for the cell growth engine. Cell 2002; 111:9–12.
12. Wullschleger S, Loewith R, Hall MN. TOR signaling in growth and metabolism. Cell 2006; 124:471–84.
13. Inoki K, Li Y, Xu T, Guan KL. Rheb GTPase is a direct target of TSC2 GAP activity and regulates mTOR signaling. Genes Dev 2003; 17:1829–34.
14. Inoki K, Li Y, Zhu T, Wu J, Guan KL. TSC2 is phosphorylated and inhibited by Akt and suppresses mTOR signalling. Nat Cell Biol 2002; 4:648–57.
15. Manning BD, Tee AR, Logsdon MN, Blenis J, Cantley LC. Identification of the tuberous sclerosis complex-2 tumor suppressor gene product tuberin as a target of the phosphoinositide 3-kinase/akt pathway. Mol Cell 2002; 10:151–62.
16. Tee AR, Manning BD, Roux PP, Cantley LC, Blenis J. Tuberous sclerosis complex gene products, tuberin and hamartin, control mTOR signaling by acting as a GTPase activating protein complex toward. Rheb Curr Biol 2003; 13:1259–68.
17. Hyun T, Yam A, Pece S, et al. Loss of PTEN expression leading to high Akt activation in human multiple myelomas. Blood 2000; 96:3560–8.
18. Corradetti MN, Inoki K, Bardeesy N, DePinho RA, Guan KL. Regulation of the TSC pathway by LKB 1: Evidence of a molecular link between tuberous sclerosis complex and Peutz-Jeghers syndrome. Genes Dev 2004; 18:1533–8.

19. Nobukuni T, Joaquin M, Roccio M, et al. Amino acids mediate mTOR/raptor signaling through activation of class 3 phosphatidylinositol 30H-kinase. Proc Natl Acad Sci USA 2005; 102:14238–43.

20. Hsu J, Shi Y, Krajewski S, et al. The AKT kinase is activated in multiple myeloma tumor cells. Blood 2001; 98:2853–5.

21. Qiang YW, Kopantzev E, Rudikoff S. Insulinlike growth factor-I signaling in multiple myeloma: Downstream elements, functional correlates, and pathway cross-talk. Blood 2002; 99:4138–46.

22. Hsu JH, Shi Y, Frost P, et al. Interleukin-6 activates phosphoinositol-3 kinase in multiple myeloma tumor cells by signaling through RAS-dependent and, separately, through p85-dependent pathways. Oncogene 2004; 23:3368–75.

23. Shi Y, Hsu JH, Hu L, Gera J, Lichtenstein A. Signal pathways involved in activation of p70S6K and phosphorylation of 4E-BP1 following exposure of multiple myeloma tumor cells to interleukin-6. J Biol Chem 2002; 277:15712–20.

24. Liu P, Leong T, Quam L, et al. Activating mutations of N- and K-ras in multiple myeloma show different clinical associations: Analysis of the Eastern Cooperative Oncology Group Phase III Trial. Blood 1996; 88:2699–706.

25. Neri A, Murphy JP, Cro L, et al. Ras oncogene mutation in multiple myeloma. J Exp Med 1989; 170:1715–25.

26. Yoganathan N, Yee A, Zhang Z, et al. Integrin-linked kinase, a promIsmg cancer therapeutic target: Biochemical and biological properties. Pharmacol Ther 2002; 93:23342.

27. Shi Y, Gera J, Hu L, et al. Enhanced sensitivity of multiple myeloma cells containing PTEN mutations to CCI-779. Cancer Res 2002; 62:5027–34.

28. Chang H, Qi XY, Claudio J, Zhuang L, Patterson B, Stewart AK. Analysis of PTEN deletions and mutations in multiple myeloma. Leuk Res 2006; 30:262–5.

29. Bahlis NJ, Miao Y, Koc ON, Lee K, Boise LH, Gerson SL. N-Benzoylstaurosporine (PKC412) inhibits Akt kinase inducing apoptosis in multiple myeloma cells. Leuk Lymphoma 2005; 46:899–908.

30. Dufner A, Andjelkovic M, Burgering BM, Hemmings BA, Thomas G. Protein kinase B localization and activation differentially affect S6 kinase 1 activity and eukaryotic translation initiation factor 4E-binding protein 1 phosphorylation. Mol Cell Biol 1999; 19:4525–34.

31. Brown EJ, Schreiber SL. A signaling pathway to translational control. Cell 1996; 86:51720.

32. Jefferies HB, Fumagalli S, Dennis PB, Reinhard C, Pearson RB, Thomas G. Rapamycin suppresses 5TOP mRNA translation through inhibition of p70s6k. Embo J 1997; 16:3693–704.

33. Sachs AB. Cell cycle-dependent translation initiation: IRES elements prevail. Cell 2000; 101:243–5.

34. Vagner S, Galy B, Pyronnet S. Irresistible IRES. Attracting the translation machinery to internal ribosome entry sites. EMBO Rep 2001; 2:893–8.

35. Pestova TV, Kolupaeva VG, Lomakin IB, et al. Molecular mechanisms of translation initiation in eukaryotes. Proc Natl Acad Sci USA 2001; 98:7029–36.

36. Tu Y, Gardner A, Lichtenstein A. The phosphatidylinositol 3-kinase/AKT kinase pathway in multiple myeloma plasma cells: Roles in cytokine-dependent survival and proliferative responses. Cancer Res 2000; 60:6763–70.

37. Hsu L, Shi Y, Hsu JH, Gera J, Van Ness B, Lichtenstein A. Downstream effectors of oncogenic ras in multiple myeloma cells. Blood 2003; 101:3126–35.

38. Yang YP, Liang ZQ, Gu ZL, Qin ZH. Molecular mechanism and regulation of autophagy. Acta Pharmacol Sin 2005; 26:1421–34.

39. van Sluijters DA, Dubbelhuis PF, Blommaart EF, Meijer AJ. Amino-acid-dependent signal transduction. Biochem J 2000; 351(Pt 3):545–50.

40. Codogno P, Meijer AJ. Autophagy and signaling: Their role in cell survival and cell death. Cell Death Differ 2005; 12(Supp. 12):1509–18.

41. Kamada Y, Funakoshi T, Shintani T, Nagano K, Ohsumi M, Ohsumi Y. Tor-mediated induction of autophagy via an Apgl protein kinase complex. J Cell Biol 2000; 150:150713.

42. Harada H, Andersen JS, Mann M, Terada N, Korsmeyer SJ. p70S6 kinase signals cell survival as well as growth, inactivating the pro-apoptotic molecule BAD. Proc Natl Acad Sci USA 2001; 98:9666–70.

43. Yokogami K, Wakisaka S, Avruch J, Reeves SA. Serine phosphorylation and maximal activation of ST A T3 during CNTF signaling is mediated by the rapamycin target mTOR. Curr Biol 2000; 10:47–50.

44. Kuo ML, Chuang SE, Lin MT, Yang SY. The involvement of PI 3-KJAkt-dependent upregulation of Mc1-1 in the prevention of apoptosis of Hep3B cells by interleukin-6. Oncogene 2001; 20:677–85.

45. Shi Y, Yan H, Frost P, Gera J, Lichtenstein A. Mammalian target of rapamycin inhibitors activate the AKT kinase in multiple myeloma cells by up-regulating the insulin-like growth factor receptor/insulin receptor substrate-l/phosphatidylinositol 3-kinase cascade. Mol Cancer Ther 2005; 4:1533–40.

46. Raje N, Kumar S, Hideshima T, et al. Combination of the mTOR inhibitor rapamycin and CC-5013 has synergistic activity in multiple myeloma. Blood 2004; 104:4188–93.

47. Zangari M, Cavallo F, Tricot G. Farnesyltransferase inhibitors and rapamycin in the treatment of multiple myeloma. Curr Pharm Biotechnol 2006; 7:449–53.

48. Frost P, Moatomed F, Hoang B, et al. In vivo anti-tumor effects of the mTOR inhibitor, CCI-779, against human multiple myeloma cells in a xenograft model. Blood 2004; 104:4181–4187.

49. Stromberg T, Dimberg A, Hammarberg A, et al. Rapamycin sensitizes multiple myeloma cells to apoptosis induced by dexamethasone. Blood 2004; 103:3138–47.

50. Yan H, Frost P, Shi Y, et al. Mechanism by which mammalian target of rapamycin inhibitors sensitize multiple myeloma Cells to dexamethasone-induced apoptosis. Cancer Res 2006; 66:2305–2313.

51. Frost P, Shi Y, Hoang B, Lichtenstein A. AKT activity regulates the ability of mTOR inhibitors to prevent angiogenesis and VEGF expression in multiple myeloma cells. Oncogene 2007; 26:2255–2262.

52. Ikezoe T, Nishioka C, Tasaka T, et al. The antitumor effects of sunitinib (formerly SU 11248) against a variety of human hematologic malignancies: Enhancement of growth inhibition via inhibition of mammalian target of rapamycin signaling. Mol Cancer Ther 2006; 5:2522–30.

53. Francis LK, Alsayed Y, Leleu X, et al. Combination mammalian target of rapamycin inhibitor rapamycin and HSP90 inhibitor 17-allylamino-17-demethoxygeldanamycin has synergistic activity in multiple myeloma. Clin Cancer Res 2006; 12:6826–35.

54. O'Reilly KE, Rojo F, She QB, et al. mTOR inhibition induces upstream receptor tyrosine kinase signaling and activates Akt. Cancer Res 2006; 66:1500–8.

55. Witzig TE, Geyer SM, Ghobrial I, et al. Phase II trial of single-agent temsirolimus (CCI779) for relapsed mantle cell lymphoma. J Clin Oncol 2005; 23:5347–56.

56. Bertoni F, Zucca E, Cotter FE. Molecular basis of mantle cell lymphoma. Br J Haematol 2004; 124:130–40.

57. Haritunians T, Mori A, O'Kelly J, Luong QT, Giles FJ, Koeffler HP. Antiproliferative activity of RAD001 (everolimus) as a single agent and combined with other agents in mantle cell lymphoma. Leukemia 2007; 21:333–9.

58. Farag S, Zhang S, Miller M, et al. Phase II trial of temsirolimus (CCI-779) in patients with relapsed or refractory multiple Myeloma: Preliminary results. Proc Amer Soc Clin Oncol 2006; 24(18s):450.

Chapter 22

CDK Inhibitors in Multiple Myeloma

Yun Dai and Steven Grant

Functions of Cyclin-Dependent Kinases

Regulation of the Cell Cycle

Cell cycle progression represents the mechanism by which normal and neoplastic cells proliferate and grow. Typically, the cell cycle is composed of four distinct but tightly-related phases, that is, the periods associated with DNA synthesis (S phase) and mitosis (M phase), which are separated by two gaps (G1 and G2 phases). Following mitogenic stimulation, cells traverse the cell cycle through G1→S→G2→M phases, and subsequently divide equally to produce two daughter cells. The daughter cells can then enter the G1 phase once again to begin the next cycle, or, alternatively, exit from the cell cycle into the G0 phase (a quiescent state). A transition point (known as the restriction point) exists in the G1 phase, determining whether cell cycle progression occurs in a manner independent of external stimuli. Cell cycle procession is tightly controlled by cyclin-dependent kinase (CDK) complex. CDK holoenzyme complexes consist of a catalytic subunit (CDK) and a regulatory subunit (cyclin) which exist in a 1:1 ratio. CDKs are serine/threonine kinases, which become active only in association with a regulatory partner (i.e., members of the cyclin family). The binding of cyclins induces a conformational change in the CDK structure producing a basal, active state.[1] Cyclin–CDK holoenzyme complexes can be fully activated by phosphorylation of CDKs at specific conserved threonine residues (e.g., Thr161 in cdc2/CDK1, Thr160 in CDK2, Thr172 in CDK4, and Thr177 in CDK6) catalyzed by the CDK-activator kinase (CAK), and dephosphorylated at specific conserved tyrosine and threonine residues (Thr14 and Tyr15 in CDK1 and CDK2, which are phosphorylated by mixed-lineage kinases Wee1 and/or Myt1), events catalyzed by the dual specificity phosphatases Cdc25 (A, B, C).[2,3] The activity of CDKs is negatively regulated by direct interactions with proteins referred to as endogenous CDK inhibitors. The latter proteins are divided into two families: the INK4 (inhibitor of CDK4) family including p16ink4a, p15ink4b, p18ink4c, and p19ink4d, which specifically inhibits cyclin D-associated kinases (CDK4, 6), and the Cip/Kip (kinase inhibitor protein) family including p21cip1/waf1, p27Kip1, and p57kip2, which inhibits most CDKs.[4] Expression of cyclins fluctuates periodically throughout the cell cycle, which

From: *Contemporary Hematology Myeloma Therapy*
Edited by: S. Lonial © Humana Press, Totowa, NJ

specifies the start of each phase and the transition from one phase to next. Most cyclins (e.g., cyclins B, A, and E) are regulated by a ubiquitin/proteasome-dependent degradation pathway, while cyclin D is primarily regulated by transcriptional and translational mechanisms.

More than 13 CDKs and 25 cyclin-box-containing proteins have been identified from human genome sequencing.[1] Among these, CDK1, 2, 4, and 6 and cyclins A (A1 and A2), B (B1 and B2), D (D1, D2, and D3), and E (E1 and E2) are directly involved in the cell cycle machinery. Generally, cyclin D-CDK4 and -CDK6 phosphorylate/inactivate the retinoblastoma protein (pRb, a major member of the "pocket protein" family), and thereby releases transcriptional factors E2Fs (activated) from the inactivated pRb–E2F complex. E2F binds to its heterodimeric partner DP-1 and induces expression of genes responsible for S phase entry and progression, including cyclin E. In addition, cyclin E-CDK2 also facilitates G1→S transition by further phosphorylating pRb, complete activation of which requires phosphorylation by both cyclin D-CDK4/6 (hypophosphorylation) and cyclin E-CDK2 (hyperphosphorylation).[5] Cyclin D-CDK4, but not cyclin E-CDK2, also phosphorylates p130 and p107 (additional members of the "pocket protein" family), which may interact with certain E2Fs (e.g., E2F1 and 4) and mimic the function of pRb in RB null tumor cells.[6] In the S phase, cyclin A-CDK2 phosphorylates various substrates, which allows DNA replication and also inactivates G1 transcription factors (i.e., E2Fs). Cyclin A- and cyclin B-CDK1/cdc2 govern G2→M transition. The cyclin B–CDK1 complex is also implicated in transition of cells into anaphase and completion of mitosis. Cyclin E-CDK2 maintains cyclin B-CDK1 activity during mitosis, and reduction of CDK2 activity is required to inactivate cyclin B-CDK1, leading to mitotic exit.[7] Cyclin B-CDK1 has recently been implicated in machinery of mitotic checkpoint (also termed as spindle assembly checkpoint). In addition, it has been reported that some CDK complexes, for example, cyclin A-CDK2 in the S phase and cyclin B1-CDK1 in the G2/M phase, are dynamically associated with DNA replication competent complex, which may be directly involved in the regulation of DNA replication.[8]

Cyclin H-CDK7 (also known as CAK) is involved in cell cycle regulation through activation of CDKs 1, 2, 4, and 6 via phosphorylation at specific threonine residues, which is required for full activation of these cell cycle CDKs.

CDK3, which is an active kinase in association with cyclin E or A in vitro, participates in G1→S progression at least in part by binding to E2Fs (e.g., E2F1-3) through DP-1 and enhancing their transcriptional activities.[9] Interestingly, a distinct CDK complex cyclin C-CDK3 may be responsible for G0→G1 transition by phosphorylating pRb, resulting in G0 exit and cell cycle reentry. CDK5 is able to bind to cyclin D. However, it remains uncertain whether its activity is regulated by cyclins, and little evidence is available showing that CDK5 is involved in cell cycle regulation.[10]

CDKs and Regulation of Transcription

The transcription of eukaryotic protein-encoding genes is controlled by RNA polymerase II (RNAPII) in the elongation phase. In turn, the interplay between negative and positive elongation factors (referred to as N-TEF and P-TEF, respectively) determines the elongation potential of RNAPII. P-TEFb is the first and only known component of P-TEF. Human P-TEFb is composed of a 43 kDa catalytic subunit, CDK9 (previously known as PITALRE), and an

87 kDa regulatory subunit, cyclin T (including T1, T2a, or T2b isoforms). Approximately 70% of CDK9 forms complexes with T1, and 10% and 20% with T2a and T2b. The cyclin T–CDK9 complex (P-TEFb) phosphorylates and activates the carboxy-terminal domain (CTD) of RNAPII preferentially at Ser2 and most likely at Ser5 as well,[11,12] leading to promotion of transcriptional elongation. These events are sensitive to 5,6-dichloro-1-β-D-ribofuranosyl-benzimidaloe (DRB), a well-known inhibitor of transcriptional elongation.[12] Another partner of CDK9 is cyclin K, and the cyclin K–CDK9 complex also phosphorylates the CTD of RNAPII and functionally substitutes for cyclin T–CDK9 (P-TEFb), at least in in vitro transcription reactions.[13] In contrast to most cyclin/CDK holoenzymes, CDK9 is regulated by the ubiquitination-proteasome machinery whereas cyclin T is relatively stable.[14] A small nuclear RNA (snRNA), referred to as 7SK, was recently identified as a specific P-TEFb-associated factor.[15] Dissociation of 7SK from P-TEFb enhances CDK9 activity.[16] In addition, it is noteworthy that CDK9 may act as a multifunctional kinase rather than solely as a CTD kinase (or transcriptional CDK) in multiple signal pathways involving cell differentiation, apoptosis, and cell cycle regulation.[17] For example, it has been reported that the cyclin T–CDK9 complex is able to phosphorylate pRb.[17]

Cyclin T-CDK9 (P-TEFb) is not the sole kinase that phosphorylates the CTD of RNAPII. As a component of the general transcription factor TFIIH (consisting of a complex of cyclin H–CDK7/Mat1), CDK7 phosphorylates the CTD of RNAPII preferentially at Ser5, facilitating promoter clearance and transcriptional initiation.[18] During the transcription cycle, Ser5 of CTD is initially phosphorylated by TFIIH, an event most likely required for further phosphorylation of the CTD at Ser2 by P-TEFb.[12] Consequently, CDK7 activity appears critical for control of transcriptional elongation. Indeed, in *Caenorhabditis elegans*, partial loss of CDK7 activity leads to a general decrease in CTD phosphorylation and embryonic transcription, while severe loss of CDK7 activity blocks all cell divisions.[18] However, as the Cyclin T–CDK9 complex also phosphorylates the CTD at Ser5, it may thus bypass the requirement of CDK7 at least in some circumstances such as transcription of Tat (a small protein encoded by HIV).[12] Nevertheless, cyclin H-CDK7 plays an important role in regulation of both cell cycle, acting as a CAT (see above), and transcription, acting as a CTD kinase. Interestingly, phosphorylation of cyclin H by protein kinase CK2 is critical for full kinase activity of the CDK7–cyclin H–Mat1 complex.[19] In this case, the activity of cyclin-CDK holoenzymes may be regulated through phosphorylation of CDKs as well as their partner cyclins.

Cyclin C-CDK8 and Cyclin L-CDK11 have been identified as components of the RNAPII holoenzyme complex. Cyclin C-CDK8 may function as another kinase for CTD phosphorylation, while it has also been reported that Cyclin C-CDK8 may phosphorylate cyclin H and thereby repress CTD kinase activity of TFIIH.[20,21] Cyclin L-CDK11 is functionally coupled to regulation of pre-mRNA splicing events.[22] Moreover, CDK10, a cdc2-related kinase, has been observed to associate with the transcriptional factor Ets2 and modulate its transactivation activity.[23]

Abnormalities in Human Cancers

Loss of cell cycle control is a classic characteristic of cancer and provides a growth advantage to neoplastic cells. Abnormalities in expression and/or activity of a variety of proteins that directly or indirectly involve the cell cycle machinery play essential roles in the pathogenesis of tumors, most frequently including loss/inactivation of endogenous CDK inhibitors, overexpression of CDK partner cyclins, and amplification/active mutations of CDK genes.

Aberrations in cell cycle regulatory molecules in human cancers occur most frequently in molecules associated with control of G1→S transition, a key step which determines initiation of the cell cycle. In fact, dysregulation of cyclin D/CDK4, 6/INK4/pRb/E2F signaling pathway has been identified in more than 80% of human cancers.[24] Among those, the most common alternation is p16INK4a inactivation by deletions of gene loci, loss-of-function point mutation, or epigenetic silencing (e.g., by hypermethylation at promoter region).[25–27] This leads to hyperactivation of cyclin D-CDK4/6 and uncontrolled proliferation. Overexpression of cyclin D (primarily cyclin D1) is also common in a variety of human cancers (e.g., breast cancer, mantle cell lymphoma, and multiple myeloma). Aberrant overexpression of cyclin D1 usually stems from gene rearrangement (e.g., of the chromosomes t[11p15;q13] and t[11;14][q13;q32]), gene amplification, or alternative splicing (which generates a cyclin D1b transcript with constitutively nuclear localization and enhanced transforming capacity).[28–32] Interestingly, cyclin D1 overexpression is often accompanied by loss of p16INK4a, suggesting their possible cooperation in oncogenesis.[24] Overexpression of cyclin D1 results in activation of CDK4/6 due to an inappropriate increase in the amount of cyclin D-CDK4/6 holoenzyme, and also leads to activation of cyclin E-CDK2 by sequestering Cip/Kip family CDK inhibitors (e.g., p21CIP1 and p27KIP1) in the cyclin D-dependent kinase complex.[24] Gene amplification and overexpression of cyclin D2 and D3 are also found in some cancers including B-cell malignancies.[33,34] Moreover, accumulating evidence also indicates that cyclin D may exert CDK-independent functions (e.g., by acting as a modulator of various transcriptional factors) in control of cell growth.[35,36] Amplification and point mutations (e.g., CDK4R24C with loss of INK4-binding ability) of the CDK4 gene have also been observed in human cancers.[37] The central mechanism by which dysregulation of the cyclin D/CDK4,6/INK4 pathway contributes to growth advantage of tumor cells involves "unscheduled" inactivation or inhibition of pocket proteins (e.g., pRb, and most likely p107 and p130 as well), resulting in the loss of their function as tumor suppressors. In fact, loss of pRb or hyperactivation of CDK4/6 is found in most human tumor cells.[24,38] In this regard, CDK4 and/or CDK6 seem to be critical in uncontrolled cell cycle progression, and thus represent a very attractive target for cancer therapeutics. Indeed, coexpression of CDK4 with oncogenic Ras in normal human epidermal cells induces invasive neoplasia resembling human squamous cell carcinoma.[39] Moreover, it has been found recently that kinase activity of the cyclin D1–CDK4 complex is largely dispensable for normal development, while it is critically required for the initiation and maintenance of mammary carcinoma.[40,41] These findings strongly support the notion that cell cycle-regulatory CDKs (cyclin D-dependent kinases in particular) definitely represent a very attractive therapeutic target.[42,43]

However, it should be noted that recent findings have challenged this linear model, that is, cyclin D↑ and/or p16INK4a↓→CDK4/6↑→pRb↓. For example, it has been found that the functions of the cyclin D–CDK4/6 complex can be recapitulated by either cyclin D-CDK2 or cyclin E-CDK2, both of which are able to phosphorylate pRb and induce cell proliferation.[44] In contrast, loss of CDK2 can also be recapitulated by CDK4, which can phosphorylate pRb even at CDK2-preferred sites, and cyclin E-CDK1 as well.[45] In this context, overexpression or constitutive activation of CDK2 has been observed in some types of human cancers.[46–48] In addition, overexpression of cyclin A or cyclin E, overexpression/activated mutation of CDK1 or CDK7, and loss of Cip1/Kip family CDK inhibitors (e.g., p27Kip1, and most likely p21Cip1 as well) have also been reported in many types of human malignancies.[24] Furthermore, loss of endogenous CDK inhibitors (e.g., p27Kip1, p16INK4a, and possibly p21Cip1) is associated with poor outcome in patients with various cancers.[49]

Anticancer Mechanisms of Clinically Relevant CDK Inhibitors

Cyclin-dependent kinases and related molecules represent very promising targets in the development of cancer therapeutics. Among a variety of CDK inhibitors under development and evaluation, several (e.g., flavopiridol, CYC202, UCN-01, and BMS-387032) are currently undergoing clinical evaluation based upon preclinical evidence of antitumor activity.[24,50–52] Flavopiridol, as a pan-CDK inhibitor, exerts multiple actions in tumor cells, including inhibition of both cell cycle and transcriptional CDKs (both CDK9 and CDK7), induction of apoptosis, and antiangiogenesis. UCN-01 was initially developed as a PKC inhibitor, and later found to act as a CDK inhibitor. However, its antitumor effects appear to be more closely related to inhibition of Chk1 (checkpoint kinase 1), leading to "unscheduled" activation of cdc2/CDK1 and abrogation of G2/M- and S-checkpoints, as well as inhibition of the prosurvival PDK1/Akt pathway. CYC-202 and BMS-387032 have been developed as CDK2 inhibitors, but like most relatively specific inhibitors of CDK2, also inhibit CDK1. In addition, CYC-202 has been also found to inhibit cyclin T-CDK9 and cyclin H-CDK7, thereby blocking phosphorylation of RNAPII CTD, which is associated with transcriptional repression of proteins with short half-lives. It is noteworthy that genetic evidence suggests that inhibition of a single CDK (e.g., CDK2) may be insufficient to induce cell death or even prevent cell growth,[53] and that inhibition of transcriptional and cell cycle regulatory CDKs may cooperate to induce lethality in tumor cells.[54] Such findings suggest that highly specific CDK inhibitors may be suboptimal as anticancer agents, and that factors other than or in addition to CDK inhibition very likely contribute to the lethal actions of these compounds.[55]

Flavopiridol (Alvocidib™)

Flavopiridol is a semisynthetic small molecular derivative of rohitukine, an alkaloid isolated from *Dysoxylum binectariferum* (a plant indigenous to India). In preclinical studies, flavopiridol potently inhibited cell proliferation ($IC_{50} = 66nM$) in all 60 NCI human tumor cell lines, with no obvious tumor-type selectivity.[56] As the first clinically relevant CDK inhibitor, initial trials used a schedule of 24- or 72-h continuous infusion every 2 weeks. These schedules achieved concentrations capable of producing preclinical effects. For example, a 72-h infusion regimen produced 271–415 nM steady- state plasma concentration (Css).[57] However, prolonged infusion of flavopiridol proved largely inactive in trials involving several hematopoietic malignancies.

Consequently, a bolus administration (1-h infusions for 1–5 days every 21 days) was designed to achieve higher plasma concentrations. Indeed, the 1-h infusion regimen resulted in 1.7–3.8 µM median Cmax levels, reflecting postinfusion peak concentrations,[57] and a limited number of response in certain settings. Notably, clinically achievable concentrations by either continuous or bolus infusion exceeded the threshold for inhibition of CDKs and cell growth, and induction of apoptosis in preclinical studies. However, in striking contrast to its impressive activity in vitro and in various xenograft models,[58] outcomes of most clinical trials were disappointing.[59–62] The failure of flavopiridol to recapitulate its in vitro activity may stem from >90% plasma protein binding and inadequate plasma concentrations of free drug. In contrast, a variety of clinical trials have demonstrated that combinations of flavopiridol and either conventional chemotherpeutic agents (e.g., paclitaxel, fludarabine, cytosine arabinoside/ara-C, and irinotecan/CPT-11) or novel signal transduction modulators may be more promising.[63]

Very recently, a pharmacologically directed infusion schedule has been developed in which half of the flavopiridol dose is administered over 30 min and the other half over 4 h. This schedule was associated with very promising activity in patients with refractory CLL.[64] In fact, the major dose-limiting toxicity was tumor lysis syndrome. Trials are currently underway to evaluate this schedule in patients with other hematologic malignancies.

Cell Cycle Arrest

Flavopiridol induces cell cycle arrest by targeting cell cycle-regulatory CDKs. In in vitro studies using purified CDKs, flavopiridol has been shown to inhibit cyclin B-CDK1 (IC50 = 30–40 nM), cyclin A- and cyclin E-CDK2 (IC50 = 100 nM), cyclin D-CDK4 (IC50 = 20–40 nM), cyclin D-CDK6 (IC50 = 60 nM), and cyclin H-CDK7 (IC50 = 110–300 nM).[65,66] X-ray crystallographic analysis reveals that L868276 (a deschlorophenyl derivative of flavopiridol with approximately a tenfold reduction in inhibitory activity toward CDKs) binds to the ATP-binding pocket of CDK2.[56,66] In the structure of flavopiridol, the chloro group on the phenyl ring is able to make additional contacts with CDK2, which may explain the tenfold greater potency of flavopiridol compared to L868276. The overall molecular structure of CDKs is quite similar, and they share 40% sequence homology, including the highly conserved catalytic core region of 300 residues. Flavopiridol directly inhibits the activity of most CDKs by occupying the ATP-binding site of these kinases, an effect that can be competitively blocked by excess ATP. Indeed, CDK1, 2, 4, and 7 in the soluble extracts from nonsmall cell lung carcinoma have been shown to bind to immobilized flavopiridol in the absence of ATP but not in its presence.[65] Furthermore, by inhibiting CAK (i.e., cyclin H-CDK7), flavopiridol also prevents phosphorylation at threonine 160 and 161 of most CDKs (e.g., CDK1, 2, 4, and 6),[56] while these phosphorylations are necessary for full activation of the CDKs.

Inhibition of CDKs by flavopiridol leads to cell cycle arrest at the G1/S phase transition and G2/M phase transitions, as well as delay in S-phase progression.[65,67] For example, flavopiridol can block G1 progression by inhibiting cyclinD-CDK4/6, retard S-phase progression, or arrest cells in the G1 phase by inhibiting cyclin E- and cyclin A-CDK2, and arrest cells in the G2 phase by inhibiting cyclin A- and cyclin B-CDK1. Moreover, flavopiridol induces cell cycle arrest also through transcriptional inhibition and downregulation of cyclin D1, although this action requires slightly higher drug concentrations (100–300 nM) than those necessary for inhibition of cell cycle-regulatory CDKs.[50] It is noteworthy that CDK6 inhibition by flavopiridol seems to play a functional role in cell cycle arrest (e.g., G1 arrest) only in tumor cells lacking CDK4.[65] Nevertheless, the patterns of cell cycle arrest (e.g., G1/S arrest, G2/M arrest, or both) induced by flavopiridol (and other pan-CDK inhibitors) appears largely cell-type dependent.

As a first-generation CDK inhibitor, flavopiridol acts as a pan-CDK inhibitor. However, its inhibitory capacity is relatively selective for most CDKs but not for a specific CDK. Subsequently, efforts have been directed at identifying either structure-based synthetic/semisynthetic compounds or natural products that act on specific CDKs, such as CDK4, CDK1, or CDK2. As a consequence, more specifically selective CDK inhibitors have been developed, for example, inhibitors of CDK4/6 (e.g., PD-0332991 and CINK4)[66,68] and inhibitors of CDK2 and CDK1 which are significantly less potent against CDK4/6 (e.g., CYC202/R-Roscovitine, BMS-387032, PNU-252808, AZ703, NU6102, and NU6140).[50,69] A number of these compounds are currently under evaluation as antitumor agents in preclinical models and for some, in early stage clinical trials. However, it is difficult to design and develop inhibitors specifically targeting only a single CDK, most likely due to conservation of amino acids lining the ATP-binding pocket and the high structural homology shared by CDKs. Three-dimensional structural analysis of CDKs, particularly the CDK-inhibitor complex, has provided useful information for the development of novel CDK inhibitors. In particular, the crystal structures of CDK2 have been well established and used extensively for the synthesis of CDK2-specific inhibitors, as well as for evaluating CDK inhibitor potency and selectivity. For example, a new purine-based inhibitor has been described which is 1,000-fold more potent than the parent compound (Ki = 6 nM for CDK2 and 9 nM for CDK1).[70] Similar strategies have been utilized to develop CDK4-specific inhibitors, by using structure-based information related to a CDK4-mimic CDK2 protein.[71,72] Moreover, new approaches (e.g., affinity chromatography of immobilized inhibitors) have been established to identify the intracellular targets (selectivity) of individual CDK inhibitors.[2] Clearly, selectivity is a key issue for the use of CDK inhibitors as pharmacological tools to demonstrate the function of CDKs. However, a key question remaining to be answered is whether inhibition of a specific CDK by an highly selective inhibitor, rather than inhibition of broad CDKs by a pan inhibitor such as flavopiridol, will be efficient in killing tumor cells in view of evidence that (a) tumor cells usually exhibit multiple genetic alterations and/or dysregulation of multiple signaling pathways related to cell cycle regulation; (b) there exists functional overlap and/or cross-talk between different CDKs as well as CDKs and other proteins (e.g., their partner cyclins). Thus, it remains possible that the broad actions of a compound like flavopiridol are beneficial for its antitumor activity.

Inhibition of Transcription

Flavopiridol very potently represses transcription (IC50 < 10 nM) in vitro by blocking transition into productive elongation mediated by RNAPII, which is controlled by P-TEFb (cyclin T-CDK9).[73] Flavopiridol inhibits CTD kinase activity of RNAPII with Ki of 3 nM, a concentration significantly lower than that required for inhibition of most other CDKs (e.g., CDK1, 2, and 4 with Ki values between 40 and 70 nM). Furthermore, unlike inhibition of other

CDKs, inhibition of CDK9 by flavopiridol is noncompetitive with respect to ATP.[74] A P-TEFb-immobilized assay demonstrates that flavopiridol (1:1 stoichiometry) remains bound even in the presence of high salt concentrations, suggesting that the apparent lack of competition with ATP could result from very tight binding between the drug and the enzyme. Indeed, recent structural information related to the binary CDK9–flavopiridol complex indicates that flavopiridol binds very tightly to the ATP-binding pocket of CDK9 with higher affinity than CDK2, even though in contrast to the case of CDK2, no additional binding site has been identified for CDK9.[75] In cells, flavopiridol inhibits transcription at concentrations far lower than those required to inhibit CDK1 and CDK2, even in the presence of physiological concentration of ATP.[50] Another potential target for transcriptional repression by flavopiridol is CDK7 (catalytic subunit of TFIIH). However, CDK7 inhibition requires higher concentrations of flavopiridol than those necessary for inhibition of CDK9.[50] Therefore, inhibition of transcription by flavopiridol primarily stems from direct inhibition of CDK9.

In mammalian cells, DNA microarrays have shown that flavopiridol inhibits gene expression broadly, similar to the actions of general transcription inhibitors (e.g., actinomycin D and DRB).[76] However, at the protein level, flavopiridol primarily downregulates the expression of short-lived proteins, such as cylcin D1 and Mcl-1, among others.

Downregulation of Cyclin D1: Cyclin D1 is a multifunctional protein that plays a critical role not only in regulation of the cell cycle (e.g., the G1/S transition) as a partner of CDK4/6 (see above), but also acts as transcriptional regulator by modulating the activity of several transcriptional factors (e.g., STAT3) which are CDK independent, and may explain why cyclin D1 is involved not only in cell cycle progression but also in cell growth and survival.[35,36] Recently, it has been shown that cyclin D1 binds to transcriptional factors STAT3 and NeuroD and inhibits their transcriptional activity, which may be related to modulation of cell differentiation.[77] It has been reported that cyclin D1 also interacts with histone deacetylases, and in so doing blocks access of transcriptional factors to the promoter and inhibits loading of the initiation complex.[78] Cyclin D1, as an oncogene, also plays an important role in carcinogenesis, probably by driving cells into the S phase and cooperating with various oncogenes (such as Myc and Ras) in malignant transformation.[79] Rearrangement of the cyclin D1 locus and/or overexpression of cyclin D1 have been reported in many human tumors.[80]

Expression of cyclin D1 is growth factor dependent, and is regulated at the levels of transcriptional activation, protein degradation, or nuclear export. Mitogen-induction of cyclin D1 generally relies on activation of the Ras/Raf/MEK/ERK pathway. Ras signaling and ERK activation promotes transcription of the cyclin D1 gene, probably through transcriptional factors.[81] In addition, the Ras signaling pathway is also necessary for associations between cyclin D1 and CDK4.[39] A variety of transcriptional factors such as AP-1, STATs (STAT3 and 5), NF-κB, Egr-1, Ets and CREB, β-catenin, and certain nuclear receptors activate the cyclin D promoter.[82] On the other hand, expression of cyclin D1 is subject to transcriptional inhibition by other factors, such as E2F-1, JunB, INI1/hSNF5, peroxisome proliferator-activated receptor (nuclear receptor), and calveolin-1.[83] In the control of cell growth rate, the TOR (target of rapamycin)/eIF4E signaling pathway may act as upstream of cyclin

D.[84] Levels of both free and CDK-bound cyclin D1 are also regulated by proteasome-dependent degradation, causing rapid turnover (an approximate half-life of 20 min) of this protein.[85] Ras signaling cascade can prevent ubiquitin/proteasome-dependent degradation of cyclin D1.[86] Following its association with CDK4, cyclin D1 is phosphorylated on Thr 286 by glycogen synthetase kinase 3β (GSK-3β), a kinase controlled by PKB/Akt through inhibitory phosphorylation.[87] This event may represent a mechanism by which cyclin D1 is exported from the nucleus to the cytoplasm, resulting in its proteasomal degradation, thereby shutting down this signaling cascade. The pharmacological inactivation of the PI-3 kinase/Akt pathway and transfection with a constitutively active form of Akt extends the half-life of cyclin D1 by two- to threefold.[88]

Flavopiridol transcriptionally downregulates expression of cyclin D1 in multiple types of cancer cells. For example, exposure of MCF-7 breast cancer cells to flavopiridol results in a decline in cyclin D1 promoter activity, leading to a decrease in mRNA and protein of cyclin D1.[89] This effect is followed by a decline in the levels of cyclin D3 but not cyclin D2 and cyclin E, as well as loss of CDK4/6 activity. In vivo, flavopiridol results in depletion of cyclin D1 in the HN12 tumor xenograft, whereas levels of cyclin D3 and cyclin E remained constant.[90] Cyclin D1 transcriptional repression may stem from inhibition of P-TEFb by flavopiridol. However, this hypothesis is not supported by observations that inhibition of cyclin D1 expression requires much higher concentrations of flavopiridol (100–1,000 nM) than that required for inhibition of P-TEFb activity. Other mechanisms may involve interruption of transcriptional regulation of cyclin D1 by a number of transcriptional factors, including positive (e.g., STAT3 and NF-κB) and negative regulators (e.g., E2F1). In addition, flavopiridol can directly bind to duplex DNA with the range of equilibrium dissociation constant values similar to that of the DNA intercalators doxorubicin and pyrazoloacridine[91] which may affect the function of DNA as a transcriptional template.

Thus, administration of flavopiridol leads to cell cycle arrest through mechanisms related to inhibition of CDK activities, that is, by direct binding to the ATP-binding sites, by preventing phosphorylation of CDKs through inhibition of CAK (cyclin H-CDK7), or by transcriptional downregulation of cyclin D1. Transcriptional repression of cyclin D1 by flavopiridol may be particularly relevant in mantle cell lymphoma, in which cyclin D1 is overexpressed in 95% of patients. Notably flavopiridol has been reported to delay disease progression in a substantial fraction of patients with mantle cell lymphoma.[92]

Repression of Mcl-1 Expression: Recently, interest has focused on the antiapoptotic protein Mcl-1 as a transcriptional target of flavopiridol. For example, in vitro treatment with flavopiridol induces declines in expression of Mcl-1 mRNA and/or protein levels, which precedes apoptosis, in a variety of cancer cells including nonsmall cell lung cancer cells, multiple myeloma cells, and freshly isolated CD5+/CD19+ cells from patients with B-cell chronic lymphocytic leukemia (B-CLL), and CD138+ cells from patients with multiple myeloma.[93,94] Downregulation of Mcl-1 has also been confirmed in vivo in primary leukemic cells from flavopiridol-treated AML patients.[63] H1299 (nonsmall cell cancer) and NIH3T3 (transformed fibroblasts) cells constitutively expressing Mcl-1 are resistant to apoptosis induced by flavopiridol.[95]

Flavopiridol induces Mcl-1 downregulation most likely by inhibition of P-TEFb.[50,96] However, expression of the Mcl-1 gene is controlled by multiple signaling pathways. For example, it is negatively regulated by E2F-1 through direct binding to the Mcl-1 promoter, and positively regulated by the PI3 kinase/Akt pathway, by the MAPK pathway, as well as by transcriptional factors like STAT3 and CREB.[97] Consequently, flavopiridol-mediated downregulation of Mcl-1 may be also related to other mechanisms, including accumulation of E2F-1 and disruption of STAT3/DNA binding.[98–100]

Induction of Apoptosis

In multicellular organisms, cells engage an intrinsic mechanism of self-destruction designated programmed cell death or apoptosis, which is essential for maintaining tissue homeostasis. Tumor cells often have defects in the apoptosis-inducing pathway, resulting in the dysregulated expansion of a population of neoplastic cells, escape of cancer cells from surveillance by the immune system, and resistance to apoptosis induced by chemo- and radiotherapy. Initiation of apoptosis involves at least two distinct pathways: the extrinsic pathway that is mediated by death receptors and the intrinsic pathway which is dependent on mitochondria.[101] In the former, apoptotic signaling is initiated by binding of members of the TNF family to death receptors (such as CD95, TRAIL-R1, and -R2). When the death receptors are activated by TNF family ligands, their death domains attract the intracellular adaptor protein FADD (Fas-associated death domain), which, in turn, recruits the inactive form of certain initiator caspases (e.g., caspase-8 and -10) to the death-inducing signaling complex (DISC). At the DISC, procaspase-8 and -10 are cleaved and converted into active forms.[102] In type I cells, the DISC-activated caspase-8 is sufficient to trigger apoptosis directly, but in type II cells, mitochondria-dependent pathway is required for amplification of initial apoptotic signals, which is linked by truncation/activation of Bid (a proapoptotic member of Bcl-2 family) by active caspase-8.[103] In the intrinsic pathway, death signals (e.g., DNA damage) lead to mitochondrial damage, probably mediated by caspase-2 activation.[104] Mitochondria release cytochrome c and other proapoptotic factors (such as AIF and smac/DIABLO) from intermembraneous space to cytosol, where cytochrome c forms a complex (known as the apoptosome) with APAF1 (apoptotic protease activating factor-1), inactive form of initiator caspase (e.g., caspase-9), and ATP.[105] In the apoptosome, procaspase-9 is cleaved and activated. For both pathways, once the initiator caspases (caspase-8 and -10 in the extrinsic pathway, and caspase-9 in the intrinsic pathway) are activated, they further cleave and activate executioner caspases (e.g., caspase-3, -6, and -7). Activation of executioner caspases can further cleave/activate other caspases (including ones lying upstream) to amplify the death-signal cascade.[106] Eventually, the activated executioner caspases cleave a number of cellular "death substrates," leading to biochemical and morphological changes of apoptosis. Apoptotic pathways are tightly controlled by various proteins. For example, processing/activation of caspase-8 is inhibited by a protein referred to as FLIP (FLICE/caspase-8 inhibitory protein) through binding to DISC.[107] Importantly, Bcl-2 family members, including antiapoptotic (e.g., Bcl-2, Bcl-xL, Bcl-w, A1, and Mcl-1) and proapoptotic proteins (e.g., multidomain family: Bax, Bak, and Bok; BH3-only family: Bid, Bim, Bik, Bad, Bmf, Hrk, Noxa, and Puma), play critical roles in regulation of both the intrinsic and extrinsic pathways, primarily at the mitochondrial level.[108] Moreover, IAP (inhibitor of apoptosis proteins; e.g., XIAP, cIAP1, cIAP2, NAIP, MLAIP, ILP2, livin/KIAP, apollon, and survivin) family members are antiapoptotic proteins that regulate apoptotic signaling mostly at downstream of mitochondria. Most members of IAPs directly bind to and inhibit the active form of both initiator (e.g., caspase-9) and executioner caspases (e.g., caspase-3, -6, and -7) by promoting their degradation through the ubiquitination/proteasome pathway.[109] In turn, IAPs are inhibited by mitochondria-releasing smac/DIABLO (second mitochondria-derived activator of caspase/direct IAP-binding protein with low pI).[110]

It has been well documented that flavopiridol induces apoptosis in broad spectrum of malignant cells. For example, in vitro, 6–48 h exposure to 100–400 nM of flavopiridol induces apoptosis in a variety of tumor cells, including leukemia, lymphoma, head and neck squamous cell carcinoma (HNSCC), breast cancer, nonsmall cell lung cancer, prostate carcinoma, gastric carcinoma, esophageal carcinoma, bladder carcinoma, etc.[67] Human leukemia cells, regardless of their origins (i.e., cultured cell lines or freshly isolated primary cells from patients) or subtypes (myeloid, B-cell, or T-cell type), are the most sensitive to induction of apoptosis by flavopiridol.[111] Notably, flavopiridol can also induce apoptosis in tumor cells that are resistant to DNA-damaging agents and radiation.[65,67] In vivo, treatment with flavopiridol (i.p. 5 mg/kg daily for 5 days) induced apoptosis in the HNSCC xenograft HN12 as detected by terminal deoxynucleotidyl transferase-mediated dUTP-biotin nick end labeling (TUNEL), with significant reduction (60–70%) in tumor size.[90]

Mechanisms by which flavopiridol induces apoptosis have been extensively studied. First, flavopiridol is able to induce apoptosis in tumor cells in which caspase-8 is absent.[112] Moreover, neither pharmacological caspase-8 inhibitor IETD-FMK nor transfection of viral caspase-8 inhibitor CrmA is able to block flavopiridol-induced cytochrome c release and apoptosis.[113] These findings suggest that the extrinsic pathway is not primarily involved in flavopiridol-induced apoptosis, despite the fact that cleavage of caspase-8 and Bid have been observed after exposure to flavopiridol.[112]

Flavopiridol induces apoptosis in resting tumor cells which exhibit similar sensitivities as proliferating cells, even in the same cell lines,[50,65] arguing against the possibility that the cytotoxicity of flavopiridol stems from inhibition of CDKs involved in cell cycle regulation. However, direct binding of flavopiridol to duplex DNA may provide an explanation for the ability of flavopiridol to kill noncycling (resting) cancer cells.[91] Moreover, no significant difference in the cytotoxic activity of flavopiridol has been found between cells expressing pRb versus those defective in pRb expression, even though flavopiridol treatment induces hypophosphorylation of pRb.[114] Moreover, certain cell lines that lack detectable pRb expression exhibit more pronounced apoptosis following flavopiridol treatment.[115] Treatment of H1299 nonsmall cell lung cancer cells with flavopiridol (200 nM) results in the rapid elevation of E2F-1 followed by apoptosis, whereas either H1299 cells with deletion of E2F-1 through RNAi or murine embryo fibroblasts deficient in E2F-1 are less susceptible but not completely resistant to the cytotoxicity of flavopiridol.[95] It is known that E2F-1 mediates cell death through both p14ARF-MDM2-p53-dependent and -independent pathways. In most cases, flavopiridol has little or no effect on p53 levels, and its cytotoxic activity appears to be independent of the genetic status of p53.[116] There is no direct evidence for the notion that transcriptional downregulation of cyclin D1 contributes to the cytotoxicity of flavopiridol although repression of cyclin D1 expression by an antisense oligonucleotide approach triggers apoptosis in carcinoma cells.[115] In contrast, overexpression of cyclin D1 sensitizes human pRb-null myeloma cells (e.g., U266) to flavopiridol.[115]

Attention has recently focused on transcriptional downregulation of proteins involved in the regulation of apoptosis, which most likely represents a central theme underlying the induction of apoptosis by flavopiridol. In this context, Mcl-1 represents an important target (see above). In addition, flavopiridol also downregulates many other antiapoptotic proteins. For example, administration of flavopiridol results in decreased expression of Bcl-2 in several cell lines, such as B-cell leukemia, ovarian carcinoma, prostate carcinoma, and multiple myeloma cells.[94] However, flavopiridol-induced apoptosis appears largely independent of Bcl-2 inasmuch as flavopiridol kills tumor cells displaying Bcl-2 overexpression, an event that confers resistance to conventional chemotherapeutic agents.[112] Moreover, neither ectopic overexpression nor antisense oligonucleotide-mediated downregulation of Bcl-2 affects flavopiridol-induced cell killing.[112] However, human leukemia cells displaying ectopic expression of N-terminal phosphorylation loop-deleted Bcl-2 (amino acids 32–80, a region known to negatively regulate its function) are highly resistant to flavopiridol-mediated cleavage of Bid, cytochrome c release, activation of caspases, degradation of PARP, and apoptosis,[117] indicating that posttranslational modification(s) (e.g., phosphorylation) of Bcl-2 rather than transcriptional regulation may be involved in flavopiridol-induced apoptosis. Exposure to flavopiridol also results in downregulation of Bcl-xL and XIAP in various types of cancer cells, events likely associated with inhibition of NF-κB.[118,119]. In addition, downregulation of other antiapoptotic molecules (e.g., BAG-1, a regulator of Hsp70 family that confers resistance to apoptosis induced by a variety of stimuli) has also been reported in B-CLL cells exposed to flavopiridol.[111]

Other Antitumor Mechanisms

In several systems, it has been reported that flavopiridol has a significant antiangiogenic activity, which indicates that inhibition of tumor angiogenesis could play a considerable role in the antitumor effects of flavopiridol.[120] The antiangiogenic activity of flavopiridol may be related to the ability of flavopiridol to induce apoptosis in both resting and proliferating endothelial cells through an unknown mechanism which is independent of CDKs (e.g., CDK1 and 2) expression.[121] Indeed, endothelial cells are more sensitive to flavopiridol than other normal cells, such as fibroblasts, bone marrow cells, and peripheral lymphocytes, but less sensitive than most tumor cells. However, inhibition of vascular endothelial growth factor (VEGF) expression could play an important role in the antiangiogenic effects of flavopiridol. VEGF is an angiogenic factor which is critical for cancer progression and metastasis. In human peripheral blood mononuclear cells and human neuroblastoma cells, it has been shown that flavopiridol completely blocks hypoxia-induced VEGF mRNA transcription and downregulates VEGF protein levels by dramatically decreasing VEGF mRNA stability.[122]

It is also been reported that flavopiridol significantly inhibits rabbit muscle glycogen phosphorylases (GPa and b).[123] Using immobilized flavopiridol, glycogen phosphorylases have been identified as flavopiridol-binding proteins.[124]

Flavopiridol treatment of A549 nonsmall cell lung cancer cells results in an increase in glycogen accumulation.[124] Further studies showed that flavopiridol inhibits GP by direct binding to inhibitor site in these proteins.[123] These findings raise the possibility that interference with glucose homeostasis may also contribute to antitumor effects of flavopiridol.

UCN-01

UCN-01 (7-hydroxystaurosporine, NSC638850 or KW-2401; Kyowa Hakka Kogyo), a derivative of the nonspecific PKC inhibitor staurosporine (a natural product isolated from *Streptomyces staurosporeus*), was originally developed as a selective PKC inhibitor. It has also been reported to inhibit several CDKs. However, recent studies have shown that UCN-01 exerts other antitumor effects, including inhibition of Chk1 (checkpoint kinase 1), which results in "inappropriate" activation of CDKs and abrogation of DNA damage-induced cell cycle checkpoints, as well as interference with the PDK1 (3-phosphoinositide-dependent protein kinase-1)/Akt survival pathway, thus promoting induction of apoptosis. These effects are largely independent of PKC inhibition. UCN-01 displays antitumor activity in in vitro systems and in vivo xenograft models involving multiple human tumor types, with greater antitumor effects observed with longer administration intervals (e.g., 72 h in in vitro systems).[50,69] Initial clinical trials of UCN-01 involved a 72-h continuous infusion schedule every 2 weeks.[125] Unexpectedly, the plasma half-life (30 days) of UCN-01 in patients was observed to be 100-fold longer than that observed in preclinical models. It was subsequently shown that UCN-01 extensively binds to plasma α1-acidic glycoprotein in humans, which accounts for the unique clinical pharmacology of UCN-01.[50,125] Based on these findings, further clinical trials are being conducted using modified UCN-01 schedules (e.g., a 36-h continuous infusion every 4 weeks). Such schedules result in a mean UCN-01 half-life of ~588 h with peak plasma concentrations of total drug ranging from 30 to 40 μM, with 100 nM concentrations of free UCN-01 detected in saliva.[125] Significantly, such concentrations are in excess of those necessary to inhibit Chk1. Several responses have been observed in patients with melanoma and refractory anaplastic large-cell lymphoma. In addition, several phase I trials with shorter schedules (e.g., 3 h infusion) are currently ongoing as combination regimens involving DNA-damaging agents.[126–128]

PKC Inhibition

UCN-01 selectively inhibits Ca^{2+}-dependent PKC isozymes (e.g., PKCα, β, and γ; $IC_{50} = 4$–30 nM), and less potently inhibits Ca^{2+}-independent PKC isozymes ($IC_{50} = 500$ nM).[129] However, it exerts no effect on the atypical PKCs (e.g., PKCζ). In clinical trials, a clear decrease in phosphorylated cytoskeletal membrane protein adducin, a specific substrate phosphorylated by PKC, was observed in tumor and bone marrow samples following UCN-01 administration.[50] However, PKC inhibition appears to be unrelated to various actions of UCN-01, including antiproliferative activity, interference with cell cycle progression, and induction of apoptosis.

CDK Inhibition

UCN-01 can either inhibit or activate CDKs. Crystal structure analysis has shown that UCN-01 binds to active phospho-CDK2/cyclin A.[130] It has been noted that UCN-01 induces G1 cell cycle arrest at low concentrations

(IC_{50} = 100–300 nM).[131] However, this effect seems unrelated to direct inhibition of CDKs, as UCN-01 inhibits cdc2/CDK1 and CDK2 in vitro only at higher concentrations (IC_{50} = 300–600 nM).[50] In HNSCC cells, UCN-01 treatment results in G1 block, a phenomenon most likely secondary to depletion of cyclin D3 and induction of the endogenous CDK inhibitors p21[waf1] and p27[kip1].[132] Similar alterations have been observed in HNSCC xenografts.[132]

Chk Inhibition

In normal cells, DNA damage generally induces G1 arrest mediated by accumulation/activation of p53, a major component of the G1 checkpoint machinery.[133,134] In contrast, p53-defective tumor cells primarily arrest in the S or G2 phase in the checkpoint response to DNA damage. As most (e.g., >50%) human tumors lack p53 function, G2 and S checkpoints play key roles in tumor cell responses to DNA damage. UCN-01 has been found to abrogate the G2 checkpoint selectively in p53-defective cells with 100,000-fold greater (IC_{50} = 50 nM) potency compared to caffeine.[50] Chk1 has been defined as a major target in UCN-01-mediated G2 abrogation.[135–137] Crystal structure analysis demonstrated that UCN-01 binds the ATP-binding pocket in the Chk1 kinase domain, and the hydroxy group in the lactam moiety of UCN-01 interacts with the ATP-binding pocket, providing a basis for the greater selectivity of UCN-01 toward Chk1 compared to staurosporine and its analogue SB218078.[138]

Pharmacological concentrations of UCN-01 inhibit the activity of both Chk1 and Chk2 immunoprecipitated from human tumor cells, which may account for the observation that UCN-01 abrogates IR-induced p53-independent G2 arrest whereas Chk1 activity remains unchanged.[139] UCN-01 was also shown to block Cdc25C phosphorylation mediated by another kinase, C-TAK1, which inhibits Cdc25C constitutively in the absence of DNA damage.[140,141] Therefore, regardless of which kinase is responsible for the phosphorylation/inactivation of Cdc25C, inhibition of this event by UCN-01 results in "inappropriate activation" of cdc2/CDK1 that drives tumor cells through mitosis prior to repair of DNA damage, resulting in apoptosis.[142,143] Plasma samples isolated from patients who received UCN-01 were found to induce a 40–70% abrogation in an ex vivo G2 checkpoint assay.[144]

UCN-01 has also been reported to abrogate the S phase checkpoint,[145] but the mechanism(s) responsible for this event appear to be complex. In p53 mutant tumor cells, low concentrations of UCN-01 causes S phase cells to progress to G2 before undergoing mitosis and cell death, whereas high concentrations (~500 nM) lead to rapid premature mitosis and death of S-phase cells. The latter event may stem from rapid Cdc25C activation by C-TAK1 (Cdc25C associated protein kinase 1) inhibition.[141] IR-induced S checkpoint response can be divided into fast (<2 h) and slow (>1–6 h) processes. The ATM-dependent pathway controls only the fast response, whereas the slow response is controlled by an ATM-independent pathway involving Chk1.[50] These results are consistent with observations that UCN-01 abolishes the UV light-induced S checkpoint response through inhibition of ATR-dependent Chk1 activation.[146]

These findings have created a theoretical basis for developing a therapeutic strategy in which UCN-01 may sensitize tumor cells (particularly p53-defective cells) to DNA-damaging agents and radiation by abrogating the G2 and/or S checkpoints. It is noteworthy that the checkpoint abrogation effects of

UCN-01 are manifested at lower drug concentrations (e.g., IC50 ~50 nM for G2 checkpoint abrogation) than those responsible for cytotoxicity or inhibition of cell proliferation.

PDK1/Akt Inhibition

The phosphophatidyliositide-3-OH kinase (PI3K)/Akt cascade represents a critical signaling pathway in cell survival mediated by many growth factors and cytokines. Phosphorylation at Thr308 of Akt is catalyzed by PDK1 and phosphorylation at Ser473 by PDK2. UCN-01 directly inhibits upstream Akt kinase PDK1 with an IC50 < 33 nM in vitro and in vivo assays, whereas enforced expression of PDK1 restores Akt kinase activity.[147] Crystal structure analysis demonstrated that UCN-01 binds to the kinase domain of PDK1 more specifically than staurosporine.[148] Overexpression of active Akt diminishes the cytotoxic effects of UCN-01, indicating that inhibition of the PDK1-Akt pathway attributes to the antitumor activity of this agent.[147]

Induction of Apoptosis

UCN-01 induces apoptosis with IC50 values of 100–1,000 nM in a panel of HNSCC cell lines in vitro and in HN12 xenograft in vivo, and exhibits enhanced cytotoxicity in cells displaying mutant p53.[132] Although the mechanism underlying UCN-01-induced apoptosis is still unknown, several potential targets have been postulated. First, inhibition of PDK1/Akt has been directly related to the cytotoxicity of UCN-01.[147] Second, as CDK1 is identified as a proapoptotic mediator,[149] Chk1/2–Cdc25C-mediated CDK1 activation, particularly under "inappropriate" circumstances, may contribute to induction of apoptosis by UCN-01 (see above). Finally, UCN-01-induced apoptosis has been associated with downregulation of antiapoptotic proteins, such as Mcl-1, XIAP, BAG-1, and Bcl-2.[111]

CYC202

CYC202 (R-roscovitine, seliciclib; Cycacel) is a substituted purine analogue derived from 6-DMAP and isopentenyladenine. In vitro kinase assays using purified recombinant kinases have revealed that CYC202 inhibits CDK2 (CDK2/cyclin E: IC50 = 100 nM; CDK7/cyclinH: IC50 = 490 nM; CDK2/cyclin A: IC50 = 710 nM), and less potently CDK1 (CDK1/cyclin B: IC50 = 2.69 μM), but neither CDK4 (CDK4/cyclin D1: IC50 = 14.21 μM) nor other kinases (e.g., PKA and PKC).[52,150] Like most of CDK inhibitors, CYC202 inhibits CDKs by competing with ATP for its CDK-binding site.[151,152] In vitro evaluation of antitumor activity demonstrated the cytotoxicity of CYC202 (average IC50 = 15.2 μM) against a panel of 19 human tumor cell lines including those with cisplatin- and doxorubincin-resistant phenotypes, independent of p53 statues and cell cycle alterations.[150] In vivo administration of CYC202 resulted in significant antitumor effect and reduction in tumor growth rate in mice xenografts bearing human colorectal carcinoma and uterine cancer.[150,153] Based on these findings, CYC202, the first oral bioavailable CDK inhibitor, has entered phase I clinical trials in patients with advanced solid tumors.[154] These studies revealed that plasma concentrations (Cmax) of >2000 ng/ml at day 1 and day 7 were achievable at 800 mg/kg twice a day for 7 days, a dose in the range of IC50 values reported for seliciclib in vitro activity and without dose-limiting toxicity (DTL).[154]

The anticancer activity of CYC202 has been related to (a) inhibition of cell cycle-regulatory CDKs (e.g., CDK1, 2, and 7) and downregulation of cyclin D1, leading to a reduction in pRb phosphorylation at multiple sites and cell cycle arrest in G1, S, and G2-M phases[155–157]; (b) inhibition of transcriptional CDKs (e.g., CDK9 in particular, and CDK7), resulting in decrease/inactivation of RNAPII and transcriptional repression of short life-time proteins such as cyclin D1, cyclin A, cyclin B1, as well as Mcl-1 and XIAP[155,156,158]; (c) more importantly, induction of apoptosis in tumor cells while largely spare normal cells,[159] which is most likely related to downregulation of antiapoptotic proteins, particularly Mcl-1[160–162]; and (d) lower the threshold of cancer cells to cytotoxic agents or other novel agents.[161,163–165]

BMS-387032

A series of compounds derived from 2-acetamido-thiazolythio acetic ester have been discovered and optimized as small molecule inhibitors of cyclin E-CDK2. Among these, compound 21 (BMS-387032) has been identified as an oral bioavailable CDK2 inhibitor. This compound selectively inhibits CDK2 (IC_{50} = 48 nM, 10- and 20-fold selective over cyclin B-CDK1 and cyclin D-CDK4, respectively).[166] X-ray crystallographic analysis demonstrated that these compounds bind to the active ATP-binding site of the CDK2 protein. BMS-387032 display marked antiproliferative activity, with IC50 values of 95 nM in A2780 ovarian carcinoma cells.[166] Similar effects were also observed in a panel of tumor cell lines in vitro. BMS-387032 has demonstrated significant antitumor activity in vivo in both murine tumor model and human tumor xenograft models.[166] This systematic investigation led to a phase I clinical trial of BMS-387032.[167] Initial results from clinical trials showed some objective tumor responses and good tolerability.

These effects in all likelihood stem from rapid induction of apoptosis and cell cycle arrest.[50,167] BMS-387032 induces E2F1 but diminishes E2F4 levels, whereas E2F1-deficient fibroblasts are less sensitive to this agent.[168] Similar phenomenon has been observed in human breast cancer cells, in which treatment with BMS-387032 leads to stabilization of E2F1 protein.[169] Moreover, this event is accompanied by significant increase in the p57 mRNA and protein, while p57-deficient cells are more sensitive to BMS-387032-induced apoptosis, indicating that this event may serve to limit E2F1-mediated cell death. In human lung carcinoma cells, BMS-387032 has been found to block IL-1 β-induced expression as well as steady-state mRNA levels of COX-2, a protein providing a survival advantage to transformed cells through the inhibition of apoptosis, increased attachment to extracellular matrix, increased invasiveness, and stimulation of angiogenesis, indicating a novel target for BMS-387032.[170]

Dysregulation of CDK-Related Proteins in Myeloma

Although its role in the pathogenesis of multiple myeloma is still unknown, cell cycle dysregulation, particularly that related to cyclin D/CDK proteins, is one of the hallmarks of multiple myeloma,[171] and represents one of the factors that makes CDK inhibitors an attractive therapeutic option in this disease. Dysregulation of this axis generally takes two forms: alterations in the expression/activity of cyclins or, alternatively, endogenous CDK inhibitors.

Cyclin D and pRb

Chromosomal abnormalities are frequently found in myeloma (e.g., t[11;14] [q13;q32] and t[4:14][p16;q32]), and often involve cyclin D1 ([11q13]).[172] Bergsagel's group has employed gene profiling to classify multiple myeloma and has observed that myeloma cells exhibit dysregulation of at least one of the three cyclins (cyclin D1 [11q13], D2 [MAF/16q23 or MAFB/20q11], or D3 [6p21]), while normal bone marrow plasma cells express low levels of cyclin D2 and D3 but a little or no cyclin D1.[173] This group has characterized the mutational status of myeloma cells in relation to overexpression of each of the cyclin D family members, and demonstrated that dysregulation of cyclin D represents an early and unifying pathogenic event in multiple myeloma. This supervised analysis of gene expression profiles provides the basis for a molecular classification of multiple myeloma based on the presence of the recurrent *IGH* chromosomal translocations and cyclin D expression, named TC classification.[174] In this context, multiple myeloma patients were classified into five groups: TC1 (11q13 [16%] and 6q21 [3%] tumors), characterized by the t(11;14) or t(6;14) translocation, with the consequent expression of high levels of either cyclin D1 or D3, and a nonhyperdiploid status; TC2 (D1 tumors [34%]), expressing low to moderate levels of cyclin D1 in the absence of a t(11;14) translocation but associated with a hyperdiploid status; TC3 (D1 + D2 tumors [6%]), a mixture of tumors that do not fall into any of the other groups, most of which express cyclin D2; TC4 (4p16 tumors [16%]), expressing high levels of cyclin D2 and also MMSET (and in most cases FGFR3) stemmed from the presence of the t(4;14) translocation; and TC5 (maf tumor [7%]), expressing the highest levels of cyclin D2 and also high levels of either c-maf or mafB, both of which are transcriptional factors upregulating cyclin D2 expresssion. This molecular classification has been further supported by the data from a study using fluorescence in situ hybridization to detect both the *cyclin D* loci arrangements and the main *IGH* translocations as well as the chromosome 13q deletion.[175] It has been postulated that this classification system may predict therapeutic outcome in patients with myeloma exhibiting specific chromosomal/genetic characteristics.[172] For example, patients whose cells exhibit dysregulation of cyclin D1 may have a particularly poor prognosis.[176]

More recently, it has been found that elevated expression of cyclin D1 or D3 alone is not sufficient to promote cell cycle progression unless CDK4 is also elevated. In contrast, cyclin D2 and CDK6 are coordinately increased, even though cyclin D2 can also bind to CDK4 in myeloma cells. Therefore, cyclin D1–CDK4 and cyclin D2–CDK6 pairing may be a critical determinant for cell cycle reentry and progression in expansion of self-renewing myeloma cells.[177] Together, these findings take on particular significance in light of evidence that CDK inhibitors such as flavopiridol downregulate cyclin D in preclinical studies.[89] In this regard, Dai et al. reported that the increased sensitivity of myeloma cells overexpressing cyclin D1 to flavopiridol reflected activation of E2F and inappropriate S-phase entry rather than cyclin D1 downregulation.[115]

In addition, abnormalities, that is, partial or complete deletions in chromosome 13 (e.g., 13q14) which harbors the RB1 locus, have been reported in up to 30% of myeloma patients and up to 70% of myeloma cell lines.[171,172] In the remaining cases, pRb is predominantly phosphorylated.[178] Abnormalities in chromosome 13 have been associated with a particularly poor prognosis in patients with multiple myeloma.[179]

INK-Family of Endogenous CDK Inhibitors

In human cancers, the main genetic alterations are deletions (bi- or monoallelic) or 5′ CpG island methylation of p15[INK4B] and p16[INK4A], while very few cases or cell lines had p18[INK4C] or p19[INK4D] deletions or hypermethylation.[180]

p16[INK4A]

Deletion of p16[INK4A] has been found in human primary myeloma cells.[181] However, a more frequent occurrence in primary myeloma cells is inactivation of p16[INK4A] and p15[INK4B] genes by methylation.[182,183] 5-CpG island hypermethylation of the p16[INK4A] locus has been reported in over 50% of patients with multiple myeloma and related disorders. However, in contrast to the case of cyclin D1 and pRb abnormalities, patients with p16[INK4A] methylation do not appear to exhibit a worse prognosis.[172] In contrast, Galm et al. reported that myeloma patients exhibiting hypermethylation of p16[INK4A] did have a worse prognosis.[184]

Deletion of p18[INK4C]

p18[INK4C] is important in the terminal differentiation of B lymphocytes into plasma cells by induction of cell cycle arrest. Deletion of p18[INK4C] is frequently found in multiple myeloma cell lines, and has been shown to contribute to the growth advantage of such cells.[185] The prognostic significance of such mutations in patients with multiple myeloma is unknown. More recently, it has been reported that human myeloma cell lines (33%) do not express normal p18[INK4C], with biallelic deletion of p18[INK4C] and expression of a mutated p18[INK4C] fragment, while biallelic deletion of p18[INK4C] appears to be a late progression event.[186] Moreover, ectopic expression of exogenous p18[INK4C] results in marked growth inhibition in multiple myeloma cells that express little or no endogenous p18[INK4C], but has no effect in multiple myeloma cells that already express a high level of p18[INK4C].

Increased Expression of p15[INK4B]

High expression of p15[INK4B] in plasma cells has been associated with diminished proliferative rate and more favorable prognosis in patients with myeloma.[187] Hypermethylation or deletion of p15[INK4B] has also been reported in 67% of patients with multiple myeloma.[182,183] Moreover, concurrent hypermethylation of p15[INK4B] and p16[INK4A] has been noted in a significant number of myeloma patients.[188]

Summary: Collectively, as summarized in Fig. 1, these findings indicate that chromosomal abnormalities and accompanying dysregulation of the cyclin D-CDK4/6-pRb-INK4 axis occur frequently in multiple myeloma, and that these events, whether they contribute to the pathogenesis of the disease, may correlate with prognosis and response to therapy. These considerations also provide a theoretical rationale for employing CDK inhibitors in this setting.

CDK Inhibitors in Myeloma

Flavopiridol

In light of the ability of flavopiridol to downregulate cyclin D1,[89] this agent represented an attractive agent to investigate in multiple myeloma. Semenov et al. reported that pharmacologically achievable concentrations of flavopiridol

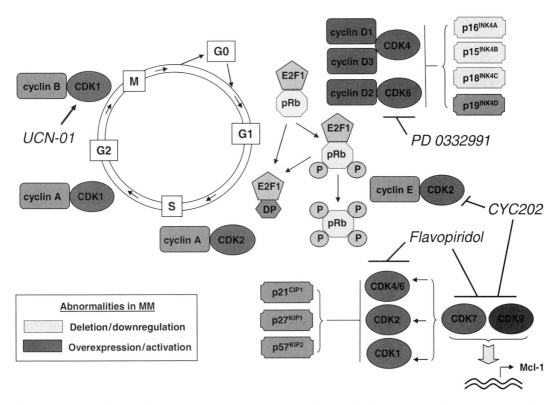

Fig. 1 Abnormalities in cell cycle regulatory proteins relevant to multiple myeloma, and potential targets for pharmacologic intervention by cyclin-dependent kinase inhibitors.

(i.e., in the 100 nM range) induced apoptosis in human multiple myeloma cell lines and primary CD38+ myeloma cells in association with CDK inhibition and downregulation of Mcl-1 and Bcl-2.[94] Interestingly, downregulation of cyclin D1 and cyclin A was not observed. Gojo et al. observed that flavopiridol-induced apoptosis in multiple myeloma cells in association with downregulation of Mcl-1 at the transcriptional level and inhibition of phosphorylation of the CTD of RNA PolII.[189] Significantly, ectopic expression of Mcl-1 protected cells from flavopiridol, indicating that Mcl-1 plays a functional role in the lethality of this compound. Using multiple myeloma cells ectopically expressing cyclin D1, Dai et al. demonstrated that upregulation of this cyclin increased flavopiridol lethality through multiple mechanisms, including interference with p21(CIP1) expression, dephosphorylation of pocket proteins, and inactivation of E2Fs culminating in S phase entry, as well as inactivation of NF-κB, leading to apoptosis rather than growth arrest.[115] Similar results were obtained with R-roscovitine. This and the previous studies suggest that the increased sensitivity of cells with cyclin D1 dysregulation to flavopiridol may result less from cyclin D1 downregulation than from further disruption of the cell cycle traverse.

In view of its pleiotropic actions, efforts to combine flavopiridol with other targeted agents in multiple myeloma have received attention. For example, synergistic interactions between flavopiridol and TRAIL (TNF-receptor apoptosis-inducing ligand) have been described by several groups. For example, Rosato et al. reported that synergism between flavopiridol and TRAIL in human leukemia cells stemmed from downregulation of XIAP.[190] Analogously, Fandy et al. found that potentiation of TRAIL lethality by flavopiridol in human multiple myeloma cells was related to downregulation of FLIP-L, but was independent of Bcl-2.[191]

Synergistic interactions between flavopiridol and small molecule Bcl-2 antagonists in multiple myeloma have also been described. Pei et al. reported that lethality of the small molecule Bcl-2/Bcl-xL inhibitor HA14-1 was markedly potentiated by flavopiridol in multiple myeloma cell lines. This effect was related to induction of oxidative injury (ROS production) and activation of the stress-related JNK pathway.[192]

Finally, synergistic interactions between flavopiridol and the proteasome inhibitor bortezomib have been described in human leukemia cells, events associated with JNK activation and inhibition of the NF-κB pathway.[193] These findings served as the basis for an ongoing trial of flavopiridol and bortezomib in patients with refractory multiple myeloma (see below).

CYC202

Several studies have shown that CYC202 (Seliciclib), the R-enantiomer of roscovitine, effectively induces apoptosis in human myeloma cells. Raje et al. reported that CYC202 rapidly induced apoptosis in multiple myeloma cells in association with diminished Mcl-1 transcription and expression. CYC202 also downregulated IL-6, and reduced Mcl-1 upregulation induced by stromal cells.[161]

McCallum et al. also reported that CYC202 induced apoptosis in myeloma cells in association with Mcl-1 transcriptional repression downregulation. This group also reported that CYC202 recapitulated the ability to inhibit phosphorylation of the CTD of RNA PolII.[194] In accord with these findings, downregulation of Mcl-1 via siRNA also induced apoptosis in these cells, consistent with the notion that Mcl-1 is a critical survival factor for myeloma cells.[160] Taken with the previous findings involving flavopiridol, these observations suggest that a major mechanism of CDK inhibitor lethality in myeloma reflects transcriptional repression of Mcl-1, rather than, or in addition to, inhibition of cell cycle traverse.

There is relatively little information available concerning interactions between CYC202 and other agents in myeloma. Raje et al. reported that CYC202 interacted synergistically with doxorubicin and bortezomib,[161] but the mechanism underlying these interactions remains to be determined.

UCN-01

Preclinical studies exploring the response of multiple myeloma cells to UCN-01 have focused on combinations with other targeted agents. As noted previously, exposure of human multiple myeloma cells to UCN-01, as in the case of human leukemia cells,[195] results in activation of MEK1/2/ERK1/2, and interference with the latter process, that is, by MEK1/2 inhibitors such as PD184352, results in a dramatic increase in apoptosis.[196] These events, which also occurred in various resistant myeloma cell lines, were associated with enhanced activation of cdc2, consistent with the ability of UCN-01 to inhibit Chk1. Lethality of the UCN-01/MEK1/2 inhibitor regimen primarily involved activation of the intrinsic, mitochondrial pathway, and was substantially blocked in cells overexpressing Bcl-2 or Bcl-xL. However, lethality of the regimen was restored in such cells by agents capable of activating the extrinsic apoptotic pathway, that is, TRAIL.[197]

Interestingly, this group also reported that inhibitors of the NF-κB pathway (e.g., Bay 11-7082) also dramatically increased UCN-01 lethality in multiple myeloma cells, but this effect was independent of interruption of the MEK1/2/ERK1/2 pathway. Instead, synergistic interactions between Bay 11-7082 and UCN-01 were associated with activation of JNK and downregulation of several NF-κB-dependent antiapoptotic proteins, for example, Bcl-xL, XIAP.[198] Taken in conjunction with the preceding findings, these studies suggest that the lethality of UCN-01 in multiple myeloma cells is regulated by both MEK1/2-dependent and MEK1/2-independent mechanisms.

Subsequent studies indicated that agents acting upstream of MEK1/2/ERK1/2 could also block ERK1/2 activation in multiple myeloma cells exposed to UCN-01. For example, Pei et al. reported that the farnesyl-transferase inhibitor L744832 dramatically increased UCN-01 lethality in myeloma cells in association of inactivation of both ERK1/2 and Akt, along with inactivation of Stat3, an important survival factor for myeloma cells.[199] Notably, enhanced lethality occurred in cells exposed to these agents in the presence of stromal cells or IL-6/IGF-1, as well as in primary CD138+ myeloma cells. Significantly, constitutively active Stat3 protected cells from this regimen, indicating that inhibition of Stat3 plays a functional role in the lethality of this regimen.

Similar results were reported in the case of the HMG CoA-reductase inhibitor lovastatin, as well as other statins, all of which markedly increased UCN-01 lethality in myeloma cells. These events were associated with inactivation of $ERK^{1/2}$, occurred in various resistant myeloma cell types, as well as in the presence of stromal or growth factors.[200] Notably, UCN-01 was shown in this study to activate Ras, and the effects of statins on UCN-01 lethality were attributed to interference with Ras farnesylation rather than geranylgeranylation.

In recent mechanistic studies, Pei et al. reported that activation of ERK1/2 by UCN-01 in multiple myeloma cells did not result from activation of cdc2, which did play an important role in lethality of the UCN-01/MEK1/2 inhibitor regimen. Collectively, these studies suggest that ERK1/2 activation represents an important compensatory response to disruption of Chk1, and that activation of the pathway originates at an upstream rather than downstream point in the cascade.[201]

Finally, very recent findings indicate that potentiation of UCN-01 lethality in myeloma cells by MEK1/2 inhibitors involves disruption of Bim-EL phosphorylation and degradation, and that upregulation of Bim-EL levels contribute functionally to the lethality of this regimen.[202]

PD 0332991

PD 0332991 is a novel, orally active CDK inhibitor that selectively targets CDK4 and CDK6, hyperactivation of which have been implicated in myeloma pathogenesis. In a NOD/SCID myeloma cell model, PD 0332991 inhibited tumor cell growth.[203] Although by itself it did not induce apoptosis in myeloma cells, when combined with another agent (e.g., dexamethasone), cell killing was substantially increased. Such findings raise the possibility that CDK inhibitors targeting CDK4/6 may have a role in myeloma therapy.

Clinical Studies

Clinical evaluation of CDK inhibitors in multiple myeloma remains relatively limited. In the one reported Phase II trial of flavopiridol in myeloma, flavopiridol was administered as a 3-h infusion daily × 3 days every 21 days. No responses were obtained, nor were consistent changes in the expression of various proteins (e.g., Mcl-1, Stat3, phospho-CTD, cyclin D1, or Bcl-2) observed.[204] The authors concluded that flavopiridol, administered by this schedule, did not have single-agent activity in myeloma.

In view of the possibility that existing schedules of flavopiridol, for example, 1- or 24-h infusions, may not yield adequate and sustained plasma flavopiridol concentrations to achieve activity, a novel pharmacodynamically driven schedule has been developed in which flavopiridol is given as a split course in which half the dose is given as a 30-min loading infusion and the other half as a 4-h infusion. This schedule has shown impressive activity in patients with refractory CLL.[64] Trials are currently underway to test the activity of this flavopiridol schedule in patients with refractory multiple myeloma and non-Hodgkin's lymphoma.

Finally, based on evidence of synergistic interactions between flavopiridol and the proteasome inhibitor bortezomib in malignant hematpoietic cells,[205] a Phase I trial has been initiated in patients with refractory multiple myeloma and indolent NHL in which escalating doses of flavopiridol and bortezomib are given as an intravenous infusion on days 1, 4, 8, and 11 every month. The regimen has proven to be well tolerated, and the MTD has not yet been reached. Notably, several patients who either did no longer responded to bortezomib have responded to the combination of bortezomib and flavopiridol.[206] Plans are underway to incorporate the 4-h flavopiridol infusion schedule into this regimen in the hope that an improvement in the activity of the regimen can be achieved.

Summary

As an anticancer strategy, targeting CDKs represents a highly attractive approach, particularly in the case of multiple myeloma, in which dysregulation of the cyclinD-CDK4/6-pRb-INK4 cascade may play an important role in disease pathogenesis and prognosis. As the first CDK inhibitor to enter clinical trials, flavopiridol has been the most extensively developed of this class of compounds. Its antitumor activity has been related to multiple mechanisms, including inhibition of CDKs, induction of apoptosis, blockade of transcription (e.g., cyclin D1, Mcl-1, and VEGF) presumably mediated through inhibition of P-TEFb (CDK9/cyclin T), and antiangiogenesis. Single-agent activity in myeloma has been disappointing to date, although the development of alternative schedules (i.e., 4-h infusion) resulting in superior pharmacokinetics may help to address this problem. UCN-01, another agent targeting CDKs and related proteins that is currently in clinical trials, exhibits its antitumor activity primarily through G2 and S checkpoint abrogation resulting from inhibition of Chk1. Interference with the PDK1/Akt survival pathway may also contribute to the cytotoxicity of UCN-01, and may be particularly relevant in the case of multiple myeloma. Significantly, the strategy of combining flavopiridol or UCN-01 with conventional chemotherapeutic drugs and importantly, other novel signal transduction modulators, for example, MEK1/2 or proteasome inhibitors, offer the potential for enhanced tumor-selective cytotoxicity and circumvention of drug resistance. In fact, the ultimate role of CDK inhibitors such as flavopiridol and UCN-01 may be as modulators of the activity of conventional and possibly more novel chemotherapeutic agents, both in multiple myeloma and in other hematologic malignancies. Finally, a variety of more novel small molecule CDK inhibitors have been developed. Among these, CYC202 and BMS-387032 have recently entered clinical trials, and others are in development. Based upon these considerations, it is likely that therapeutic strategies targeting CDKs will remain the focus of intense interest in the treatment of multiple myeloma for the foreseeable future.

Acknowledgments: This work was supported by Public Health Service grants CA-63753, CA-93738, CA-100866, and CA88906 from the National Cancer Institute, award 6045-03 from the Leukemia and Lymphoma Society of America, and a Translational Research award from the V-foundation.

References

1. Knockaert M, Greengard P, Meijer L. Pharmacological inhibitors of cyclin-dependent kinases. Trends Pharmacol Sci 2002; 23:417–425.
2. Lents NH, Keenan SM, Bellone C, Baldassare JJ. Stimulation of the Raf/MEK/ERK cascade is necessary and sufficient for activation and Thr-160 phosphorylation of a nuclear-targeted CDK2. J Biol Chem 2002; 277:47469–47475.
3. Morris MC, Gondeau C, Tainer JA, Divita G. Kinetic mechanism of activation of the Cdk2/cyclin A complex. Key role of the C-lobe of the Cdk. J Biol Chem 2002; 277:23847–23853.
4. Sandal T. Molecular aspects of the mammalian cell cycle and cancer. Oncologist 2002; 7:73–81.
5. Ezhevsky SA, Ho A, Becker-Hapak M, Davis PK, Dowdy SF. Differential regulation of retinoblastoma tumor suppressor protein by G(1) cyclin-dependent kinase complexes in vivo. Mol Cell Biol 2001; 21:4773–4784.
6. Calbo J, Parreno M, Sotillo E, et al. G1 cyclin/cyclin-dependent kinase-coordinated phosphorylation of endogenous pocket proteins differentially regulates their interactions with E2F4 and E2F1 and gene expression. J Biol Chem 2002; 277:50263–50274.
7. D'Angiolella V, Costanzo V, Gottesman ME, Avvedimento EV, Gautier J, Grieco D. Role for cyclin-dependent kinase 2 in mitosis exit. Curr Biol 2001; 11:1221–1226.
8. Frouin I, Montecucco A, Biamonti G, Hubscher U, Spadari S, Maga G. Cell cycle-dependent dynamic association of cyclin/Cdk complexes with human DNA replication proteins. EMBO J 2002; 21:2485–2495.
9. Yamochi T, Semba K, Tsuji K et al. ik31/Cables is a substrate for cyclin-dependent kinase 3 (cdk 3). Eur J Biochem 2001; 268:6076–6082.
10. Sharma P, Veeranna, Sharma M et al. Phosphorylation of MEK1 by cdk5/p35 down-regulates the mitogen-activated protein kinase pathway. J Biol Chem 2002; 277:528–534.
11. Shim EY, Walker AK, Shi Y, Blackwell TK. CDK-9/cyclin T (P-TEFb) is required in two postinitiation pathways for transcription in the C. elegans embryo. Genes Dev 2002; 16:2135–2146.
12. Price DH. P-TEFb, a cyclin-dependent kinase controlling elongation by RNA polymerase II. Mol Cell Biol 2000; 20:2629–2634.

13. Fu TJ, Peng J, Lee G, Price DH, Flores O. Cyclin K functions as a CDK9 regulatory subunit and participates in RNA polymerase II transcription. J Biol Chem 1999; 274:34527–34530.

14. Kiernan RE, Emiliani S, Nakayama K et al. Interaction between cyclin T1 and SCF(SKP2) targets CDK9 for ubiquitination and degradation by the proteasome. Mol Cell Biol 2001; 21:7956–7970.

15. Yang Z, Zhu Q, Luo K, Zhou Q. The 7SK small nuclear RNA inhibits the CDK9/cyclin T1 kinase to control transcription. Nature 2001; 414:317–322.

16. Nguyen VT, Kiss T, Michels AA, Bensaude O. 7SK small nuclear RNA binds to and inhibits the activity of CDK9/cyclin T complexes. Nature 2001; 414:322–325.

17. Simone C, Bagella L, Bellan C, Giordano A. Physical interaction between pRb and cdk9/cyclinT2 complex. Oncogene 2002; 21:4158–4165.

18. Wallenfang MR, Seydoux G. cdk-7 Is required for mRNA transcription and cell cycle progression in Caenorhabditis elegans embryos. Proc Natl Acad Sci U S A 2002; 99:5527–5532.

19. Schneider E, Kartarius S, Schuster N, Montenarh M. The cyclin H/cdk7/Mat1 kinase activity is regulated by CK2 phosphorylation of cyclin H. Oncogene 2002; 21:5031–5037.

20. Akoulitchev S, Chuikov S, Reinberg D. TFIIH is negatively regulated by cdk8-containing mediator complexes. Nature 2000; 407:102–106.

21. Barette C, Jariel-Encontre I, Piechaczyk M, Piette J. Human cyclin C protein is stabilized by its associated kinase cdk8, independently of its catalytic activity. Oncogene 2001; 20:551–562.

22. Hu D, Mayeda A, Trembley JH, Lahti JM, et al. Kidd VJ. CDK11 complexes promote pre-mRNA splicing. J Biol Chem 2003; 278:8623–8629.

23. Kasten M, Giordano A. Cdk10, a Cdc2-related kinase, associates with the Ets2 transcription factor and modulates its transactivation activity. Oncogene 2001; 20:1832–1838.

24. Shapiro GI. Cyclin-dependent kinase pathways as targets for cancer treatment. J Clin Oncol 2006; 24:1770–1783.

25. Kohno T, Yokota J. Molecular processes of chromosome 9p21 deletions causing inactivation of the p16 tumor suppressor gene in human cancer: Deduction from structural analysis of breakpoints for deletions. DNA Repair (Amst) 2006; 5:1273–1281.

26. Chakravarti A, DeSilvio M, Zhang M. Prognostic value of p16 in locally advanced prostate cancer: A study based on Radiation Therapy Oncology Group Protocol 9202. J Clin Oncol 2007; 25:3082–3089.

27. Auerkari EI. Methylation of tumor suppressor genes p16(INK4a), p27(Kip1) and E-cadherin in carcinogenesis. Oral Oncol 2006; 42:5–13.

28. Lu F, Gladden AB, Diehl JA. An alternatively spliced cyclin D1 isoform, cyclin D1b, is a nuclear oncogene. Cancer Res 2003; 63:7056–7061.

29. Carrere N, Belaud-Rotureau MA, Dubus P, Parrens M, de MA, Merlio JP. The relative levels of cyclin D1a and D1b alternative transcripts in mantle cell lymphoma may depend more on sample origin than on CCND1 polymorphism. Haematologica 2005; 90:854–856.

30. Burd CJ, Petre CE, Morey LM . Cyclin D1b variant influences prostate cancer growth through aberrant androgen receptor regulation. Proc Natl Acad Sci U S A 2006; 103:2190–2195.

31. Krieger S, Gauduchon J, Roussel M, Troussard X, Sola B. Relevance of cyclin D1b expression and CCND1 polymorphism in the pathogenesis of multiple myeloma and mantle cell lymphoma. BMC Cancer 2006; 6:238.

32. Knudsen KE, Diehl JA, Haiman CA, Knudsen ES. Cyclin D1: Polymorphism, aberrant splicing and cancer risk. Oncogene 2006; 25:1620–1628.

33. Delmer A, jchenbaum-Cymbalista F, et al. Tang R. Overexpression of cyclin D2 in chronic B-cell malignancies. Blood 1995; 85:2870–2876.

34. Sonoki T, Harder L, Horsman DE et al. Cyclin D3 is a target gene of t(6;14)(p21.1;q32.3) of mature B-cell malignancies. Blood 2001; 98:2837–2844.

35. Tashiro E, Tsuchiya A, Imoto M. Functions of cyclin D1 as an oncogene and regulation of cyclin D1 expression. Cancer Sci 2007; 98:629–635.

36. Fu M, Wang C, Li Z, Sakamaki T, Pestell RG. Minireview: Cyclin D1: Normal and abnormal functions. Endocrinology 2004; 145:5439–5447.

37. Wolfel T, Hauer M, Schneider J et al. A p16INK4a-insensitive CDK4 mutant targeted by cytolytic T lymphocytes in a human melanoma. Science 1995; 269:1281–1284.

38. van Deursen JM. Rb loss causes cancer by driving mitosis mad. Cancer Cell 2007; 11:1–3.

39. Lazarov M, Kubo Y, et al. Cai T . CDK4 coexpression with Ras generates malignant human epidermal tumorigenesis. Nat Med 2002; 8:1105–1114.

40. Landis MW, Pawlyk BS, Li T, Sicinski P, Hinds PW. Cyclin D1-dependent kinase activity in murine development and mammary tumorigenesis. Cancer Cell 2006; 9:13–22.

41. Yu Q, Sicinska E, Geng Y . Requirement for CDK4 kinase function in breast cancer. Cancer Cell 2006; 9:23–32.

42. Lee YM, Sicinski P. Targeting cyclins and cyclin-dependent kinases in cancer: Lessons from mice, hopes for therapeutic applications in human. Cell Cycle 2006; 5:2110–2114.

43. Deshpande A, Sicinski P, Hinds PW. Cyclins and cdks in development and cancer: A perspective. Oncogene 2005; 24:2909–2915.

44. Malumbres M, Sotillo R, Santamaria D . Mammalian cells cycle without the D-type cyclin-dependent kinases Cdk4 and Cdk6. Cell 2004; 118:493–504.

45. Ortega S, Prieto I, Odajima J et al. Cyclin-dependent kinase 2 is essential for meiosis but not for mitotic cell division in mice. Nat Genet 2003; 35:25–31.

46. Kohzato N, Dong Y, Sui L . Overexpression of cyclin E and cyclin-dependent kinase 2 is correlated with development of hepatocellular carcinomas. Hepatol Res 2001; 21:27–39.

47. Li KK, Ng IO, Fan ST, Albrecht JH, Yamashita K, Poon RY. Activation of cyclin-dependent kinases CDC2 and CDK2 in hepatocellular carcinoma. Liver 2002; 22:259–268.

48. Dong Y, Sui L, Tai Y, Sugimoto K, Tokuda M. The overexpression of cyclin-dependent kinase (CDK) 2 in laryngeal squamous cell carcinomas. Anticancer Res 2001; 21:103–108.

49. Senderowicz AM, Sausville EA. Preclinical and clinical development of cyclin-dependent kinase modulators. J Natl Cancer Inst 2000; 92:376–387.

50. Dai Y, Grant S. Small molecule inhibitors targeting cyclin-dependent kinases as anticancer agents. Curr Oncol Rep 2004; 6:123–130.

51. Schwartz GK, Shah MA. Targeting the cell cycle: A new approach to cancer therapy. J Clin Oncol 2005; 23:9408–9421.

52. Benson C, Kaye S, Workman P, Garrett M, Walton M, de BJ. Clinical anticancer drug development: Targeting the cyclin-dependent kinases. Br J Cancer 2005; 92:7–12.

53. Tetsu O, McCormick F. Proliferation of cancer cells despite CDK2 inhibition. Cancer Cell 2003; 3:233–245.

54. Cai D, Latham VM, Jr., Zhang X, Shapiro GI. Combined depletion of cell cycle and transcriptional cyclin-dependent kinase activities induces apoptosis in cancer cells. Cancer Res 2006; 66:9270–9280.

55. Sausville EA. Complexities in the development of cyclin-dependent kinase inhibitor drugs. Trends Mol Med 2002; 8:S32–S37.

56. Senderowicz AM. The cell cycle as a target for cancer therapy: Basic and clinical findings with the small molecule inhibitors flavopiridol and UCN-01. Oncologist 2002; 7, Suppl 3:12–19.

57. Colevas D, Blaylock B, Gravell A. Clinical trials referral resource. Flavopiridol Oncology (Williston Park) 2002; 16:1204–1202, 1214.

58. Zhai S, Senderowicz AM, Sausville EA, Figg WD. Flavopiridol, a novel cyclin-dependent kinase inhibitor, in clinical development. Ann Pharmacother 2002; 36:905–911.

59. Shapiro GI, Supko JG, Patterson A et al. A phase II trial of the cyclin-dependent kinase inhibitor flavopiridol in patients with previously untreated stage IV non-small cell lung cancer. Clin Cancer Res 2001; 7:1590–1599.

60. Schwartz GK, Ilson D, Saltz L . et al. Phase II study of the cyclin-dependent kinase inhibitor flavopiridol administered to patients with advanced gastric carcinoma. J Clin Oncol 2001; 19:1985–1992.

61. Lin TS, Howard OM, Neuberg DS, Kim HH, Shipp MA. Seventy-two hour continuous infusion flavopiridol in relapsed and refractory mantle cell lymphoma. Leuk Lymphoma 2002; 43:793–797.

62. Tan AR, Headlee D, Messmann R et al. Phase I clinical and pharmacokinetic study of flavopiridol administered as a daily 1-hour infusion in patients with advanced neoplasms. J Clin Oncol 2002; 20:4074–4082.

63. Karp JE, Passaniti A, Gojo I et al. Phase I and pharmacokinetic study of flavopiridol followed by 1-beta-D-arabinofuranosylcytosine and mitoxantrone in relapsed and refractory adult acute leukemias. Clin Cancer Res 2005; 11:8403–8412.

64. Byrd JC, Lin TS, Dalton JT et al. Flavopiridol administered using a pharmacologically derived schedule is associated with marked clinical efficacy in refractory, genetically high-risk chronic lymphocytic leukemia. Blood 2007; 109:399–404.

65. Sedlacek HH. Mechanisms of action of flavopiridol. Crit Rev Oncol Hematol 2001; 38:139–170.

66. Hardcastle IR, Golding BT, Griffin RJ. Designing inhibitors of cyclin-dependent kinases. Annu Rev Pharmacol Toxicol 2002; 42:325–348.

67. Shapiro GI. Preclinical and clinical development of the cyclin-dependent kinase inhibitor flavopiridol. Clin Cancer Res 2004; 10:4270s–4275s.

68. Fry DW, Bedford DC, Harvey PH et al. Cell cycle and biochemical effects of PD 0183812. A potent inhibitor of the cyclin D-dependent kinases CDK4 and CDK6. J Biol Chem 2001; 276:16617–16623.

69. Dai Y, Grant S. Cyclin-dependent kinase inhibitors. Curr Opin Pharmacol 2003; 3:362–370.

70. Davies TG, Bentley J, Arris CE et al. Structure-based design of a potent purine-based cyclin-dependent kinase inhibitor. Nat Struct Biol 2002; 9:745–749.

71. Ikuta M, Kamata K, Fukasawa K et al. Crystallographic approach to identification of cyclin-dependent kinase 4 (CDK4)-specific inhibitors by using CDK4 mimic CDK2 protein. J Biol Chem 2001; 276:27548–27554.

72. Honma T, Hayashi K, Aoyama T et al. Structure-based generation of a new class of potent Cdk4 inhibitors: New de novo design strategy and library design. J Med Chem 2001; 44:4615–4627.

73. Chao SH, Fujinaga K, Marion JE et al. Flavopiridol inhibits P-TEFb and blocks HIV-1 replication. J Biol Chem 2000; 275:28345–28348.

74. Chao SH, Price DH. Flavopiridol inactivates P-TEFb and blocks most RNA polymerase II transcription in vivo. J Biol Chem 2001; 276:31793–31799.

75. De AW, Jr., Canduri F, da Silveira NJ. Structural basis for inhibition of cyclin-dependent kinase 9 by flavopiridol. Biochem Biophys Res Commun 2002; 293:566–571.

76. Lu X, Burgan WE, Cerra MA et al. Transcriptional signature of flavopiridol-induced tumor cell death. Mol Cancer Ther 2004; 3:861–872.

77. Coqueret O. Linking cyclins to transcriptional control. Gene 2002; 299:35–55.

78. Fu M, Rao M, Bouras T et al. Cyclin D1 inhibits peroxisome proliferator-activated receptor gamma-mediated adipogenesis through histone deacetylase recruitment. J Biol Chem 2005; 280:16934–16941.

79. Rodriguez-Bravo V, Guaita-Esteruelas S, Florensa R, Bachs O, Agell N. Chk1-and Claspin-Dependent but ATR/ATM- and Rad17-Independent DNA Replication Checkpoint Response in HeLa Cells. Cancer Res 2006; 66:8672–8679.

80. Hosokawa Y, Arnold A. Mechanism of cyclin D1 (CCND1, PRAD1) overexpression in human cancer cells: Analysis of allele-specific expression. Genes Chromosomes Cancer 1998; 22:66–71.

81. Jirmanova L, Afanassieff M, Gobert-Gosse S, Markossian S, Savatier P. Differential contributions of ERK and PI3-kinase to the regulation of cyclin D1 expression and to the control of the G1/S transition in mouse embryonic stem cells. Oncogene 2002; 21:5515–5528.

82. Lavoie JN, Rivard N, L'Allemain G, Pouyssegur J. A temporal and biochemical link between growth factor-activated MAP kinases, cyclin D1 induction and cell cycle entry. Prog Cell Cycle Res 1996; 2:49–58.

83. Hulit J, Bash T, Fu M et al. The cyclin D1 gene is transcriptionally repressed by caveolin-1. J Biol Chem 2000; 275:21203–21209.

84. Shi Y, Sharma A, Wu H, Lichtenstein A, Gera J. Cyclin D1 and c-myc internal ribosome entry site (IRES)-dependent translation is regulated by AKT activity and enhanced by rapamycin through a p38. J Biol Chem 2005; 280:10964–10973.

85. Diehl JA, Zindy F, Sherr CJ. Inhibition of cyclin D1 phosphorylation on threonine-286 prevents its rapid degradation via the ubiquitin-proteasome pathway. Genes Dev 1997; 11:957–972.

86. Shao J, Sheng H, DuBois RN, Beauchamp RD. Oncogenic Ras-mediated cell growth arrest and apoptosis are associated with increased ubiquitin-dependent cyclin D1 degradation. J Biol Chem 2000; 275:22916–22924.

87. Takahashi-Yanaga F, Mori J, Matsuzaki E . Involvement of GSK-3beta and DYRK1B in differentiation-inducing factor-3-induced phosphorylation of cyclin D1 in HeLa cells. J Biol Chem 2006; 281:38489–38497.

88. Radu A, Neubauer V, Akagi T, Hanafusa H, Georgescu MM. PTEN induces cell cycle arrest by decreasing the level and nuclear localization of cyclin D1. Mol Cell Biol 2003; 23:6139–6149.

89. Carlson B, Lahusen T, Singh S et al. Down-regulation of cyclin D1 by transcriptional repression in MCF-7 human breast carcinoma cells induced by flavopiridol. Cancer Res 1999; 59:4634–4641.

90. Patel V, Senderowicz AM, Pinto D, Jr. et al. Flavopiridol, a novel cyclin-dependent kinase inhibitor, suppresses the growth of head and neck squamous cell carcinomas by inducing apoptosis. J Clin Invest 1998; 102:1674–1681.

91. Bible KC, Bible RH, Jr., Kottke TJ et al. Flavopiridol binds to duplex DNA. Cancer Res 2000; 60:2419–2428.

92. Kouroukis CT, Belch A, Crump M et al. Flavopiridol in untreated or relapsed mantle-cell lymphoma: Results of a phase II study of the National Cancer Institute of Canada Clinical Trials Group. J Clin Oncol 2003; 21:1740–1745.

93. Pepper C, Thomas A, Hoy T, Fegan C, Bentley P. Flavopiridol circumvents Bcl-2 family mediated inhibition of apoptosis and drug resistance in B-cell chronic lymphocytic leukaemia. Br J Haematol 2001; 114:70–77.

94. Semenov I, Akyuz C, Roginskaya V, Chauhan D, Corey SJ. Growth inhibition and apoptosis of myeloma cells by the CDK inhibitor flavopiridol. Leuk Res 2002; 26:271–280.

95. Ma Y, Cress WD, Haura EB. Flavopiridol-induced apoptosis is mediated through up-regulation of E2F1 and repression of Mcl-1. Mol Cancer Ther 2003; 2:73–81.

96. Blagosklonny MV. Flavopiridol, an inhibitor of transcription: Implications, problems and solutions. Cell Cycle 2004; 3:1537–1542.

97. Wang JM, Chao JR, Chen W, Kuo ML, Yen JJ, Yang-Yen HF. The antiapoptotic gene mcl-1 is up-regulated by the phosphatidylinositol 3-kinase/Akt signaling pathway through a transcription factor complex containing CREB. Mol Cell Biol 1999; 19:6195–6206.

98. Croxton R, Ma Y, Song L, Haura EB, Cress WD. Direct repression of the Mcl-1 promoter by E2F1. Oncogene 2002; 21:1359–1369.

99. Lee YK, Isham CR, Kaufman SH, Bible KC. Flavopiridol disrupts STAT3/DNA interactions, attenuates STAT3-directed transcription, and combines with the Jak kinase inhibitor AG490 to achieve cytotoxic synergy. Mol Cancer Ther 2006; 5:138–148.

100. Aggarwal BB, Sethi G, Ahn KS et al. Targeting signal-transducer-and-activator-of-transcription-3 for prevention and therapy of cancer: Modern target but ancient solution. Ann N Y Acad Sci 2006; 1091:151–169.

101. Strasser A, O'Connor L, Dixit VM. Apoptosis signaling. Annu Rev Biochem 2000; 69:217–245.

102. Fulda S, Debatin KM. Extrinsic versus intrinsic apoptosis pathways in anticancer chemotherapy. Oncogene 2006; 25:4798–4811.

103. Scaffidi C, Fulda S, Srinivasan A et al. Two CD95 (APO-1/Fas) signaling pathways. EMBO J 1998; 17:1675–1687.

104. Lassus P, Opitz-Araya X, Lazebnik Y. Requirement for caspase-2 in stress-induced apoptosis before mitochondrial permeabilization. Science 2002; 297:1352–1354.

105. Zou H, Li Y, Liu X, Wang X. An APAF-1.cytochrome c multimeric complex is a functional apoptosome that activates procaspase-9. J Biol Chem 1999; 274:11549–11556.

106. Green DR, Kroemer G. The pathophysiology of mitochondrial cell death. Science 2004; 305:626–629.

107. Micheau O. Cellular FLICE-inhibitory protein: An attractive therapeutic target? Expert Opin Ther Targets 2003; 7:559–573.

108. Zamzami N, Kroemer G. The mitochondrion in apoptosis: How Pandora's box opens. Nat Rev Mol Cell Biol 2001; 2:67–71.

109. Vaux DL, Silke J. IAPs, RINGs and ubiquitylation. Nat Rev Mol Cell Biol 2005; 6:287–297.

110. Verhagen AM, Vaux DL. Cell death regulation by the mammalian IAP antagonist Diablo/Smac. Apoptosis 2002; 7:163–166.

111. Kitada S, Zapata JM, Andreeff M, Reed JC. Protein kinase inhibitors flavopiridol and 7-hydroxy-staurosporine down-regulate antiapoptosis proteins in B-cell chronic lymphocytic leukemia. Blood 2000; 96:393–397.

112. Achenbach TV, Muller R, Slater EP. Bcl-2 independence of flavopiridol-induced apoptosis. Mitochondrial depolarization in the absence of cytochrome c release. J Biol Chem 2000; 275:32089–32097.

113. Decker RH, Dai Y, Grant S. The cyclin-dependent kinase inhibitor flavopiridol induces apoptosis in human leukemia cells (U937) through the mitochondrial rather than the receptor-mediated pathway. Cell Death Differ 2001; 8:715–724.

114. Yu C, Rahmani M, Dai Y et al. The lethal effects of pharmacological cyclin-dependent kinase inhibitors in human leukemia cells proceed through a phosphatidylinositol 3-kinase/Akt-dependent process. Cancer Res 2003; 63:1822–1833.

115. Dai Y, Hamm TE, Dent P, Grant S. Cyclin D1 overexpression increases the susceptibility of human U266 myeloma cells to CDK inhibitors through a process involving p130-, p107- and E2F-dependent S phase entry. Cell Cycle 2006; 5:437–446.

116. Reed JC. Apoptosis-targeted therapies for cancer. Cancer Cell 2003; 3:17–22.

117. Decker RH, Wang S, Dai Y, Dent P, Grant S. Loss of the Bcl-2 phosphorylation loop domain is required to protect human myeloid leukemia cells from flavopiridol-mediated mitochondrial damage and apoptosis. Cancer Biol Ther 2002; 1:136–144.

118. Rosato RR, Almenara JA, Kolla SS et al. Mechanism and functional role of XIAP and Mcl-1 down-regulation in flavopiridol/vorinostat antileukemic interactions. Mol Cancer Ther 2007; 6:692–702.

119. Gao N, Dai Y, Rahmani M, Dent P, Grant S. Contribution of disruption of the nuclear factor-kappaB pathway to induction of apoptosis in human leukemia cells by histone deacetylase inhibitors and flavopiridol. Mol Pharmacol 2004; 66:956–963.

120. Newcomb EW. Flavopiridol: Pleiotropic biological effects enhance its anti-cancer activity. Anticancer Drugs 2004; 15:411–419.

121. Brusselbach S, Nettelbeck DM, Sedlacek HH, Muller R. Cell cycle-independent induction of apoptosis by the anti-tumor drug Flavopiridol in endothelial cells. Int J Cancer 1998; 77:146–152.

122. Newcomb EW, Ali MA, Schnee T et al. Flavopiridol downregulates hypoxia-mediated hypoxia-inducible factor-1alpha expression in human glioma cells by a proteasome-independent pathway: Implications for in vivo therapy. Neuro Oncol 2005; 7:225–235.

123. Oikonomakos NG, Schnier JB, Zographos SE, Skamnaki VT, Tsitsanou KE, Johnson LN. Flavopiridol inhibits glycogen phosphorylase by binding at the inhibitor site. J Biol Chem 2000; 275:34566–34573.

124. Kaiser A, Nishi K, Gorin FA, Walsh DA, Bradbury EM, Schnier JB. The cyclin-dependent kinase (CDK) inhibitor flavopiridol inhibits glycogen phosphorylase. Arch Biochem Biophys 2001; 386:179–187.

125. Fuse E, Kuwabara T, Sparreboom A, Sausville EA, Figg WD. Review of UCN-01 development: A lesson in the importance of clinical pharmacology. J Clin Pharmacol 2005; 45:394–403.

126. Dees EC, Baker SD, O'Reilly S et al. A phase I and pharmacokinetic study of short infusions of UCN-01 in patients with refractory solid tumors. Clin Cancer Res 2005; 11:664–671.

127. Edelman MJ, Bauer KS, Jr., Wu S, Smith R, Bisacia S, Dancey J. Phase I and pharmacokinetic study of 7-hydroxystaurosporine and carboplatin in advanced solid tumors. Clin Cancer Res 2007; 13:2667–2674.

128. Sampath D, Cortes J, Estrov Z et al. Pharmacodynamics of cytarabine alone and in combination with 7-hydroxystaurosporine (UCN-01) in AML blasts in vitro and during a clinical trial. Blood 2006; 107:2517–2524.

129. Hofmann J. Protein kinase C isozymes as potential targets for anticancer therapy. Curr Cancer Drug Targets 2004; 4:125–146.

130. Johnson LN, De ME, Brown NR et al. Structural studies with inhibitors of the cell cycle regulatory kinase cyclin-dependent protein kinase 2. Pharmacol Ther 2002; 93:113–124.

131. Akiyama T, Yoshida T, Tsujita T et al. G1 phase accumulation induced by UCN-01 is associated with dephosphorylation of Rb and CDK2 proteins as well as induction of CDK inhibitor p21/Cip1/WAF1/Sdi1 in p53-mutated human epidermoid carcinoma A431 cells. Cancer Res 1997; 57:1495–1501.

132. Patel V, Lahusen T, Leethanakul C et al. Antitumor activity of UCN-01 in carcinomas of the head and neck is associated with altered expression of cyclin D3 and p27(KIP1). Clin Cancer Res 2002; 8:3549–3560.

133. Zhou BB, Bartek J. Targeting the checkpoint kinases: Chemosensitization versus chemoprotection. Nat Rev Cancer 2004; 4:216–225.

134. Bartek J, Lukas J. Chk1 and Chk2 kinases in checkpoint control and cancer. Cancer Cell 2003; 3:421–429.

135. Tse AN, Carvajal R, Schwartz GK. Targeting checkpoint kinase 1 in cancer therapeutics. Clin Cancer Res 2007; 13:1955–1960.

136. Reinhardt HC, Aslanian AS, Lees JA, Yaffe MB. p53-deficient cells rely on ATM- and ATR-mediated checkpoint signaling through the p38MAPK/MK2 pathway for survival after DNA damage. Cancer Cell 2007; 11:175–189.

137. Vogel C, Hager C, Bastians H. Mechanisms of mitotic cell death induced by chemotherapy-mediated G2 checkpoint abrogation. Cancer Res 2007; 67:339–345.

138. Zhao B, Bower MJ, McDevitt PJ et al. Structural basis for Chk1 inhibition by UCN-01. J Biol Chem 2002; 277:46609–46615.

139. Yu Q, La RJ, Zhang H, Takemura H, Kohn KW, Pommier Y. UCN-01 inhibits p53 up-regulation and abrogates gamma-radiation-induced G(2)-M checkpoint independently of p53 by targeting both of the checkpoint kinases, Chk2 and Chk1. Cancer Res 2002; 62:5743–5748.

140. Karlsson-Rosenthal C, Millar JB. Cdc25: Mechanisms of checkpoint inhibition and recovery. Trends Cell Biol 2006; 16:285–292.

141. Kohn EA, Ruth ND, Brown MK, Livingstone M, Eastman A. Abrogation of the S phase DNA damage checkpoint results in S phase progression or premature mitosis depending on the concentration of 7-hydroxystaurosporine and the kinetics of Cdc25C activation. J Biol Chem 2002; 277:26553–26564.

142. Callegari AJ, Kelly TJ. Shedding light on the DNA damage checkpoint. Cell Cycle 2007; 6:660–666.

143. Harrison JC, Haber JE. Surviving the breakup: The DNA damage checkpoint. Annu Rev Genet 2006; 40:209–235.

144. Kawabe T. G2 checkpoint abrogators as anticancer drugs. Mol Cancer Ther 2004; 3:513–519.

145. Gottifredi V, Prives C. The S phase checkpoint: When the crowd meets at the fork. Semin Cell Dev Biol 2005; 16:355–368.

146. Heffernan TP, Simpson DA, Frank AR et al. An ATR- and Chk1-dependent S checkpoint inhibits replicon initiation following UVC-induced DNA damage. Mol Cell Biol 2002; 22:8552–8561.

147. Sato S, Fujita N, Tsuruo T. Interference with PDK1-Akt survival signaling pathway by UCN-01 (7-hydroxystaurosporine). Oncogene 2002; 21:1727–1738.

148. Komander D, Kular GS, Bain J, Elliott M, Alessi DR, Van Aalten DM. Structural basis for UCN-01 (7-hydroxystaurosporine) specificity and PDK1 (3-phosphoinositide-dependent protein kinase-1) inhibition. Biochem J 2003; 375:255–262.

149. Castedo M, Perfettini JL, Roumier T, Kroemer G. Cyclin-dependent kinase-1: Linking apoptosis to cell cycle and mitotic catastrophe. Cell Death Differ 2002; 9:1287–1293.

150. McClue SJ, Blake D, Clarke R et al. In vitro and in vivo antitumor properties of the cyclin dependent kinase inhibitor CYC202 (R-roscovitine). Int J Cancer 2002; 102:463–468.

151. Tang L, Li MH, Cao P et al. Crystal structure of pyridoxal kinase in complex with roscovitine and derivatives. J Biol Chem 2005; 280:31220–31229.

152. Bach S, Knockaert M, Reinhardt J et al. Roscovitine targets, protein kinases and pyridoxal kinase. J Biol Chem 2005; 280:31208–31219.

153. Raynaud FI, Whittaker SR, Fischer PM et al. In vitro and in vivo pharmacokinetic-pharmacodynamic relationships for the trisubstituted aminopurine cyclin-dependent kinase inhibitors olomoucine, bohemine and CYC202. Clin Cancer Res 2005; 11:4875–4887.

154. Benson C, White J, de BJ et al. A phase I trial of the selective oral cyclin-dependent kinase inhibitor seliciclib (CYC202; R-Roscovitine), administered twice daily for 7 days every 21 days. Br J Cancer 2007; 96:29–37.

155. Whittaker SR, Walton MI, Garrett MD, Workman P. The Cyclin-dependent kinase inhibitor CYC202 (R-roscovitine) inhibits retinoblastoma protein phosphorylation, causes loss of Cyclin D1, and activates the mitogen-activated protein kinase pathway. Cancer Res 2004; 64:262–272.

156. Lacrima K, Valentini A, Lambertini C et al. In vitro activity of cyclin-dependent kinase inhibitor CYC202 (Seliciclib, R-roscovitine) in mantle cell lymphomas. Ann Oncol 2005; 16:1169–1176.

157. Lacrima K, Rinaldi A, Vignati S et al. Cyclin-dependent kinase inhibitor seliciclib shows in vitro activity in diffuse large B-cell lymphomas. Leuk Lymphoma 2007; 48:158–167.

158. Hahntow IN, Schneller F, Oelsner M et al. Cyclin-dependent kinase inhibitor Roscovitine induces apoptosis in chronic lymphocytic leukemia cells. Leukemia 2004; 18:747–755.

159. Alvi AJ, Austen B, Weston VJ et al. A novel CDK inhibitor, CYC202 (R-roscovitine), overcomes the defect in p53-dependent apoptosis in B-CLL by down-regulation of genes involved in transcription regulation and survival. Blood 2005; 105:4484–4491.

160. Zhang B, Gojo I, Fenton RG. Myeloid cell factor-1 is a critical survival factor for multiple myeloma. Blood 2002; 99:1885–1893.

161. Raje N, Kumar S, Hideshima T et al. Seliciclib (CYC202 or R-roscovitine), a small-molecule cyclin-dependent kinase inhibitor, mediates activity via down-regulation of Mcl-1 in multiple myeloma. Blood 2005; 106:1042–1047.

162. Rossi AG, Sawatzky DA, Walker A et al. Cyclin-dependent kinase inhibitors enhance the resolution of inflammation by promoting inflammatory cell apoptosis. Nat Med 2006; 12:1056–1064.

163. Coley HM, Shotton CF, Thomas H. Seliciclib (CYC202; r-roscovitine) in combination with cytotoxic agents in human uterine sarcoma cell lines. Anticancer Res 2007; 27:273–278.

164. Coley HM, Shotton CF, Kokkinos MI, Thomas H. The effects of the CDK inhibitor seliciclib alone or in combination with cisplatin in human uterine sarcoma cell lines. Gynecol Oncol 2007; 105:462–469.

165. Ribas J, Boix J, Meijer L. (R)-roscovitine (CYC202, Seliciclib) sensitizes SH-SY5Y neuroblastoma cells to nutlin-3-induced apoptosis. Exp Cell Res 2006; 312:2394–2400.

166. Misra RN, Xiao HY, Kim KS et al N-(cycloalkylamino)acyl-2-aminothiazole inhibitors of cyclin-dependent kinase 2. N-[5-[[[5-(1,1-dimethylethyl)-2-oxazolyl]methyl]thio]-2-thiazolyl]-4- piperidinecarboxamide (BMS-387032), a highly efficacious and selective antitumor agent. J Med Chem 2004; 47:1719–1728.

167. Senderowicz AM. Small-molecule cyclin-dependent kinase modulators. Oncogene 2003; 22:6609–6620.

168. Ma Y, Freeman SN, Cress WD. E2F4 deficiency promotes drug-induced apoptosis. Cancer Biol Ther 2004; 3:1262–1269.

169. Ma Y, Cress WD. Transcriptional upregulation of p57 (Kip2) by the cyclin-dependent kinase inhibitor BMS-387032 is E2F dependent and serves as a negative feedback loop limiting cytotoxicity. Oncogene 2007; 26:3532–3540.

170. Mukhopadhyay P, Ali MA, Nandi A, Carreon P, Choy H, Saha D. The cyclin-dependent kinase 2 inhibitor down-regulates interleukin-1beta-mediated induction of cyclooxygenase-2 expression in human lung carcinoma cells. Cancer Res 2006; 66:1758–1766.

171. Kramer A, Schultheis B, Bergmann J et al. Alterations of the cyclin D1/pRb/p16(INK4A) pathway in multiple myeloma. Leukemia 2002; 16:1844–1851.

172. Lesage D, Troussard X, Sola B. The enigmatic role of cyclin D1 in multiple myeloma. Int J Cancer 2005; 115:171–176.

173. Bergsagel PL, Kuehl WM, Zhan F, Sawyer J, Barlogie B, Shaughnessy J, Jr. Cyclin D dysregulation: An early and unifying pathogenic event in multiple myeloma. Blood 2005; 106:296–303.

174. Bergsagel PL, Kuehl WM. Molecular pathogenesis and a consequent classification of multiple myeloma. J Clin Oncol 2005; 23:6333–6338.

175. Agnelli L, Bicciato S, Mattioli M . Molecular classification of multiple myeloma: A distinct transcriptional profile characterizes patients expressing CCND1 and negative for 14q32 translocations. J Clin Oncol 2005; 23:7296–7306.

176. Perez-Simon JA, Garcia-Sanz R, Tabernero MD et al. Prognostic value of numerical chromosome aberrations in multiple myeloma: A FISH analysis of 15 different chromosomes. Blood 1998; 91:3366–3371.

177. Ely S, Di LM, Niesvizky R . Mutually exclusive cyclin-dependent kinase 4/cyclin D1 and cyclin-dependent kinase 6/cyclin D2 pairing inactivates retinoblastoma protein and promotes cell cycle dysregulation in multiple myeloma. Cancer Res 2005; 65:11345–11353.

178. Urashima M, Ogata A, Chauhan D . Interleukin-6 promotes multiple myeloma cell growth via phosphorylation of retinoblastoma protein. Blood 1996; 88:2219–2227.

179. Tricot G, Barlogie B, Jagannath S et al. Poor prognosis in multiple myeloma is associated only with partial or complete deletions of chromosome 13 or abnormalities involving 11q and not with other karyotype abnormalities. Blood 1995; 86:4250–4256.

180. Drexler HG. Review of alterations of the cyclin-dependent kinase inhibitor INK4 family genes p15, p16, p18 and p19 in human leukemia-lymphoma cells. Leukemia 1998; 12:845–859.

181. Tasaka T, Berenson J, Vescio R et al. Analysis of the p16INK4A, p15INK4B and p18INK4C genes in multiple myeloma. Br J Haematol 1997; 96:98–102.

182. Chen-Kiang S. Cell-cycle control of plasma cell differentiation and tumorigenesis. Immunol Rev 2003; 194:39–47.

183. Ng MH, Chung YF, Lo KW, Wickham NW, Lee JC, Huang DP. Frequent hypermethylation of p16 and p15 genes in multiple myeloma. Blood 1997; 89:2500–2506.

184. Galm O, Wilop S, Reichelt J et al. DNA methylation changes in multiple myeloma. Leukemia 2004; 18:1687–1692.

185. Kulkarni MS, Daggett JL, Bender TP, Kuehl WM, Bergsagel PL, Williams ME. Frequent inactivation of the cyclin-dependent kinase inhibitor p18 by homozygous deletion in multiple myeloma cell lines: Ectopic p18 expression inhibits growth and induces apoptosis. Leukemia 2002; 16:127–134.

186. Dib A, Peterson TR, Raducha-Grace L et al. Paradoxical expression of INK4c in proliferative multiple myeloma tumors: Bi-allelic deletion vs increased expression. Cell Div 2006; 1:23.

187. Sarasquete ME, Garcia-Sanz R, Armellini A et al. The association of increased p14ARF/p16INK4a and p15INK4a gene expression with proliferative activity and the clinical course of multiple myeloma. Haematologica 2006; 91:1551–1554.

188. Chim CS, Fung TK, Liang R. Disruption of INK4/CDK/Rb cell cycle pathway by gene hypermethylation in multiple myeloma and MGUS. Leukemia 2003; 17:2533–2535.

189. Gojo I, Zhang B, Fenton RG. The cyclin-dependent kinase inhibitor flavopiridol induces apoptosis in multiple myeloma cells through transcriptional repression and down-regulation of Mcl-1. Clin Cancer Res 2002; 8:3527–3538.

190. Rosato RR, Dai Y, Almenara JA, Maggio SC, Grant S. Potent antileukemic interactions between flavopiridol and TRAIL/Apo2L involve flavopiridol-mediated XIAP downregulation. Leukemia 2004; 18:1780–1788.

191. Fandy TE, Ross DD, Gore SD, Srivastava RK. Flavopiridol synergizes TRAIL cytotoxicity by downregulation of FLIPL. Cancer Chemother Pharmacol 2007; 60:313–319.

192. Pei XY, Dai Y, Grant S. The small-molecule Bcl-2 inhibitor HA14–1 interacts synergistically with flavopiridol to induce mitochondrial injury and apoptosis in human myeloma cells through a free radical-dependent and Jun NH2-terminal kinase-dependent mechanism. Mol Cancer Ther 2004; 3:1513–1524.

193. Dai Y, Rahmani M, Grant S. Proteasome inhibitors potentiate leukemic cell apoptosis induced by the cyclin-dependent kinase inhibitor flavopiridol through a SAPK/JNK- and NF-kappaB-dependent process. Oncogene 2003; 22:7108–7122.

194. MacCallum DE, Melville J, Frame S et al. Seliciclib (CYC202, R-Roscovitine) induces cell death in multiple myeloma cells by inhibition of RNA polymerase II-dependent transcription and down-regulation of Mcl-1. Cancer Res 2005; 65:5399–5407.

195. Dai Y, Yu C, Singh V et al. Pharmacological inhibitors of the mitogen-activated protein kinase (MAPK) kinase/MAPK cascade interact synergistically with UCN-01 to induce mitochondrial dysfunction and apoptosis in human leukemia cells. Cancer Res 2001; 61:5106–5115.

196. Dai Y, Landowski TH, Rosen ST, Dent P, Grant S. Combined treatment with the checkpoint abrogator UCN-01 and MEK1/2 inhibitors potently induces apoptosis in

drug-sensitive and -resistant myeloma cells through an IL-6-independent mechanism. Blood 2002; 100:3333–3343.

197. Dai Y, Dent P, Grant S. Tumor necrosis factor-related apoptosis-inducing ligand (TRAIL) promotes mitochondrial dysfunction and apoptosis induced by 7-hydroxystaurosporine and mitogen-activated protein kinase kinase inhibitors in human leukemia cells that ectopically express Bcl-2 and Bcl-xL. Mol Pharmacol 2003; 64:1402–1409.

198. Dai Y, Pei XY, Rahmani M, Conrad DH, Dent P, Grant S. Interruption of the NF-kappaB pathway by Bay 11–7082 promotes UCN-01-mediated mitochondrial dysfunction and apoptosis in human multiple myeloma cells. Blood 2004; 103:2761–2770.

199. Pei XY, Dai Y, Rahmani M, Li W, Dent P, Grant S. The farnesyltransferase inhibitor L744832 potentiates UCN-01-induced apoptosis in human multiple myeloma cells. Clin Cancer Res 2005; 11:4589–4600.

200. Dai Y, Khanna P, Chen S, Pei XY, Dent P, Grant S. Statins synergistically potentiate 7-hydroxystaurosporine (UCN-01) lethality in human leukemia and myeloma cells by disrupting Ras farnesylation and activation. Blood 2007; 109:4415–4423.

201. Pei XY, Li W, Dai Y, Dent P, Grant S. Dissecting the roles of checkpoint kinase 1/CDC2 and mitogen-activated protein kinase kinase 1/2/extracellular signal-regulated kinase 1/2 in relation to 7-hydroxystaurosporine-induced apoptosis in human multiple myeloma cells. Mol Pharmacol 2006; 70:1965–1973.

202. Pei XY, Dai Y, Tenorio S et al . MEK1/2 inhibitors potentiate UCN-01 lethality in human multiple myeloma cells through a Bim-dependent mechanism. Blood 2007

203. Baughn LB, Di Liberto M, Wu K et al. A novel orally active small molecule potently induces G1 arrest in primary myeloma cells and prevents tumor growth by specific inhibition of cyclin-dependent kinase 4/6. Cancer Res 2006; 66:7661–7667.

204. Dispenzieri A, Gertz MA, Lacy MQ et al. Flavopiridol in patients with relapsed or refractory multiple myeloma: A phase 2 trial with clinical and pharmacodynamic end-points. Haematologica 2006; 91:390–393.

205. Dai Y, Rahmani M, Pei XY, Dent P, Grant S. Bortezomib and flavopiridol interact synergistically to induce apoptosis in chronic myeloid leukemia cells resistant to imatinib mesylate through both Bcr/Abl-dependent and -independent mechanisms. Blood 2004; 104:509–518.

206. S, Grant Sullivan D,. et al. Phase I Trial of Bortezomib (NSC 681239) and Flavopiridol (NSC 649890) in Patients with Recurrent or Refractory Indolent B-cell Neoplasms. Blood 2005; 104.

Chapter 23

Fibroblast Growth Factor Receptor 3 and Multiple Myeloma

Victor Hugo Jiménez-Zepeda and A. Keith Stewart

Introduction

Chromosomal translocations involving the immunoglobulin heavy chain (IgH) gene locus are found in 40% of patients with multiple myeloma (MM), a malignancy of terminally differentiated B cells.[1–3] One of the most common translocations, t(4;14), seen in 15% of cases, is associated with a poor prognosis.[4–7] The molecular pathogenesis of t(4;14) is thought to involve aberrant immunoglobulin class-switching recombination, leading to a reciprocal translocation between chromosomes 14q32 and 4p16.3 that repositions fibroblast growth factor receptor 3 (FGFR3) to der(14) and creates a fusion gene with MM SET domain containing protein (MMSET) on der(4) under the influence of strong enhancers from the IgH region.[8,9] FGFR3 is one of a family of five tyrosine kinases through which fibroblast growth factors signal. These receptors are characterized by an extracellular domain with two or three immunoglobulin-like domains, a transmembrane domain, and a cytoplasmic tyrosine kinase domain. On ligand binding, FGFR3 undergoes dimerization and tyrosine autophosphorylation, resulting in cell proliferation and differentiation. In MM, FGFR3 dysregulation appears to occur exclusively as a consequence of translocation.[10,11] Plowright et al. and others[12,13] have demonstrated that aberrant FGFR3 expression induces lymphoid malignancies in mice and that aberrant expression in myeloma cell lines result in cell proliferation and survival.[2,14–16] Recent studies suggest that the inhibition of FGFR3 by small molecules or antibodies induces differentiation and apoptosis of myeloma cell lines and primary MM cells, suggesting FGFR3 is a therapeutic target.[15–17]

t(4;14) can be detected by fluorescence in situ hybridization (FISH), reverse transcriptase-polymerase chain reaction (RT-PCR), or gene-expression profiling,[18,19] and FGFR3 expression has been assessed by flow cytometry (FC) or immunohistochemistry[6,20] (Table 1).

Table 1 FGFR3 expression associated to t(4;14).

Clinical study	Assay	FGFR3 and t(4;14) (%)
Chesi et al.[8]	RT-PCR	3/8 (40)a
Nakazawa et al.[85]	RT-PCR	6/7 (86)
Sibley et al.[46]	RT-PCR	7/7 (100)
Keats et al.[6]	RT-PCR	23/31 (74)
Santra et al.[18]	RT-PCR	22/32 (68)
Chang et al.[7]	IHC	12/16 (75)
Fabris et al.[25]	RT-PCR	4/6 (67)
Rasmussen et al.[86]	RT-PCR	2/3 (67)
Chandesris et al.[53]	FC	20/24 (84)

aCell lines and primary tumors

IHC immunohistochemistry, *FC* flow cytometry, *RT-PCR* reverse transcriptase-polymerase chain reaction, *FGFR3* fibroblast growth factor receptor 3

t(4;14) (p16;q32)

The first comprehensive analysis of t(4;14) was published by Chesi et al.[8] Sequencing of cloned switch translocation breakpoints from four t(4;14)-positive cell lines and one patient sample identified a common breakpoint region on 4p16, situated just centromeric of FGFR3. This observation led to the hypothesis that FGFR3 was the target gene of t(4;14) because the identified breakpoints would create a der(14) on which FGFR3 would be brought into close proximity with the 3′ regulatory regions (Ea1 and Ea2) of the IgH locus. To test this hypothesis, a panel of cell lines and patient samples were screened for FGFR3 expression by RT-PCR. This assay showed that FGFR3 was ectopically expressed at a very high level in t(4;14)-positive samples. Although one t(4;14)-positive cell line (JIM3) did not express FGFR3, it was noted that the tumor sample from which the line was derived expressed FGFR3. Further strengthening the argument of FGFR3 as the target gene, two positive cell lines and one patient sample expressed a mutated allele of FGFR3, known to cause hyperactivation of the FGFR3 signaling cascade. All three missense mutations were previously identified in thanatophoric dysplasia (type I and II) and therefore represented somatic mutation events because none of the samples originated from an individual with a skeletal disorder.[21] The t(4;14) translocation is undetectable by conventional cytogenetics (G-banding) or spectral karyotyping (SKY) because of the telomeric localization of both chromosomal partner domains. It was first identified by Southern Blotting and has subsequently been detected by FISH and RT-PCR in MM, monoclonal gammopathy of undetermined significance (MGUS), and primary amyloidosis.[22–25] The genomic locations of t(4;14) breakpoints are almost exclusively in or near switch regions of the IgH loci.[19] The breakpoints on chromosome 4 occur within an ~113 kb region between FGFR3 and MMSET exon 5. This breakpoint region is a small part of a conserved gene cluster including the transforming acidic coiled-coil protein 3 (TACC3), FGFR3, and MMSET, also known as WHSCI and NSD2. FGFR3 and TACC3 may be dysregulated by the strong 3′ enhancers on der(14), whereas MMSET and REIIBP may be dysregulated by the intronic Eu enhancer on der(4).[26]

FGFR3

The FGFR family, represented by four major transmembrane receptors, plays an important role in normal angiogenesis and embryonic development. Germline-activating mutations of FGFRs[27–30] are associated with a range of skeletal disorders including the common forms of dwarfism. Changes in expression of FGFRs are implicated in tumor development in many organs, and recent results indicate an important role for mutant FGFR3 in certain tumor types (bladder and breast cancer).[31,32]

FGFR3 Expression and Its Biological Significance

Although there is overlapping expression of the FGFRs in different tissues, there is also specificity and temporal variation of the expression during embryonic development.[33,34] FGFR3 is expressed in adult kidney, lung, and brain,[35] whereas in embryos it is also present in glial cells and astrocytes.[36] Expression has also been detected in cartilage (proliferating and hypertrophic chondrocytes), intestine,[33,36] pancreas, and testis. Additionally, in mouse embryos, FGFR3 has been shown to be expressed in the cochlear duct and in the lens,[37] where it is involved in differentiation.[38] Knowing where and when FGFR3 is expressed can give some clues to function, but more enlightening information has come from the generation of FGFR3 null mice.[39] These mice show bone dysplasia with longer vertebral bodies and overgrowth of the long bones, associated with an increased number of proliferating chondrocytes during embryogenesis. This indicates that FGFR3 is a negative regulator of bone growth. It follows that the FGFR3 mutations associated with dwarfism must be activating mutations. Interestingly, such activating mutations, which clearly provide negative regulatory signals in the chondrocyte, are found not only in skeletal disorders but also in MM.

FGFR3 Mutations Associated with Multiple Myeloma

Some of the missense mutations observed in achondroplasia are also associated with human MM[8,40] and carcinomas of bladder and cervix.[41] Additionally, in colon carcinoma, two novel mutations have been identified: E322K and a nonsense mutation at nucleotide 849.[42] No mutations in FGFR3 have yet been found in prostate, skin, lung, stomach, brain, or renal tumors,[43–46] indicating that FGFR3 mutations seem to be specific to a few cancers.

MM, a B-cell entity, provided the first indication that FGFR3 could act as oncogene. Here, the chromosomal translocation t(4;14) (p16.3;q32), which results in ectopic expression of FGFR3 (from der[4]) and IgH–MMSET transcripts (from der[4][8,25]), has been described in 15% of patients. These translocations are found not only in MM but also in MGUS, which is a precursor for MM.[47] Thus, the translocation is considered to be an early genetic alteration in MM development. However, the role of FGFR3 expression in these conditions is not entirely clear. MMSET (from der[4]) is universally expressed in tumors with the translocation, but FGFR3 is not expressed in ~25% of cases with t(4;14) presumably since der(l4) is lost during tumor progression as part of clonal evolution.[18,26] Clearly, this does not indicate that FGFR3 is irrelevant, but it does raise the intriguing possibility that the role of FGFR3 may change during MM progression. Where FGFR3 is expressed in MM,

FGFR3 IIIc appears to be the major isoform, but some tumors express FGFR3 IIIb or both isoforms.[45,48] So far, neither isoform has been associated with specific characteristics of MM tumors or cell lines.

In some cases of MM, the translocated FGFR3 is on occasion mutated, mostly in late-stage disease. However, it should be noted that FGFR3 has also been found mutated in an MM tumor not showing t(4;14).[49] In that case, it is possible that constitutive activation of FGFR3 would compensate for the absence of overexpression. One study of 150 newly diagnosed cases reported that FGFR3 overexpression was present in 16% but mutated only in 1.3% at diagnosis.[50] Sibley et al.[48] analyzed samples taken 13 months apart from the same patient, and identified a K650E mutation only in the later sample, reinforcing the concept that FGFR3 mutations contribute late in the multistage disease process. FGFR3 mutations found in MM tumors include R248C,[49] K650E, K650M,[8] and Y241C,[51] which have not been seen in chondrodysplasia. In MM cell lines, mutations include K650E in OPM2, Y373C in KMS-11,[8,40] and G384D in KMS-18. It seems, then, that overexpression of wild-type FGFR3 is therefore required but by itself is not sufficient to lead to aggressive MM. Its constitutive activation or secondary mutations are likely to promote a stronger proliferative signal. This is in agreement with experimental transformation systems, in which wild-type FGFR3 is less potent than mutant receptor. For example, overexpression of wild-type FGFR3 in NIH3T3 cells does not induce focus formation in vitro or tumorigenicity in nude mice in contrast to the constitutively active kinase K650E mutant.[51] However, in vitro transduction of mouse bone marrow (BM) cells with a retrovirus encoding the wild-type FGFR3 followed by transplantation into mice does lead to delayed lymphoma/leukemias after ~1 year. Again, the mutant receptor is more potent in this assay.[52] It is possible that in MM, overexpression of other oncogenes or a predisposition to any one secondary genetic mutation in other pathways could compensate for the weak proliferative or transforming signal from the wild-type receptor. Interestingly, oncogenic mutations of RAS genes (KRAS and NRAS) have been observed in 40% of MM. These and FGFR3 mutations appear to be mutually exclusive, suggesting that there may be an overlapping function.[52]

Detection of FGFR3 Expression

Identification of t(4;14) translocation and FGFR3 expression is an important step in the management of patients with MM, given its associated poor prognosis and the potential development of targeted therapy against FGFR3 tyrosine kinase activity. To recognize this subgroup of MM, analysis of BM plasma cells by FISH is the current method of choice[62]. As previously suggested (Chesi et al., 1999), polymerase chain reaction for detection of IgH/MMSET is also useful for the diagnosis and characterization of t(4;14) MM. The detection of FGFR3 protein, by immunohistochemistry on decalcified, paraffin-embedded BM biopsies, has also been proposed by Chang et al.[20]). Chandesris et al. (2007) reported the usefulness of FC analysis for FGFR3 expression in BM and peripheral blood samples of MM patients.[53] This approach is quick to perform and is easily applied to routine laboratory practice. In addition, it provides results in real time, which is convenient for clinical decision-making. In this series of 200 patients, FC detection of FGFR3-positive cells was consistently associated with the presence of t(4;14) translocation, by FISH and/or by real-time quantitative polymerase chain reaction (RQ-PCR) for IgH/MMSET and FGFR3 transcripts.

RAS/MAPK Signaling in t(4;14) MM: Role of MIP-lα/CCL3

Masih-Khan et al.[54] found that MIP-lα/CCL3 was one of only ten genes whose expression was consistently and significantly decreased in t(4;14) myeloma cells when constitutively active FGFR3 was inhibited by small molecular tyrosine kinase inhibitors and more specifically with FGFR3 siRNA. MIP-lα is a low molecular weight monokine with inflammatory and chemokinetic properties and has been characterized to be a potent osteoclast stimulatory factor in MM.[55,56] It is elevated in the BM plasma cells of patients with active MM and correlates with the presence of lytic bone lesions.[55] More recently, serum MIP-lα was reported to correlate with survival and bone resorption markers, suggesting that MIP-lα contributes to the pathogenesis of bone disease in MM and possibly in tumor growth as reflected by its impact on survival.[54,57] MIP-lα/CCL3 may be regulated by the RAS/MAPK pathway, downstream of FGFR3. These results confirm that the RAS/ERK pathway is relevant for FGFR3-mediated signaling and is involved in upregulation of a number of critical genes that may be involved in disease severity. These findings are further supported by gene expression profiling results of FGFR3 RNAi knockdown[58] and a comparison of t(4;14)-positive versus -negative cell lines[19] in which activation of the RAS/MAPK pathway is evident. Interestingly, levels of MIP-lα on gene expression profiling have also been correlated with poor outcome in diffuse large B-cell lymphoma, suggesting a broader role for this gene in cell proliferation.[59]

Cyclin D Dysregulation

Two oncogenic pathways have been hypothesized for MM and premalignant MGUS tumors: a nonhyperdiploid pathway associated with a high prevalence of IgH translocations and a hyperdiploid pathway associated with multiple trisomies of chromosomes.[60,61] Both myeloma variants are unified by cyclin Dl, D2, or D3 expression, which appears to be increased and/or dysregulated in virtually all tumors. Translocations can directly dysregulate CCNDI (11q13) or CCND3 (6p21), while FGFR3, MAF (16q23), or MAFB (20q11) all upregulate CCND2.[62] Using gene expression profiling to identify five recurrent translocations, specific trisomies, and expression of cyclin D genes, MM tumors can be divided into eight TC (translocation/cyclin D) groups (11q13, 6p21, 4p16, maf, Dl, D1 + D2, D2, and none) that appear to be defined by early, and perhaps initiating, oncogenic events. Thus, cyclin D2 upregulation may contribute to the pathogenesis of t(4;14).

Association with Other High-Risk Features and Poor Clinical Outcome

The two most common IgH translocations are t(4;14) and t(11;14). These translocations result from illegitimate IgH rearrangements.[63] The presence of these rearrangements has been correlated with morphology (plasmablastic with t[4;14] and lymphoplasmacytic or small mature with t[11;14]) and with tumor mass.

In addition, a close relationship between t(4;14) and chromosome 13 abnormalities has been generally reported (up to 73% of t[4;14] also has deletion of chromosome 13).[3–5,64,65] Some studies have shown a higher prevalence of IgA isotype and elevated B2-microglobulin concentrations in patients with t(4;14).[3–5] Notably, in a recent study,[66] resistance to alkylating agents after posttransplant relapse has been identified as a potential factor contributing to the poor prognosis of t(4;14) patients treated with autologous stem cell transplantation. Interestingly the poor prognosis is due to early relapse as response rates are actually higher than in other subtypes. Jaksic et al.[67] reported a very nice response rate in the group of t(4;14) (19 cases) after induction therapy and autologous stem cell transplantation, but early relapse was frequent (Table 2).

Patients with t(4;14) overall have an inferior outcome, regardless of the mode of treatment (conventional or high dose).[6,68] Gertz et al.[69] reported the clinical implications of t(4;14) translocations in a series of patients. This chromosome translocation had a profound effect on both time to progression and overall survival (OS). Time to progression for patients with and without t(4;14) was 8.2 versus 17.8 months ($p = 0.001$), and OS was 18.8 versus 43.9 months ($p = 0.001$). Patients with t(4;14) translocation had a higher C-reactive protein, PCLI, and percentage of BM plasma cells (all $p = 0.04$). Age, creatinine, lactate dehydrogenase, and B2-microglobulin were not significantly different between both groups. When the analysis is restricted to the 70 patients who had transplantation upfront after first response, t(4;14) retained its significance. The median survival rates were 29 months for patients with t(4;14) and 75 months for those without this translocation. When both t(4;14) and -13/13q- were present, OS was 18.8 months, significantly worse than for patients who had -13/13q- but not t(4;14) (26.8 months, $p = 0.001$). Avet-Loiseau et al. recently reported in a multivariate analysis that patients with t(4;14) translocation and a high level of B2-microglobulin have a median OS of only 19 months compared to 84% at 4 years for those without the translocation.[70] Recently, Moreau et al.[66] designed a simple staging system in t(4;14) patients able to identify a group of patients with a better prognosis: those presenting at diagnosis with both low B2-microglobulin (<4 mg/dl) and high hemoglobin (>l0 g/l) had a median survival of 54.6 months, and a median event-free survival (EFS) of 26 months, respectively; conversely patients with only one adverse prognostic factor (either B2-microglobulin or low hemoglobin (>4 mg/dl)) had a median OS and EFS of 37 and 19 months, respectively, and patients with both high B2-microglobulin and low hemoglobin had a median OS and EFS of 19 and 11 months, respectively ($p = 0.0003$).

Novel Agents and t(4;14)

Whether the adverse impact of t(4;14) can be overcome by novel agents remains to be elucidated. Unfortunately, most studies are hampered by small numbers and short follow-up. Chang et al. reported in a small series of relapsed/refractory MM patients that bortezomib therapy response is independent of cytogenetic abnormalities.[71] This data was similar to that of Mateos

Table 2 t(4;14), FGFR3, and MMSET in multiple myeloma.

Author	Year	No. of patients	Treatment	OS (months)	EFS (months)	P	Assay	HR
Avet-Loiseau[70]	2007	100/714 (14%)	HDCTX	41.3 vs 79	20.6 vs 65.5	5.10–11, 0.5<0.0001, PFS<0.001	FISH	2.79
Gutierrez et al.[68]	2007	29/260 (11%)	HDCTX	24 vs 48	NA	<0.0001	FISH	2.6
Gertz et al.[59]	2005	26/153	HDCTX	18.8 vs 43.9	NA	0.001	FISH	2.1
Fonseca et al.[5]	2003	42/332 RR69 vs 62	CCTX	26 vs 45	17 vs 31	<0.01, <0.01	FISH	1.78
Moreau et al.[4]	2002	22/168	HDCTX	22.8 vs 66	20.7 vs 28.5	<0.0001, 0.002	FISH	NA
Keats et al.[6]	2003	31/208 (14.9%)	CCTX/HDCTX	21.1	NA	0.003	RT-PCR, IgH/ MMSET	2.0
Chang et al.[7]	2004	15/120 (12.5%)	HDCTX	18.3 vs 48.1	9.9 vs 25.8	<0.0001, 0.0003	FISH	NA
Dewald et al.[83]	2005	10/154 (6.5%)	NS	13.3 vs 45	NA	<0.01	IgH, FGFR3	NA
Jaksic et al.[67]	2005	19/124	HDCTX	24.2 vs NA	14.1 vs 25.8	0.003	clg FISH	NA
Cavo et al.[64]	2006	17/63 (27%)	HDCTX	NA	23 vs 30	0.01	RT-PCR, IgH, FISH	NA
Chieccio et al.[84]	2006	28/535 (5%)	NS	9 vs 41	NA	<0.001	CC	NA
		85/729		19 vs NR	NA	0.004	FISH	NA
		59/490		19 vs 44	NA	0.002	Combined	NA
Chang et al.[71]	2006	41 (15%)	Velcade	9.4 vs 15.1	10.5 vs 6.8	NS	FISH	NA
Chang et al.[20]	2005	16/85 (19%)	HDCTX	19.2 vs 46.3	11.5 vs 25.8	<0.01, <0.01	FISH/IHC, FGFR3	NA

HDCTX high-dose therapy, *CCTX* conventional chemotherapy, *CC* conventional cytogenetic technique, *NA* not available, *RR* response rate, *MA* multivariate analysis, *HR* hazard ratio, *CCA* complex chromosome abnormalities, *IHC* immunohistochemistry, *NS* not specified or not significant, *NR* not reached, *FISH* fluorescence in situ hybridization, *OS* overall survival, *EFS* event-free survival, *IgH* immunoglobulin heavy chain, *FGFR3* fibroblast growth factor receptor 3, *MMSET* MM SET domain g-containing protein et al. in a series of elderly patients not eligible for BM transplantation.[72] The role of thalidomide and immunomodulatory drugs (IMIDs) in FGFR3 and t(4;14) translocation remains uncertain. Avet-Loiseau et al. reported that the poor prognosis associated with high B2-microglobulin level, t(4;14), and del(17p) seemed not to be modified by the administration of thalidomide as maintenance therapy. However, because the Intergroupe Francophone du Myélome (IFM) 99-02 trial was dedicated to patients with 0 or 1 poor-prognosis factor, these abnormalities were underrepresented in this trial.[70] Bahlis et al.[73] reported the preliminary results of the use of lenalidomide and dexamethasone in nine patients with chromosome 13 deletion and seven patients with t(4;14) treated previously. The overall response rate to Lenalidomide (LD) was similar for both groups with and without t(4;14). Unfortunately, follow-up in all of these studies is short and the number of cases is small.

FGFR3 as a Therapeutic Target

As t(4;14) dysregulates a receptor tyrosine kinase which apparently regulates MM survival, FGFR3 is a potential therapeutic target (Table 3).

CHIR-258

CHIR-258 now called TK1258, a novel benzimidazole-quinolinone, is a potent inhibitor of FGFR3 and class III, IV, and V receptor tyrosine kinases (RTKs), including FGFR1, VEGFRII2I3, PDGFR, FLT3, c-KIT, and CSF-1R. Trudel et al. identified CHIR-258 as a highly active inhibitor of both wild type (WT) and mutant FGFR3 tyrosine kinases.[17] The activity of this inhibitor against a broad spectrum of RTKs implies that CHIR-258 requires less stringent conformation requirements for binding to the kinase domain and is consistent with the retained activity of CHIR-258 against many FGFR3 mutants. CHIR-258 treatment selectively induced apoptotic cell death of MM cell lines and

Table 3 FGFR3 inhibitors.

Inhibitor	Characteristic
SU5402	Y373C mutation is highly sensitive
PRO-001	It is an FGFR3-neutralizing antibody. PRO-001 binds to FGFR3-expressed and inhibits FGF ligand-mediated activation of FGFR3 signaling
PD173074	Inhibition of Src, EGF, VEGF, and PDGF as well as several serine/threonine kinases
PKC412	Inhibition of FLT3, PKC, KDR, c-Kit, PDGFRA, and PDGFRB
Short hairpin RNAs	RNA interference effect by using vector-based expression of short hairpin RNA
TKI-258	It is a potent inhibitor of FGFR3 and class III, IV, and V RTKs, including FGFR1, VEGFR1-3, PDGFR, FL T3, c-KIT, and CSF-1R

PDGFR platelet-derived growth factor receptor, *FGFR3* fibroblast growth factor receptor 3, *RTKs* receptor tyrosine kinases, *VEGF* vascular endothelial growth factor, *PDGF* platelet-derived growth factor, *EGF* epidermal growth factor primary patient samples that harbor FGFR3. The potential clinical application of CHIR-258 for the treatment of MM was further validated using a xenograft mouse model in which CHIR-258 treatment inhibited activity in vivo and produced tumor regression. It is important to note that OPM2 cells responded to this broadly active RTK inhibitor when they did not respond to more selectively FGFR3 inhibitor PD173074.[15,16] Patterson and others[15,74] have demonstrated that the multitargeted RTK inhibitor SU5402 induced cytotoxic responses in OPM2 cells, whereas PD173074 failed to induce apoptosis. These findings therefore raise the possibility that CHIR-258 is targeting other, as yet to be defined, targets important for myeloma cell viability, a fact that is of further relevance given the demonstration that FGFR3 is sometimes lost during disease progression and may therefore be supplanted by other downstream signaling mediators.

PRO-001

PRO-001 is a high-affinity fully human, anti-FGFR3-neutralizing antibody. The antibody is highly selective, inhibiting FGF-stimulated proliferation of FGFR3-expressing Factor dependent cell progenitor cell line (FDCP) cells but not the growth of FDCP cell expressing FGFR1 or FGFR2 within the effective range of antibody concentration. PRO-001 binds to FGFR3 expressed on the surface of t(4;14) myeloma cells and inhibits FGF ligand-mediated activation of FGFR3 signaling in cell lines and primary myeloma cells. The data show that PRO-001 can selectively induce apoptosis of UTMC2 cells and can overcome the protective effects of myeloma–Bone marrow stormal cells (BMSC) interactions and IL-6 and IGF-1. Most importantly, primary myeloma cells expressing WT FGFR3 were also susceptible to PRO-001-induced cell death. The effect on primary t(4;14) myeloma cells was particularly impressive,[75] with all patients demonstrating sensitivity to PRO-001 and one sample with up to 80% induction of apoptosis. The potential clinical application of PRO-001 was further evaluated in a xenograft mouse model in which PRO-001 treatment inhibited FGFR3-mediated tumor growth demonstrating in vivo efficacy with a favorable therapeutic window.

PKC412

PKC412 is a potent inhibitor of several kinases including FLT3, PKC, KDR, cKit, PDGFRcL, and PDGFBR, [76–78] and is currently being evaluated in Phase II clinical trials for acute myelogenous leukemia patients with and without FLT3-activating mutations.[79,80] Chen et al. demonstrated[81] that PKC412 also has inhibitory activity for FGFR family members, such as FGFR1, and was therefore tested for activity to inhibit FGFR3 TDII mutant, as well as a TEL–FGFR3 (Fusion of 2 Kinases) tyrosine kinase in vitro and in vivo.[82] They tested the inhibitory effects of PKC412 by performing a dose–response analysis using t(4;14)-positive primary MM cell lines, including OPM-1, LPI, and KMS-11. PKC412 effectively inhibited the growth of OPM-1 and KMS-11 cells. PKC412 also inhibits LPI cells with relatively higher cellular IC50, and such difference of drug sensitivity might be due to the lower expression level of FGFR3 protein in LPI cells than in OPM-1 cells. In contrast, no significant event was observed in a t(4;14)-negative MM cell line (OCI-My5) in which no expression of FGFR3 was detected. These data suggest that PKC412 effectively inhibits proliferation of FGFR3-positive t(4;14) MM cells and that FGFR3 is the molecular target for inhibition of the t(4;14) MM cells by PKC412. Moreover, PKC412 has minimal nonspecific cytotoxicity in all tested MM cell lines and does not inhibit the control t(4;14)-negative OCl-My5 MM cells. These data also correlate with the observation that PKC412 effectively inhibited FGFR3 tyrosine autophosphorylation as well as phosphorylation and activation of signaling intermediate, such as PLCy, in OPM-1 cells.

Conclusions

FGFR3 is dysregulated by mutation in a number of tumor systems and inherited conditions associated with abnormal bone growth and development. These mutations are associated with constitutive activation of the tyrosine kinase activity of the gene; however, in myeloma patients such mutations are rare and deregulation seems to occur exclusively as a consequence of the t(4;14) translocation. The oncogenic nature of FGFR3 in myeloma has been extensively evaluated. These studies demonstrate that FGFR3 is capable of producing lymphoid malignancies in mice and that overexpression in myeloma cell lines result in increased cell proliferation and survival. Recent studies also suggest that the inhibition of FGFR3 by a small molecule induces differentiation and apoptosis of t(4;14) myeloma cell lines, suggesting that FGFR3 may be a possible therapeutic target. Given its association with inferior outcomes, the possible role of newer drugs in overcoming this poor prognosis and its potential as a therapeutic target routine testing for t(4;14) is necessary.

References

1. Bergsagei PL, Chesi M, Nardini E, et al. Promiscuous translocation into immunoglobulin heavy chain switch regions in multiple myeloma. Proc Natl Acad Sci USA. 1996;93:13931–13936.
2. Konigsberg R, Zojer N, Ackermann J, et al. Predictive role of interphase cytogenetics for survival of patients with multiple myeloma. J Clin Oncol. 2000;18:804–812.
3. Avet-Loiseau H, Facon T, Grosbois B, et al. Oncogenesis of multiple myeloma: 14q32 and 13 q chromosomal abnormalities are not randomly distributed, but correlate with natural history, immunological features, and clinical presentation. Blood. 2002;99:2185–2191.
4. Moreau P, Facon T, Leleu X, et al. Recurrent 14q32 translocations determine the prognosis of multiple myeloma, especially in patients receiving intensive chemotherapy. Blood. 2002;100:1579–1583.
5. Fonseca R, Blood E, Rue M, et al. Clinical biologic implications of recurrent genomic aberrations in myeloma. Blood. 2003;101:4569–4575.
6. Keats JJ, Reiman T, Maxwell CA, et al. In multiple myeloma, t(4;14) (p16;32) is an adverse prognostic factor irrespective of FGFR3 expression. Blood. 2003;101:1520–1529.
7. Chang H, Sloan S, Li D, et al. The t(4;14) is associated with poor prognosis in myeloma patients undergoing autologous stem cell transplant. Br J Haematol. 2004;125:64–68.
8. Chesi M, Nardini E, Brents LA, et al. Frequent translocation t(4;14) (p16.3;q32.3) in multiple myeloma is associated with increased expression and activating mutations of fibroblast growth factor receptor 3. Nat Genet. 1997;16:260–264.
9. Chesi M, Nardini E, Urn RS, et al. The t(4;14) translocation in myeloma dysregulates both FGFR3 and a novel gene MMSET, resulting in lgH/MMSET hybrid transcripts. Blood. 1998;92:3025–3034.

10. Bergsagel PL and Kuehl WM. Chromosome translocations in multiple myeloma. Oncogene. 2001;20:5611–5622.

11. Hallek M, Bergsagel PL and Anderson KC. Multiple myeloma: increasing evidence for a multistep transformation process. Blood. 1998;91:3.

12. Plowright EE, Li Z, Bergsagel PL, et al. Ectopic expression of fibroblast growth factor receptor 3 promotes myeloma cell proliferation and prevents apoptosis. Blood. 2000;95:992–998.

13. Cheng J, Ifor R, Lee B, et al. Constitutively activated FGFR3 mutants signal through PLC7-dependent and -independent pathways for hematopoietic transformation. Blood. 2005;106:328–337.

14. Colvin JS, Bohne BA, Harding GW, McEwan DG and Ornitz DM. Skeletal overgrowth and deafness in mice lacking fibroblast growth factor receptor 3. Nat Genet. 1996;12:390.

15. Paterson JL, Li Z, Wen XY, et al. Preclinical studies of fibroblast growth factor receptor 3 as a therapeutic target in multiple myeloma. Br J Haematol. 2004;124:595–603.

16. Trudel S, Ely S, Farooqi Y, et al. Inhibition of fibroblast growth factor receptor 3 induces differentiation and apoptosis in t(4;14) myeloma. Blood. 2004;103:3521–3528.

17. Trudel S, Li ZH, Wei E, et al. CHIR 258, a novel, multitargeted tyrosine kinase inhibitor for the potential treatment of t(4;14) multiple myeloma. Blood. 2005;105:2941–2948.

18. Santra M, Zhan F, Tian E, et al. A subset of multiple myeloma harboring the t(4;14) (p16;q32) translocation lacks FGFR3 expression but maintains an lgH/MMSET fusion transcript. Blood. 2003;101:2374–2376.

19. Dring AM, Davies FE, Fenton JA, et al. A global expression-based analysis of the consequences of the t(4;14) translocation in myeloma. Clin Cancer Res. 2004;10: 5692–5701.

20. Chang H, Stewart AK, Ying-Qi X, et al. Immunohistochemistry accurately predicts FGFR3 aberrant expression and t(4;14) in multiple myeloma. Blood. 2005;106:353–355.

21. Passos-Bueno MR, Wilcox JR, Jabs EW, et al. Clinical spectrum of fibroblast growth factor receptor mutations. Hum Mutat. 1999;14:115–125.

22. Boersma-Vreugdenhil GR, Kuipers J, Van Stralen E, et al. The recurrent translocation t(14;20) (q32;q12) in multiple myeloma results in aberrant expression of MAFB: a molecular and genetic analysis of the chromosomal breakpoint. Br J Haematol. 2004;126:355–363.

23. Smadja NV, Leroux D, Soulier J, et al. Further cytogenetic characterization of multiple myeloma confirms that 14q32 translocations are a very rare event in hyperdiploid cases. Genes Chromosomes Cancer. 2003;38:234–239.

24. Malgeri U, Baldini L, Perfetti V, et al. Detection of t(4;14) (p16.3;q32) chromosomal translocation in multiple myeloma by reverse transcription polymerase chain reaction analysis of lgH-MMSET fusion transcripts. Cancer Res. 2000;60:4058–4061.

25. Fabris S, Agnelli L, Mattioli M, et al. Characterization of oncogene dysregulation in multiple myeloma by combined FISH and DNA microarray analyses. Genes Chromosomes Cancer. 2005;42:117–127.

26. Keats JJ, Reiman T, Belch AR, et al. Ten years and counting: so what do we know about t(4;14) (p16;q32) multiple myeloma. Leuk Lymphoma. 2006;47:2289–2300.

27. Webster MK and Donoghue DJ. FGFR activation in skeletal disorders: too much of a good thing. Trends Genet. 1997;13:178–182.

28. Ishikawa H, Tsuyama N, Liu S, et al. Accelerated proliferation of myeloma cells by interleukin-6 cooperating with fibroblast growth factor receptor 3-mediated signals. Oncogene. 2005;24(41):6328–6332.

29. Firme L and Bush AB. FGF signaling inhibits the proliferation of human myeloma cells and reduces c-myc expression. BMC Cell Biol. 2003;4:17.

30. Sleeman M, Fraser J, McDonald M, et al. Identification of a new fibroblast growth factor receptor, FGFR5. Gene. 2001;271:171–182.

31. Elsheikh E, Green AR, Lambros MB, et al . FGFR1 amplification in breast carcinomas: a chromogenic in situ hybridisation analysis. Breast Cancer Res. 2007;9(2):R23.

32. Hernadez S, Toll A, Baselga E, et al. Fibroblast growth factor receptor 3 mutations in epidermal nevi and associated low grade bladder tumors. J Invest Dermatol. 2007;127(7):1664–1666.

33. Patstone G, Pasquale EB and Maher PA. Different members of the fibroblast growth factor receptor family are specific to distinct cell types in the developing chicken embryo. Dev Biol. 1993;155:107–123.

34. Vidrich A, Buzan JM, Lb C, et al. Fibroblast growth factor receptor-3 is expressed in undifferentiated intestinal epithelial cells during murine crypt morphogenesis. Dev Dyn. 2004;230:114–123.

35. Chellaiah AT, McEwen DG, Werner S, et al. Fibroblast growth factor receptor (FGFR) 3. Alternative splicing in immunoglobulin-like domain Ill creates a receptor highly specific for acidic FGF/FGF-1. J Biol Chem. 1994;269:11620–11627.

36. Pringle NP, Yu WP, Howell M, et al. Fgfr3 expression by astrocytes and their precursors: evidence that astrocytes and oligodendrocytes originate in distinct neuroepithelial domains. Development. 2003;130:93–102.

37. Peters K, Ornitz D, Werner S and Williams L. Unique expression pattern of the FGF receptor 3 gene during mouse organogenesis. Dev Biol. 1993;155:423–430.

38. Govindarajan V and Overbeek PA. Secreted FGFR3, but not FGFR1, inhibits lens fiber differentiation. Development. 2001;128:1617–1627.

39. Deng C, Wynshaw-Boris A, Zhou F, et al. Fibroblast growth factor receptor 3 is a negative regulator of bone growth. Cell. 1996;84:911–921.

40. Richelda R, Ronchetti D, Baldini L, et al. A novel chromosomal translocation t(4;14) (p16.3;q32) in multiple myeloma involves the fibroblast growth factor receptor 3 gene. Blood. 1997;90:4062–4070.

41. Cappeflen D, De Oliveira C, Ricol D, et al. Frequent activating mutations of FGFR3 in human bladder and cervix carcinomas. Nat Genet. 1999;23:18–20.

42. Hata H. Bone lesions and macrophage inflammatory protein-1 alpha (MIP-1a) in human multiple myeloma. Leuk Lymphoma. 2005;46:967–972.

43. Jang H, Shin KH and Park JG. Mutations in fibroblast growth factor receptor 2 and fibroblast growth factor receptor 3 genes associated with human gastric and colorectal cancers. Cancer Res. 2001;65:3541–3543.

44. Naimi B, Latil A, Berthon P and Cussenot O. No evidence for fibroblast growth factor receptor 3 (FGFR-3) R248C/S249C mutations in human prostate cancer. Int J Cancer. 2000;87:455–456.

45. Karoui M, Hofmann-Radvanyi H, Zimmermann U, et al. No evidence of somatic FGFR3 mutation in various types of carcinoma. Oncogene. 2001;20:5059–5061.

46. Sibley K, Stern P and Knowles MA Frequency of fibroblast growth factor receptor 3 mutations in sporadic tumours. Oncogene. 2001;20:4416–4418.

47. Avet-Loiseau H, Facon T, Daviet A, et al. 14q32 translocations and monosomy 13 observed in monoclonal gammopathy of undetermined significance delineate a multistep process for the oncogenesis of multiple myeloma. lntergroupe Francophone du Myelome. Cancer Res. 1999;59:4546–4550.

48. Sibley K, Fenton JA, Dring AM, et al. A molecular study of the t(4;14) in multiple myeloma. Br J Haematol. 2002;118:514–520.

49. Soverini S, Terragna C, Testoni N, et al. Novel mutation and RNA splice variant of fibroblast growth factor receptor 3 in multiple myeloma patients at diagnosis. Haematologica. 2002;87:1036–1040.

50. Onwuazor ON, Wen XY, Wang DY, et al. Mutation, SNP, and isoform analysis of fibroblast growth factor receptor 3 (FGFR3) in 150 newly diagnosed multiple myeloma patients. Blood. 2003;102:772–773.

51. Chesi M, Brents LA, Ely SA, et al. Activated fibroblast growth factor receptor 3 is an oncogene that contributes to tumor progression in multiple myeloma. Blood. 2001;98:1271–1272.

52. Li Z, Zhu YX, Plowright EE, et al. The myeloma-associated oncogene fibroblast growth factor receptor 3 is transforming in hematopoietic cells. Blood. 2001;97:2413–2419.

53. Chandesris MO, Soulier J, Labaume S, et al. Detection and follow-up of fibroblast growth factor receptor 3 expression on bone marrow and circulating plasma cells by flow cytometry in patients with t(4;14) multiple myeloma. Br J Haematol. 2007;36(4):609–614.

54. Masih-Khan E, Trudel S, Heise C, et al. MIP-lalpha (CCL3) is a downstream target of FGFR3 signalling in multiple myeloma. Blood. 2006;108(10): 3465–3471.

55. Roodman GD and Choi SJ. MIP-1 alpha and myeloma bone disease. Cancer Treat Res. 2004;118:83–100.

56. Terpos E, Politou M, Szydlo R, Goldman JM, Apperley JF and Rahemtulla A. Serum levels of macrophage inflammatory protein-1 alpha (MIP-l alpha) correlate with the extent of bone disease and survival in patients with multiple myeloma. Br J Haematol. 2003;123:106–109.

57. Lentzsch S, Chatterjee M, Gries M, et al. P13-K'AKT/FKHR and MAPK signaling cascades are redundantly stimulated by a variety of cytokines and contribute independently to proliferation and survival of multiple myeloma cells. Leukemia. 2004;18:1883–1890.

58. Zhu L, Somlo G, Zhou B, et al. Fibroblast growth factor receptor 3 inhibition by short hairpin RNAs leads to apoptosis in multiple myeloma. Mol Cancer Ther. 2005;4:787–798.

59. Lossos IS, Czerwinski DK, Alizadeh AA, et al. Prediction of survival in diffuse large-B-cell lymphoma based on the expression of six genes. N Engl J Med. 2004;350:1828–1837.

60. Kuehl WM and Bergsagel PL. Multiple myeloma: evolving genetic events and host interactions. Nat Rev Cancer. 2002;2:175–187.

61. Fonseca R, Barlogie B,Bataille R, et al. Genetics and cytogenetics of multiple myeloma: a workshop report. Cancer Res. 2004;64:1546–1558.

62. Bergsaget PL, Kuehl WM, Zhan F, et al. Cyclin D dysregulation: an early unifying pathogenic event in multiple myeloma. Blood. 2005;106:296–303.

63. Poulsen TS, Silahtaroglu AN, Gisselo CG, et al. Detection of illegitimate rearrangements within the immunoglobulin light chain loci in B cell malignancies using end sequenced probes. Leukemia. 2002;16:2148–2155.

64. Cavo M, Terragna C, Renzulli M, et al. Poor outcome with front-line autologous transplantation in t(4;14) multiple myeloma: low complete remission rate and short duration of remission. J Clin Oncol. 2006Jan 20;24(3):e4–e5.

65. Mulligan G, Mitsiades C, Bryant B, et al. Gene expression profiling and correlation with outcome in clinical trials of the proteasome inhibitor bortezomib. Blood. 2007;109:3177–3188.

66. Moreau P, Attal M, Garban F, et al. Heterogeneity of t(4;14) in multiple myeloma. Long-term follow-up of 100 cases treated with tandem transplantation in IFM99 trials. Leukemia. 2007 July 12; [Epub ahead of print].

67. Jaksic W, Trudel S,Chang H, et al. Clinical outcomes in t(4;14) multiple myeloma: a chemotherapy-sensitive disease characterized by rapid relapse and alkylating agent resistance. J Clin Oncol. 2005 Oct 1;23(28):7069–7073.

68. Gutierrez NC, Castellanos MV, MartIn ML, et al. Prognostic implications of genetic abnormalities in multiple myeloma undergoing autologous stem cell transplantation: t(4;14) is the most relevant adverse prognostic factor, whereas RB deletion as a unique abnormality is not associated with adverse prognosis. Leukemia. 2007;21:143–150.

69. Gertz MA, Lacy MQ, Dispenzieri A, et al. Clinical implications of t(11;14) (q13;q32), t(4;14) (p16.2,q32), and -17p13 in myeloma patients treated with high-dose therapy. Blood. 2005;106:2837–2840.

70. Avet-Loiseau H, Attal M, Moreau P, et al. Genetic abnormalities and survival in multiple myeloma: the experience of the Intergroupe Francophone du Myelome. Blood. 2007 Apr 15;109(8):3489–3495.

71. Chang H, Tribu Y, Qi X, et al. Bortezomib therapy response is independent of cytogenetic abnormalities in relapsed/refractory multiple myeloma. Leuk Res. 2006 Sep 20; [Epub ahead of print].

72. Mateos MV, Hernández JM, Hernández MT, et al. Bortezomib plus melphalan and prednisone in elderly untreated patients with multiple myeloma: results of a multi-center phase I/II study. Blood. 2006;108:2165–2172.

73. Bahlis NJ, Mansoor A, Lategan JC, et al. Lenalidomide overcomes poor prognosis conferred by deletion of chromosome 13 and t(4;14) in multiple myeloma: MMOI6 Trial. Blood. 2006;108:(Abstract).

74. Grand EK, Chase AJ, Heath C, et al. Targeting FGFR3 in multiple myeloma: inhibition of t(4;14)-positive cells by SU5402 and PD173074. Leukemia. 2004;18:962–966.

75. Trudel S, Stewart AK, Rom E, et al. The inhibitory anti-FGFR3 antibody, PRO-001, is cytotoxic to t(4;14) multiple myeloma cells. Blood. 2006 May 15;107(10):4039–4046.

76. Andrejauskas-Buchdunger E and Regenass U. Differential inhibition of the epidermal growth factor-, platelet-derived growth factor-, and protein kinase C-mediated signal transduction pathways by the staurosporine derivative CGP 41251. Cancer Res. 1992;52(19):5353–5358.

77. Fabbro D, Ruetz S, Bodis S, et al. PKC412—a protein kinase inhibitor with a broad therapeutic potential. Anticancer Drug Des. 2000;15:17–28.

78. Weisberg E, Boulton C, Kelly LM, et al. Inhibition of mutant FLT3 receptors in leukemia cells by the small molecule tyrosine kinase inhibitor PKC4I 2. Cancer Cell. 2002;1:433–443.

79. Estey EH, Fisher T, Giles F, et al. Effect of circulating blasts at time of complete remission on subsequent relapse-free survival time in newly diagnosed AML. Blood. 2003;102:3097–3099.

80. Stone RM, DeAngelo DJ, KIlmek V, et al. Patients with acute myeloid leukemia and an activating mutation in FLT3 respond to a small-molecule FLT3 tyrosine kinase inhibitor, PKC412. Blood. 2005 Jan 1;105(1):54–60.

81. Chen J, DeAngelo DJ, Kutok JL, et al. PKC412 inhibits the zinc finger 198-fibroblast growth factor receptor 1 fusion tyrosine kinase and is active in treatment of stem cell myeloproliferative disorder. Proc Natl Acad Sci USA. 2004;101:14479–14484.

82. Chen J, Lee BH, Williams IR, et al. FGFR3 as a therapeutic target of the small molecule inhibitor PKC4I2 in hematopoietic malignancies. Oncogene. 2005 Dec 15; 24(56):8259–8267.

83. Dewald GW, Therneau T, Larson D, Relationship of patient survival and chromosome anomalies detected in metaphase and/or interphase cells at diagnosis of myeloma. Blood. 2005 Nov 15; 106(10):3553–3558.

84. Chiecchio L, Protheroe RK, Ibrahim AH, Deletion of chromosome 13 detected by conventional cytogenetics is a critical prognostic factor in myeloma. Leukemia. 2006 Sep; 20(9):1610–1617.

85. Nakazawa N, Nishida K, Tamura A, Interphase detection of t(4;14) (p16.3;q32) by in situ hybridization and FGFR3 overexpression in plasma cell malignancies. Cancer Genet Cytogenet. 2000;117:89–96.

86. Rasmussen T, Theligaard-Monch K, Hudlebusch HR, Occurrence of dysregulated oncogenes in primary plasma cells representing consecutive stages of myeloma pathogenesis: indications for different disease entities. Br J Haematol. 2003; 123:253–262.

Chapter 24

Histone Deacetylase Inhibitors in Multiple Myeloma

Teru Hideshima

Histones and Histone Decaetylases

Histones are the main protein components of chromatin and have been found in the nuclei of all eukaryotic cells where they are complexed to DNA in chromatin and chromosomes. Histones are of relatively low molecular weight (10–20 kD) and can be grouped into five major classes. Two copies of H2A, H2B, H3, and H4 bind to about 200 base pairs of DNA to form the repeating structure of chromatin, the nucleosome, with H1 binding to the linker sequence. During transcription, the transcription factors have to bind to their specific binding site in the promoter region of DNA. When the DNA is in compact form, it is often difficult for proteins to access DNA, thereby limiting transcription. In contrast, when DNA is bundled into chromosomes, histones play a major role in restricting the binding of transcription factors to DNA. In activation of histones, the acetylation status of amino-terminus is crucial in their binding process to DNA. It is regulated by the balance of activities of two key enzymes, histone acetyltransferase (HAT) and histone deacetylase (HDAC).

HDACs, depending on sequence identity and domain organization, are divided into four classes. In class I, HDAC1, 2, 3, and 8; in class II, HDAC 4, 5, 6, 7, 9, and 10; in class III, SIR1, 2, 3, 4, 5, 6, and 7; and in class IV, HDAC11 (Table 1). Importantly, class I and IV HDACs are constitutively localized in the nucleus, whereas class II HDACs can shuttle between the nucleus and the cytoplasm interacting with 14-3-3 protein[1,2] (Fig. 1). In general, class I HDACs are widely expressed, whereas class II and IV HDACs show various degrees of tissue specificity. HDACs catalyze the removal of the acetyl modification on lysine residues of proteins, including the core nucleosomal histones H2A, H2B, H3, and H4. Hypoacetylation of histones is associated with a condensed chromatin structure resulting in the repression of gene transcription, whereas acetylated histones are associated with a more open chromatin structure and activation of transcription. Therefore, histone acetyltransferases allow transcription to occur, whereas HDACs prevent transcription. HDAC inhibitors therefore trigger transcription (Fig. 1). In addition to histones, other acetylated proteins have also been shown to be substrates for the HDACs.

From: *Contemporary Hematology Myeloma Therapy*
Edited by: S. Lonial © Humana Press, Totowa, NJ

Table 1 Classification of histone deacetylase.

Class I	Class II	Class III[a]	Class IV
HDAC1	HDAC4	SIRT1	HDAC11
HDAC2	HDAC5	SIRT2	
HDAC3	HDAC6	SIRT3	
HDAC8	HDAC7	SIRT4	
	HDAC9	SIRT5	
	HDAC10	SIRT6	
		SIRT7	

HDCA histone deacetylase
[a] Class III HDACS are homologues of the yeast protein SIR2

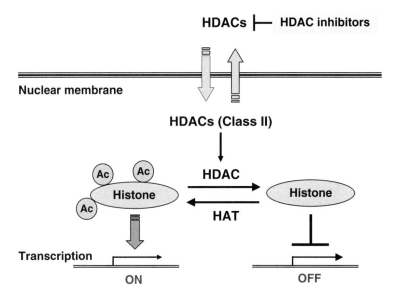

Fig. 1 Among histone deacetylases (HDACs), only class II HDACs can shuttle between cytoplasm and nucleus. HDAC inhibitors block HDACs activity, thereby accumulating acetylated histones, which facilitates transcriptional activity (*see* Plate 5).

HDAC Inhibitors

HDAC inhibitors are members of novel class of antitumor agents for malignancies, and a large number of structurally diverse HDAC inhibitors have been purified from natural sources or synthetically developed. HDAC inhibitors can be divided into six classes based on their chemical structure. These classes are short-chain fatty acid, hydroxamate, benzamide, cyclic tetrapeptide, electrophilic ketone, and others[3] (Table 2). Accumulated histone acetylation by HDAC inhibitors attenuates their electrostatic interaction with the negatively charged DNA backbone, promoting the unfolding of histone–DNA complex, thereby modulating access of transcription factors to their binding sites of action and transcription of their target genes.[4–6] Previous studies have shown that deletions or inactivating mutations of histone acetyltransferases which decrease histone acetylation are involved in the development of human neoplasms.[7,8] In contrast, inhibition of HDAC activity triggers growth arrest and/or apoptosis of tumor

Table 2 HDAC Inhibitors in clinical trials.

Compound	Clinical trial
Short-chain fatty acid	
Butylate	I, II
Valporoic acid	I, II
AN-9	I, II
Hydroxamate	
SAHA	I, II, III
PXD101	I
LAQ824	I
LBH589	I
Pyroxamide	I
Benzamide	
MS-275	I, II
CI-994	I, II, III
Cyclic peptide	
Depsipeptide	I, II
Others	
MGCD-0103	I

HDAC histone deacetylase, SAHA suberoylanilide hydroxamic acid

cells. Although possible mechanisms of action of HDAC inhibitor for antitumor activities have recently been comprehensively described by Bolden et al.,[3] their mechanisms of action in growth inhibitory effects in multiple myeloma (MM) cells have not yet been fully characterized.

As described above, inhibition of histone deacetylation triggers gene transcription, and HDAC inhibitors therefore could induce transcription of both positive and negative regulators of cell proliferation/survival. In other words, the cytotoxicity/growth inhibition induced by HDAC is the result of relative imbalance of downregulation of prosurvival factors and upregulation of proapoptotic (tumor suppressive) factors. However, many reports have demonstrated that upregulation of histone acetylation in tumor cells predominantly causes growth inhibition and/or apoptosis, and many HDAC inhibitors are currently under evaluation in clinical trials in different types of cancers (Table 2).

Suberoylanilide Hydroxamic Acid

Suberoylanilide hydroxamic acid (SAHA), a class I, II HDAC inhibitor, has been extensively studied for its antitumor activities in many types of cancers. SAHA directly interacts with the catalytic site of HDAC-like protein and inhibits its enzymatic activity. Inhibition of HDAC activity by SAHA results in alteration of gene expression in various cell lines, including MM.[9] Like other HDAC inhibitors,[10–14] SAHA also increases p21^{WAF1} expression,[15,16] thereby inhibiting tumor cell growth.

In MM, SAHA modulates gene expression and inhibits tumor cell growth at low micromolar concentrations.[9,17] It induces upregulation of p21^{WAF1} and p53 protein expression, as well as dephosphorylation of Rb followed by apoptosis. Importantly, upregulation of p21^{WAF1} occurs prior to p53 induction, suggesting that p21^{WAF1} upregulation is independent of p53 activity.[9] SAHA-induced apoptosis in MM cells is associated with

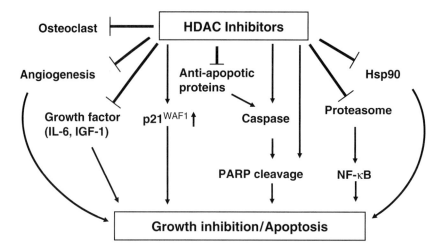

Fig. 2 Molecular mechanisms of action of histone deacetylase inhibitors. Histone deacetylase inhibitors induce upregulation of p21^{WAF1}; trigger apoptosis via caspase-dependent and/or -independent pathway; inhibit effects of growth factors (i.e., IL-6, IGF-1); inhibit angiogenesis; downregulate proteasome activity; and block osteoclastogenesis.

Bcl-2 interacting protein Bid; conversely, overexpression of Bcl-2 abrogates SAHA-induced apoptosis, suggesting that Bcl-2 plays a crucial role in regulating SAHA-induced apoptosis in MM cells. Interestingly, SAHA does not trigger caspase activation, and the caspase inhibitor does not protect against SAHA-induced cytotoxicity. However, poly(ADP)ribose polymerase (PARP) is significantly cleaved by SAHA, suggesting that SAHA triggers atypical PARP cleavage in MM cells.[9] SAHA enhances the anti-MM activity of other proapoptotic agents including dexamethasone, cytotoxic chemotherapy, and thalidomide analogues. Importantly, SAHA suppresses the expression and activity of the proteasome and its subunits, providing the rationale for its use in combination with bortezomib to enhance cytotoxicity.[17] It has also been shown that SAHA enhances tumour necrosis factor-related apoptosis-inducing ligand (TRAIL)-induced cytotoxicity associated with upregulation of the proapoptotic proteins (Bim, Bak, Bax, Noxa, and PUMA) and downregulation of antiapoptotic proteins (Bcl-2 and Bcl-xL)[18] (Fig. 2).

Clinical trials of SAHA in different type of malignancies have been published.[19–22] In these studies, the maximum concentration of SAHA in plasma (C^{max}) was 1631–1649 ng/ml and 2339–2963 ng/ml after 150 mg/m^2 and 300 mg/m^2 administration, respectively.[19] The maximum tolerated dose (MTD) of SAHA in patients with solid tumors and hematologic malignancies treated with oral SAHA was 400 mg once a day and 200 mg twice a day for continuous daily dosing, respectively, and 300 mg twice a day for three consecutive days per week. The major dose-limiting toxicities (DLTs) were anorexia, dehydration, diarrhea, and fatigue.[20] The most common grade 3 or 4 adverse affects were thrombocytopenia and dehydration, and the 400 mg daily regimen has the most favorable safety profile.[22] In MM, a phase I clinical trial of SAHA is ongoing.

MVP-LAQ824 (LAQ824)

LAQ824 is a member of hydroxamate HDAC inhibitor which blocks class I and II HDAC activity. LAQ824 blocks HDAC activity with an IC50 of 32 nM and inhibits proliferation of cancer cell lines with IC50s of 10–150 nM ranges in vitro, indicating that antiproliferative potency of LAQ824 is up to 200-fold higher than that of SAHA.[23,24] Antitumor activity of LAQ824 has been extensively studied in leukemia cells. It downregulates human enhancer of zeste 2 (EZH2) protein, which belongs to the multiprotein polycomb repressive complex 2 and embryonic ectoderm development,[25] as well as antiapoptotic proteins (Bcl-2, Bcl-xL, XIAP).[26,27] LAQ is also effective in an in vivo mouse model; however, BCR/ABL kinase activity may not be a direct target of NVP-LAQ824.[28] Interestingly, NVP-LAQ824 inhibited angiogenesis, associated with downregulation of angiogenesis-related genes such as angiopoietin-2, Tie-2, and survivin in endothelial cells.[14]

LAQ824 induces apoptosis at IC50 of 100 nM at 24 h in most MM cell lines and patient tumor cells. Importantly, LAQ824 is effective in cells which are resistant to conventional therapies (dexamethasone, doxorubicin, melphalan). Paracrine MM cell proliferation in the presence of BMSCs is also inhibited by LAQ824. Moreover, LAQ824 inhibits cell growth in vivo in a preclinical murine myeloma model. Unlike SAHA, LAQ824-induced apoptosis is associated with caspase activation.[29]

LBH589

LBH589 is also a hydroxamic acid analogue which blocks class I and II HDAC activity. LBH589 has been studied in many malignancies as a single agent, as well as combined with other anticancer agents.[30–33] LBH589 has been shown to inhibit angiogenesis in vitro.[34] Molecular mechanisms of LBH589 triggering cytotoxicity are similar to LAQ824; however, one distinct feature of LBH589 is its inhibitory effect of HDAC6 activity. HDAC6 is a member of class II HDAC and, unlike other HDACs, it has potent tubulin, but not HDAC, activity.[35] HDAC6 has been shown to play a crucial role in the aggresome/autophagy protein degradation system[36] (please see below in the "Tubacin" section). Importantly, recent studies have also shown that inhibition of HDAC6 by LBH589 leads to acetylation of heat shock protein 90 and disruption of its chaperone function, resulting in polyubiquitylation and depletion of progrowth and prosurvival heat shock protein 90 client proteins.[37] Therefore, inhibition of HDAC6 by LBH589 may indicate significant biologic sequelae in tumor cells.

In MM, LBH589 blocks cell cycle progression associated with upregulation of p21[WAF1], p53, and p57. LBH589 also induces cytotoxicity through an increase in mitochondrial outer membrane permeability.[38] The IC50 of LBH589 is 40–80 nM in most MM cell lines, including those resistant cells to conventional therapeutic agents,[38,39] associated with caspase/PARP cleavage. Interestingly, LBH589 triggers a caspase-independent apoptotic pathway through the release of AIF from mitochondria.[38] Importantly, synergistic cytotoxicity against MM cells is observed with LBH589 in combination with bortezomib[39] (Fig. 3). Based on preclinical studies, an international multicenter clinical trial of LBH589 with bortezomib in MM has just begun.

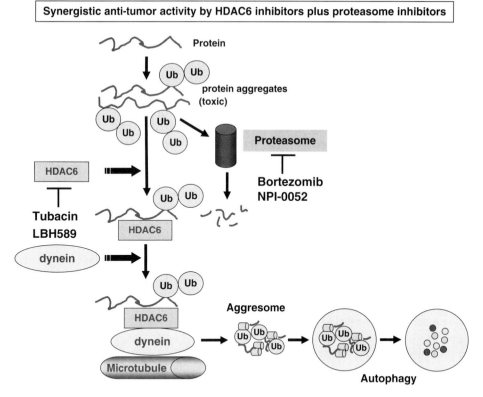

Fig. 3 Possible ubiquitinated protein catabolism in tumor cells and rationale for combination treatment of HDAC6 inhibitors with proteasome inhibitors. Misfolded proteins become polyubiquitinated and normally degraded by proteasomes. However, misfolded proteins can escape degradation due to abnormal or pathological conditions and form toxic aggregates. These misfolded and aggregated proteins are recognized and bound by HDAC6 through the presence of polyubiquitin chains. This allows for the loading of polyubiquitinated misfolded protein cargo onto the dynein motor complex by HDAC6. The polyubiquitinated cargo-HDAC6-dynein motor complex then travels to the aggresome, where the misfolded and aggregated proteins are processed and degraded, clearing the cell of cytotoxic protein aggregates. Inhibition of both proteasomal and aggresomal protein degradation pathway by bortezomib/NPI0052 and tubacin/LBH589, respectively, induces endoplasmic reticulum stress, followed by synergistic cytotoxicity. *HDAC* histone deacetylase (*see* Plate 6).

Depsipeptide (FR901228, FK228)

Depsipeptide is a natural (isolated from *Chromobacterium violaceum*) or synthetic compound with sequences of amino and hydroxy carboxylic acid residues. Depsipeptide is in a class of cyclic tetrapeptide and inhibits only class I HDAC activity.[40] A number of studies of antitumor activities of depsipeptide in various types of cancer have already been reported.[41–47] These studies show that depsipeptide induces apoptosis, associated with caspase activation associated with downregulation of Bcl-2 and Bcl-xL mRNA, through de novo protein synthesis, and thereby suppressing the expression of Bcl-2 and Bcl-xL proteins.[42] In MM, depsipeptide induces apoptosis in MM cell lines and in primary patient tumor cells, associated with downregulation of Bcl-2, Bcl-xL, and Mcl-1 expression.[48]

Clinical trials of depsipeptide for different cancer types have been reported.[49–53] In a phase I study, depsipeptide was administrated by a 4-h intravenous infusion on days 1 and 5 of a 21-day cycle. The starting dose was 1 mg/m^2, and dose escalations proceeded through a total of eight dose levels to a maximum of 24.9 mg/m^2. The MTD of depsipeptide given on a day 1 and 5 schedule every 21 days is 17.8 mg/m^2. The DLTs are fatigue, nausea, vomiting, transient thrombocytopenia, and neutropenia. Although cardiac toxicity was a potential concern based on preclinical data, there was no clinical toxicity.[49] Similar results were also reported from phase I study in which MTD was defined as 13.3 mg/m^2, with DLTs being grade 3 thrombocytopenia and fatigue.[50] In a phase II trial in renal cell cancer, patients received 13 mg/m^2 of depsipeptide intravenously on days 1, 8, and 15 of a 28-day cycle, and overall response rate was 7%.[53] Interestingly, multidrug-resistance gene 1 level was up to a sixfold increase in normal peripheral blood mononuclear cells and up to a eightfold increase in circulating tumor cells after depsipeptide administration providing the basis for clinical trials evaluating depsipeptide in combination with a P-glycoprotein inhibitors.[52] A phase II clinical trial of FR901228 for relapsed refractory MM is ongoing.

PXD101

PXD101 is a hydroxamate class HDAC inhibitor[54] which demonstrates broad antitumor activity in vitro and in vivo.[54,55] PXD101 has antiproliferative activity in MM cell lines, and shows additive and/or synergistic effects with conventional agents used in MM. PXD101 is being tested as monotherapy and also in combination with standard agents for treatment of MM. In a phase II trial, PXD101 was administered intravenously on days 1–5 of a 3-week cycle at a dose of 1,000 mg/m^2/day (900 mg/m^2/day in earlier patients). Among 24 enrolled patients, 1 patient had a minimal response (duration 6 weeks) and 5 patients had stable disease.[56]

MS-275

MS-275 belongs to the benzamide class and inhibits class I and II HDACs. MS-275 shows antitumor activity in various types of cancers both in vitro and in vivo.[57–61] Like other HDAC inhibitors, MS-275 induces caspase-dependent apoptosis, associated with downregulation of Bcl-2 in chronic lymphocytic leukemia cells in vitro.[62] MS-275 synergistically enhances the cytotoxicity induced by proteasome inhibitor NPI-0052[63] or fludarabine[60] in vitro. Clinical trials of MS-275 have also been reported.[64,65] In these studies, the MTD was 10 mg/m^2 in patients treated with MS-275 orally, initially on a once daily × 28 every-6-weeks (daily) and later on once every-14-days (q14-day) schedules. The DLTs were nausea, vomiting, anorexia, and fatigue.[65]

Tubacin

Tubacin is a hydroxamic acid HDAC inhibitor; however, it specifically inhibits only HDAC6 activity.[35] Previous studies have characterized the aggresome as an alternative system to the proteasome for degradation of polyubiquitinated misfolded/unfolded proteins. The aggresome pathway therefore likely provides a novel system for delivery of aggregated proteins from cytoplasm to lysosomes for degradation.[66] In this aggresomal protein degradation pathway, HDAC6 has an essential role, since it can bind both polyubiquitinated proteins and dynein motors, thereby acting to recruit protein cargo to dynein motors for transport to aggresomes.[36] We have demonstrated that blockade of both proteasomal and aggresomal protein degradation by their specific inhibitors bortezomib and tubacin, respectively, synergistically enhances cytotoxicity in MM cells in vitro[67] (Fig. 3); however, in vivo activity of tubacin is not yet defined.

Other HDAC Inhibitors

KD5170 is a nonhydroxamate, orally bioavailable HDAC inhibitor which significantly inhibits osteoclast formation at lower micromolar range and triggers apoptosis in MM cells.[68] Suberoyl-3-aminopyridineamide hydroxamic acid (pyroxamide) belongs to the hydroxamate class and has shown its antitumor activities against prostate cancer and rhabdomyosarcoma in vitro.[69,70] CI-994 is a substituted benzamide derivative that has demonstrated significant antitumor activity in vitro and in vivo in a broad spectrum of tumor models.[71–74] Although CI-994 (*N*-acetyldinaline) is a pan-HDAC inhibitor, its specificity and molecular mechanisms whereby it induced cytotoxicity in tumor cells are unclear.

Future Direction

Although HDAC inhibitors demonstrate significant antitumor activities with minimal toxicity to normal cells as single agents, their cytotoxicity can be enhanced by combination with other agents. In MM, HDAC inhibitors can be combined with conventional therapeutic agents. For example, dexamethasone enhances LAQ824-induced cytotoxicity in MM[29] since LAQ824 triggers extrinsic (caspase-8)-dependent apoptosis, whereas dexamethasone triggers intrinsic (caspase-9)-dependent apoptosis; combining these agents induces dual apoptotic signaling cascades. The other rationally based combination treatment option is HDAC inhibitors and proteasome inhibitors.[38,63,75–78] Synergistic antitumor activity of SAHA plus bortezomib[9] and LAQ824 plus bortezomib[29] has been reported in MM.

References

1. Verdin, E., Dequiedt, F., and Kasler, H. G. Class II histone deacetylases: Versatile regulators. Trends Genet, *19*: 286–293, 2003.
2. Minucci, S. and Pelicci, P. G. Histone deacetylase inhibitors and the promise of epigenetic (and more) treatments for cancer. Nat Rev Cancer, *6*: 38–51, 2006.
3. Bolden, J. E., Peart, M. J., and Johnstone, R. W. Anticancer activities of histone deacetylase inhibitors. Nat Rev Drug Discov, *5*: 769–784, 2006.
4. Finnin, M. S., Donigian, J. R., Cohen, A., Richon, V. M., Rifkind, R. A.., Marks, P. A., Breslow, R., and Pavletich, N. P., Structures of a histone deacetylase homologue bound to the TSA and SAHA inhibitors. Nature, *401*: 188–1893, 1999.
5. Marks, P. A. and Jiang, X. Histone deacetylase inhibitors in programmed cell death and cancer therapy. Cell Cycle, *4*: 549–551, 2005.

6. Marks, P. A. and Dokmanovic, M. Histone deacetylase inhibitors: Discovery and development as anticancer agents. Expert Opin Investig Drugs, *14*: 1497–1511, 2005.

7. Lin, R. J., Nagy, L., Inoue, S., Shao, W., Miller, W. H., Jr., and Evans, R. M. Role of the histone deacetylase complex in acute promyelocytic leukaemia. Nature, *391*: 811–814, 1998.

8. Marks, P., Rifkind, R. A., Richon, V. M., Breslow, R., Miller, T., and Kelly, W. K. Histone deacetylases and cancer: Causes and therapies. Nat Rev Cancer, *1*: 194–202, 2001.

9. Mitsiades, N., Mitsiades, C. S., Richardson, P. G., McMullan, C., Poulaki, V., Fanourakis, G., Schlossman, R., Chauhan, D., Munshi, N. C., Hideshima, T., Richon, V. M., Marks, P. A., and Anderson, K. C. Molecular sequelae of histone deacetylase inhibition in human malignant B cells. Blood, *101*: 4055–4062, 2003.

10. Sowa, Y., Orita, T., Minamikawa, S., Nakano, K., Mizuno, T., Nomura, H., and Sakai, T. Histone deacetylase inhibitor activates the WAF1/Cip1 gene promoter through the Sp1 sites. Biochem Biophys Res Commun, *241*: 142–150, 1997.

11. Archer, S. Y., Meng, S., Shei, A., and Hodin, R. A. p21(WAF1) is required for butyrate-mediated growth inhibition of human colon cancer cells. Proc Natl Acad Sci USA, *95*: 6791–6796, 1998.

12. Sandor, V., Senderowicz, A., Mertins, S., Sackett, D., Sausville, E., Blagosklonny, M. V., and Bates, S. E. P21-dependent g(1)arrest with downregulation of cyclin D1 and upregulation of cyclin E by the histone deacetylase inhibitor FR901228. Br J Cancer, *83*: 817–825, 2000.

13. Burgess, A. J., Pavey, S., Warrener, R., Hunter, L. J., Piva, T. J., Musgrove, E. A., Saunders, N., Parsons, P. G., and Gabrielli, B. G. Up-regulation of p21(WAF1/CIP1) by histone deacetylase inhibitors reduces their cytotoxicity. Mol Pharmacol, *60*: 828–837, 2001.

14. Qian, D. Z., Wang, X., Kachhap, S. K., Kato, Y., Wei, Y., Zhang, L., Atadja, P., and Pili, R. The histone deacetylase inhibitor NVP-LAQ824 inhibits angiogenesis and has a greater antitumor effect in combination with the vascular endothelial growth factor receptor tyrosine kinase inhibitor PTK787/ZK222584. Cancer Res, *64*: 6626–6634, 2004.

15. Huang, L., Sowa, Y., Sakai, T., and Pardee, A. B. Activation of the p21WAF1/CIP1 promoter independent of p53 by the histone deacetylase inhibitor suberoy-lanilide hydroxamic acid (SAHA) through the Sp1 sites. Oncogene, *19*: 5712–5719, 2000.

16. Richon, V. M., Sandhoff, T. W., Rifkind, R. A., and Marks, P. A. Histone deacety-lase inhibitor selectively induces p21WAF1 expression and gene-associated histone acetylation. Proc Natl Acad Sci U S A, *97*: 10014–10019, 2000.

17. Mitsiades, C. S., Mitsiades, N. S., McMullan, C. J., Poulaki, V., Shringarpure, R., Hideshima, T., Akiyama, M., Chauhan, D., Munshi, N., Gu, X., Bailey, C., Joseph, M., Libermann, T. A., Richon, V. M., Marks, P. A., and Anderson, K. C. Transcriptional signature of histone deacetylase inhibition in multiple myeloma: Biological and clini-cal implications. Proc Natl Acad Sci USA, *101*: 540–545, 2004.

18. Fandy, T. E., Shankar, S., Ross, D. D., Sausville, E., and Srivastava, R. K. Interactive effects of HDAC inhibitors and TRAIL on apoptosis are associated with changes in mitochondrial functions and expressions of cell cycle regulatory genes in multiple myeloma. Neoplasia, *7*: 646–657, 2005.

19. Kelly, W. K., Richon, V. M., O'Connor, O., Curley, T., MacGregor-Curtelli, B., Tong, W., Klang, M., Schwartz, L., Richardson, S., Rosa, E., Drobnjak, M., Cordon-Cordo, C., Chiao, J. H., Rifkind, R., Marks, P. A., and Scher, H. Phase I clinical trial of histone deacetylase inhibitor: Suberoylanilide hydroxamic acid administered intravenously. Clin Cancer Res, *9*: 3578–3588, 2003.

20. Kelly, W. K., O'Connor, O. A., Krug, L. M., Chiao, J. H., Heaney, M., Curley, T., MacGregore-Cortelli, B., Tong, W., Secrist, J. P., Schwartz, L., Richardson, S.,

Chu, E., Olgac, S., Marks, P. A., Scher, H., and Richon, V. M. Phase I study of an oral histone deacetylase inhibitor, suberoylanilide hydroxamic acid, in patients with advanced cancer. J Clin Oncol, *23*: 3923–3931, 2005.

21. Krug, L. M., Curley, T., Schwartz, L., Richardson, S., Marks, P., Chiao, J., and Kelly, W. K. Potential role of histone deacetylase inhibitors in mesothelioma: Clinical experience with suberoylanilide hydroxamic acid. Clin Lung Cancer, *7*: 257–261, 2006.

22. Duvic, M., Talpur, R., Ni, X., Zhang, C., Hazarika, P., Kelly, C., Chiao, J. H., Reilly, J. F., Ricker, J. L., Richon, V. M., and Frankel, S. R. Phase 2 trial of oral vorinostat (suberoylanilide hydroxamic acid, SAHA) for refractory cutaneous T-cell lymphoma (CTCL). Blood, *109*: 31–39, 2007.

23. Remiszewski, S. W., Sambucetti, L. C., Bair, K. W., Bontempo, J., Cesarz, D., Chandramouli, N., Chen, R., Cheung, M., Cornell-Kennon, S., Dean, K., Diamantidis, G., France, D., Green, M. A., Howell, K. L., Kashi, R., Kwon, P., Lassota, P., Martin, M. S., Mou, Y., Perez, L. B., Sharma, S., Smith, T., Sorensen, E., Taplin, F., Trogani, N., Versace, R., Walker, H., Weltchek-Engler, S., Wood, A., Wu, A., and Atadja, P. N-hydroxy-3-phenyl-2-propenamides as novel inhibitors of human histone deacetylase with in vivo antitumor activity: Discovery of (2E)-N-hydroxy-3-[4-[[(2-hydroxyethyl)[2-(1H-indol-3-yl)eth yl]amino]methyl]phenyl]-2-propenamide (NVP-LAQ824). J Med Chem, *46*: 4609–4624, 2003.

24. Atadja, P., Gao, L., Kwon, P., Trogani, N., Walker, H., Hsu, M., Yeleswarapu, L., Chandramouli, N., Perez, L., Versace, R., Wu, A., Sambucetti, L., Lassota, P., Cohen, D., Bair, K., Wood, A., and Remiszewski, S. Selective growth inhibition of tumor cells by a novel histone deacetylase inhibitor, NVP-LAQ824. Cancer Res, *64*: 689–695, 2004.

25. Fiskus, W., Pranpat, M., Balasis, M., Herger, B., Rao, R., Chinnaiyan, A., Atadja, P., and Bhalla, K. Histone deacetylase inhibitors deplete enhancer of zeste 2 and associated polycomb repressive complex 2 proteins in human acute leukemia cells. Mol Cancer Ther, *5*: 3096–3104, 2006.

26. Guo, F., Sigua, C., Tao, J., Bali, P., George, P., Li, Y., Wittmann, S., Moscinski, L., Atadja, P., and Bhalla, K. Cotreatment with histone deacetylase inhibitor LAQ824 enhances Apo-2L/tumor necrosis factor-related apoptosis inducing ligand-induced death inducing signaling complex activity and apoptosis of human acute leukemia cells. Cancer Res, *64*: 2580–2589, 2004.

27. Rosato, R. R., Maggio, S. C., Almenara, J. A., Payne, S. G., Atadja, P., Spiegel, S., Dent, P., and Grant, S. The histone deacetylase inhibitor LAQ824 induces human leukemia cell death through a process involving XIAP down-regulation, oxidative injury, and the acid sphingomyelinase-dependent generation of ceramide. Mol Pharmacol, *69*: 216–225, 2006.

28. Weisberg, E., Catley, L., Kujawa, J., Atadja, P., Remiszewski, S., Fuerst, P., Cavazza, C., Anderson, K., and Griffin, J. D. Histone deacetylase inhibitor NVP-LAQ824 has significant activity against myeloid leukemia cells in vitro and in vivo. Leukemia, *18*: 1951–1963, 2004.

29. Catley, L., Weisberg, E., Tai, Y. T., Atadja, P., Remiszewski, S., Hideshima, T., Mitsiades, N., Shringarpure, R., LeBlanc, R., Chauhan, D., Munshi, N., Schlossman, R., Richardson, P., Griffin, J., and Anderson, K. C. NVP-LAQ824 is a potent novel histone deacetylase inhibitor with significant activity against multiple myeloma. Blood, *102*: 2615–2622, 2003.

30. George, P., Bali, P., Annavarapu, S., Scuto, A., Fiskus, W., Guo, F., Sigua, C., Sondarva, G., Moscinski, L., Atadja, P., and Bhalla, K. Combination of the shistone deacetylase inhibitor LBH589 and the hsp90 inhibitor 17-AAG is highly active against human CML-BC cells and AML cells with activating mutation of FLT-3. Blood, 105: 1768–1776, 2005.

31. Fiskus, W., Pranpat, M., Bali, P., Balasis, M., Kumaraswamy, S., Boyapalle, S., Rocha, K., Wu, J., Giles, F., Manley, P. W., Atadja, P., and Bhalla, K. Combined effects of novel tyrosine kinase inhibitor AMN107 and histone deacetylase inhibitor LBH589 against Bcr-Abl-expressing human leukemia cells. Blood, *108*: 645–652, 2006.

32. Geng, L., Cuneo, K. C., Fu, A., Tu, T., Atadja, P. W., and Hallahan, D. E. Histone deacetylase (HDAC) inhibitor LBH589 increases duration of gamma-H2AX foci and confines HDAC4 to the cytoplasm in irradiated non-small cell lung cancer. Cancer Res, *66*: 11298–11304, 2006.

33. Yu, C., Friday, B. B., Lai, J. P., McCollum, A., Atadja, P., Roberts, L. R., and Adjei, A. A. Abrogation of MAPK and Akt signaling by AEE788 synergistically potentiates histone deacetylase inhibitor-induced apoptosis through reactive oxygen species generation. Clin Cancer Res, *13*: 1140–1148, 2007.

34. Qian, D. Z., Kato, Y., Shabbeer, S., Wei, Y., Verheul, H. M., Salumbides, B., Sanni, T., Atadja, P., and Pili, R. Targeting tumor angiogenesis with histone deacetylase inhibitors: The hydroxamic acid derivative LBH589. Clin Cancer Res, *12*: 634–642, 2006.

35. Haggarty, S. J., Koeller, K. M., Wong, J. C., Grozinger, C. M., and Schreiber, S. L. Domain-selective small-molecule inhibitor of histone deacetylase 6 (HDAC6)-mediated tubulin deacetylation. Proc Natl Acad Sci U S A, *100*: 4389–4394, 2003.

36. Kawaguchi, Y., Kovacs, J. J., McLaurin, A., Vance, J. M., Ito, A., and Yao, T. P. The deacetylase HDAC6 regulates aggresome formation and cell viability in response to misfolded protein stress. Cell, 115: 727–738, 2003.

37. Bali, P., Pranpat, M., Bradner, J., Balasis, M., Fiskus, W., Guo, F., Rocha, K., Kumaraswamy, S., Boyapalle, S., Atadja, P., Seto, E., and Bhalla, K. Inhibition of histone deacetylase 6 acetylates and disrupts the chaperone function of heat shock protein 90: A novel basis of antileukemia activity of histone deacetylase inhibitors. J Biol Chem, *280*: 26729–26734, 2005.

38. Maiso, P., Carvajal-Vergara, X., Ocio, E. M., Lopez-Perez, R., Mateo, G., Gutierrez, N., Atadja, P., Pandiella, A., and San Miguel, J. F. The histone deacetylase inhibitor LBH589 is a potent antimyeloma agent that overcomes drug resistance. Cancer Res, *66*: 5781–5789, 2006.

39. Catley, L., Weisberg, E., Kiziltepe, T., Tai, Y. T., Hideshima, T., Neri, P., Tassone, P., Atadja, P., Chauhan, D., Munshi, N. C., and Anderson, K. C. Aggresome induction by proteasome inhibitor bortezomib and alpha-tubulin hyperacetylation by tubulin deacetylase (TDAC) inhibitor LBH589 are synergistic in myeloma cells. Blood, *108*: 3441–3449, 2006.

40. Furumai, R., Matsuyama, A., Kobashi, N., Lee, K. H., Nishiyama, M., Nakajima, H., Tanaka, A., Komatsu, Y., Nishino, N., Yoshida, M., and Horinouchi, S. FK228 (depsipeptide) as a natural prodrug that inhibits class I histone deacetylases. Cancer Res, *62*: 4916–4921, 2002.

41. Rajgolikar, G., Chan, K. K., and Wang, H. C. Effects of a novel antitumor depsipeptide, FR901228, on human breast cancer cells. Breast Cancer Res Treat, *51*: 29–38, 1998.

42. Doi, S., Soda, H., Oka, M., Tsurutani, J., Kitazaki, T., Nakamura, Y., Fukuda, M., Yamada, Y., Kamihira, S., and Kohno, S. The histone deacetylase inhibitor FR901228 induces caspase-dependent apoptosis via the mitochondrial pathway in small cell lung cancer cells. Mol Cancer Ther, *3*: 1397–1402, 2004.

43. Zhang, Y., Adachi, M., Zhao, X., Kawamura, R., and Imai, K. Histone deacetylase inhibitors FK228, N-(2-aminophenyl)-4-[N-(pyridin-3-yl-methoxycarbonyl)amino-methyl]benzamide and m-carboxycinnamic acid bis-hydroxamide augment radiation-induced cell death in gastrointestinal adenocarcinoma cells. Int J Cancer, *110*: 301–308, 2004.

44. Sakimura, R., Tanaka, K., Nakatani, F., Matsunobu, T., Li, X., Hanada, M., Okada, T., Nakamura, T., Matsumoto, Y., and Iwamoto, Y. Antitumor effects of histone deacetylase inhibitor on Ewing's family tumors. Int J Cancer, *116*: 784–792, 2005.

45. Konstantinopoulos, P. A., Vandoros, G. P., and Papavassiliou, A. G. FK228 (depsipeptide): A HDAC inhibitor with pleiotropic antitumor activities. Cancer Chemother Pharmacol, *58*: 711–715, 2006.s

46. Kano, Y., Akutsu, M., Tsunoda, S., Izumi, T., Kobayashi, H., Mano, H., and Furukawa, Y. Cytotoxic effects of histone deacetylase inhibitor FK228 (depsipeptide, formally named FR901228) in combination with conventional anti-leukemia/lymphoma agents against human leukemia/lymphoma cell lines. Invest New Drugs, *25*: 31–40, 2007.

47. Karam, J. A., Fan, J., Stanfield, J., Richer, E., Benaim, E. A., Frenkel, E., Antich, P., Sagalowsky, A. I., Mason, R. P., and Hsieh, J. T. The use of histone deacetylase inhibitor FK228 and DNA hyspomethylation agent 5-azacytidine in human bladder cancer therapy. Int J Cancer, *120*: 1795–1802, 2007.

48. Khan, S. B., Maududi, T., Barton, K., Ayers, J., and Alkan, S. Analysis of histone deacetylase inhibitor, depsipeptide (FR901228), effect on multiple myeloma. Br J Haematol, *125*: 156–161, 2004.

49. Sandor, V., Bakke, S., Robey, R. W., Kang, M. H., Blagosklonny, M. V., Bender, J., Brooks, R., Piekarz, R. L., Tucker, E., Figg, W. D., Chan, K. K., Goldspiel, B., Fojo, A. T., Balcerzak, S. P., and Bates, S. E. Phase I trial of the histone deacetylase inhibitor, depsipeptide (FR901228, NSC 630176), in patients with refractory neoplasms. Clin Cancer Res, *8*: 718–728, 2002.

50. Marshall, J. L., Rizvi, N., Kauh, J., Dahut, W., Figuera, M., Kang, M. H., Figg, W. D., Wainer, I., Chaissang, C., Li, M. Z., and Hawkins, M. J. A phase I trial of depsipeptide (FR901228) in patients with advanced cancer. J Exp Ther Oncol, *2*: 325–332, 2002.

51. Byrd, J. C., Marcucci, G., Parthun, M. R., Xiao, J. J., Klisovic, R. B., Moran, M., Lin, T. S., Liu, S., Sklenar, A. R., Davis, M. E., Lucas, D. M., Fischer, B., Shank, R., Tejaswi, S. L., Binkley, P., Wright, J., Chan, K. K., and Grever, M. R. A phase 1 and pharmacodynamic study of depsipeptide (FK228) in chronic lymphocytic leukemia and acute myeloid leukemia. Blood, *105*: 959–967, 2005.

52. Robey, R. W., Zhan, Z., Piekarz, R. L., Kayastha, G. L., Fojo, T., and Bates, S. E. Increased MDR1 expression in normal and malignant peripheral blood mononuclear cells obtained from patients receiving depsipeptide (FR901228, FK228, NSC630176). Clin Cancer Res, *12*: 1547–1555, 2006.

53. Stadler, W. M., Margolin, K., Ferber, S., McCulloch, W., and Thompson, J. A. A phase II study of depsipeptide in refractory metastatic renal cell cancer. Clin Genitourin Cancer, *5*: 57–60, 2006.

54. Plumb, J. A., Finn, P. W., Williams, R. J., Bandara, M. J., Romero, M. R., Watkins, C. J., La Thangue, N. B., and Brown, R. Pharmacodynamic response and inhibition of growth of human tumor xenografts by the novel histone deacetylase inhibitor PXD101. Mol Cancer Ther, *2*: 721–728, 2003.

55. Qian, X., LaRochelle, W. J., Ara, G., Wu, F., Petersen, K. D., Thougaard, A., Sehested, M., Lichenstein, H. S., and Jeffers, M. Activity of PXD101, a histone deacetylase inhibitor, in preclinical ovarian cancer studies. Mol Cancer Ther, *5*: 2086–2095, 2006.

56. Sullivan, D., Singhal, S., Schuster, M., Berenson, J., Gimsing, P., Wislö, F., Waage, A., Alsina, M., Gerwien, R., Clarke, A., Moller, K., and Ooi, C. E. A phase II study of PXD101 in advanced multiple myeloma. Blood, 108: 1023a, 2006.

57. Suzuki, T., Ando, T., Tsuchiya, K., Fukazawa, N., Saito, A., Mariko, Y., Yamashita, T., and Nakanishi, O. Synthesis and histone deacetylase inhibitory activity of new benzamide derivatives. J Med Chem, 42: 3001–3003, 1999.

58. Saito, A., Yamashita, T., Mariko, Y., Nosaka, Y., Tsuchiya, K., Ando, T., Suzuki, T., Tsuruo, T., and Nakanishi, O. A synthetic inhibitor of histone deacetylase, MS-27–275, with marked in vivo antitumor activity against human tumors. Proc Natl Acad Sci USA, *96*: 4592–4597, 1999.

59. Jaboin, J., Wild, J., Hamidi, H., Khanna, C., Kim, C. J., Robey, R., Bates, S. E., and Thiele, C. J. MS-27–275, an inhibitor of histone deacetylase, has marked in vitro and in vivo antitumor activity against pediatric solid tumors. Cancer Res, *62*: 6108–6115, 2002.

60. Maggio, S. C., Rosato, R. R., Kramer, L. B., Dai, Y., Rahmani, M., Paik, D. S., Czarnik, A. C., Payne, S. G., Spiegel, S., and Grant, S. The histone deacetylase inhibitor MS-275 interacts synergistically with fludarabine to induce apoptosis in human leukemia cells. Cancer Res, *64*: 2590–2600, 2004.

61. Qian, D. Z., Wei, Y. F., Wang, X., Kato, Y., Cheng, L., and Pili, R. Antitumor activity of the histone deacetylase inhibitor MS-275 in prostate cancer models. Prostate, *67*: 1182–1193, 2007.

62. Lucas, D. M., Davis, M. E., Parthun, M. R., Mone, A. P., Kitada, S., Cunningham, K. D., Flax, E. L., Wickham, J., Reed, J. C., Byrd, J. C., and Grever, M. R. The histone deacetylase inhibitor MS-275 induces caspase-dependent apoptosis in B-cell chronic lymphocytic leukemia cells. Leukemia, *18*: 1207–1214, 2004.

63. Miller, C. P., Ban, K., Dujka, M. E., McConkey, D. J., Munsell, M., Palladino, M., and Chandra, J. NPI-0052, a novel proteasome inhibitor, induces caspase-8 and ROS-dependent apoptosis alone and in combination with HDAC inhibitors in leukemia cells. Blood, *110*: 267–277, 2007.

64. Gojo, I., Jiemjit, A., Trepel, J. B., Sparreboom, A., Figg, W. D., Rollins, S., Tidwell, M. L., Greer, J., Chung, E. J., Lee, M. J., Gore, S. D., Sausville, E. A., Zwiebel, J., and Karp, J. E. Phase 1 and pharmacologic study of MS-275, a histone deacetylase inhibitor, in adults with refractory and relapsed acute leukemias. Blood, 109: 2781–2790, 2007.

65. Ryan, Q. C., Headlee, D., Acharya, M., Sparreboom, A., Trepel, J. B., Ye, J., Figg, W. D., Hwang, K., Chung, E. J., Murgo, A., Melillo, G., Elsayed, Y., Monga, M., Kalnitskiy, M., Zwiebel, J., and Sausville, E. A. Phase I and pharmacokinetic study of MS-275, a histone deacetylase inhibitor, in patients with advanced and refractory solid tumors or lymphoma. J Clin Oncol, *23*: 3912–3922, 2005.

66. Garcia-Mata, R., Gao, Y. S., and Sztul, E. Hassles with taking out the garbage: Aggravating aggresomes. Traffic, *3*: 388–396, 2002.

67. Hideshima, H., Bradner, J. E., Wong, J., D., C., Richardson, P., Schreiber, S. L., and Anderson, K. C. Small molecule inhibition of proteasome and aggresome function induces synergistic anti-tumor activity in multiple myeloma. Proc Natl Acad Sci USA, *102*: 8567–8572, 2005.

68. Feng, R., Hager, J. H., Hassig, C. A., Scranton, S. A., Payne, J. E., Mapara, M. Y., Roodman, D., and Lentzsch, S. A novel, mercaptoketone-based HDAC inhibitor, KD5170 exerts marked inhibition of osteoclast formation and anti-Myeloma activity in vitro. Blood, *108*: 991a, 2006.

69. Butler, L. M., Webb, Y., Agus, D. B., Higgins, B., Tolentino, T. R., Kutko, M. C., LaQuaglia, M. P., Drobnjak, M., Cordon-Cardo, C., Scher, H. I., Breslow, R., Richon, V. M., Rifkind, R. A., and Marks, P. A. Inhibition of transformed cell growth and induction of cellular differentiation by pyroxamide, an inhibitor of histone deacetylase. Clin Cancer Res, 7: 962–870, 2001.

70. Kutko, M. C., Glick, R. D., Butler, L. M., Coffey, D. C., Rifkind, R. A., Marks, P. A., Richon, V. M., and LaQuaglia, M. P. Histone deacetylase inhibitors induce growth suppression and cell death in human rhabdomyosarcoma in vitro. Clin Cancer Res, 9: 5749–5755, 2003.

71. LoRusso, P. M., Demchik, L., Foster, B., Knight, J., Bissery, M. C., Polin, L. M., Leopold, W. R., 3rd, and Corbett, T. H. Preclinical antitumor activity of CI-994. Invest New Drugs, 14: 349–356, 1996.

72. Graziano, M. J., Pilcher, G. D., Walsh, K. M., Kasali, O. B., and Radulovic, L. Preclinical toxicity of a new oral anticancer drug, CI-994 (acetyldinaline), in rats and dogs. Invest New Drugs, 15: *295*–310, 1997.

73. Piekarz, R. and Bates, S. A review of depsipeptide and other histone deacetylase inhibitors in clinical trials. Curr Pharm Des, *10*: 2289–2298, 2004.

74. Loprevite, M., Tiseo, M., Grossi, F., Scolaro, T., Semino, C., Pandolfi, A., Favoni, R., and Ardizzoni, A. In vitro study of CI-994, a histone deacetylase inhibitor, in non-small cell lung cancer cell lines. Oncol Res, *15*: 39–48, 2005.

75. Yu, C., Rahmani, M., Conrad, D., Subler, M., Dent, P., and Grant, S. The proteasome inhibitor bortezomib interacts synergistically with histone deacetylase inhibitors to induce apoptosis in Bcr/Abl+ cells sensitive and resistant to STI571. Blood, *102*: 3765–3774, 2003.

76. Denlinger, C. E., Keller, M. D., Mayo, M. W., Broad, R. M., and Jones, D. R. Combined proteasome and histone deacetylase inhibition in non-small cell lung cancer. J Thorac Cardiovasc Surg, *127*: 1078–1086, 2004.

77. Sutheesophon, K., Kobayashi, Y., Takatoku, M. A., Ozawa, K., Kano, Y., Ishii, H., and Furukawa, Y. Histone deacetylase inhibitor depsipeptide (FK228) induces apoptosis in leukemic cells by facilitating mitochondrial translocation of Bax, which is enhanced by the proteasome inhibitor bortezomib. Acta Haematol, *115*: 78–90, 2006.

78. Emanuele, S., Lauricella, M., Carlisi, D., Vassallo, B., D'Anneo, A., Di Fazio, P., Vento, R., and Tesoriere, G. SAHA induces apoptosis in hepatoma cells and synergistically interacts with the proteasome inhibitor Bortezomib. Apoptosis, *12*(7): 1327–1338, 2007.

Chapter 25

Death Receptors in Multiple Myeloma and Therapeutic Opportunities

Faustino Mollinedo

Introduction

Multiple myeloma (MM) is a malignancy of terminally differentiated B-lymphocytes, also known as plasma cells, that accounts for about 10% of all hematologic cancers,[1] ranking as the second most common blood cancer, after non-Hodgkin lymphoma.[2] MM is characterized by a clonal expansion and accumulation of malignant plasma cells within the bone marrow (BM), serum and/or urine monoclonal immunoglobulin, and osteolytic lesions. Because of the infiltration and growth of myeloma cells in the local BM microenvironment, MM patients commonly develop osteolytic bone disease, which predominantly affects the skull, ribs, vertebrae, pelvis, and proximal long bones. The interaction of myeloma cells with cells of the BM microenvironment leads to disruption of normal hematopoiesis, neutropenia, anemia, bone destruction, and hipercalcemia. Thus, most patients with MM will have pathological fractures or develop some form of osteolytic bone disease during the course of their disease, making this a major cause of morbidity. The lytic bone disease observed in most MM patients results from an unbalanced bone turnover with enhanced resorption related to increased osteoclast recruitment and activity and low bone formation. Myeloma cells grow predominantly in the local BM microenvironment, where the tumor cells interact with a range of cells including BM stromal cells, hematopoietic cells, and the cells of bone.[3] This interaction between MM cells and BM microenvironment is essential for maintenance and progression of the disease process. Thus, the reciprocal relationship between MM cells and osteoclasts leads to the induction of osteoclastogenesis and the activation of bone resorption, as well as to the inhibition of osteoblasts, thus preventing lesion repair.[4–6]

MM, currently an incurable disease, is characterized as a tumor composed of long-surviving rather than fast-growing malignant plasma cells,[7] which leads to accumulation of these cells within the BM due to a loss of critical apoptotic controls. Because resistance to apoptosis may play a crucial role in pathogenesis and resistance to treatment of MM, a therapeutic potential lies in circumventing antiapoptotic signals and/or potentiating apoptosis. Despite new insights into the pathogenesis of MM and novel targeted therapies, the

From: *Contemporary Hematology Myeloma Therapy*
Edited by: S. Lonial © Humana Press, Totowa, NJ

median survival remains 3–5 years. Thus, there is a need to overcome the deadlock in the present clinical state of MM treatment with further developments of new therapeutic drugs and approaches.

Death Receptors as Proapoptotic Targets in Cancer Therapy

Apoptosis is a genetically programmed cell death and a controlled cellular mechanism that is required for morphogenesis during embryonic development and for tissue homeostasis in adult organisms. Failure to undergo apoptosis has been implicated in tumor development and resistance to cancer therapy, and therefore strategies for overcoming resistance to apoptosis are an attractive approach in cancer treatment, and in MM in particular. Molecular insights into the apoptotic machinery present in tumor cells will provide new targets and approaches for rational therapeutic intervention to direct tumor cells to self-destruction.

There are two major signaling pathways leading to apoptosis in mammalian cells: the intrinsic pathway, initiated at the mitochondrial level, and the extrinsic pathway, initiated through death receptor-mediated signals at the cell surface. Although different molecules participate in the core machinery of both apoptosis signaling pathways, cross-talk exists at multiple levels, and in most cases the extrinsic signaling activation is followed by the onset of an intrinsic mitochondrial signaling route.

Death receptors are members of the tumor necrosis factor (TNF) receptor gene superfamily, which consists of more than 20 proteins with a broad range of biological functions, including the modulation of cell death and survival, differentiation, or immune regulation.[8–10] Death receptors share a number of high homology regions, including cysteine-rich extracellular domains and a cytoplasmic domain of about 80 amino acids called "death domain," which is critical for transducing apoptotic signals from the cell's surface to intracellular signaling pathways through the interaction of death receptors with their cognate ligands. Fas/CD95 ligand (FasL/CD95L) and TNF-related apoptosis-inducing ligand (TRAIL) as well as their corresponding receptors are the most important death receptor signaling systems promoting apoptosis. The best characterized death receptors to date comprise TNF receptor 1 (TNF-R1), Fas (CD95/APO-1), TRAIL receptor 1 (TRAIL-R1) (death receptor 4, DR4), and TRAIL receptor 2 (TRAIL-R2) (death receptor 5, DR5), while the roles of DR3[11] and DR6[12] have not exactly been defined. Additional known TRAIL receptors are decoy receptor (DcR) 1 (TRAIL-R3) and DcR2 (TRAIL-R4), which lack intact cytoplasmic death domains, and the soluble osteoprotegerin (OPG). These receptors sequester TRAIL from DR4 and DR5, thereby antagonizing TRAIL-mediated apoptosis. Some structural features of these receptors are summarized in Fig. 1 and Table 1. Fas/CD95 and TRAIL receptors are the most potent proapoptotic members of the death receptor family and seem to be of major clinical relevance.

Innate and acquired resistance to chemotherapy and radiation therapy has been a major obstacle for clinical oncology. One potential adjunct to conventional treatment is direct induction of cell death by activation of death receptor-mediated apoptosis. Death receptor-targeted therapy is also attractive since it is not dependent on the p53 tumor suppressor gene, known as

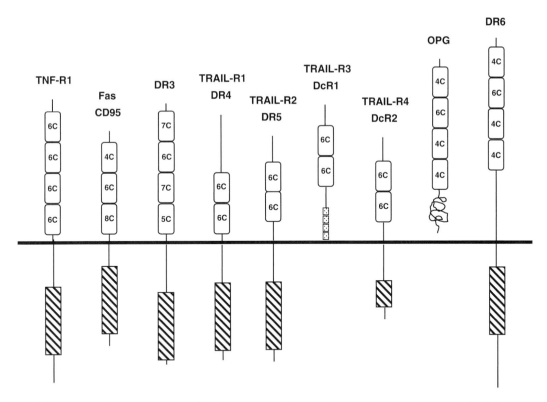

Fig. 1 Diagrammatic representation of death receptors. The cysteine-rich domains characteristic of the extracellular ligand-binding portion of the tumor necrosis factor receptor family are shown as open boxes with the number of cysteines indicated. The cytoplasmic "death domains" are shown as striped boxes. The glycosylphosphatidylinositol anchor attaching TRAIL-R3/DcR1 to the cell surface is illustrated as small-dotted boxes. *TRAIL* TNF-related apoptosis-inducing ligand.

"the gatekeeper" of cellular integrity, which is the most frequently mutated protein in human cancer, being deleted or inactivated in more than half of human tumors,[13] and therefore it should be effective in p53-deficient tumors.[14] The prevalence of p53 mutations, however, differs considerably between tumor types and stages of cancer.[15] In MM, mutation or deletion of the gene for p53 is rarely detected at diagnosis, although both become more frequent in advanced disease.[16–19] Activation of p53 by using nutlin-3, a small-molecule activator of p53, induces apoptosis in MM cells,[20] and an additive effect of TRAIL and Adeno-p53 was observed in the induction of apoptosis in MM cell lines expressing nonfunctional p53.[21]

Fas/CD95 and TRAIL Signaling in Apoptosis

Mature Fas/CD95 (Fig. 1, Table 1) is a 48-kDa type I transmembrane receptor of 319 amino acids with a single transmembrane domain of 17 amino acids, an N-terminal cysteine-rich extracellular domain, and a C-terminal cytoplasmic domain of 145 amino acids that is relatively abundant in charged amino acids (24 basic and 19 acidic amino acids). The cytoplasmic portion of Fas/CD95 contains a domain of 85 amino acids termed "death domain," which plays a

Table 1 Death receptors.

Name	Protein name	Synonyms	Entry name/ abbreviations	Amino acid sequence	MW (unprocessed precursor, derived from sequence)/ SDS-PAGE
TNF-R1	Tumor necrosis factor receptor superfamily member 1A (TNFRSF1A)	p60; TNFR1; TNF-RI; TNFR-I; p55; tumor necrosis factor-binding protein 1 (TBPI); CD120a antigen	TNR1A_HUMAN/ TNFAR, TNFR1	455 (signal, 21 aas) Mature protein: Extracellular: 190 Transmembrane: 23 Cytoplasmic: 221 (DD, 86 aas)	50,495 Da/60 kDa
DR3	Tumor necrosis factor receptor superfamily member 25 (TNFRSF25)	WSL-1 protein; apoptosis-mediating receptor DR3; apoptosis-mediating receptor TRAMP; death domain receptor 3; WSL protein; apoptosis-inducing receptor AIR; Apo-3; lymphocyte-associated receptor of death; LARD	TNR25_HUMAN/ APO3, DDR3, DR3, TNFRSF12, WSL, WSL1	417 (signal, 24 aas) Mature protein: Extracellular: 175 Transmembrane: 21 Cytoplasmic: 197 (DD, 82 aas)	45,385 Da/47 kDa
FAS	Tumor necrosis factor receptor superfamily member 6 (TNFRSF6)	FASLG receptor; apoptosis-mediating surface antigen FAS; Apo-1 antigen; CD95 antigen	TNR6_HUMAN/ APT1, FAS1	335 (signal, 16 aas) Mature protein: Extracellular: 157 Transmembrane: 17 Cytoplasmic: 145 (DD, 85 aas)	37,732 Da/48 kDa

TRAIL-R1	Tumor necrosis factor receptor superfamily member 10A (TNFRSF10A)	Death receptor 4; TNF-related apoptosis-inducing ligand receptor 1; TRAIL receptor 1; CD261 antigen	TR10A_HUMAN/ APO2, DR4, TRAILR1	468 (signal, 23 aas) Mature protein: Extracellular: 216 Transmembrane: 23 Cytoplasmic: 206 (DD, 84 aas)	50,061 Da/60 kDa
TRAIL-R2	Tumor necrosis factor receptor superfamily member 10B (TNFRSF10B)	Death receptor 5; TNF-related apoptosis-inducing ligand receptor 2; TRAIL receptor 2; CD262 antigen	TR10B_HUMAN/ DR5, KILLER, TRAILR2, TRICK2, ZTNFR9	440 (signal, 55 aas) Mature protein: Extracellular: 155 Transmembrane: 21 Cytoplasmic: 209 (DD, 84 aas)	47,850 Da/56 kDa
TRAIL-R3	Tumor necrosis factor receptor superfamily member 10C (TNFRSF10C)	Decoy receptor 1; DcR1; Decoy TRAIL receptor without death domain; TNF-related apoptosis-inducing ligand receptor 3; TRAIL receptor 3; Trail receptor without an intracellular domain; lymphocyte inhibitor of TRAIL; antagonist decoy receptor for TRAIL/ Apo-2L; CD263 antigen	TR10C_HUMAN/ DCR1, LIT, TRAILR3, TRID	259 (signal, 23 aas) Mature protein: Extracellular: 236	27,395 Da/65 kDa

(continued)

Table 1 (continued)

Name	Protien name	Synonyms	Entry name/ abbreviations	Amino acid sequence	MW (unprocessed precursor, derived from sequence)/ SDS-PAGE
TRAIL-R4	Tumor necrosis factor receptor superfamily member 10D (TNFRSF10D)	Decoy receptor 2; DcR2; TNF-related apoptosis-inducing ligand receptor 4; TRAIL receptor 4; TRAIL receptor with a truncated death domain; CD264 antigen	TR10D_HUMAN/ DCR2, TRAILR4, TRUNDD	386 (signal, 55 aas) Mature protein: Extracellular: 156 Transmembrane: 21 Cytoplasmic: 154 (DD, 27 aas; truncated domain)	41,823 Da/35 kDa
DR6	Tumor necrosis factor receptor superfamily member 21 (TNFRSF21)	TNFR-related death receptor 6; death receptor 6	TNR21_HUMAN/ DR6	655 (signal, 41 aas) Mature protein: Extracellular: 308 Transmembrane: 21 Cytoplasmic: 285 (DD, 84 aas)	71,845 Da/66 kDa
Osteoprotegerin	Tumor necrosis factor receptor superfamily member 11B (TNFRSF11B)	Osteoclastogenesis inhibitory factor	TR11B_HUMAN/ OPG, OCIF	401 (signal, 21 aas) Mature protein: Extracellular: 380	46,040 Da/55 kDa

DD death domain, *aas* amino acids, *Da* dalton, *kDa* kilodalton, *TRAIL* TNF-related apoptosis-inducing ligand crucial role in transmitting the death signal from the cell's surface to intracellular pathways.[22–24] Unlike the intracellular regions of other transmembrane receptors involved in signal transduction, the "death domain" does not possess enzymatic activity, but mediates signaling through protein–protein interactions. The "death domain" has the propensity to self-associate and form large aggregates in solution.[25] The presence of a high number of charged amino acids in the surface of the death domain is probably responsible for mediating the interactions between death domains. Stimulation of Fas/CD95 by FasL/CD95L results in receptor aggregation,[26,27] previously assembled in trimers,[28,29] and recruitment of the adaptor molecule Fas-associated death domain-containing protein (FADD) (208 amino acids, 29 kDa)[30] through interaction between its own "death domain" and the clustered receptor death domains. FADD also contains a "death effector domain" that binds to an analogous domain repeated in tandem within the zymogen form of caspase-8 (479 amino acids, 55 kDa).[31] Upon recruitment by FADD, procaspase-8 oligomerization drives its activation through self-cleavage, activating downstream effector caspases and leading to apoptosis.[32] Thus, activation of Fas/CD95 results in receptor aggregation and formation of the so-called "death-inducing signaling complex" (DISC),[33] containing trimerized Fas/CD95, FADD, and procaspase-8 (Fig. 2). Recent evidence suggests that activation of Fas/CD95-mediated apoptotic signaling ensues Fas/CD95 clustering in lipid rafts and DISC formation in a process likely mediated by ezrin and actin cytoskeleton[34–36] (Fig. 2). Fas/CD95 activation can proceed independently of its interaction with FasL/CD95L.[36–40] Signaling through Fas can be negatively regulated by the cellular FLICE-like inhibitory protein (c-FLIP)[41] (caspase-8 was formerly called FLICE), which is a "death effector domain"-containing protein acting as a catalytically inactive procaspase-8 molecule. c-FLIP comes in two main isoforms, c-FLIP-long (480 amino acids, 55 kDa) and c-FLIP-short (221 amino acids, 28 kDa). Both proteins possess two "death effector domain" motifs that are very similar to the "death effector domain" on procaspase-8. The short c-FLIP isoform consists of only these "death effector domains," whereas the long c-FLIP isoform also has a domain that is homologous to the catalytic domain of caspase-8, but devoid of enzymaytic activity due to the substitution of the active-center cysteine residue by a tyrosine residue. Both c-FLIP proteins were originally thought to be inhibitors of death receptor-induced apoptosis by competing with procaspase-8 for binding to FADD at the DISC. In agreement with this notion, increased levels of c-FLIP are associated with cancer and confer protection against FasL/CD95L- or TRAIL-induced apoptosis.[42] However, unlike c-FLIP-short, the long form of c-FLIP has been shown to promote caspase-8 activation and therefore has a proapoptotic function.[43,44] This new notion is strengthened by the fact that c-FLIP-deficient mice show the same phenotype as caspase-8 and FADD-deficient mice, characterized by heart failure resulting in death at day 10.5 of embryonic development.[45–47] Thus, differences in the relative levels of c-FLIP-long, c-FLIP-short, and procaspase-8 might activate or inhibit caspase-8 activity depending on the relative abundance of these molecules at the DISC.

TRAIL-R1/DR4 and TRAIL-R2/DR5 share the cysteine-rich extracellular domain and the cytoplasmic "death domain" with Fas/CD95, and trigger an apoptotic signaling upon interaction with their ligand TRAIL through the formation of DISC.[48] Recent data suggest that TRAIL-R2/DR5 may contribute

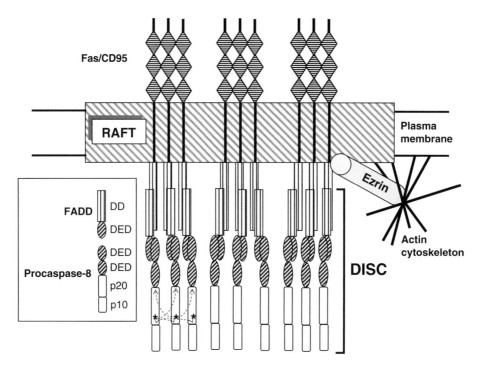

Fig. 2 Schematic representation of Fas/CD95 activation through its aggregation in membrane rafts. Fas/CD95 molecules are brought together and concentrated in membrane rafts facilitating the formation of the death-inducing signaling complex, following protein–protein interactions between Fas/CD95-FADD (Fas-associated death domain-containing protein) through their respective "death domains", and FADD-procaspase-8 through their respective "death effector domains." Death-inducing signaling complex formation leads to activation of unprocessed procaspase-8 by driving its dimerization and autoproteolysis, resulting in the release of mature, active caspase-8 (composed of a p20/p10 heteromer) into the cytoplasm. The asterisks represent the active-site cysteine residues of caspase-8, the dash lines indicate proteolytic processing in trans, and the arrowheads point to the sites of proteolytic cleavage. Actin cytoskeleton through ezrin is involved in the clustering of Fas in lipid rafts. From Mollinedo and Gajate.[40] © Elsevier, used with permission.

more than TRAIL-R1/DR4 to TRAIL-induced apoptosis in cancer cells that express both death receptors.[49] Differential expression of TRAIL-R1/DR4 and TRAIL-R2/DR5 has been described for various tumor types, usually with TRAIL-R2/DR5 being the most prevalent.

Death Receptor Ligands as Potential Anticancer Agents

Death receptor ligands TNFα, FasL/CD95L, and TRAIL might be interesting candidates to promote tumor cell killing as they are able to induce apoptosis by binding to their cell membrane receptors.[50] However, for the clinical application of these molecules, it is of primary importance that their safety be guaranteed. The therapeutic potential of TNFα is tempered by the demonstration that the systemic administration of recombinant human TNFα has shown low antitumor activity and higher doses induce a severe inflammatory response syndrome that resembles septic shock. Systemic recombinant human FasL administration in humans is not yet feasible because of observed severe liver damage in mice due to Fas/CD95-mediated apoptosis of hepatocytes. Intraperitoneal administration of agonistic antibody to Fas/CD95 in tumor-bearing mice was rapidly lethal with severe damage of the liver, apparently through apoptosis induction in hepatocytes that express abundant Fas/CD95.[51] Ligands of the TNF family and their cognate receptors play a key role in liver pathogenesis,[52] and this seems to be a major challenge and concern for the clinical application of death receptor-targeted therapy.

Interestingly, TRAIL seems to be unique, because it has been reported to be nontoxic to normal cells while killing a broad range of tumor cells,[53–56] making this molecule a promising anticancer therapeutic agent. Nevertheless, several reports have shown apoptotic activity of TRAIL toward a number of normal cells, including primary human hepatocytes,[57] keratinocytes,[58] prostate epithelial cells,[59] and brain tissue.[60] Despite these observations, new ways to activate TRAIL receptors by either recombinant forms of TRAIL and by agonistic anti-TRAIL-R1/DR4 and anti-TRAIL-R2/DR5 antibodies are being generated and assayed as potential clinical options for cancer treatment, lacking apparently toxicity.[61,62] TRAIL and anti-TRAIL-R1/DR4 and anti-TRAIL-R2/DR5 agonistic antibodies are currently in clinical trials.[63]

Native TRAIL is expressed as a homotrimeric type II transmembrane protein that can be proteolytically cleaved into soluble homotrimeric TRAIL.[53–56] Both membrane and soluble TRAIL can interact with the agonistic TRAIL receptors TRAIL-R1/DR4 and TRAIL-R2/DR5, which initiate apoptosis via their intracellular death domains. TRAIL can also interact with two antagonist receptors TRAIL-R3 (DcR1) and TRAIL-R4 (DcR2) (Fig. 1, Table 1), which are unable to engage apoptosis due to the lack or truncation of the cytoplasmic death domain.[32] The different TRAIL receptors are widely expressed on a variety of normal tissues and malignant cell types. The decoy receptors TRAIL-R3/DcR1 and TRAIL-R4/DcR2 were thought to be predominantly expressed in normal cells, hence sparing normal cells from apoptosis. However, there is no correlation between TRAIL sensitivity and expression of either TRAIL-R3/DcR1 or TRAIL-R4/DcR2.[64,65] Thus, the mechanism for the tumor-selective activity of TRAIL remains elusive.

Osteoprotegerin

Although TRAIL predominantly interacts with death receptors triggering and decoy receptors inhibiting TRAIL-induced apoptosis, this ligand can also bind to OPG at low affinity.[66,67] Thus, OPG can act as a receptor for TRAIL, inhibiting TRAIL-mediated apoptosis.[66] OPG was first described as a secreted member of the TNF receptor family that regulates bone resorption.[68] Unlike other members of the TNF receptor family, OPG does not possess a transmembrane domain (Fig. 1; Table 1). The effects of OPG on bone result from its ability to inhibit osteoclastogenesis, through its interaction with another member of the TNF family, named OPG ligand (OPGL),[69] aka receptor activator of NF-κB ligand (RANKL), osteoclast differentiation factor, or TNF-related activation induced cytokine (TRANCE). RANKL has been shown to be expressed by stromal cells and osteoblasts in the local BM microenvironment, where it can bind to its receptor RANK on the surface of osteoclast precursors. The interaction between RANKL and RANK plays a critical role in promoting osteoclast differentiation (osteoclastogenesis) and is responsible for activating mature osteoclasts to increase bone resorption.[70–73] The soluble decoy receptor OPG binds to RANKL, inhibiting its interaction with RANK and blocking osteoclast formation. Overexpression of OPG in mice, or mice deficient in

RANKL, has been reported to reduce osteoclast formation and results in the development of osteopetrosis.[68,71] In contrast, mice deficient in OPG develop osteoporosis.[74,75]

Activation of Fas/CD95 Through Clustering in Lipid Rafts

A novel framework on the regulation of apoptosis has been set up since the seminal observation in 2001 that Fas/CD95 activation proceeded through Fas/CD95 translocation and clustering in aggregated lipid rafts, and disruption of lipid rafts blocked both Fas/CD95 activation and Fas/CD95-mediated apoptosis.[76] This led to unravel a novel regulatory mechanism for Fas/CD95-mediated apoptosis through lipid rafts. Lipid rafts are membrane microdomains highly enriched in cholesterol and sphingolipids varying in size from 50 to 70 nm, and the proteins located in these microdomains are severely limited in their ability to freely diffuse over the plasma membrane.[77] Subsequent studies using different cell types and activators, including the natural ligand FasL/CD95L, confirmed that coclustering of Fas/CD95 into lipid rafts was required for the onset of Fas/CD95-mediated apoptosis and demonstrated the formation of DISC in these membrane microdomains.[35,36,40,78–80] Actin cytoskeleton, likely through ezrin[34,35] (Fig. 2), as well as palmitoylation of Fas/CD95[81] seem to be involved in both Fas/CD95 clustering and localization in lipid rafts. Recent evidence suggests that translocation and aggregation of Fas/CD95 and downstream signaling molecules into lipid rafts[35,38,76] constitutes a novel and promising target in cancer therapy[40] and in FasL/CD95L-independent activation of Fas/CD95.[37,39,40]

Fas/CD95 and MM

Programmed cell death through the Fas/CD95-FasL/CD95L system has been implicated in the elimination of activated B cells both during ontogeny and in immune physiology.[82] Thus, the loss of function of the Fas/CD95 antigen might contribute to the pathogenesis and progression of MM, by allowing susceptible cells to evade immune surveillance and the prolonged survival might allow the cell to accumulate mutations leading to malignancy. In an analysis of BM samples from 48 MM patients, only 5 of them showed point mutations in Fas/CD95 that led to a change in the amino acid sequence,[83] all of them located at the "death domain." (Fig. 3) Thus, Fas antigen mutations may contribute to the pathogenesis and progression of myeloma in some patients, but it is not a widespread feature.

Fas/CD95 is present in most of MM cell lines and malignant cells derived from myeloma patients.[84,85] However, not all the MM cells identified as positive for Fas/CD95 expression underwent apoptosis when challenged with agonistic anti-Fas/CD95 antibody.[84–86] Thus, there is no correlation between Fas/CD95 antigen expression and susceptibility to Fas/CD95-mediated apoptosis in MM. The reasons for this apparent resistance remain largely unknown. In this regard, both MM cell lines RPM18226 and U266 express cell surface Fas/CD95 at similar levels, but only RPM18226 cells are killed upon anti-Fas/CD95 agonistic antibody treatment. The sequence of the cDNA for Fas/CD95 in U266 appears to be wild-type,[85] and the resistance of U266 cells to anti-Fas/CD95 antibodies did not appear to reflect dysregulation of

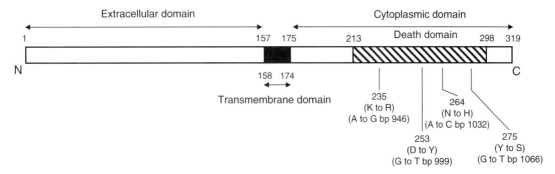

Fig. 3 Diagrammatic representation of Fas/CD95 mutations identified in myeloma patients. The protein and cDNA sequence changes are indicated. Numbers show the amino acid position in the extracellular, transmembrane (solid box), and cytoplasmic domains of mature Fas/CD95. The striped box represents the "death domain" of the protein.

antiapoptotic Bcl-2 or Bcl-XL, and proapoptotic Bax because these proteins were expressed in both RPMI-8226 and U266 cells to similar levels. mRNA levels of the endogenous inhibitor of Fas/CD95 signaling c-FLIP were constitutively elevated in U266 cells.[87] Consistent with this observation, U266 cells expressed both c-FLIP-long protein and its truncated 43 kDa product which is seen in c-FLIP-long-overexpressing cells. The truncated form of c-FLIP-long protein was not detected in RPM18226. Moreover, the levels of truncated c-FLIP-long in U266 cells were considerably higher than those present in RPM18226, suggesting that c-FLIP-long may play a role in the intrinsic resistance of U266 cells to the apoptotic action of Fas/CD95.[87] In this regard, microarray studies have shown that c-FLIP was highly expressed in MM patient cells as compared to normal counterparts.[88] In addition, constitutively activated signal transducer and activator of transcription 3 (Stat3) signaling has been shown to contribute to the pathogenesis of MM by preventing apoptosis, in particular Fas/CD95-mediated cell death.[89] Furthermore, interleukin-6 (IL-6) is a well-known growth factor for MM,[90,91] which inhibits plasma cell apoptosis[92,93] and stimulates MM cells to proliferate.[94] IL-6 has been shown to inhibit Fas/CD95-induced apoptosis, likely through its inhibitory effects on c-jun N-terminal kinase (JNK)/c-jun signaling.[95,96] The antiapoptotic activity of IL-6 is mediated, at least in part, through the activation of Stat3 in myeloma cells.[89] IL-6 induces intracellular signaling through Stat activation, but does not affect c-FLIP levels. However, it has also been reported that the presence of the major survival factor IL-6 in myeloma does not affect the responses of the IL-6-dependent cell lines to the anti-Fas/CD95 agonistic monoclonal antibody, but does prevent these cell lines from undergoing spontaneous cell death as a result of growth factor withdrawal.[85] Thus, it is not fully defined why despite the expression of Fas/CD95, some clones of myeloma cells are resistant to Fas-mediated apoptosis.

Antitumor Agents Promoting Fas/CD95-Mediated Apoptosis in MM Cells

As stated above, there is a lack of correlation between Fas expression in myeloma cells and their respective sensitivity to Fas-mediated apoptosis. Nevertheless, this Fas-mediated signaling can be potentiated by a number of agents, leading to the framework of novel therapeutic approaches.

Interferon Potentiates Fas/CD95-Induced Apoptosis

The benefits of interferon (IFN) in MM treatment are under debate due to the diverse response to therapy in different patients and reports on adverse effects.[97–100] However, an important therapeutic potential of IFN may be achieved in combination with other therapeutic agents. IFN-α and IFN-γ have been shown to enhance Fas/CD95 antigen expression and increase the Fas/CD95-induced apoptosis in MM cell lines.[101] Thus, MM cells might be resensitized to Fas/CD95-mediated apoptosis by pretreatment with IFN.

IFN treatment in addition activates the transcription factor Stat1 and attenuates Stat3 activation in MM cells.[102] This is of interest, as Stat3 is a crucial prosurvival mediator in many cancers,[103] IL-6-induced activation of Stat3 has been associated with resistance to apoptosis, including Fas/CD95-mediated apoptosis,[89] and Stat3, in complex with c-Jun, suppresses Fas/CD95 transcription.[104]Thus, IFN treatment interferes with Stat3 survival signaling, which has been linked with resistance to Fas/CD95-mediated apoptosis, and has been implicated as a crucial mediator of the survival functions of IL-6 in MM cells, inducing the antiapoptotic protein Bcl-XL.[89,105] Conversely, Fas/CD95 can be positively regulated by Stat1-dependent mechanisms in response to IFN treatment.[106] Interestingly, Stat3 and Stat1 may counteract the effects of each other,[107,108] and have been shown to exert opposing effects on the transcription of the antiapoptotic Bcl-2 family members Bcl-2 and Bcl-XL.[109] Both IFN-α and IFN-γ upregulated fourfold Fas mRNA expression, which was translated into an elevated Fas protein expression, and highly increased TRAIL mRNA expression (>100 times for IFN-α and sixfold for IFN-γ) and protein, whereas the mRNA levels of FasL, caspase-8, DR4, and DR5 remained unchanged during IFN treatment in the U-266-1970 MM cell line.[102] These observations were extended to additional MM cell lines. However, reflecting the known heterogeneity of primary MM cells, the above results could be confirmed only in some of patient-derived MM cells.[102] By using recombinant human DR4:Fc, consisting of the extracellular domain of human DR4 fused to the Fc portion of human IgG1, which inhibited TRAIL-induced apoptosis, no inhibition was observed in the sensitizing effect of IFN on Fas/CD95-mediated apoptosis indicating that TRAIL was not involved in the IFN-mediated Fas/CD95 potentiating process.[102]

The above data on the sensitizing effect of IFN on Fas/CD95-mediated apoptosis following an increase in Fas/CD95 expression suggest that the level of Fas/CD95 expression is of importance in the apoptotic response induced by Fas/CD95. In accordance with this notion, elevated Fas/CD95 expression in MM cells and ectopic expression of Fas/CD95 in these cells sensitize MM cells to Fas/CD95-mediated apoptosis.[36,102] In this regard, a clonal variability in Fas/CD95 expression has been shown to determine sensitivity to Fas/CD95-mediated apoptosis in RPMI 8226 MM cells.[110]

Alkyl-lysophospholipids Trigger Fas/CD95-Induced Apoptosis

Interestingly, edelfosine (1-O-octadecyl-2-O-methyl-rac-glycero-3-phosphocholine) and perifosine (octadecyl-(1,1-dimethyl-piperidinio-4-yl)-phosphate), two major members of a new family of promising anticancer agents collectively known as synthetic alkyl-lysophospholipids (ALPs) or antitumor lipids (ATLs),[14,111,112] induce apoptosis efficiently in MM cell lines and malignant cells derived from MM patients, sparing normal untransformed cells.[36]

This apoptotic response is triggered by the translocation of Fas/CD95, DR4, and DR5, as well as downstream signaling molecules, into lipid rafts, leading to the clustering of Fas/CD95 in aggregated lipid rafts in MM cells, with Fas/CD95 playing a crucial role in the apoptotic response[36] (Fig. 4). Translocation of Fas/CD95 together with downstream signaling molecules led to the formation of DISC, made up of Fas/CD95, FADD, and caspase-8[36] (Fig. 5). Fas/CD95 retrovirus transduction bestowed edelfosine and perifosine sensitivity in Fas/CD95-deficient and drug-resistant MM cells, indicating a major role of Fas/CD95 in ALP-induced apoptosis in MM cells.[36] In addition, disruption of lipid rafts inhibited ALP-induced formation of Fas/CD95 clustering and apoptosis[36] (Fig. 6). This indicates that Fas/CD95 clustering in lipid rafts plays an important role in ALP-induced apoptosis in MM cells. ALP-induced apoptosis in MM cells through Fas/CD95 translocation and clustering in lipid rafts was independent of FasL and involved a subsequent mitochondria signaling.[36] In addition, the ALP-elicited recruitment of death receptors in lipid rafts potentiated apoptosis by death receptor ligands, such as TRAIL or FasL/CD95L.[36]

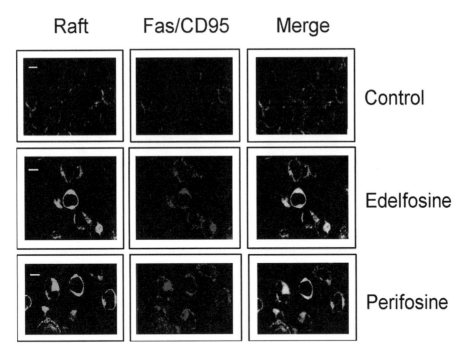

Fig. 4 Edelfosine and perifosine induce coclustering of membrane rafts and Fas/CD95 in multiple myeloma (MM) cells. MM cell line MM144 was either untreated (Control) or treated with 10 μM edelfosine or perifosine for 12 h, and then stained with fluorescein isothiocyanate (FITC)-cholera toxin B subunit to identify membrane rafts (green fluorescence), due to its binding to ganglioside GM1 mainly found in lipid rafts, and with an anti-Fas/CD95 monoclonal antibody, followed by CY3-conjugated antimouse immunoglobulin antibody (red fluorescence). Areas of colocalization between membrane rafts and Fas/CD95 in the merge panels are yellow. Fas/CD95 was homogenously distributed in the cell membrane prior to alkyl-lysophospholipid treatment and formed clusters after stimulation. The FITC-cholera toxin B subunit staining shows profound reorganization of membrane rafts leading to aggregates that contain clustered Fas/CD95, as evidenced in the merge picture. Bar, 10 μm. From Gajate and Mollinedo.[36] © American Society of Hematology, used with permission (*see* Plate 7).

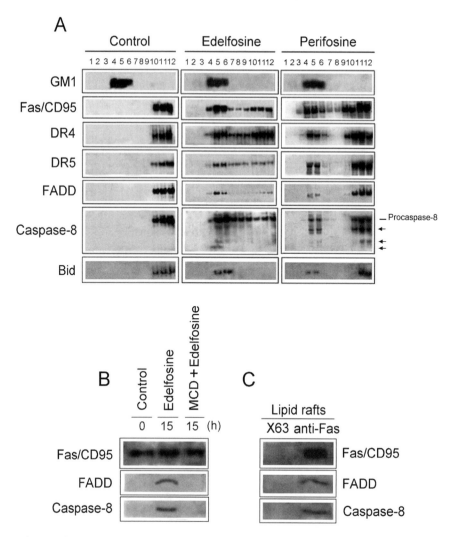

Fig. 5 Recruitment of death receptors and downstream signaling molecules, and death-inducing signaling complex formation in membrane rafts following alkyl-lysophospholipid treatment of MM cells. **a** Untreated MM144 cells (Control) and MM144 cells treated with 10 μM edelfosine or perifosine for 15 h were fractionated by discontinuous sucrose density gradient centrifugation to isolate lipid rafts, and samples from each fraction were subjected to Western blot for protein identification. Location of GM1-containing lipid rafts (fractions 4–6) was determined using cholera toxin B subunit conjugated to horseradish peroxidase. The migration positions of the 55-kDa procaspase-8 as well as of the cleavage products (arrows) are denoted. **b** Fas/CD95 was immunoprecipitated from untreated control or edelfosine-treated (15 h) MM144 cell extracts. Fas/CD95 was also immunoprecipitated from MM144 cells pretreated with methyl-β-cyclodextrin (MCD) to disrupt lipid rafts and then treated for 15 h with edelfosine. As shown in the figure, Fas/CD95 coimmunoprecipitated with FADD (Fas-associated death domain-containing protein) and caspase-8, forming the death-inducing signaling complex , upon edelfosine treatment. **c** Fas/CD95 was immunoprecipitated from a pool of membrane raft-enriched fractions 4–6 from sucrose gradients of edelfosine-treated MM144 cells. Immunoprecipitates were subjected to Western blot using Fas/CD95, FADD-, and caspase-8-specific antibodies. Membrane raft-enriched fractions were also immunoprecipitated with P3X63 (X63) myeloma supernatant as a negative control. From Gajate and Mollinedo.[36]© American Society of Hematology, used with permission.

This is of particular importance for TRAIL, because this ligand shows a promising and selective antitumor action in different cancer cells[113] as well as antimyeloma activity.[114,115] Thus, edelfosine and perifosine are not only effective in the killing of MM cells, but they might also be valuable drugs in

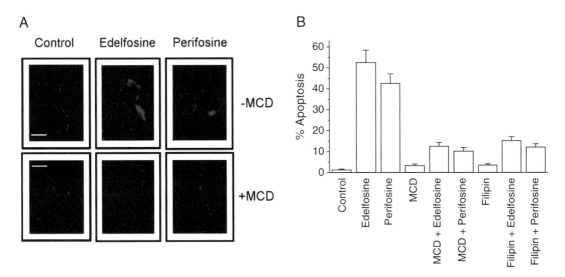

Fig. 6 Disruption of membrane rafts inhibits alkyl-lysophospholipid-induced Fas/CD95 clustering and apoptosis. MM144 cells were untreated (Control) or pretreated with methyl-β-cyclodextrin (MCD) or filipin to disrupt lipid rafts, and then incubated with 10 μM edelfosine or perifosine for 12 h and analyzed for Fas/CD95 clustering by confocal microscopy (**a**), or for 24 h and examined for the percentage of apoptotic cells by flow cytometry (**b**). Bar, 10 μm. From Gajate and Mollinedo.[36] © American Society of Hematology, used with permission (*see* Plate 8).

combination therapy. In addition, ALPs have been shown to induce cell killing in MM cells resistant to dexamethasone, doxorubicin, melphalan, mitoxantrone, VP-16, cytoxan, and vincristine,[36,116,117] suggesting that these agents could circumvent drug resistance in MM. Interestingly, edelfosine induces apoptosis through the intracellular activation of Fas/CD95 once the drug is taken up by the tumor cell.[38] Furthermore, the ALPs edelfosine and perifosine induced apoptosis in MM cells lines and patient MM cells, whereas normal B and T lymphocytes were spared.[36] In addition, edelfosine and perifosine have been shown to be efficient in killing MM cells in vivo in animal models.[117,118] Akt signaling has been reported to mediate survival and drug resistance in myeloma,[119] and perifosine has been shown to inhibit Akt activation in MM cells.[117] Thus, perifosine is able to trigger apoptosis signaling (Fas/CD95) and inhibit survival signaling (Akt). Ongoing clinical trials conducted by Æterna Zentaris and Keryx Biopharmaceuticals indicate that perifosine alone or in combination with dexamethasone shows activity in patients with advanced, relapsed/refractory MM.[112] Figure 7 depicts a schematic view of Fas/CD95 modulation in MM.

TRAIL and MM

TRAIL induces apoptosis in malignant cells derived from MM patients and in most MM cell lines, including cells sensitive or resistant to dexamethasone, doxorubicin, melphalan, and mitoxantrone, sparing normal hematopoietic stem cells.[114,115,120] TRAIL also overcame the survival effect of IL-6 on MM cells, did not affect normal cells, and inhibited tumor growth in a xenograft in vivo model.[115] Furthermore, the synergistic action of TRAIL in concert with

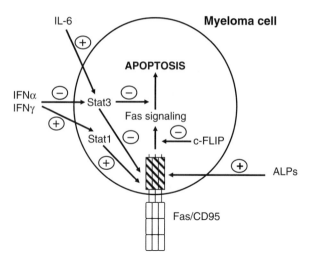

Fig. 7 Regulation of Fas/CD95-mediated apoptosis in multiple myeloma (MM). This scheme depicts major endogenous and exogenous modulators of Fas/CD95 signaling. The transcription factors Stat1 and Stat3 show opposing effects on Fas/CD95 expression. Stat3 also induces antiapoptotic Bcl-xL, inhibiting Fas/CD95-mediated apoptotic signaling. IL-6 promotes resistance of MM cells to undergo apoptosis through Stat3 activation. c-FLIP, highly expressed in MM cells, inhibits Fas/CD95-induced apoptosis acting as a catalytically inactive procaspase-8 and competing for DISC formation. IFNs potentiate Fas/CD95-mediated apoptosis by activating Stat1 and inhibiting Stat3, thus leading to Fas/CD95 upregulation. Alkyl-lysophospholipids (ALPs) edelfosine and perifosine activate Fas/CD95 through coclustering of the death receptor and membrane rafts.

cytotoxic drugs such as doxorubicin or the proteasome inhibitor PS-341 (bortezomib, VELCADE®) also suggested its clinical value in MM.[115]

In analogy with Fas, the presence of TRAIL receptors, either proapoptotic DR4 and DR5 or decoy receptors DcR1 and DcR2, could not reliably predict TRAIL sensitivity or resistance of MM cells.[115] Thus, IM-9 and U266 MM cell lines express both DR4 and DR5, but they are resistant to TRAIL-induced apoptosis.[121] However, some MM cells resistant to Fas were shown to be sensitive to TRAIL.[114,122,123] The sensitivity to TRAIL has been reported to be dependent of c-FLIP and caspase-8, but this remains controversial.[123,124] Doxorubicin upregulated the expression of DR5 and synergistically enhanced the effect of TRAIL not only against MM cells sensitive to dexamethasone- or doxorubicin-induced apoptosis but also against those resistant to dexamethasone- or doxorubicin-induced apoptosis.[115] IFN-α and IFN-β have been shown to induce TRAIL and to kill MM U266 cells through a TRAIL/DR5 system.[122] The mechanism by which IFN-α induces TRAIL in MM cells is currently unknown, but it seems to be mediated by the promyelocytic leukemic (PML) gene.[125] Despite the fact that DR5 seems to contribute more than DR4 to TRAIL-induced apoptosis in cancer cells that express both receptors,[49] B-chronic lymphocytic leukemic cells exhibit apoptotic signaling via DR4.[126] In line with this, preclinical experiments carried out to evaluate the ability of two human monoclonal antibodies directed against TRAIL-R1/DR4 (HGS-ETR1) and TRAIL-R2/DR5 (HGS-ETR2) to kill human myeloma cells rendered the killing of 15 and 9 human myeloma cell lines, respectively, out of 22 MM cell lines assayed.[127] This killing was not prevented by IL-6. In addition, HGS-ETR1 and, to a lesser extent, the HGS-ETR2 monoclonal antibodies were able to induce the killing of primary myeloma cells from patients.[127] Thus, preclinical evidence suggests that agonistic antibodies to TRAIL receptors 1 and 2 have significant potential to provide novel therapeutic options to patients with MM. The above data prompted Human Genome Sciences, Inc. (HGS), to announce on July 2006 that it has initiated dosing of patients in a randomized Phase 2 clinical trial of anti-TRAIL-R1/DR4 antibody HGS-ETR1 (mapatumumab) in combination with the proteasome inhibitor bortezomib (VELCADE®) in advanced MM. HGS-ETR1 is an agonistic human monoclonal antibody that specifically binds to the TRAIL-R1/DR4 protein and triggers apoptosis in cancer cells. HGS-ETR1 does this by mimicking the activity of the natural protein TRAIL. HGS-ETR1 was generated through a collaboration between Human Genome Sciences and Cambridge Antibody Technology.

TRAIL and Osteoblasts

Bone destruction is a hallmark of MM[128,129] that results from increased formation and activity of osteoclasts, the bone-resorbing cells, occurring in close proximity to myeloma cells, and from a lower number of osteoblasts. Thus, in MM patients with bone lesions there is uncoupled or severely imbalanced bone remodeling with increased bone resorption and decreased or absent bone formation. This leads to lytic bone lesions, severe bone pain, and pathological fractures. The breakdown of bone also leads to release of calcium into the blood, leading to hypercalcemia. Osteoclastogenesis is positively or negatively regulated by a complex signaling system that involves the receptor activator of nuclear factor (NF)-κB (RANK), OPG, and RANKL, all belonging to the TNF family.[130,131] In normal bone remodeling, osteoclasts resorb old or damaged bone leaving space for osteoblasts to form new bone. Disturbances of this balance in patients with MM are further characterized by a marked impairment of bone formation by osteoblasts.[132] MM cells stimulate RANKL in T lymphocytes, thus supporting the formation, activation, and longer survival of osteoclasts.[131,133] MM cells also upregulate production of OPG and TRAIL, in addition to RANKL, in MM T cells as well as TRAIL decoy receptor DcR2 in osteoclatsts.[134] The high production of OPG may lead to the formation of OPG–TRAIL complexes, and then MM T cells would support osteoclast formation and survival by RANKL generation and unbalanced osteoclast expression of TRAIL death and decoy receptors.[134]

Despite the fact that FasL and TRAIL are potent ligands in the induction of apoptosis of tumor cells, there is accumulating evidence that death receptor ligands might also be used by tumor cells themselves to kill bystander cells, a mechanism called "the tumor counter-attack."[135] In this regard, it has been shown that myeloma cells express functional FasL[136] and TRAIL.[137,138] Erythroblasts have been identified as alternate targets for FasL- and/or TRAIL-mediated suppression by FasL+/TRAIL+ highly malignant myeloma cells as a major pathogenic mechanism of anemia in MM.[137,139] In MM, neoplastic plasma cells accumulate in the BM where their survival, proliferation, and apoptosis are controlled by interaction with the BM microenvironment. Myeloma cells actively control these interactions by activating stromal and endothelial cells for production of important survival factors for MM cells, such as IL-6, insulin-like growth factor-1, and vascular endothelial growth factor,[140] and suppressing other cell types such as erythroblasts, normal B cell progenitors, and T-cells. In addition, it has been shown that primary osteoblasts are additional potential targets for myeloma cell-mediated suppression which was partially dependent on the death receptor ligand TRAIL.[138] Besides killing of osteoblasts, MM cell lines sensitized osteoblasts to cell death mediated by recombinant TRAIL, whereas primary osteoblasts protected myeloma cells from TRAIL-mediated apoptosis via OPG.[138] Thus, increase of osteoclastogenesis and osteoclast activity, together with suppression of bone-forming cells by myeloma cells, might contribute to bone loss in MM patients. On these grounds, clinical development of recombinant TRAIL as antimyeloma therapy should include evaluation of potential side effects on viability of normal bone cells.

The nature of inhibitors of osteoblast viability and activity in MM, however, has remained unclear although a role of cytokines and death receptor ligands has been postulated.[141,142] Myeloma cells express FasL[136] and TRAIL,[137,138] and osteoblasts express Fas/CD95[143] and DR5.[144] However, in coculture with myeloma cells, significant killing of osteoblats resulted independent of FasL/CD95L, but partly dependent of TRAIL.[138] In view of the rapid convergence of Fas and TRAIL-R signaling into a common effector pathway of cell death, the change of sensitivity from Fas to TRAIL receptor observed in osteoblasts might be the result of changes at the very early stages of death receptor activation or in molecules present in the DISC. The ability of the neoplastic cells to kill bone-forming cells by TRAIL might allow them to gain ground within bone necessary for their expansion. Expression of TRAIL in myeloma cells is not part of the neoplastic transformation process, since TRAIL expression has also been demonstrated in normal IL-6-differentiated plasma cells.[145]

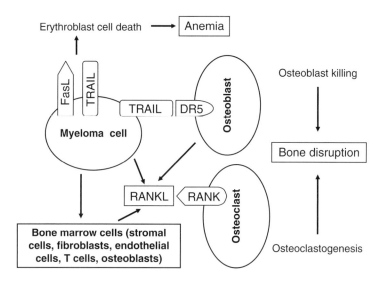

Fig. 8 Schematic representation of the interaction of myeloma cells with bone marrow cells leading to anemia and bone disruption.

In these cells, TRAIL-induced killing in an autocrine manner.[145] However, MM cells protect themselves in vivo by constitutive activation of NF-κB signaling pathway and by their interaction with BM stromal cells.[146] In this regard, as mentioned above, primary osteoblasts protected myeloma cells from TRAIL-mediated apoptosis that was mediated by OPG. Figure 8 shows a schematic view of the interactions between myeloma cells and BM cells through death receptors that lead to anemia and bone disruption.

OPG and MM

Unlike human MM cells, the human osteoblast-like cell line MG63 and primary BM stromal cells produce OPG. OPG binds to RANKL, inhibits bone resorption, and prevents TRAIL-induced apoptosis in myeloma cells, suggesting that OPG may function as a paracrine survival factor in the BM microenvironment in MM.[147] Myeloma cells alter the local regulation of bone metabolism by increasing RANKL and decreasing OPG expression within the BM microenvironment, thereby inducing an imbalance in the BM environment of the RANKL/OPG ratio in favor of RANKL, which triggers the central pathway for osteoclast formation and activation leading to bone destruction. Myeloma cells express RANKL, and can promote osteoclastogenesis and bone resorption in a stromal cell-independent manner in vitro.[148–150] Myeloma cells can also upregulate the expression of RANKL in cells found in the BM, including osteoblasts, fibroblasts, stromal cells, and endothelial cells,[151,152] and downregulate the production of OPG in osteoblasts and endothelial cells,[131,153,154] thereby promoting bone resorption. In addition, myeloma cells produce the chemokines MIP-1α, MIP-1β, and SDF-1α, which also increase osteoclast activity. Furthermore, myeloma cells suppress osteoblast function by the secretion of osteoblast-inhibiting factors, for example, Dickkopf (DKK)-1. The resulting bone destruction releases several cytokines, which, in turn, promote myeloma cell growth. Therefore, the inhibition of bone resorption could stop this vicious circle and decrease not only myeloma bone disease but also the tumor progression. On these grounds, targeting RANKL offers the possibility of developing therapeutical approaches to treat myeloma bone disease. Recombinant Fc-OPG has been shown to decrease osteoclast number and prevent the development of lytic bone disease in the 5T2MM murine model of myeloma.[155] Fc-OPG also decreases tumor burden and increases survival in the 5T33MM murine model for myeloma.[156] Preclinical studies have provided strong evidence that the suppression of the osteoclast activity using bisphosphonates,[157,158] RANKL blockade, or inhibition of MIP-1α or MIP-1β is effective in reducing both myeloma bone disease and tumor growth and therefore may offer an important treatment strategy in MM.[159] An OPG-like peptidomimetic (OP3-4) (YCEIEFCYLIR) was designed to block the RANKL–RANK interaction. OP3-4 inhibited osteoclast formation and bone resorption in vitro, whereas it had no effect on TRAIL-induced apoptosis of RPMI-8226 myeloma cells. Treatment of 5T2MM myeloma-bearing mice with OP3-4 decreased osteoclast number and the proportion of bone surface covered by osteclasts, preventing development of osteolytic lesions, and also reduced tumor burden.[160]

References

1. Rajkumar SV, Gertz MA, Kyle RA, Greipp PR. Current therapy for multiple myeloma. Mayo Clin Proc2002; 77:813–22.
2. Hussein MA, Juturi JV, Lieberman I. Multiple myeloma: Present and future. Curr Opin Oncol 2002; 14:31–5.
3. Mundy GR. Myeloma bone disease. Eur J Cancer 1998; 34:246–51.
4. Barille-Nion S, Bataille R. New insights in myeloma-induced osteolysis. Leuk Lymphoma 2003; 44:1463–7.
5. Epstein J, Yaccoby S. Consequences of interactions between the bone marrow stroma and myeloma. Hematol J 2003; 4:310–4.
6. Tian E, Zhan F, Walker R, et al. The role of the Wnt-signaling antagonist DKK1 in the development of osteolytic lesions in multiple myeloma. N Engl J Med 2003; 349:2483–94.
7. Kuehl WM, Bergsagel PL. Multiple myeloma: Evolving genetic events and host interactions. Nat Rev Cancer 2002; 2:175–87.
8. Walczak H, Krammer PH. The CD95 (APO-1/Fas) and the TRAIL (APO-2L) apoptosis systems. Exp Cell Res 2000; 256:58–66.
9. Wajant H. The Fas signaling pathway: More than a paradigm. Science 2002; 296:1635–6.
10. Debatin KM, Krammer PH. Death receptors in chemotherapy and cancer. Oncogene 2004; 23:2950–66.
11. Marsters SA, Sheridan JP, Donahue CJ, et al. Apo-3, a new member of the tumor necrosis factor receptor family, contains a death domain and activates apoptosis and NF-kappa B. Curr Biol 1996; 6:1669–76.
12. PanG, Bauer JH, Haridas V, et al. Identification and functional characterization of DR6, a novel death domain-containing TNF receptor. FEBS Lett 1998; 431:351–6.
13. El-DeiryWS. Insights into cancer therapeutic design based on p53 and TRAIL receptor signaling. Cell Death Differ 2001; 8:1066–75.
14. Mollinedo F, Gajate C, Martin-Santamaria S, Gago F. ET-18-OCH3 (edelfosine): A selective antitumour lipid targeting apoptosis through intracellular activation of Fas/CD95 death receptor. Curr Med Chem 2004; 11:3163–84.
15. Hainaut P, Hollstein M. p53 and human cancer: The first ten thousand mutations. Adv Cancer Res 2000; 77:81–137.
16. Mazars GR, Portier M, Zhang XG, et al. Mutations of the p53 gene in human myeloma cell lines. Oncogene1992; 7:1015–8.
17. Neri A, Baldini L, Trecca D, Cro L, Polli E, Maiolo AT. p53 gene mutations in multiple myeloma are associated with advanced forms of malignancy. Blood 1993; 81:128–35.
18. Avet-Loiseau H, Li JY, Godon C, et al. P53 deletion is not a frequent event in multiple myeloma. Br J Haematol 1999; 106:717–9.
19. Chang H, Qi C, Yi QL, Reece D, Stewart AK. p53 gene deletion detected by fluorescence in situ hybridization is an adverse prognostic factor for patients with multiple myeloma following autologous stem cell transplantation. Blood 2005; 105:358–60.
20. Stuhmer T, ChatterjeeM, Hildebrandt M, et al. Nongenotoxic activation of the p53 pathway as a therapeutic strategy for multiple myeloma. Blood 2005; 106:3609–17.
21. Liu Q, El-Deiry WS, Gazitt Y. Additive effect of Apo2L/TRAIL and Adeno-p53 in the induction of apoptosis in myeloma cell lines. Exp Hematol 2001; 29:962–70.
22. Itoh N, Yonehara S, Ishii A, et al. The polypeptide encoded by the cDNA for human cell surface antigen Fas can mediate apoptosis. Cell 1991; 66:233–43.
23. Itoh N, Nagata S. A novel protein domain required for apoptosis. Mutational analysis of human Fas antigen. J Biol Chem 1993; 268:10932–7.
24. Nagata S. Apoptosis by death factor. Cell 1997; 88:355–65.
25. Huang B, Eberstadt M, Olejniczak ET, Meadows RP, Fesik SW. NMR structure and mutagenesis of the Fas (APO-1/CD95) death domain. Nature 1996; 384:638–41.

26. Siegel RM, Chan FK, Chun HJ, Lenardo MJ. The multifaceted role of Fas signaling in immune cell homeostasis and autoimmunity. Nat Immunol 2000; 1:469–74.

27. Chan FK, Chun HJ, Zheng L, Siegel RM, Bui KL, Lenardo MJ. A domain in TNF receptors that mediates ligand-independent receptor assembly and signaling. Science 2000; 288:2351–4.

28. Papoff G, Hausler P, Eramo A, et al. Identification and characterization of a ligand-independent oligomerization domain in the extracellular region of the CD95 death receptor. J Biol Chem 1999; 274:38241–50.

29. Siegel RM, Frederiksen JK, Zacharias DA, et al. Fas preassociation required for apoptosis signaling and dominant inhibition by pathogenic mutations. Science 2000; 288:2354–7.

30. Chinnaiyan AM, O'Rourke K, Tewari M, Dixit VM. FADD, a novel death domain-containing protein, interacts with the death domain of Fas and initiates apoptosis. Cell 1995; 81:505–12.

31. Boldin MP, Goncharov TM, Goltsev YV, Wallach D. Involvement of MACH, a novel MORT1/FADD-interacting protease, in Fas/APO-1- and TNF receptor-induced cell death. Cell 1996; 85:803–15.

32. Ashkenazi A, Dixit VM. Death receptors: Signaling and modulation. Science 1998; 281:1305–8.

33. Kischkel FC, Hellbardt S, Behrmann I, et al. Cytotoxicity-dependent APO-1 (Fas/CD95)-associated proteins form a death-inducing signaling complex (DISC) with the receptor. Embo J 1995; 14:5579–88.

34. Parlato S, Giammarioli AM, Logozzi M, et al. CD95 (APO-1/Fas) linkage to the actin cytoskeleton through ezrin in human T lymphocytes: A novel regulatory mechanism of the CD95 apoptotic pathway. Embo J 2000; 19:5123–34.

35. Gajate C, Mollinedo F. Cytoskeleton-mediated Death Receptor and Ligand Concentration in Lipid Rafts Forms Apoptosis-promoting Clusters in Cancer Chemotherapy. J Biol Chem 2005; 280:11641–7.

36. Gajate C, Mollinedo F. Edelfosine and perifosine induce selective apoptosis in multiple myeloma by recruitment of death receptors and downstream signaling molecules into lipid rafts. Blood 2007; 109:711–9.

37. Gajate C, Fonteriz RI, Cabaner C, et al. Intracellular triggering of Fas, independently of FasL, as a new mechanism of antitumor ether lipid-induced apoptosis. Int J Cancer 2000; 85:674–82.

38. Gajate C, Del Canto-Janez E, Acuna AU, et al. Intracellular Triggering of Fas Aggregation and Recruitment of Apoptotic Molecules into Fas-enriched Rafts in Selective Tumor Cell Apoptosis. J Exp Med 2004; 200:353–65.

39. Mollinedo F, Gajate C. FasL-independent activation of Fas. In: Wajant H, ed. Fas Signaling. Georgetown, TX: Landes Bioscience and Springer Science, 2006: Chapter 2, pp. 13–27.

40. Mollinedo F, Gajate C. Fas/CD95 death receptor and lipid rafts: New targets for apoptosis-directed cancer therapy. Drug Resist Updat 2006; 9:51–73.

41. Irmler M, Thome M, Hahne M, et al. Inhibition of death receptor signals by cellular FLIP. Nature 1997; 388:190–5.

42. Kataoka T. The caspase-8 modulator c-FLIP. Crit Rev Immunol 2005; 25:31–58.

43. Chang DW, Xing Z, Pan Y, et al. c-FLIP(L) is a dual function regulator for caspase-8 activation and CD95-mediated apoptosis. Embo J 2002; 21:3704–14.

44. Micheau O, Thome M, Schneider P, et al. The long form of FLIP is an activator of caspase-8 at the Fas death-inducing signaling complex. J Biol Chem 2002; 277:45162–71.

45. Rasper DM, Vaillancourt JP, Hadano S, et al. Cell death attenuation by 'Usurpin', a mammalian DED-caspase homologue that precludes caspase-8 recruitment and activation by the CD-95 (Fas, APO-1) receptor complex. Cell Death Differ 1998; 5:271–88.

46. Yeh WC, Pompa JL, McCurrach ME, et al. FADD: Essential for embryo development and signaling from some, but not all, inducers of apoptosis. Science 1998; 279:1954–8.

47. Yeh WC, Itie A, Elia AJ, et al. Requirement for Casper (c-FLIP) in regulation of death receptor-induced apoptosis and embryonic development. Immunity 2000; 12:633–42.

48. Falschlehner C, Emmerich CH, Gerlach B, Walczak H. TRAIL signalling: Decisions between life and death. Int J Biochem Cell Biol 2007.

49. Kelley RF, Totpal K, Lindstrom SH, et al. Receptor-selective mutants of apoptosis-inducing ligand 2/tumor necrosis factor-related apoptosis-inducing ligand reveal a greater contribution of death receptor (DR) 5 than DR4 to apoptosis signaling. J Biol Chem 2005; 280:2205–12.

50. de Vries EG, Timmer T, Mulder NH, et al. Modulation of death receptor pathways in oncology. Drugs Today (Barc) 2003; 39 (Suppl C):95–109.

51. Ogasawara J, Watanabe-Fukunaga R, Adachi M, et al. Lethal effect of the anti-Fas antibody in mice. Nature 1993; 364:806–9.

52. Faubion WA, Gores GJ. Death receptors in liver biology and pathobiology. Hepatology 1999; 29:1–4.

53. Wiley SR, Schooley K, Smolak PJ, et al. Identification and characterization of a new member of the TNF family that induces apoptosis. Immunity 1995; 3:673–82.

54. Pitti RM, Marsters SA, Ruppert S, Donahue CJ, Moore A, Ashkenazi A. Induction of apoptosis by Apo-2 ligand, a new member of the tumor necrosis factor cytokine family. J Biol Chem 1996; 271:12687–90.

55. Walczak H, Miller RE, Ariail K, et al. Tumoricidal activity of tumor necrosis factor-related apoptosis-inducing ligand in vivo. Nat Med 1999; 5:157–63.

56. Ashkenazi A, Pai RC, Fong S, et al. Safety and antitumor activity of recombinant soluble Apo2 ligand. J Clin Invest 1999; 104:155–62.

57. Jo M, Kim TH, Seol DW, et al. Apoptosis induced in normal human hepatocytes by tumor necrosis factor-related apoptosis-inducing ligand. Nat Med 2000; 6:564–7.

58. Leverkus M, Neumann M, MenglingT, et al. Regulation of tumor necrosis factor-related apoptosis-inducing ligand sensitivity in primary and transformed human keratinocytes. Cancer Res 2000; 60:553–9.

59. Nesterov A, Ivashchenko Y, Kraft AS. Tumor necrosis factor-related apoptosis-inducing ligand (TRAIL) triggers apoptosis in normal prostate epithelial cells. Oncogene 2002; 21:1135–40.

60. Nitsch R, Bechmann I, Deisz RA, et al. Human brain-cell death induced by tumour-necrosis-factor-related apoptosis-inducing ligand (TRAIL). Lancet 2000; 356:827–8.

61. Takeda K, Stagg J, Yagita H, Okumura K, Smyth MJ. Targeting death-inducing receptors in cancer therapy. Oncogene 2007; 26:3745–57.

62. Kelley SK, Harris LA, Xie D, et al. Preclinical studies to predict the disposition of Apo2L/tumor necrosis factor-related apoptosis-inducing ligand in humans: Characterization of in vivo efficacy, pharmacokinetics, and safety. J Pharmacol Exp Ther 2001; 299:31–8.

63. Fesik SW. Promoting apoptosis as a strategy for cancer drug discovery. Nat Rev Cancer 2005; 5:876–85.

64. Clodi K, Wimmer D, Li Y, et al. Expression of tumour necrosis factor (TNF)-related apoptosis-inducing ligand (TRAIL) receptors and sensitivity to TRAIL-induced apoptosis in primary B-cell acute lymphoblastic leukaemia cells. Br J Haematol 2000; 111:580–6.

65. Lincz LF, Yeh TX, Spencer A. TRAIL-induced eradication of primary tumour cells from multiple myeloma patient bone marrows is not related to TRAIL receptor expression or prior chemotherapy. Leukemia 2001; 15:1650–7.

66. EmeryJG, McDonnell P, Burke MB, et al. Osteoprotegerin is a receptor for the cytotoxic ligand TRAIL. J Biol Chem 1998; 273:14363–7.

67. Truneh A, Sharma S, Silverman C, et al. Temperature-sensitive differential affinity of TRAIL for its receptors. DR5 is the highest affinity receptor. J Biol Chem 2000; 275:23319–25.

68. Simonet WS, Lacey DL, Dunstan CR, et al. Osteoprotegerin: A novel secreted protein involved in the regulation of bone density. Cell 1997; 89:309–19.

69. Lacey DL, Timms E, Tan HL, et al. Osteoprotegerin ligand is a cytokine that regulates osteoclast differentiation and activation. Cell 1998; 93:165–76.

70. Nakagawa N, Kinosaki M, Yamaguchi K, et al. RANK is the essential signaling receptor for osteoclast differentiation factor in osteoclastogenesis. Biochem Biophys Res Commun 1998; 253:395–400.

71. Kong YY, Yoshida H, Sarosi I, et al. OPGL is a key regulator of osteoclastogenesis, lymphocyte development and lymph-node organogenesis. Nature 1999; 397:315–23.

72. Burgess TL, Qian Y, Kaufman S, et al. The ligand for osteoprotegerin (OPGL) directly activates mature osteoclasts. J Cell Biol 1999; 145:527–38.

73. De Leenheer E, Mueller GS, Vanderkerken K, Croucher PI. Evidence of a role for RANKL in the development of myeloma bone disease. Curr Opin Pharmacol 2004; 4:340–6.

74. Bucay N, Sarosi I, Dunstan CR, et al. osteoprotegerin-deficient mice develop early onset osteoporosis and arterial calcification. Genes Dev 1998; 12:1260–8.

75. Mizuno A, Amizuka N, Irie K, et al. Severe osteoporosis in mice lacking osteoclastogenesis inhibitory factor/osteoprotegerin. Biochem Biophys Res Commun1998; 247:610–5.

76. Gajate C, Mollinedo F. The antitumor ether lipid ET-18-OCH3 induces apoptosis through translocation and capping of Fas/CD95 into membrane rafts in human leukemic cells. Blood 2001; 98:3860–3.

77. Varma R, Mayor S. GPI-anchored proteins are organized in submicron domains at the cell surface. Nature1998; 394:798–801.

78. Hueber AO, Bernard AM, Herincs Z, Couzinet A, He HT. An essential role for membrane rafts in the initiation of Fas/CD95-triggered cell death in mouse thymocytes. EMBO Rep 2002; 3:190–6.

79. Scheel-Toellner D, Wang K, Singh R, et al. The death-inducing signalling complex is recruited to lipid rafts in Fas-induced apoptosis. Biochem Biophys Res Commun 2002; 297:876–9.

80. Delmas D, Rebe C, Lacour S, et al. Resveratrol-induced apoptosis is associated with Fas redistribution in the rafts and the formation of a death-inducing signaling complex in colon cancer cells. J Biol Chem 2003; 278:41482–90.

81. Chakrabandhu K, Herincs Z, Huault S, et al. Palmitoylation is required for efficient Fas cell death signaling. Embo J 2007; 26:209–20.

82. Krammer PH. CD95's deadly mission in the immune system. Nature 2000; 407:789–95.

83. Landowski TH, Qu N, Buyuksal I, Painter JS, Dalton WS. Mutations in the Fas antigen in patients with multiple myeloma. Blood 1997; 90:4266–70.

84. ShimaY, Nishimoto N, Ogata A, Fujii Y, Yoshizaki K, Kishimoto T. Myeloma cells express Fas antigen/APO-1 (CD95) but only some are sensitive to anti-Fas antibody resulting in apoptosis. Blood 1995; 85:757–64.

85. Westendorf JJ, Lammert JM, Jelinek DF. Expression and function of Fas (APO-1/CD95) in patient myeloma cells and myeloma cell lines. Blood 1995; 85:3566–76.

86. Hata H, Matsuzaki H, Takeya M, et al. Expression of Fas/Apo-1 (CD95) and apoptosis in tumor cells from patients with plasma cell disorders. Blood 1995; 86:1939–45.

87. Kim DK, Cho ES, Yoo JH, Um HD. FLIP is constitutively hyperexpressed in Fas-resistant U266 myeloma cells, but is not induced by IL-6 in Fas-sensitive RPM18226 cells. Mol Cells 2000; 10:552–6.

88. Munshi NC, Hideshima T, Carrasco D, et al. Identification of genes modulated in multiple myeloma using genetically identical twin samples. Blood 2004; 103:1799–806.

89. Catlett-Falcone R, Landowski TH, Oshiro MM, et al. Constitutive activation of Stat3 signaling confers resistance to apoptosis in human U266 myeloma cells. Immunity 1999; 10:105–15.

90. Kawano M, Hirano T, Matsuda T, et al. Autocrine generation and requirement of BSF-2/IL-6 for human multiple myelomas. Nature 1988; 332:83–5.

91. Zhang XG, Klein B, Bataille R. Interleukin-6 is a potent myeloma-cell growth factor in patients with aggressive multiple myeloma. Blood 1989; 74:11–3.
92. Hardin J, MacLeod S, Grigorieva I, et al. Interleukin-6 prevents dexamethasone-induced myeloma cell death. Blood 1994; 84:3063–70.
93. Lichtenstein A, Tu Y, Fady C, Vescio R, Berenson J. Interleukin-6 inhibits apoptosis of malignant plasma cells. Cell Immunol 1995; 162:248–55.
94. Barut BA, Zon LI, Cochran MK, et al. Role of interleukin 6 in the growth of myeloma-derived cell lines. Leuk Res1992; 16:951–9.
95. Chauhan D, Kharbanda S, Ogata A, et al. Interleukin-6 inhibits Fas-induced apoptosis and stress-activated protein kinase activation in multiple myeloma cells. Blood 1997; 89:227–34.
96. Xu FH, Sharma S, Gardner A, et al. Interleukin-6-induced inhibition of multiple myeloma cell apoptosis: Support for the hypothesis that protection is mediated via inhibition of the JNK/SAPK pathway. Blood 1998; 92:241–51.
97. Blade J, Lopez-Guillermo A, Tassies D, Montserrat E, Rozman C. Development of aggressive plasma cell leukaemia under interferon-alpha therapy. Br J Haematol 1991; 79:523–5.
98. Shustik C. Interferon in the Treatment of Multiple Myeloma. Cancer Control 1998; 5:226–34.
99. Tu KL, Bowyer J, Schofield K, Harding S. Severe interferon associated retinopathy. Br J Ophthalmol 2003; 87:247–8.
100. Schaar CG, Kluin-Nelemans HC, Te Marvelde C, et al. Interferon-alpha as maintenance therapy in patients with multiple myeloma. Ann Oncol2005; 16:634–9.
101. Spets H, Georgii-Hemming P, Siljason J, Nilsson K, Jernberg-Wiklund H. Fas/APO-1 (CD95)-mediated apoptosis is activated by interferon-gamma and interferon- in interleukin-6 (IL-6)-dependent and IL-6-independent multiple myeloma cell lines. Blood 1998; 92:2914–23.
102. Dimberg LY, DimbergAI, Ivarsson K, et al. Ectopic and IFN-induced expression of Fas overcomes resistance to Fas-mediated apoptosis in multiple myeloma cells. Blood 2005; 106:1346–54.
103. Bowman T, Garcia R, Turkson J, Jove R. STATs in oncogenesis. Oncogene 2000; 19:2474–88.
104. Ivanov VN, Bhoumik A, Krasilnikov M, et al. Cooperation between STAT3 and c-jun suppresses Fas transcription. Mol Cell 2001; 7:517–28.
105. Alas S, Bonavida B. Inhibition of constitutive STAT3 activity sensitizes resistant non-Hodgkin's lymphoma and multiple myeloma to chemotherapeutic drug-mediated apoptosis. Clin Cancer Res 2003; 9:316–26.
106. Xu X, Fu XY, Plate J, Chong AS. IFN-gamma induces cell growth inhibition by Fas-mediated apoptosis: Requirement of STAT1 protein for up-regulation of Fas and FasL expression. Cancer Res 1998; 58:2832–7.
107. Shen Y, Devgan G, Darnell JE, Jr., Bromberg JF. Constitutively activated Stat3 protects fibroblasts from serum withdrawal and UV-induced apoptosis and antagonizes the proapoptotic effects of activated Stat1. Proc Natl Acad Sci USA 2001; 98:1543–8.
108. Hong F, Jaruga B, Kim WH, et al. Opposing roles of STAT1 and STAT3 in T cell-mediated hepatitis: Regulation by SOCS. J Clin Invest 2002; 110:1503–13.
109. Stephanou A, Brar BK, Knight RA, Latchman DS. Opposing actions of STAT-1 and STAT-3 on the Bcl-2 and Bcl-x promoters. Cell Death Differ 2000; 7:329–30.
110. Shain KH, Landowski TH, Buyuksal I, Cantor AB, Dalton WS. Clonal variability in CD95 expression is the major determinant in Fas-medicated, but not chemotherapy-medicated apoptosis in the RPMI 8226 multiple myeloma cell line. Leukemia 2000; 14:830–40.
111. Gajate C, Mollinedo F. Biological activities, mechanisms of action and biomedical prospect of the antitumor ether phospholipid ET-18-OCH3 (edelfosine), a proapoptotic agent in tumor cells. Curr Drug Metab 2002; 3:491–525.

112. Mollinedo F. Antitumor ether lipids: Proapoptotic agents with multiple therapeutic indications. Expert Opin Ther Patents 2007; 17:385–405.

113. Yagita H, Takeda K, Hayakawa Y, Smyth MJ, OkumuraK. TRAIL and its receptors as targets for cancer therapy. Cancer Sci 2004; 95:777–83.

114. Gazitt Y. TRAIL is a potent inducer of apoptosis in myeloma cells derived from multiple myeloma patients and is not cytotoxic to hematopoietic stem cells. Leukemia 1999; 13:1817–24.

115. Mitsiades CS, Treon SP, Mitsiades N, et al. TRAIL/Apo2L ligand selectively induces apoptosis and overcomes drug resistance in multiple myeloma: Therapeutic applications. Blood 2001; 98:795–804.

116. Glasser L, Dalton WS, Fiederlein RL, Cook P, Powis G, Vogler WR. Response of human multiple myeloma-derived cell lines to alkyl-lysophospholipid. Exp Hematol 1996; 24:253–7.

117. Hideshima T, Catley L, Yasui H, et al. Perifosine, an oral bioactive novel alkyl-phospholipid, inhibits Akt and induces in vitro and in vivo cytotoxicity in human multiple myeloma cells. Blood 2006; 107:4053–62.

118. Berdel WE, Bausert WR, Fink U, Rastetter J, Munder PG. Anti-tumor action of alkyl-lysophospholipids (review). Anticancer Res 1981; 1:345–52.

119. Mitsiades CS, Mitsiades N, Poulaki V, et al. Activation of NF-kappaB and upregulation of intracellular anti-apoptotic proteins via the IGF-1/Akt signaling in human multiple myeloma cells: Therapeutic implications. Oncogene 2002; 21:5673–83.

120. Chen Q, Ray S, Hussein MA, Srkalovic G, Almasan A. Role of Apo2L/TRAIL and Bcl-2-family proteins in apoptosis of multiple myeloma. Leuk Lymphoma 2003; 44:1209–14.

121. Gomez-Benito M, Martinez-Lorenzo MJ, Anel A, Marzo I, Naval J. Membrane expression of DR4, DR5 and caspase-8 levels, but not Mcl-1, determine sensitivity of human myeloma cells to Apo2L/TRAIL. Exp Cell Res 2007; 313:2378–88.

122. Chen Q, Gong B, Mahmoud-Ahmed AS, et al. Apo2L/TRAIL and Bcl-2-related proteins regulate type I interferon-induced apoptosis in multiple myeloma. Blood 2001; 98:2183–92.

123. Mitsiades N, Mitsiades CS, Poulaki V, Anderson KC, Treon SP. Intracellular regulation of tumor necrosis factor-related apoptosis-inducing ligand-induced apoptosis in human multiple myeloma cells. Blood 2002; 99:2162–71.

124. Spencer A, Yeh SL, Koutrevelis K, Baulch-Brown C. TRAIL-induced apoptosis of authentic myeloma cells does not correlate with the procaspase-8/cFLIP ratio. Blood 2002; 100:3049; author reply 3050–1.

125. Crowder C, Dahle O, Davis RE, Gabrielsen OS, Rudikoff S. PML mediates IFN-alpha-induced apoptosis in myeloma by regulating TRAIL induction. Blood 2005; 105:1280–7.

126. MacFarlane M, Inoue S, Kohlhaas SL, et al. Chronic lymphocytic leukemic cells exhibit apoptotic signaling via TRAIL-R1. Cell Death Differ2005; 12:773–82.

127. Menoret E, Gomez-Bougie P, Geffroy-Luseau A, et al. Mcl-1L cleavage is involved in TRAIL-R1- and TRAIL-R2-mediated apoptosis induced by HGS-ETR1 and HGS-ETR2 human mAbs in myeloma cells. Blood 2006; 108:1346–52.

128. Roodman GD. Mechanisms of bone lesions in multiple myeloma and lymphoma. Cancer1997; 80:1557–63.

129. Kyle RA, Rajkumar SV. Multiple myeloma. N Engl J Med 2004; 351:1860–73.

130. Boyle WJ, Simonet WS, Lacey DL. Osteoclast differentiation and activation. Nature 2003; 423:337–42.

131. Giuliani N, Colla S, Rizzoli V. New insight in the mechanism of osteoclast activation and formation in multiple myeloma: Focus on the receptor activator of NF-kappaB ligand (RANKL). Exp Hematol 2004; 32:685–91.

132. Hjorth-Hansen H, Seifert MF, Borset M, et al. Marked osteoblastopenia and reduced bone formation in a model of multiple myeloma bone disease in severe combined immunodeficiency mice. J Bone Miner Res 1999; 14:256–63.

133. Giuliani N, Colla S, Sala R, et al. Human myeloma cells stimulate the receptor activator of nuclear factor-kappa B ligand (RANKL) in T lymphocytes: A potential role in multiple myeloma bone disease. Blood 2002; 100:4615–21.

134. Colucci S, Brunetti G, Rizzi R, et al. T cells support osteoclastogenesis in an in vitro model derived from human multiple myeloma bone disease: The role of the OPG/TRAIL interaction. Blood 2004; 104:3722–30.

135. O'Connell J, Bennett MW, O'Sullivan GC, Collins JK, Shanahan F. The Fas counterattack: Cancer as a site of immune privilege. Immunol Today 1999; 20:46–52.

136. Villunger A, Egle A, Marschitz I, et al. Constitutive expression of Fas (Apo-1/CD95) ligand on multiple myeloma cells: A potential mechanism of tumor-induced suppression of immune surveillance. Blood 1997; 90:12–20.

137. Silvestris F, Cafforio P, Tucci M, Dammacco F. Negative regulation of erythroblast maturation by Fas-L(+)/TRAIL(+) highly malignant plasma cells: A major pathogenetic mechanism of anemia in multiple myeloma. Blood 2002; 99:1305–13.

138. Tinhofer I, Biedermann R, Krismer M, Crazzolara R, Greil R. A role of TRAIL in killing osteoblasts by myeloma cells. Faseb J 2006; 20:759–61.

139. Silvestris F, Tucci M, Cafforio P, Dammacco F. Fas-L up-regulation by highly malignant myeloma plasma cells: Role in the pathogenesis of anemia and disease progression. Blood 2001; 97:1155–64.

140. Menu E, Kooijman R, Van Valckenborgh E, et al. Specific roles for the PI3K and the MEK-ERK pathway in IGF-1-stimulated chemotaxis, VEGF secretion and proliferation of multiple myeloma c ells: Study in the 5T33MM model. Br J Cancer 2004; 90:1076–83.

141. Silvestris F, Cafforio P, Tucci M, Grinello D, Dammacco F. Upregulation of osteoblast apoptosis by malignant plasma cells: A role in myeloma bone disease. Br J Haematol 2003; 122:39–52.

142. Silvestris F, Cafforio P, Calvani N, Dammacco F. Impaired osteoblastogenesis in myeloma bone disease: Role of upregulated apoptosis by cytokines and malignant plasma cells. Br J Haematol2004; 126:475–86.

143. Leithauser F, Dhein J, Mechtersheimer G, et al. Constitutive and induced expression of APO-1, a new member of the nerve growth factor/tumor necrosis factor receptor superfamily, in normal and neoplastic cells. Lab Invest1993; 69:415–29.

144. Atkins GJ, Bouralexis S, Evdokiou A, et al. Human osteoblasts are resistant to Apo2L/TRAIL-mediated apoptosis. Bone 2002; 31:448–56.

145. Ursini-Siegel J, Zhang W, Altmeyer A, et al. TRAIL/Apo-2 ligand induces primary plasma cell apoptosis. J Immunol2002; 169:5505–13.

146. HideshimaT, ChauhanD, RichardsonP, et al. NF-kappa B as a therapeutic target in multiple myeloma. J Biol Chem2002; 277:16639–47.

147. Shipman CM, Croucher PI. Osteoprotegerin is a soluble decoy receptor for tumor necrosis factor-related apoptosis-inducing ligand/Apo2 ligand and can function as a paracrine survival factor for human myeloma cells. Cancer Res 2003; 63:912–6.

148. Sezer O, Heider U, Jakob C, Eucker J, Possinger K. Human bone marrow myeloma cells express RANKL. J Clin Oncol 2002; 20:353–4.

149. Sezer O, Heider U, Jakob C, et al. Immunocytochemistry reveals RANKL expression of myeloma cells. Blood 2002; 99:4646–7; author reply 4647.

150. Heider U, Langelotz C, Jakob C, et al. Expression of receptor activator of nuclear factor kappaB ligand on bone marrow plasma cells correlates with osteolytic bone disease in patients with multiple myeloma. Clin Cancer Res 2003; 9:1436–40.

151. Pearse RN, Sordillo EM, Yaccoby S, et al. Multiple myeloma disrupts the TRANCE/ osteoprotegerin cytokine axis to trigger bone destruction and promote tumor progression. Proc Natl Acad Sci U S A 2001; 98:11581–6.

152. Okada T, Akikusa S, Okuno H, Kodaka M. Bone marrow metastatic myeloma cells promote osteoclastogenesis through RANKL on endothelial cells. Clin Exp Metastasis 2003; 20:639–46.

153. Giuliani N, Bataille R, Mancini C, Lazzaretti M, Barille S. Myeloma cells induce imbalance in the osteoprotegerin/osteoprotegerin ligand system in the human bone marrow environment. Blood 2001; 98:3527–33.
154. Seidel C, HjertnerO, Abildgaard N, et al. Serum osteoprotegerin levels are reduced in patients with multiple myeloma with lytic bone disease. Blood 2001; 98:2269–71.
155. Croucher PI, Shipman CM, Lippitt J, et al. Osteoprotegerin inhibits the development of osteolytic bone disease in multiple myeloma. Blood 2001; 98:3534–40.
156. Vanderkerken K, De Leenheer E, Shipman C, et al. Recombinant osteoprotegerin decreases tumor burden and increases survival in a murine model of multiple myeloma. Cancer Res 2003; 63:287–9.
157. Croucher PI, Shipman CM, Van CampB, Vanderkerken K. Bisphosphonates and osteoprotegerin as inhibitors of myeloma bone disease. Cancer 2003; 97:818–24.
158. Croucher PI, De Hendrik R, Perry MJ, et al. Zoledronic acid treatment of 5T2MM-bearing mice inhibits the development of myeloma bone disease: Evidence for decreased osteolysis, tumor burden and angiogenesis, and increased survival. J Bone Miner Res 2003; 18:482–92.
159. Sezer O. Myeloma bone disease. Hematology 2005; 10(Suppl 1):19–24.
160. Heath DJ, Vanderkerken K, Cheng X, et al. An osteoprotegerin-like peptidomimetic inhibits osteoclastic bone resorption and osteolytic bone disease in myeloma. Cancer Res2007; 67:202–8.

Chapter 26

Proteasome Inhibitors as Therapy in Multiple Myeloma

Dharminder Chauhan, Ajita, Singh, and Kenneth Anderson

Ubiquitin-Proteasome System: Constitution and Function

Normal cellular homeostasis requires balanced regulation of protein synthesis and degradation. Intracellular protein degradation occurs majorly via a multi-subunit complex called the proteasome.[1–4] Initial studies by Ciechanover, Hershko, and Rose demonstrated that ATP-dependent conjugation of proteins with polypeptide (ubiquitin) mediates protein degradation.[5–11] The role of ubiquitin in cellular protein turnover was further established in later studies.[6,11]

Proteolysis is mediated via the 26S multi-subunit proteasome complex[12–15] consisting of 19S units flanking a barrel-shaped 20S proteasome core.[16–18] The 19S units of the 26S proteasome complex regulate entry of ubiquitinated proteins into the 20S core chamber.[2,19,20] Protein ubiquitination is facilitated through several enzymatic reactions: E1 ubiquitin enzyme first activates ubiquitin and then links it to the ubiquitin-conjugating enzyme E2, followed by binding of this complex to the target protein via E3 ubiquitin ligases.[21,22] Repeated cycles of this process result in the formation of polyubiquitinated proteins which are eventually degraded by the proteasomes into small peptides, and free ubiquitin is recycled.[23–26] E3 ubiquitin ligases confer specificity in the ubiquitin-proteasome system pathway by selectively tagging protein substrates for proteasomal degradation,[21] and this attribute of E3 ligases makes them attractive therapeutic targets. Once the ubiquitinated proteins are recognized by the 19S regulatory subunits of the proteasome complex, they are degraded into small peptides via three major proteasomal activities residing within the 20S core complex, that is, chymotrypsin-like (CT-L), trypsin-like (T-L), and caspase-like (C-L) activities (also known as β5, β2, and β1 activities, respectively).[27–30]

Proteasome Inhibitor as Anticancer Agents

As noted above, protein degradation is a normal cellular process, and therefore many proteins with normal cellular functions are substrates for proteasomes, for example, proteins involved in the maintenance of normal cell cycle progression,

From: *Contemporary Hematology Myeloma Therapy*
Edited by: S. Lonial © Humana Press, Totowa, NJ

growth, and survival.[1,2,6,31–33] Deregulation of proteasome function disrupts the normal elimination process of misfolded and functionally redundant proteins from the cells. This results in buildup of unwanted proteins within the cells, thereby causing toxicity and eventual cell death.[34–36] These observations provided the rationale for potential utility of proteasome inhibitors as anticancer agents. However, since the proteasome regulates normal cellular functions, its inhibition may also cause toxicity even against normal cells. Nonetheless, it was later established that proteasome inhibitors are more cytotoxic to proliferating malignant cells than the quiescent normal cells, suggesting a favorable therapeutic index.[37–42]

Proteasome inhibitors, either naturally occurring or synthesized in the laboratory, are classified as peptide aldehydes, peptide boronates, nonpeptide inhibitors, peptide vinyl sulfones, and peptide epoxyketones.[4,43–45] Importantly, these inhibitors differentially affect both proteasome and proteases. For example, peptide aldehydes (MG-132, MG-115, ALLN, or PSI, initially generated at ProScript, formerly known as Myogenics, Cambridge, MA) potently, but reversibly, block the CT-L activity of the proteasome; however, they also inhibit lysosomal cysteine and serine proteases as well as calpains, thereby limiting their clinical utility.[46] Lactacystin is a natural, irreversible, nonpeptide inhibitor which was originally identified by Omura at the Kitasato Institute, Tokyo, as an inducer of neuritogenesis in neuroblastoma cells[47] and later reported as capable of blocking the proteasome and inducing cell cycle arrest.[48,49] The dipeptidyl boronic acid bortezomib/PS-341 (developed by Julian Adams at ProScript, later Millenium, Inc., Cambridge, MA) is a potent and reversible inhibitor of CT-L activity.[35] Initial National Cancer Institute (NCI) screening showed remarkable antitumor activity of bortezomib in a panel of 60 tumor cell lines.[4,50]

Rationale for Proteasome Inhibitor bortezomib/PS-341 as Therapy in Multiple Myeloma

As noted above, a broad spectrum of intracellular proteins are substrates of proteasome and one among these is nuclear factor-kappa B (NF-κB). NF-κB is a transcription factor that plays a pivotal role in inflammatory response and carcinogenesis by regulating genes involved in growth, survival, cell cycle progression, angiogenesis, and invasion.[51–54] Activation of NF-κB occurs through phosphorylation of IκB-α whose activity is triggered by an upstream IκB-α kinase (IKK). Ubiquitination and degradation of phosphorylated IκB-α result in the disassociation of p50/p65 NF-κB complex, which then translocates from the cytoplasm to the nucleus. Once in the nucleus p50/p65 heterodimers bind to the promoters of various growth and survival genes and trigger their transcription and secretion. For example, NF-κB activation promotes the secretion of cytokines, such as interleukin-6 (IL-6), TNF-α, inhibitors of apoptosis protein XIAP, antiapoptotic protein Bcl-xL, and several cell adhesion molecules.[51–54] In 1996, Palombella et al. showed that the ubiquitin-proteasome pathway is required for processing the NF-κB1 precursor protein and activation of NF-κB[55]; conversely, inhibition of proteasome by proteasome inhibitor MG-132 blocked NF-κB activity.[56]

In the context of multiple myeloma (MM), our earlier study showed that adhesion of MM cells to the bone marrow stromal cells (BMSCs) triggers transcription and secretion of various cytokines that confer growth, survival, and drug resistance in MM cells.[57,58] Various later studies further confirmed the role of NF-κB as a major growth and survival signaling pathway in MM.[59–62] Given the protective role of NF-κB in MM, coupled with the ability of proteasome inhibitors to block NF-κB, provided initial support for clinical utility of proteasome inhibitors in MM. In 1998, Palobmbella et al. in their study developed a series of peptide boronic acid inhibitors of the proteasome, in particular PS-341/bortezomib, and demonstrated their inhibitory activity on NF-κB.[56] In 1999–2000, we started evaluating the effects of PS-341/bortezomib in MM cells. Our in vitro studies showed that bortezomib downregulates NF-κB, induces apoptosis in both MM cell lines and freshly isolated MM cells from patients, downregulates adhesion molecules, and inhibits constitutive and MM cell adhesion-induced cytokine secretion in BMSCs.[41,60] In vivo studies using animal models showed potent anti-MM activity of bortezomib.[42,63]

Importantly, we completed laboratory and animal studies showing the mechanisms whereby bortezomib overcomes drug resistance in MM. These data, coupled with phase I data demonstrating safety and early anti-MM activity,[64] provided the rationale for a multicenter phase II trial of bortezomib in patients with relapsed refractory MM which achieved marked responses, even complete responses, which were both durable and associated with clinical benefit.[65,66] This clinical data, along with another randomized phase II trial,[67] provided the basis for the expedited Food and Drug Administration (FDA) approval of bortezomib for treatment of refractory-relapsed MM in 2003, with translation of preclinical studies from the bench to the bedside and FDA approval in less than 3 years. This efficacy was subsequently confirmed in another phase II trial,[68,69] and a phase III trial comparing bortezomib versus dexamethasone treatment in relapsed MM rapidly demonstrated prolonged time to progression in the bortezomib arm[70] leading to FDA approval for these patients in 2005. Further studies have defined the clinical parameters for its optimal clinical use.[71–74]

Despite the success of bortezomib therapy, treatment can be associated with toxicity and the development of drug resistance.[75] In addition, many MM patients with advanced MM do not respond to bortezomib therapy.[76] To address this issue, extensive laboratory efforts are focused on delineating molecular mechanisms mediating bortezomib-induced cytotoxicity and drug resistance.

Molecular Mechanisms Mediating Bortezomib-Induced Apoptosis in MM Cells

Bortezomib-triggered apoptosis in MM cells is associated with inhibition of NF-κB. We examined the effects of PS-1145, a specific inhibitor of IKK-β, and bortezomib on NF-κB blockade and consequent biological response (cell death) in MM cells. Both PS-1145 and bortezomib block TNF-α-induced NF-κB activation by inhibiting phosphorylation and degradation of IκB-α; in contrast to bortezomib, however, PS-1145 only partially inhibits MM cell growth.[77] These findings showed that NF-κB inhibition alone is unlikely to account for the total anti-MM activity of bortezomib.

Indeed, besides NF-κB, bortezomib trigger pleiotropic intracellular signaling pathways. For example, bortezomib-triggered cell death correlates with (1) activation of stress response proteins such as heat shock proteins Hsp27, Hsp70, and Hsp90[78,79], (2) upregulation of c-Jun N-terminal kinase,[80] (3) variation of mitochondrial membrane potential and production of reactive oxygen species,[81] (4) release of mitochondrial proteins cytochrome-c/Smac into cytosol and activation of downstream caspase-9 and caspase-3,[82] (5) activation of Bid, Bim, and caspase-8,[78] (6) inactivation of DNA-dependent protein kinase (DNA-PK),[83] a kinase required for DNA repair, (7) inhibition of MM to BMSCs interaction,[84] (8) inhibition of MM cell growth factor-triggered signaling: MAPK and PI3-kinase/Akt,[85] and (9) induction of ER stress/UPR.[86-88]

Mechanistic Studies Provide Rationale for Combination Therapies

Gene profiling, proteomic, and cell signaling studies have helped to identify in vivo mechanisms of action and drug resistance, as well as aided in the clinical application of combination therapies. For example, our microarray studies showed that Hsp-27 gene and protein expression was associated with bortezomib resistance.[79] To confirm its functional significance, we showed that forced overexpression of Hsp27 in sensitive tumor cells confers bortezomib resistance; conversely, blocking Hsp27 activity in bortezomib-resistant tumor cells using Hsp27 antisense strategy or small inhibitory RNA restores sensitivity. These studies support targeting Hsp27 to sensitize or overcome resistance to bortezomib, and we have already completed a clinical trial of p38MAPK inhibitor (to block downstream Hsp27) and bortezomib to overcome clinical resistance. Bcl-2 protein family members also confer drug resistance in many cell types,[89] and bortezomib-triggered apoptosis in MM cells is partially abrogated by overexpression of wild-type Bcl-2.[78] In a later study, we showed that specific Bcl-2/Bcl-xL/Bcl-w inhibitor ABT-737 enhances the anti-MM activity of bortezomib.[90] Upregulated expression of inhibitors of apoptosis proteins, such as XIAP, may also contribute to bortezomib resistance,[78] and we recently demonstrated that Smac mimetics (which bind and block XIAP function) increase bortezomib anti-MM activity.[91]

Outcome to proteasome inhibitor bortezomib has recently been correlated with gene profile of treated patients.[92] In addition, gene microarray profiling of bortezomib-treated MM cells reveals induction of Hsp90 stress response,[78,93] providing the rationale for the combined clinical use of bortezomib and the Hsp90 inhibitor 17-AAG to enhance anti-MM activity; clinical trials of 17-AAG alone and combined with bortezomib are ongoing which show that addition of 17-AAG can overcome bortezomib resistance, and a phase III trial for FDA approval of this combination will begin this year. Proteomics also provides insight into possible applications of novel agents. For example, protein profiling of bortezomib-treated MM cells demonstrated cleavage of DNA repair enzymes,[83] providing the rationale for clinical trials combining bortezomib with DNA-damaging agents to enhance sensitivity or overcome resistance to these conventional therapies. These preclinical studies provided the basis for the recent FDA approval of bortezomib plus liposomal doxorubicin combination treatment in MM. Cell signaling studies suggested that combining lenalidomide with bortezomib would trigger dual activation of both extrinsic and intrinsic apoptotic signaling,[94] and an ongoing clinical trial has shown responses to the combination in 68% patients, many of whom were refractory to either agent alone.

Finally, our preclinical studies showed that the simultaneous targeting of lysosomal and proteasomal (nonlysosomal mechanism) protein degradation triggers synergistic anti-MM activity. For example, we have recently shown that the histone deacetylase (HDAC) inhibitors tubacin and LBH589 can inhibit protein degradation in the aggresome-autophagy pathway.[95,96] A recent study in pancreatic cancer cells showed that bortezomib triggered the formation of aggresomes (aggregates of ubiquitin-conjugated proteins), which are cytoprotective, whereas their disruption by HDAC 6 (small interfering RNA) induce synergistic apoptosis.[97] These findings set the stage for evaluation of combined bortezomib with HDAC inhibitors treatment protocols in both hematologic malignancies and solid tumors. Ultimately, it may be possible to carry out gene and protein profiling both to select cocktails of targeted therapies for specific patients[98] and to define targets of sensitivity versus resistance in order to develop next generation, more potent and less toxic, therapeutics. For example, our ability to perform qualitative and quantitative assessment of inhibition of the proteasome in patient tumor samples may allow us to develop more potent and selective proteasome inhibitors.[42,99,100]

Discovery of Novel Proteasome Inhibitors NPI-0052 and PR-171

Our recent study showed that a novel proteasome inhibitor NPI-0052 (Salinosporamide A) can overcome bortezomib resistance in MM cells. It is a small molecule derived from fermentation of Salinospora, a new marine gram-positive actinomycete.[42,101,102] NPI-0052 is a nonpeptide proteasome inhibitor with structural similarity to Omuralide.[101-103] NPI-0052 has a uniquely methylated carbon 3 ring juncture, chlorinated alkyl group at carbon 2, and cyclohexene ring at carbon 5. It inhibits proteasome activity by covalently modifying the active site thereonine residue of the 20S proteasome. Initial screening of NPI-0052 against the NCI panel of 60 tumor cell lines showed GI50 of less than 10 nM in all cases. Importantly, NPI-0052 similarly triggered apoptosis in purified tumor cells from several MM patients relapsing after prior therapies including bortezomib and thalidomide.[42] In vivo efficacy of NPI-0052 was shown using a human plasmacytoma xenograft mouse model: specifically, NPI-0052 inhibited MM tumor growth and prolonged survival of these mice at concentrations, which were well tolerated without significant weight loss or neurological changes. Analysis at day 300 showed no recurrence of tumor in 57% of NPI-0052-treated mice.[42] In agreement with our study in MM cells, recent studies showed that NPI-0052 is a more effective inducer of apoptosis than bortezomib in leukemic cells.[104,105]

Examination of signal transduction pathways in MM cells showed that (1) NPI-0052 is a more potent inhibitor of NF-κB than is bortezomib, (2) NPI-0052-induced MM cell death predominantly relies on FADD-caspase-8 activation, whereas bortezomib-induced apoptosis requires both caspase-8 and caspase-9 activation,[42,105] and (3) ectopic expression of antiapoptotic protein Bcl-2 provided more protection against bortezomib than NPI-0052.[42] Importantly, NPI-0052 and bortezomib differentially affect 20S proteasomal activities: NPI-0052 inhibits all three proteasomal activities, that is, CT-L, T-L, and C-L, whereas bortezomib blocks CT-L and C-L, but not T-L activities.[42] An earlier study showed that simultaneous inhibition (>93%) of all three proteasomal activities blocked cystic fibrosis transmembrane conductance regulator degradation by ~90%, and inhibition of both protease and ATPase activities was required to completely prevent the generation of small peptide fragments.[106] A recent study showed that simultaneous inhibition of multiple proteasome activities is a prerequisite for significant (i.e.,>50%) proteolysis.[29] Whether blocking all three activities is therapeutically advantageous is being evaluated in phase I clinical trial of NPI-0052. Nonetheless, the mechanistic differences between NPI-0052 and bortezomib, that is, their differential effect on proteasome activities and their dependence on specific apoptotic signal transduction pathways, provide a rationale for combining two proteasome inhibitors as therapeutic strategy to enhance MM cytotoxicity and overcome drug resistance. Indeed, in vitro data suggest that the combination of NPI-0052 with bortezomib induces synergistic anti-MM activity, without significantly affecting the viability of normal lymphocytes.[42] These data provide the preclinical framework for clinical trials of combined proteasome inhibitors to reduce toxicity, enhance cytotoxicity, and overcome bortezomib resistance.

Another novel proteasome inhibitor PR-171[107,108] is under evaluation in a phase I clinical trial. PR-171 is a novel epoxy ketone-based irreversible proteasome inhibitor which, like bortezomib, primarily targets CT-L activity. In vitro studies have shown potent antitumor activity.[107,108] It remains to be examined whether similar to NPI-0052, PR-171 can be combined with bortezomib synergistically to reduce toxicity and to enhance cytotoxicity. Ongoing studies are defining a correlation between specific antitumor activity and the extent of inhibition of each and/or all three proteasomal activities in response to combined treatment with two proteasome inhibitors.

Conclusions

Bortezomib therapy is a major advance in the treatment of MM; however, it is associated with toxicity and the development of drug resistance. Preclinical studies have delineated the molecular mechanisms of bortezomib-induced apoptosis,[109] thereby providing the rationale for combining bortezomib with many conventional (dexamethasone , doxorubicin, or melphalan) and novel (lenalidomide, Hsp inhibitors, or HDAC inhibitors) agents to reduce toxicity, enhance cytotoxicity, and overcome drug resistance. Many of these combination regimens have already shown promise in clinical trials. Even though bortezomib and NPI-0052 fall in the same class of drugs, our data show that they are distinct in their mechanism of action on MM cells[42,109] and therefore can be rationally combined as therapy. While the definitive demonstration of increased efficacy with decreased toxicity of combined bortezomib and NPI-0052 therapy requires clinical trials, the synergy observed in our studies suggests an increased therapeutic index of combined therapy.

Acknowledgments: This investigation was supported by NIH grants CA 50947, CA 78373, and CA10070; the Myeloma Research Fund; and LeBow Family Fund to Cure Myeloma.

References

1. Rock K, Gramm C, Rothstein L, et al. Inhibitors of the proteasome block the degradation of most cell proteins and the generation of peptides presented on MHC class I molecules. Cell 1994;78(5):761–71.
2. Goldberg AL. Protein degradation and protection against misfolded or damaged proteins. Nature 2003;426(6968):895–9.
3. Goldberg AL. Functions of the proteasome: from protein degradation and immune surveillance to cancer therapy. Biochem Soc Trans 2007;35(Pt. 1):12–7.
4. Adams J. The proteasome: a suitable antineoplastic target. Nat Rev Cancer 2004;4(5):349–60.
5. Ciechanover A, Elias S, Heller H, Ferber S, Hershko A. Characterization of the heat-stable polypeptide of the ATP-dependent proteolytic system from reticulocytes. J Biol Chem 1980;255(16):7525–8.
6. Ciechanover A, Finley D, Varshavsky A. The ubiquitin-mediated proteolytic pathway and mechanisms of energy-dependent intracellular protein degradation. J Cell Biochem 1984;24(1):27–53.
7. Ciechanover A, Heller H, Elias S, Haas AL, Hershko A. ATP-dependent conjugation of reticulocyte proteins with the polypeptide required for protein degradation. Proc Natl Acad Sci U S A 1980;77(3):1365–8.
8. Ciechanover A, Schwartz AL. The ubiquitin-proteasome pathway: the complexity and myriad functions of proteins death. Proc Natl Acad Sci U S A 1998;95(6):2727–30.
9. Ciehanover A, Hod Y, Hershko A. A heat-stable polypeptide component of an ATP-dependent proteolytic system from reticulocytes. Biochem Biophys Res Commun 1978;81(4):1100–5.
10. Hershko A, Ciechanover A, Heller H, Haas AL, Rose IA. Proposed role of ATP in protein breakdown: conjugation of protein with multiple chains of the polypeptide of ATP-dependent proteolysis. Proc Natl Acad Sci U S A 1980;77(4):1783–6.
11. Hershko A, Ciechanover A. Mechanisms of intracellular protein breakdown. Annu Rev Biochem 1982;51:335–64.
12. Wilk S, Orlowski M. Evidence that pituitary cation-sensitive neutral endopeptidase is a multicatalytic protease complex. J Neurochem 1983;40(3):842–9.
13. Hough R, Pratt G, Rechsteiner M. Purification of two high molecular weight proteases from rabbit reticulocyte lysate. J Biol Chem 1987;262(17):8303–13.
14. Waxman L, Fagan JM, Goldberg AL. Demonstration of two distinct high molecular weight proteases in rabbit reticulocytes, one of which degrades ubiquitin conjugates. J Biol Chem 1987;262(6):2451–7.
15. Eytan E, Ganoth D, Armon T, Hershko A. ATP-dependent incorporation of 20S protease into the 26S complex that degrades proteins conjugated to ubiquitin. Proc Natl Acad Sci U S A 1989;86(20):7751–5.
16. Ganoth D, Leshinsky E, Eytan E, Hershko A. A multicomponent system that degrades proteins conjugated to ubiquitin. Resolution of factors and evidence for ATP-dependent complex formation. J Biol Chem 1988;263(25):12412–9.
17. Arrigo A-P, Suhan JP, Welch WJ. Dynamic changes in the structure and intracellular locale of the mammalian low-molecular-weight heat shock protein. Mol Cell Biol 1988;8:5059–71.
18. Arrigo AP, Tanaka K, Goldberg AL, Welch WJ. Identity of the 19S 'prosome' particle with the large multifunctional protease complex of mammalian cells (the proteasome). Nature 1988;331(6152):192–4.

19. Peters J, Franke W, Kleinschmidt J. Distinct 19 S and 20 S subcomplexes of the 26 S proteasome and their distribution in the nucleus and the cytoplasm. J Biol Chem 1994;269(10):7709–18.

20. Gray C, Slaughter C, DeMartino G. PA28 activator protein forms regulatory caps on proteasome stacked rings. J Mol Biol 1994;236(1):7–15.

21. Hershko A. The ubiquitin system for protein degradation and some of its roles in the control of the cell division cycle. Cell Death Differ 2005;12(9):1191–7.

22. Hershko A, Heller H, Elias S, Ciechanover A. Components of ubiquitin-protein ligase system. Resolution, affinity purification, and role in protein breakdown. J Biol Chem 1983;258(13):8206–14.

23. Wilkinson K, Urban M, Haas A. Ubiquitin is the ATP-dependent proteolysis factor I of rabbit reticulocytes. J Biol Chem 1980;255(16):7529–32.

24. Hough R, Pratt G, Rechsteiner M. Ubiquitin-lysozyme conjugates. Identification and characterization of an ATP-dependent protease from rabbit reticulocyte lysates. J Biol Chem 1986;261(5):2400–8.

25. Swaminathan S, Amerik A, Hochstrasser M. The Doa4 deubiquitinating enzyme is required for ubiquitin homeostasis in yeast. Mol Biol Cell 1999;10(8):2583–94.

26. Pickart CM. Back to the future with ubiquitin. Cell 2004;116(2):181–90.

27. Arendt C, Hochstrasser M. Identification of the yeast 20S proteasome catalytic centers and subunit interactions required for active-site formation. Proc Natl Acad Sci U S A 1997;94(14):7156–61.

28. Heinemeyer W, Fischer M, Krimmer T, Stachon U, Wolf D. The active sites of the eukaryotic 20 S proteasome and their involvement in subunit precursor processing. J Biol Chem 1997;272(40):25200–9.

29. Kisselev AF, Callard A, Goldberg AL. Importance of the different proteolytic sites of the proteasome and the efficacy of inhibitors varies with the protein substrate. J Biol Chem 2006;281(13):8582–90.

30. Kisselev AF, Goldberg AL. Proteasome inhibitors: from research tools to drug candidates. Chem Biol 2001;8(8):739–58.

31. Glotzer M, Murray A, Kirschner M. Cyclin is degraded by the ubiquitin pathway. Nature 1991;349(6305):132–8.

32. Pagano M, Tam S, Theodoras A, et al. Role of the ubiquitin-proteasome pathway in regulating abundance of the cyclin-dependent kinase inhibitor p27. Science 1995;269(5224):682–5.

33. Zhao J, Tenev T, Martins L, Downward J, Lemoine N. The ubiquitin-proteasome pathway regulates survivin degradation in a cell cycle-dependent manner. J Cell Sci 2000;113(Pt. 23):4363–71.

34. Finley D, Sadis S, Monia B, et al. Inhibition of proteolysis and cell cycle progression in a multiubiquitination-deficient yeast mutant. Mol Cell Biol 1994;14(8):5501–9.

35. Adams J, Palombella VJ, Sausville EA, et al. Proteasome inhibitors: a novel class of potent and effective antitumor agents. Cancer Res 1999;59(11):2615–22.

36. Dantuma N, Lindsten K, Glas R, Jellne M, Masucci M. Short-lived green fluorescent proteins for quantifying ubiquitin/proteasome-dependent proteolysis in living cells. Nat Biotechnol 2000;18(5):538–43.

37. Masdehors P, Omura S, Merle-Beral H, et al . Increased sensitivity of CLL-derived lymphocytes to apoptotic death activation by the proteasome-specific inhibitor lactacystin. Br J Haematol 1999;105(3):752–7.

38. Drexler HC, Risau W, Konerding MA. Inhibition of proteasome function induces programmed cell death in proliferating endothelial cells. Faseb J 2000;14(1):65–77.

39. Kudo Y, Takata T, Ogawa I, et al. p27Kip1 accumulation by inhibition of proteasome function induces apoptosis in oral squamous cell carcinoma cells. Clin Cancer Res 2000;6(3):916–23.

40. Bogner C, Schneller F, Hipp S, Ringshausen I, Peschel C, Decker T. Cycling B-CLL cells are highly susceptible to inhibition of the proteasome: involvement of p27, early D-type cyclins, Bax, and caspase-dependent and -independent pathways. Exp Hematol 2003;31(3):218–25.

41. Hideshima T, Richardson P, Chauhan D, et al. The proteasome inhibitor PS-341 inhibits growth, induces apoptosis, and overcomes drug resistance in human multiple myeloma cells. Cancer Res 2001;61(7):3071–6.

42. Chauhan D, Catley L, Li G, et al. A novel orally active proteasome inhibitor induces apoptosis in multiple myeloma cells with mechanisms distinct from Bortezomib. Cancer Cell 2005;8(5):407–19.

43. Adams J. Potential for proteasome inhibition in the treatment of cancer. Drug Discov Today 2003;8(7):307–15.

44. Chauhan D, Hideshima T, Anderson KC. Proteasome inhibition in multiple myeloma: therapeutic implication. Annu Rev Pharmacol Toxicol 2005;45:465–76.

45. Chauhan D, Hideshima T, Mitsiades C, Richardson P, Anderson KC. Proteasome inhibitor therapy in multiple myeloma. Mol Cancer Ther 2005;4(4):686–92.

46. Vinitsky A, Michaud C, Powers JC, Orlowski M. Inhibition of the chymotrypsin-like activity of the pituitary multicatalytic proteinase complex. Biochemistry 1992;31 (39):9421–8.

47. Omura S, Fujimoto T, Otoguro K, et al. Lactacystin, a novel microbial metabolite, induces neuritogenesis of neuroblastoma cells. J Antibiot (Tokyo) 1991;44(1):113–6.

48. Fenteany G, Standaert R, Lane W, Choi S, Corey E, Schreiber S. Inhibition of proteasome activities and subunit-specific amino-terminal threonine modification by lactacystin. Science 1995;268(5211):726–31.

49. Fenteany G, Standaert R, Reichard G, Corey E, Schreiber S. A beta-lactone related to lactacystin induces neurite outgrowth in a neuroblastoma cell line and inhibits cell cycle progression in an osteosarcoma cell line. Proc Natl Acad Sci U S A 1994;91(8):3358–62.

50. Adams J, Kauffman M. Development of the proteasome inhibitor Velcade (Bortezomib). Cancer Invest 2004;22(2):304–11.

51. Karin M, Yamamoto Y, Wang QM. The IKK NF-kappa B system: a treasure trove for drug development. Nat Rev Drug Discov 2004;3(1):17–26.

52. Van WC. Nuclear factor-kappaB in development, prevention, and therapy of cancer. Clin Cancer Res 2007;13(4):1076–82.

53. Stancovski I, Baltimore D. NF-κB activation: the I κB kinase revealed? Cell 1997;91:299–302.

54. Haefner B. NF-kappa B: arresting a major culprit in cancer. Drug Discov Today 2002;7(12):653–63.

55. Palombella VJ, Rando OJ, Goldberg AL, Maniatis T. The ubiquitin proteasome pathway is required for processing the NF-kB1 precursor protein and the activation of NF-kB. Cell 1994;78:773–85.

56. Jensen TJ, Loo MA, Pind S, Williams DB, Goldberg AL, Riordan JR. Multiple proteolytic systems, including the proteasome, contribute to CFTR processing. Cell 1995;83(1):129–35.

57. Chauhan D, Uchiyama H, Urashima M, Yamamoto K, Anderson KC. Regulation of interleukin 6 in multiple myeloma and bone marrow stromal cells. Stem Cells 1995;13(Suppl 2):35–9.

58. Chauhan D, Uchiyama H, Akbarali Y, et al. Multiple myeloma cell adhesion-induced interleukin-6 expression in bone marrow stromal cells involves activation of NF-kappa B. Blood 1996;87(3):1104–12.

59. Ni H, Ergin M, Huang Q, et al. Analysis of expression of nuclear factor kappa B (NF-kappa B) in multiple myeloma: downregulation of NF-kappa B induces apoptosis. Br J Haematol 2001;115(2):279–86.

60. Mitsiades N, Mitsiades CS, Poulaki V, et al. Biologic sequelae of nuclear factor-kappaB blockade in multiple myeloma: therapeutic applications. Blood 2002;99(11):4079–86.

61. Landowski TH, Olashaw NE, Agrawal D, Dalton WS. Cell adhesion-mediated drug resistance (CAM-DR) is associated with activation of NF-kappa B (RelB/p50) in myeloma cells. Oncogene 2003;22(16):2417–21.

62. Bharti AC, Donato N, Singh S, Aggarwal BB. Curcumin (diferuloylmethane) down-regulates the constitutive activation of nuclear factor-kappa B and Ikappa

Balpha kinase in human multiple myeloma cells, leading to suppression of proliferation and induction of apoptosis. Blood 2003;101(3):1053–62.

63. LeBlanc R, Catley LP, Hideshima T, et al. Proteasome inhibitor PS-341 inhibits human myeloma cell growth in vivo and prolongs survival in a murine model. Cancer Res 2002;62(17):4996–5000.

64. Orlowski RZ, Stinchcombe TE, Mitchell BS, et al. Phase I trial of the proteasome inhibitor PS-341 in patients with refractory hematologic malignancies. J Clin Oncol 2002;20(22):4420–7.

65. Richardson P, Blood E, Mitsiades CS, et al. A randomized phase 2 trial of lenalidomide therapy for patients with relapsed or relapsed and refractory multiple myeloma. Blood 2006;15:3458–64.

66. Richardson PG, Barlogie B, Berenson J, et al. Extended follow-up of a phase II trial in relapsed, refractory multiple myeloma: final time-to-event results from the SUMMIT trial. Cancer 2006;106(6):1316–9.

67. Jagannath S, Durie B, Wolf JL, et al. A phase 2 study of Bortezomib as first line therapy in patients with multiple myeloma. Blood 2004;104:abstr 333.

68. Jagannath S, Barlogie B, Berenson J, et al. A phase 2 study of two doses of bortezomib in relapsed or refractory myeloma. Br J Haematol 2004;127(2):165–72.

69. Jagannath S, Barlogie B, Berenson JR, et al. Bortezomib in recurrent and/or refractory multiple myeloma: initial experience in patients with impaired renal function. Cancer 2005;103:1195–200.

70. Richardson PG, Sonneveld P, Schuster MW, et al. Bortezomib or high-dose dexamethasone for relapsed multiple myeloma. N Engl J Med 2005;352(24):2487–98.

71. Richardson P, Barlogie B, Berenson JR, et al. Clinical factors predictive of outcome with Bortezomib in patients with relapsed, refractory multiple myeloma. Blood 2005;106:2977–81.

72. Berenson J, Jagannath S, Barlogie B, et al. Safety of prolonged therapy with Bortezomib in relapsed or refractory multiple myeloma. Cancer 2005;104:2141–8.

73. Lonial S, Waller EK, Richardson P, et al. Risk factors and kinetics of thrombocytopenia associated with bortezomib for relapsed, refractory multiple myeloma. Blood 2005;106:3777–84.

74. Richardson PG, Briemberg H, Jagannath S, et al. Frequency, characteristics, and reversibility of peripheral neuropathy during treatment of advanced multiple myeloma with bortezomib. J Clin Oncol 2006;24(19):3113–20.

75. Richardson PG, Hideshima T, Mitsiades C, Anderson KC. The emerging role of novel therapies for the treatment of relapsed myeloma. J Natl Compr Canc Netw 2007;5(2):149–62.

76. Richardson PG, Sonneveld P, Schuster M, et al. Extended follow-up of a phase 3 trial in relapsed multiple myeloma: final time-to-event results of the APEX trial. Blood 2007;110(10):3557–60.

77. Hideshima T, Chauhan D, Richardson P, et al. NF-kappa B as a therapeutic target in multiple myeloma. J Biol Chem 2002;28:28.

78. Mitsiades N, Mitsiades CS, Poulaki V, et al. Molecular sequelae of proteasome inhibition in human multiple myeloma cells. Proc Natl Acad Sci U S A 2002;99(22):14374–9.

79. Chauhan D, Li G, Shringarpure R, et al. Blockade of Hsp27 overcomes Bortezomib/proteasome inhibitor PS-341 resistance in lymphoma cells. Cancer Res 2003;63(19):6174–7.

80. Chauhan D, Li G, Hideshima T, et al. JNK-dependent release of mitochondrial protein, Smac, during apoptosis in multiple myeloma (MM) cells. J Biol Chem 2003;278(20):17593–6.

81. Chauhan D, Guilan L, Sattler M, et al. Superoxide-dependent and independent mitochondrial signaling during apoptosis in multiple myeloma (MM) cells. Oncogene 2003;22(40):6296–300.

82. Chauhan D, Anderson KC. Mechanisms of cell death and survival in multiple myeloma (MM): therapeutic implications. Apoptosis 2003;8(4):337–43.

83. Mitsiades N, Mitsiades CS, Richardson PG, et al. The proteasome inhibitor PS-341 potentiates sensitivity of multiple myeloma cells to conventional chemotherapeutic agents: therapeutic applications. Blood 2003;101(6):2377–80.

84. Hideshima T, Anderson KC. Molecular mechanisms of novel therapeutic approaches for multiple myeloma. Nat Rev Cancer 2002;2(12):927–37.

85. Hideshima T, Mitsiades C, Akiyama M, et al. Molecular mechanisms mediating antimyeloma activity of proteasome inhibitor PS-341. Blood 2003;101(4):1530–4.

86. Obeng EA, Boise LH. Caspase-12 and caspase-4 are not required for caspase-dependent endoplasmic reticulum stress-induced apoptosis. J Biol Chem 2005;280(33):29578–87.

87. Obeng EA, Carlson LM, Gutman DM, Harrington WJ, Jr., Lee KP, Boise LH. Proteasome inhibitors induce a terminal unfolded protein response in multiple myeloma cells. Blood 2006;107(12):4907–16.

88. Nawrocki ST, Carew JS, Dunner K, Jr., et al. Bortezomib inhibits PKR-like endoplasmic reticulum (ER) kinase and induces apoptosis via ER stress in human pancreatic cancer cells. Cancer Res 2005;65(24):11510–9.

89. Cory S, Adams JM. The Bcl2 family: regulators of the cellular life-or-death switch. Nat Rev Cancer 2002;2(9):647–56.

90. Chauhan D, Velankar M, Brahmandam M, et al. A novel Bcl-2/Bcl-X(L)/Bcl-w inhibitor ABT-737 as therapy in multiple myeloma. Oncogene 2007;26(16):2374–80.

91. Chauhan D, Neri P, Velankar M, et al. Targeting mitochondrial factor Smac/DIABLO as therapy for multiple myeloma (MM). Blood 2007;109(3):1220–7.

92. Mulligan G, Mitsiades C, Bryant B, et al. Gene expression profiling and correlation with outcome in clinical trials of the proteasome inhibitor bortezomib. Blood 2007;109(8):3177–88.

93. Mitsiades CS, Mitsiades NS, McMullan CJ, et al. Antimyeloma activity of heat shock protein-90 inhibition. Blood 2006;107(3):1092–100.

94. Mitsiades N, Mitsiades CS, Poulaki V, et al. Apoptotic signaling induced by immunomodulatory thalidomide analogs in human multiple myeloma cells: therapeutic implications. Blood 2002;99(12):4525–30.

95. Hideshima T, Bradner JE, Wong J, et al. Small-molecule inhibition of proteasome and aggresome function induces synergistic antitumor activity in multiple myeloma. Proc Natl Acad Sci U S A 2005;102(24):8567–72.

96. Catley L, Weisberg E, Kiziltepe T, et al. Aggresome induction by proteasome inhibitor bortezomib and {alpha}-tubulin hyperacetylation by tubulin deacetylase (TDAC) inhibitor LBH589 are synergistic in myeloma cells. Blood 2006;108(10):3441–9.

97. Nawrocki ST, Carew JS, Pino MS, et al. Aggresome disruption: a novel strategy to enhance bortezomib-induced apoptosis in pancreatic cancer cells. Cancer Res 2006;66(7):3773–81.

98. Munshi NC, Hideshima T, Carrasco D, et al. Identification of genes modulated in multiple myeloma using genetically identical twin samples. Blood 2004;103(5):1799–806.

99. Berkers CR, Verdoes M, Lichtman E, . Activity probe for in vivo profiling of the specificity of proteasome inhibitor bortezomib. Nat Methods 2005;2(5):357–62.

100. Altun M, Galardy P, Shringapure R, et al. Effects of PS 341 on the activity and composition of proteasomes in multiple myeloma cells. Cancer Res 2005;65:7896–901.

101. Feling RH, Buchanan GO, Mincer TJ, Kauffman CA, Jensen PR, Fenical W. Salinosporamide A: a highly cytotoxic proteasome inhibitor from a novel microbial source, a marine bacterium of the new genus salinospora. Angew Chem Int Ed Engl 2003;42(3):355–7.

102. Macherla VR, Mitchell SS, Manam RR, et al. Structure-activity relationship studies of salinosporamide A (NPI-0052), a novel marine derived proteasome inhibitor. J Med Chem 2005;48(11):3684–7.

103. Groll M, Huber R, Potts BC. Crystal structures of Salinosporamide A (NPI-0052) and B (NPI-0047) in complex with the 20S proteasome reveal important consequences of beta-lactone ring opening and a mechanism for irreversible binding. J Am Chem Soc 2006;128(15):5136–41.

104. Ruiz S, Krupnik Y, Keating M, Chandra J, Palladino M, McConkey D. The proteasome inhibitor NPI-0052 is a more effective inducer of apoptosis than bortezomib in lymphocytes from patients with chronic lymphocytic leukemia. Mol Cancer Ther 2006;5(7):1836–43.

105. Miller CP, Ban K, Dujka ME, et al. NPI-0052, a novel proteasome inhibitor, induces caspase-8 and ROS-dependent apoptosis alone and in combination with HDAC inhibitors in leukemia cells. Blood 2007;110(1):267–77.

106. Oberdorf J, Carlson EJ, Skach WR. Redundancy of mammalian proteasome beta subunit function during endoplasmic reticulum associated degradation. Biochemistry 2001;40(44):13397–405.

107. Demo SD, Kirk CJ, Aujay MA, et al. Antitumor activity of PR-171, a novel irreversible inhibitor of the proteasome. Cancer Res 2007;67(13):6383–91.

108. Stapnes C, Doskeland AP, Hatfield K, et al. The proteasome inhibitors bortezomib and PR-171 have antiproliferative and proapoptotic effects on primary human acute myeloid leukaemia cells. Br J Haematol 2007;136(6):814–28.

109. Chauhan D, Hideshima T, Anderson KC. A novel proteasome inhibitor NPI-0052 as an anticancer therapy. Br J Cancer 2006;95(8):961–5.

Section 6

Supportive Care

Chapter 27

Pathophysiology of Bone Disease in Multiple Myeloma

Tomer M. Mark and Roger N. Pearse

Introduction

Multiple myeloma (MM) is a malignancy of plasma cells characterized by growth in the bone marrow (BM) environment and the development of lytic lesions in the skeleton. These lytic lesions are responsible for many of the clinical sequelae of progressive disease, including pathologic fractures, severe pain, and hypercalcemia.[1] Historically, the burden of skeletal disease has been used to predict MM prognosis and survival, as outlined in the Salmon-Durie staging system.[2] However, this correlation is weakened by the finding of increased prevalence of bone disease in MM with favorable cytogenetics.[3] As a result, bone disease has been omitted from recent staging schema.[4] Nonetheless, bone destruction remains a major source of morbidity.[5]

The hallmark of MM bone disease is the development of osteolytic lesions without associated osteoblastic activity. The absence of reactive bone formation renders MM-associated skeletal lesions silent on bone scan, and helps to explain the delayed healing that is frequently observed. This paucity of osteoblastic activity suggests a disruption of homeostatic mechanisms that normally couple bone remodeling, where osteoclastic bone resorption triggers new bone formation by osteoblasts (OBL).[6] In fact, it is the uncoupling of osteoblast from osteoclast activity that is the pathophysiologic theme of MM-associated bone disease. Recent studies have shed light on various potential mechanisms by which MM can both activate osteoclasts (OC) and inhibit OBL, leading to a state of uncompensated additive bone destruction. Elucidation of molecular signaling pathways by which MM plasma cells communicate within the BM milieu provides insight into the nature of this lytic bone disease as well as illustrates potential therapeutic targets in the future.

This chapter will review the basic physiology of both OC and OBL function in bone remodeling with a description of the molecular signals which drive both their differentiation and activity. There will then be a description of the mechanisms by which MM influences these pathways to cause bone destruction.

From: *Contemporary Hematology Myeloma Therapy*
Edited by: S. Lonial © Humana Press, Totowa, NJ

Bone Physiology

Bone is mineralized connective tissue. Bone shape, strength, and resilience is determined by an organic matrix composed predominantly (90%) of type-1 collagen, with osteocalcin, osteopontin (OPN), osteonectin, proteoglycans, glycosaminoglycans, and lipids. Bone hardness is provided by crystallization of hydroxyapatite $Ca_{10}(PO4)_6(OH)_2$ within this matrix. While hardness significantly improves weight-bearing capability, the inherent brittleness of hydroxyapatite results in the accumulation of microfractures after repeated stress to the skeleton. Repair of these microfractures requires resorption of the existing bone, followed by deposition and mineralization of new bone, a process known as remodeling. Understanding the regulation of bone remodeling is critical to understanding MM, as this malignancy uses these same pathways to enhance tumor growth as it causes bone destruction. At least three cell types participate in bone remodeling: OC, hematopoietic cells responsible for bone resorption; OBL, mesenchymal cells responsible for the synthesis of new bone matrix and the regulation of its mineralization; *osteocytes*, derived from OBL, sense microfractures and initiate the remodeling process.

Osteoclasts

Bone is resorbed by OC, multinucleated giant cells of the monocyte–macrophage lineage.[7] OC dissolve bone by secreting acid to leach the hydroxyapatite and lysosomal proteases, such as cathepsin B, to dissolve the underlying collagen matrix. To generate high concentrations of acid and enzymes at the bone surface, OC use adhesion molecules, such as integrin $\alpha_v\beta_3$, to seal their perimeter to the bone. The bone degradation products are then endocytosed by the OC, which possesses a ruffled cell border at its basal surface to increase the area available for uptake. Within the OC, the endocytic vesicles fuse with vesicles containing tartrate-resistant acid phosphatase isoform 5b (TRACP-5b) to facilitate further degradation of the bone matrix. The vesicles then transit the OC to release their contents via the apical surface. In this fashion, bone breakdown products enter the systemic circulation, and can be measured either in serum or urine to give a relative measure of overall bone resorptive activity.[8] Markers of bone resorption include *N*-telopeptide cross-links (NTx) of collagen type 1, C-telopeptide of collagen type 1 (ICTP), deoxypyridoline (DPD) and pyridinoline, as well as TRACP-5b.

OC arise from hematopoietic cells that have committed to the myelomonocytic lineage. A number of growth factors regulate this development, including macrophage-colony stimulating factor (M-CSF), which is necessary for the generation of precursor OC from the granulocyte–macrophage colony-forming unit (CFU-GM). It has been shown using the *M-CSF* knockout mouse that absence of this growth factor leads to inhibition of bone resorption and osteopetrosis due to lack of OC differentiation.[9,10] The chemokine macrophage inflammatory protein-1α (MIP-1α) has been shown to be chemotactic for monocytes as well as OC precursors and can by itself induce differentiation of OC.[11] Other factors that stimulate the generation of OC precursors include interleukin 3 (IL-3), IL-6, granulocyte–macrophage colony-stimulating factor (GM-CSF), and vascular endothelial growth factor (VEGF).[8,12]

OC precursors develop into activated OC under the influence of RANKL (receptor activator for nuclear factor κB ligand, also known as tumor necrosis factor superfamily member 11: TNFSF11 and tumor necrosis factor [TNF]-related activation-induced cytokine: TRANCE).[13,14] RANKL is a TNF family member that is expressed both as a secreted and as a membrane-bound trimeric ligand by several cell types, including activated T cells, immature OBL, and marrow stromal cells.[15] Additional cytokines, including TNF, IL-1, IL-6, IL-11 as well as chemokines such as MIP-1α and stromal-derived factor-1α (SDF-1α), contribute to OC differentiation.[16–18] However, RANKL is the dominant cytokine responsible for the differentiation, activation, and survival of OC, and the major osteoclastogenic mediator of factors responsible for bone homeostasis, such as parathyroid hormone (PTH), IL-11, glucocorticoids, and 1,25-dihydroxyvitamin D3 (vitD3).[19] The necessity of RANKL for normal OC development is confirmed by the lack of OC and profound osteopetrosis exhibited by *RANKL*-deficient mice.[20]

RANKL acts by binding to and thereby trimerizing its receptor RANK (receptor activator of nuclear factor κB [NF-κB], also known as TNF receptor superfamily member 11a: TNFRSF11a), which is expressed on the surface of immature and mature OC.[13] RANK trimerization leads to the recruitment of TRAF2 (TNF receptor associated factor2) and TRAF6, and the initiation of intracellular signal cascades that are critical for OC formation.[21] The ultimate targets for these signaling pathways are several transcription factors that coordinate OC differentiation and activation, including NF-κB, NFATc1 (nuclear factor of activated T-cells), cFOS, and MITF (microthalmia transcription factor).[22–24] The importance of RANKL–RANK signaling to normal OC development is confirmed by the lack of OC and profound osteopetrosis exhibited by *RANK*-deficient mice, a similar phenotype to that of the *RANKL*-knockout mouse.[25]

RANK signaling is regulated by several mechanisms that provide control over OC development and activation. RANKL expression is determined by factors responsible for bone homeostasis, including PTH, IL-11, glucocorticoids, and vitD3.[26] Additional control over RANKL availability is provided by osteoprotegerin (OPG; also known as TNFRSF11b), a soluble decoy receptor for RANKL that prevents RANKL–RANK signaling.[27] Osteoclastogenesis is thus regulated by the opposing effects of RANKL and OPG, and it is the relative ratio of RANKL to OPG that determines RANK signaling activity.[7] This has been confirmed using knockout animals: mice that lack *RANKL* or *RANK* exhibit profound osteopetrosis, whereas mice that lack *OPG* exhibit increased OC activity and severe osteoporosis.[28,29] The expression of OPG by OBL and BM stromal cells is controlled by many of the factors that regulate RANKL expression. Importantly, OPG expression is regulated by TGF-β in an autocrine feedback loop that serves to limit bone resorption. TGF-β, in an inactive complex with latency-associated peptide, is synthesized by OBL and deposited with osteoid in developing bone (bone matrix is the largest source of TGF-β in the body).[30] OC-mediated bone resorption releases active TGF-β, which stimulates OBL to increase OPG and decrease RANKL expression, thereby limiting further OC activity.[31,32] A third mechanism involves regulation of RANK signaling within OC. Negative regulation of RANK signaling is exerted by interferon gamma (IFN-γ), which triggers ubiquinization and degradation of TRAF6.[33] In contrast, positive regulation is achieved by costimulation of RANK with an immunoglobulin-like receptor such as TREM2 (triggering receptors expressed by myeloid cells), RAGE (receptor for advanced glycation end products), or OSCAR (OC-associated receptor).[34–36] These immunoglobulin-like receptors activate ITAM (immunoreceptor tyrosine-based activation motif) containing adaptor proteins DAP12 (DNAX activating protein 12) and FcR-γ (Fc receptor common γ subunit). Activation of DAP12 or FcR-γ is necessary for RANK to activate the critical transcription factor NFAT1c.[37]

Relevance to MM-associated bone disease: MM disrupts the RANKL/OPG balance by triggering increased RANKL and decreased OPG expression by surrounding stromal cells and infiltrating lymphocytes.[38] As will be discussed in the Section "Osteoclast Activation by Multiple Myeloma" below, the resulting increase in RANKL–RANK signaling by myeloid precursors drives the heightened osteoclastogenesis seen in MM. It is currently unknown whether MM also influences DAP12 or FcR-γ–mediated signals within these precursors to further augment RANK signaling. However, MM does amplify the number of OC by secreting osteoclastogeneic factors such as TNFα, thus creating more targets for these signals.[39]

Osteoblasts

OBL are responsible for the production of new bone. They secrete a mix of bone matrix proteins, termed osteoid, into the resorption pits that have been created by OC, and then direct the incorporation of hydroxyapatite into that matrix. Total OBL activity is thus reflected by systemic levels of osteoid components, including OPN, osteocalcin, and osteonectin, as well as by levels of bone-specific alkaline phosphatase (BSAP), a marker of OBL maturation. In addition to their role in bone formation, OBL serve as supportive environment for quiescent hematopoietic stem cells (HSCs). This support is mediated by OBL-expressed cytokines and chemokines, such as IL-6, c-KitL, MIP-1α, and SDF1α, and by direct OBL–HSC interactions mediated by Notch1/Jagged1 and N-cadherin. Osteogenic agents, such as PTH, have been shown to regulate the HSC pool by regulating OBL expression of N-cadherin and Jag1. These molecules trigger Notch1 and β-catenin signaling in HSCs, and therefore determine HSC survival and self-renewal.[40–42]

OBL are derived from a pool of mesenchymal stem cells (MSCs) with the capacity to differentiate into OBL, chondrocytes, adipocytes, or fibroblasts. Commitment to the OBL lineage requires MSC expression of the Runx2/Cbfa1 (runt-related transcription factor 2/core-binding factor α1) transcription factor complex.[43] The critical role of Runx2/Cbfa1 in OBL development is illustrated by *Cbfa1*-deficient mice, which fail to generate OBL and thus develop normally patterned skeletons of nonossified cartilage.[44] Expression of Runx2/Cbfa1 is induced by bone morphogenic proteins (BMPs) and Indian hedgehog (Ihh).[45] Additional factors, including transforming growth factor-beta (TGF-β), fibroblast growth factors (FGFs), insulin-like growth factor (IGF), and platelet-derived growth factor (PDGF), are produced by OBL to facilitate their own transition from MSC.[8] OBL differentiation is thus regulated by autocrine as well as paracrine signaling.

OBL development is also driven by wingless-type glycoproteins (Wnts). The first indication that Wnt signaling is important for OBL activation came from two spontaneous mutations involving the Wnt coreceptor lipoprotein-related protein 5 (LRP5). A loss of function mutation of *LRP5* is the cause of osteoporosis–pseudoglioma syndrome.[46] By the same token, a gain of function mutation (G171V) in *LRP5* results in a familial syndrome characterized by increased OBL activity and abnormally high bone mass.[47] Experimentally, β-catenin-dependent Wnts (Wnt1, Wnt2, or Wnt3a) cooperate with BMPs to stimulate OBL differentiation and function in vitro.[45,48] In vivo, genetic ablation of Wnt signaling in developing mesenchyme results in chondrocyte accumulation at the expense of OBL development. Conversely, constitutive activation of Wnt signaling in the same mesenchymal precursors inhibits chondrocyte differentiation and promotes bone formation.[45,49–51]

Wnt ligands trigger multiple intracellular signals, grouped into canonical (β-catenin dependent) and noncanonical pathways. The importance of LRP5 and β-catenin to Wnt osteogenic activity indicates use of the canonical pathway, which functions to allow β-catenin-mediated transcription of genes involved in cell proliferation and development. In the absence of Wnt signaling, β-catenin is phosphorylated at residues S33, S37, and T41 by a complex composed of adenomatous polyposis coli protein (APC), Axin, and glycogen synthase kinase (GSK)-3β. Phosphorylated β-catenin is targeted for degradation by the proteosome. In the presence of canonical Wnt signaling, Wnt complexes with LRP5 to activate frizzled (Fz) cell surface receptors. Fz then activates the serine/threonine kinase CK1γ. CK1γ phosphorylates the cytosolic protein disheveled (Dsh), which recruits Axin from the APC–Axin–Gsk-3β complex, thereby disrupting its negative control over β-catenin. Unphosphorylated β-catenin accumulates in the cytoplasm, translocates to the cell nucleus, and activates gene transcription by binding to the transcription factors lymphoid enhancer-binding factor (LEF) and T-cell transcription factor (TCF).[52] Negative control over canonical Wnt signaling is mediated by Dickkopf (DKK) and secreted Fz-related proteins (sFRPs). DKK proteins are soluble factors which block canonical Wnt signaling by binding and sequestering LRP5/6. sFRPs bind directly to Wnts to prevent receptor engagement (see Fig. 1).

Relevance to MM-associated bone disease: Canonical Wnt signaling is necessary for OBL development. MM inhibits canonical Wnt signaling by secreting DKK1 and sFRP2. As will be discussed in the Section "Osteoblast Inhibition by Multiple Myeloma," this inhibition is believed to be responsible for the OBL defect in MM.

Osteocytes

Osteocytes are terminally differentiated OBL that assist in the coordination of bone resorption with formation. The transition from OBL to osteocyte occurs as OBL become trapped within the growing bone matrix.[53] Osteocytes are believed to act as mechanosensors that survey and maintain skeletal integrity. Osteocytes remain in communication with each other and with the bone surface via dendritic processes that extend through interconnecting canaliculi. Through these dendrites they are able to trigger the remodeling process and influence the development and activity of both OBL and OC.[54]

Osteoclast–Osteoblast Coupling

Skeletal homeostasis requires that bone loss and gain be balanced during bone remodeling. This is achieved by active communication between OBL and OC,

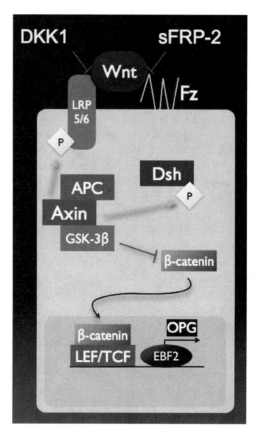

Fig. 1 Regulation of the canonical Wnt signaling pathway in osteoblasts (OBL) (adapted from Pearse[6]). APC/Axin/glycogen synthase 3-beta (GSK-3β) form a complex which phosphorylates β-catenin. Phosphorylated beta-catenin is then degraded by the proteosome (not shown above). Binding of Wnt glycoproteins to the frizzled (*Fz*)/lipoprotein-related protein (*LRP*) receptor complex triggers the phosphorylation of Disheveled (*Dsh*) and LRP. Phosphorylated Dsh and LRP recruit and bind Axin, which disrupts the APC/Axin/GSK-3β complex, thereby preventing the degradation of β–catenin. As a result, β-catenin is allowed to translocate to the nucleus, where it is associated with lymphoid enhancer-binding factor (*LEF*)/T-cell transcription factor (*TCF*) to facilitate transcription of their target genes. In mature OBL, β-catenin complexes with TCF1 and TCF4 to facilitate the transcription of osteoprotegerin (*OPG*), in cooperation with early B cell factor 2 (*EBF2*). Inhibition of Wnt signaling in OBL leads to reduced expression of OPG, which results in heightened osteoclastogenesis, and increased bone resorption. Myeloma inhibits Wnt signaling through the secretion of Wnt antagonists, Dickkopf1 (*DKK*1), and secreted frizzled-related proteins2 (*sFRP*-2) (DKK1 binds to the Wnt core-ceptors, LRP5/6, to block activation of the receptor complex; sFRP-2 is a decoy receptor for Wnts). Secretion of DKK1 and sFRP-2 may therefore contribute to the dysregulation of RANKL/OPG expression seen in multiple myeloma (*MM*1) (*see* Plate 9).

a process known as coupling.[55] In balance, coupling appears to favor mutual stimulation, that is, increased OC activity leads to increased OBL activity, and vice versa. As an example, OC express ephrinB2, which binds and stimulates EphB4 on MSC and immature OBL. Once activated, EphB4 triggers expression of Dlx5, Osx, and Runx2, osteogenic transcription factors that stimulate OBL development and increase bone formation.[56] Further, OC secrete TRAP and release IGF from the bone matrix. Both TRAP and IGF are OBL growth factors.[57-59] Similarly, increased OBL activity leads to increased OC activity. OBL are the main source of M-CSF, RANKL, and OPG within the marrow, and thus regulate both the CFU-GM precursor pool, and the maturation and activation of OC from that pool.[60] Agents that stimulate OBL activity, such as PTH and vitD3, also increase RANKL and decrease OPG expression, thereby increasing OC activity.

However, coupling also employs inhibitory signaling between OBL and OC. TGF-β, released from the bone matrix by OC activity, acts on immature OBL to induce their expression of OPG while inhibiting their maturation to functional OBL. TGF-β thus acts as a bidirectional signal to inhibit both OC (via OPG) and OBL activity.[31] In contrast, the interaction of ephrinB2 (on OC) with EphB4 (on OBL) acts as a unidirectional inhibitory signal, initiating a reverse signal to the OC that suppresses OC activation.[56] Similarly, canonical Wnt signaling, which is necessary for MSC to OBL commitment and for OBL activation by BMPs, acts as a unidirectional inhibitor of OC activity by increasing OPG expression. The role of canonical Wnt signaling in OBL to OC coupling was demonstrated using conditional knockout mice.[61] As Wnt signaling is necessary for MSC to OBL commitment, the authors targeted Wnt signaling components in committed OBL. Mice whose OBL had constitutive expression of β-catenin, and therefore active canonical Wnt signaling, had lack of eruption of lower incisors and a relative increase in bone mass. Histologic sections and chemical markers revealed that these findings were due to *lack of OC activity* rather than hyperactive OBL. As a complimentary finding, mice whose OBL lacked β-*catenin* showed a decrease in bone mass due to OC hyperactivity. Upon further investigation, it was discovered that canonical Wnt signaling regulates OPG expression. The work of Holmen et al. corroborates the critical role of canonical Wnt signaling in bone remodeling.[62] Targeting the *APC* gene in order to generate a mouse with constitutive β-catenin signaling, they confirmed that active canonical Wnt signaling leads to increased OPG expression, resulting in decreased osteoclastogenesis and osteopetrosis.

Relevance to MM-Associated Bone Disease

Canonical Wnt signaling appears necessary for OPG expression by OBL. As will be discussed in the Section "Osteoclast Activation by Multiple Myeloma," MMC inhibit canonical Wnt signaling by secreting DKK1 and sFRP2. Therefore, Wnt inhibition may be responsible for the decreased expression of OPG seen in MM patients.

Osteoclast Activation by Multiple Myeloma

The hallmark of MM bone disease is the development of osteolytic lesions without associated osteoblastic activity. This is evidenced biochemically by a disproportionate increase in systemic markers of bone turnover, such as NTX and DPD, compared with markers of OBL activity, such as osteocalcin and BSAP.[63,64] Histomorphometric analysis of bone biopsy specimens from patients with advanced MM confirm this imbalance, showing OC accumulation at bone-resorbing surfaces with no evidence of bone regeneration within the skeletal lesions.[65] The level of bone destruction and appearance of bone turnover markers in the serum has been correlated with overall prognosis, tumor burden, and survival in MM.[66,67]

MM has been shown to influence the activity of OC through several mechanisms, including cell–cell contact activation, dysregulation of the RANKL/OPG ratio, and through manipulation of the chemokines MIP-1α and SDF-1.[68] Paracrine signaling among malignant plasma cells, marrow stromal cells, OC, and the bone matrix fuels the linked processes of bone destruction and MM tumor growth. What follows is a discussion of each of these mechanisms of action.

Multiple Myeloma Disrupts the Balance of RANKL/OPG

RANKL is the major promoter of OC differentiation and activation. Animal models of RANKL hyperactivity, created by either increasing RANKL or decreasing OPG expression, display severe bone loss. Thus, it is surmised that the RANKL/OPG ratio in the BM milieu determines OC activity. Prior laboratory investigation has shown that MM alters the RANKL/OPG ratio by coordinating an increase in RANKL with a decrease in OPG production by BM stromal cells.[38] Interestingly, in this study it did not appear that the MMC themselves were a significant source of RANKL. The pathogenic role of RANKL in myelomatous bone destruction was confirmed using a recombinant decoy receptor, RANK-Fc, which blocked MM-associated osteolysis. RANK-Fc treatment also blocked MM tumor progression, suggesting that OC activity contributes to MMC growth. While this study found that the source of RANKL was BM stromal cells, induced in the presence of MMC, other groups have shown that MM plasma cells themselves may be capable of RANKL expression and secretion.[69,70]

The OPG decrease seen in MM may occur through several mechanisms. CD138, often highly expressed on the surface of MM plasma cells, binds to the heparin-binding domain of OPG. Such interaction may induce internalization of the OPG–CD138 complex, and clearance of OPG from the BM microenvironment.[71] It has also been shown that cell–cell contact between MM and BM stromal cells leads to a decrease in OPG gene transcription in OBL and stromal cells.[72] This decrease in OPG production may be secondary to inhibitory effects of MM on the differentiation of OBL, since mature OBL are the major source of OPG. In contrast, immature OBL express little OPG, but considerable RANKL. Thus, maintenance of a relatively immature OBL population promotes a higher RANKL/OPG ratio. This concept will be expanded in the Section "Osteoblast Inhibition by Multiple Myeloma" of this chapter.

Chemokines

MIP-1α is a C-C chemokine that acts as a chemoattractant for phagocytes, including OC, and functions to recruit leukocytes to areas of inflammation.[73] MIP-1α is also a MM-associated OC activating factor, its role in osteolysis having been identified during a functional screen of MM cDNA libraries.[74] MIP-1α is present in BM supernatants of patients with active myelomatous bone disease, and absolute levels of MIP-1α appear to correlate with OC activity.[75,76] Further, it has been shown that antisense blockade of MIP-1α expression can inhibit bone destruction in MM xenograft models.[77] Recombinant MIP-1α has been shown to increase the development of OC from human marrow cultures in a manner independent of RANKL. Thus, it is likely that MIP-1α mediates osteolysis via direct enhancement of OC activation, working at a later stage of OC differentiation than RANKL.[78]

MMC produce both MIP-1α and MIP-1β, and express the receptors for these chemokines, CCR1 and CCR5. Thus, MIP-1α and MIP-1β are potential autocrine growth factors for MM.[79] In addition, MIP-1α–CCR5 signaling has recently been implicated in the homing of MMC to the BM.[80] MIP-1α has also been shown to increase the adhesion of MMC to marrow stromal cells, which, in turn, stimulates production of RANKL and IL-6, fostering the vicious cycle of osteolytic activity and MM growth.[81]

SDF-1α is a CXC chemokine that aids in the localization and support of HSCs within their BM niche. Several lines of evidence suggest that SDF-1α participates in MM-associated bone disease. Akin to MIP-1α, SDF-1α is a chemoattractant for OC precursors and has been implicated in the homing of MMC to bone.[82] Increased plasma levels of SDF-1α are demonstrable in MM patients with active bone disease. Further, in vitro data suggests that blocking the receptor for SDF-1α, CXCR4, may inhibit the OC formation that is induced by coculture of BM with MMC.[83]

Direct Contact with Multiple Myeloma Cells Facilitates Osteoclast Development and Activation

The characteristic nature of MM to grow in the BM environment implies that cell–cell interactions contribute to MM growth and survival. Data from several groups suggest that cell–cell contact may also be critical for the development of osteolytic lesions. Abe et al. have shown that contact between MMC and OC can enhance MMC growth, protect MMC from chemotherapy, and increase the production of autocrine growth factors, such as IL-6.[84] The prosurvival effect of OC on MMC is bidirectional as coculture can increase OC resistance to apoptosis as well as bone resorption activity. Direct cell contact is necessary, as these effects were lost on addition of blocking antibodies against adhesion molecules VLA-4 (expressed by MMC) and $\alpha_1\beta_3$ integrin (expressed by OC). Similarly, Michigami et al. have shown that direct interaction between vascular cell adhesion molecule, VCAM-1 (expressed by marrow stromal cells), and $\alpha_4\beta_1$-integrin (expressed by MMC) leads to increased expression of RANKL and heightened osteoclastogenesis.[85] Further, disruption of this interaction was shown to reduce both tumor growth and bone destruction in MM xenograft models.[86] Thus, it appears that the MM BM niche fosters direct cellular interactions between MMC, BM stromal cells, and OC that promote MMC growth and osteoclastogenesis.

The Vicious Cycle of Myeloma Growth and Bone Destruction

Inhibitors of OC activation prevent bone destruction and block tumor progression when tested in MM xenograft models.[38,87,88] These results support the clinical observation that bisphosphonates reduce tumor burden in progressive MM and improve the survival of patients with advanced stages of MM.[89,90] Together, these findings suggest that OC and or OC-mediated bone resorption support MMC growth, and promote a vicious cycle of MM expansion and osteolysis.

Osteoclasts Support Multiple Myeloma Cells

OC have been shown to enhance the growth and survival of MMC in culture, and to rescue MMC from apoptosis induced by serum depletion or doxorubicin treatment.[91] This support is mediated by direct OC–MMC contact (Section "Direct Contact with Multiple Myeloma Cells Facilitates Osteoclast Development and Activation"), as well as by the secretion of IL-6, OPN, B-cell activating factor (BAFF), a proliferation-inducing ligand (APRIL), and chondroitin synthase 1 (CHSY1).

OPN is a noncollagenous bone matrix protein that is expressed at high level by OC. OPN is a ligand for $\alpha_v\beta_3$ integrins (expressed by vascular endothelial cells as well as OC), and has been shown to cooperate with VEGF to enhance MM-associated angiogenesis.[92] The resulting endothelial cell expansion leads to increased expression of RANKL, IL-8, and IL-6, thereby expanding OC and MMC growth. Thus, neoangiogenesis may arise from and contribute to the vicious cycle of heightened OC development, bone resorption, and MM tumor progression.

BAFF and APRIL, members of the TNF superfamily, are growth and survival factors for MMC. They have been shown to increase MMC expression of Bcl-2, and to protect MMC from the proapoptotic effects of IL-6 deprivation and dexamethasone treatment.[93] Their importance is highlighted by the ability of a BAFF/APRIL decoy receptor to block OC support of MMC in culture.[94] APRIL may be the more significant of the pair, as it is secreted at very high levels by OC, and is concentrated by MMC through its interaction with CD138. BAFF and APRIL share two receptors that are expressed by MMC, transmembrane activator and calcium modulator and cyclophilin ligand interactor (TACI) and B-cell maturation antigen (BCMA). TACI overexpression has been shown to predict MMC dependence on the BM microenvironment, again highlighting the significance of BAFF/APRIL signaling in MMC survival.[95]

CHSY1 was identified as a potential MM survival factor because its expression by OC is markedly increased on coculture with MMC, and because knockdown of CHSY1 abrogates OC support of MMC survival.[96] CHSY1 is a type-II membrane protein with a DDD motif that allows it to glycosylate Notch receptors and thereby modulate Notch signaling. MMC express four Notch receptors and BM stromal cells express six Notch ligands: Delta (1–4) and Jagged (1 and 2). Their interactions are believed critical to stromal cell support of MMC growth and survival.[97,98] The binding of Delta or Jagged results in proteolytic cleavage of Notch, followed by translocation of its intracellular domain to the nucleus, where it modulates transcription. Glycosylation by CHSY1 potentiates signaling by Notch2 but inhibits signaling by Notch1. In other cell systems, Notch activation has been found to promote and inhibit differentiation, increase and decrease proliferation, promote survival, and induce apoptosis. Similarly, in MM Notch activation has been shown to both promote proliferation and induce cell cycle arrest as a means of permitting cell survival. The pleiotropic effects of Notch signaling appear to reflect both the intrinsic potential of the cell receiving the Notch signal and its microenvironmental context. Notch signaling between MMC and stromal cells appears to be bidirectional, as MMC, but not benign plasma cells, secrete Jagged 1 and 2, and BM stromal cells express Notch. Further, Notch signaling promotes production of IL-6, IGF, and VEGF by BM stromal cells, thus providing additional growth signals for MM.[99] Together, these results are consistent with the notion that Notch signaling plays an important role in the growth and survival of MMC in the BM microenvironment; however, it is currently unclear how CHSY1 modulation fits into this complex network.

Bone Resorption Contributes to Multiple Myeloma Cell Growth and Survival

OC-mediated bone resorption results in the release of bioactive factors, including IGF-1 and TGF-β, which contribute to MM progression.[100,101] IGF-1 acts directly on MMC, stimulating growth, chemotaxis, and survival.[102,103] In contrast, TGF–β acts indirectly, stimulating BM stromal cells to express IL-6 and VEGF, which then act as growth and survival factors for OC and MMC.[104] In fact, increased levels of TGF-β are responsible for the increased levels of IL-6 and VEGF seen in MM. The importance of this activity is highlighted by the ability of TGF-β signaling inhibitors to block MM tumor progression in xenograft models.[105] Thus, while TGF-β acts to enhance OPG production, thereby tempering OC activation, the overall impact of TGF-β release is to foster MM tumor growth and bone destruction. TGF-β is also a potent suppressor of normal B-cell proliferation and immunoglobulin production, and is responsible for the reciprocal suppression and functional immune impairment seen in MM.[106,107] In contrast to normal plasma cells, MMC do not express a cell surface receptor for TGF-β, and thus escape its antiproliferative effects.[104,108]

Osteoblast Inhibition by Multiple Myeloma

Recruitment and activation of both OBL and OC is a common histological feature of early stage MM.[109] However, this picture evolves with disease progression, until OBL inhibition becomes the dominant hallmark. As a consequence, lytic lesions are not repaired despite effective OC inhibition by bisphosphonates. In vitro investigations have confirmed OBL suppression by MMC.[110] MMC suppression of Wnt signaling (previously described in the Section "Osteoblasts"), direct MMC–OBL contact, and other mechanisms are now beginning to be elucidated as potential mechanisms for OBL inhibition by MM.[111]

Multiple Myeloma Inhibition of Wnt Signaling

Tian et al. provided the first link between Wnt-signaling and MM-associated bone disease.[112] Comparing the transcriptional profiles of MMC isolated from patients with different disease characteristics, they found that *DKK1*, encoding a soluble inhibitor of canonical Wnt signaling, was highly expressed only in samples taken from patients with active bone disease. Because canonical Wnt signaling was known to be critical to OBL development, they confirmed that addition of recombinant DKK1 would blunt OBL differentiation in vitro. They then demonstrated that the OBL inhibitory effect of MM BM plasma could be abrogated by anti-DKK1 antibody, demonstrating for the first time a clear role for a Wnt signaling inhibitor in the pathogenesis of malignant bone disease. Further work has extended these observations to in vivo systems. The use of anti-DKK1 antibody in SCID mice implanted with rabbit bones injected with primary human MM samples (SCID-rab model) has shown actual *increases* in bone mineral density of both the implanted myelomatous bone and the non-involved mouse bones. There was also a concomitant decrease in MM tumor mass, as measured by paraprotein production.[113] These observations confirm a critical role for DKK1 in MM bone disease (both OC activation and OBL inhibition), and also suggest that active OBL inhibition may contribute to MMC survival. However, DKK1 overexpression is not universal among MM patients with bone disease. Rather, it appears to be restricted to MM with a mature plasma cell phenotype.[3,112] Plasma cells with aggressive features, including plasma cell leukemia, do not express DKK1, but frequently express a second soluble inhibitor of canonical Wnt signaling, sFRP-2.[114] sFRP-2 also blocks OBL differentiation in vitro, and may contribute to the OBL dysfunction seen in patients with high-grade MM.

Inadequate bone repair is the obvious clinical manifestation of canonical Wnt signal inhibition. However, preventing OBL maturation may be equally important, as mature OBL express high levels of OPG and little RANKL, thus limiting OC formation and, presumably, MM tumor progression.[115] In contrast, immature OBL are strong producers of RANKL and produce relatively little OPG, thus altering the RANKL/OPG ratio in favor of OC development and activation. Furthermore, mature OBL may block the prosurvival effects of OC on MM.[116]

Several recent discoveries concerning the role of Wnt signaling in MM add complexity to the above picture. Qiang et al. found that Wnt-3a acts as a chemokine to induce the migration of MMC through activation of PKC and the noncanonical Wnt/RhoA pathway.[117] This pathway directs actin reorganization to regulate cell cytoskeletal structure, motility, and migration.[118] MMC have also been shown to overexpress β-catenin in both active and inactive forms, and to be stimulated to proliferate through activation of canonical Wnt signaling.[119] Furthermore, MMC have been shown to express Wnt 5a, Wnt 10b, and Wnt 16, suggesting possible autocrine growth loops. Wnts control multiple aspects of cellular development, including establishment of cell polarity, cell migration, hematopoietic stem cell regeneration, and B-cell proliferation.[120–122] Thus, it is not surprising that Wnts influence MMC (and likely OC), as well as OBL. The evolution of Wnt-3a as chemoattractant for MMC might be explained as a signal for healthy (non-infiltrated) BM for MM to exploit. Noncanonical Wnt signaling will not be inhibited by DKK1 or sFRP-2. However, the role of Wnts as potential growth factors for MM and the paradoxical findings that MMC produce both Wnts and Wnt inhibitors remains to be clarified. Wnt signals are the subject of dysregulation in other human cancers as well, which further substantiates its importance in cell growth and development.[123,124] A well-known example of a Wnt-signaling pathway disturbance is the mutation of the APC gene found in 80% of colorectal cancers. Therefore, consequences of targeting Wnt signaling for therapeutic benefit in MM or destructive bone disease should be evaluated carefully for possible oncogenic consequences.

Multiple Myeloma Suppression of Runx2/Cbfa1

The Runx2/Cbfa1-signaling pathway, critical to the transition of MSC to mature OBL (Section "Osteoblasts"), is also suppressed by MM.[125] Suppression appears to be mediated through direct cell contact (via VLA-4 on MM and VCAM on osteoprogenitors) and through the secretion of IL-7 by MMC. Previous work had shown that IL-7 decreases Runx2/Cbfa1 expression in osteoprogenitors, resulting in reduced maturation reflected by reduced expression of mature OBL markers, such as osteocalcin.[126] Runx2/Cbfa1 suppression may also reflect inhibition of canonical Wnt signaling by MM, as it has recently been shown in a murine model that Wnt signaling leads to increased Runx2/Cbfa1 activity and thus to increased bone formation.[127] However, the full impact of MM on the complex interplay that exists between β-catenin, LEF, and Runx2 remains to be determined.[128–130] As described previously, blocking OBL maturation favors increased RANKL (from OBL progenitors) and decreased OPG expression (from mature OBL). Blockade of Runx2/Cbfa1 represents yet another method of RANKL/OPG dysregulation by MM.[131]

Additional Mechanisms that May Underlie Osteoblast Inhibition

Normal bone remodeling is coordinated by an OBL network that is maintained through homophilic NCAM binding (Neural cell adhesion molecule: CD56). MMC also express NCAM, and strong expression has been found to correlate with radiographically evident bone disease.[132] In vitro, MMC have been shown to bind OBL via NCAM, and it has been proposed that MM uses NCAM to disrupt intra-OBL communication in vivo, thereby decreasing OBL activity.

IL-3 may also contribute to OBL inhibition in MM. Produced by MMC and tumor infiltrating T lymphocytes, IL-3 levels are elevated in the BM plasma of most (70%) patients with MM compared to normal controls or patients with monoclonal gammopathy of undetermined significance (MGUS). IL-3 has been shown to directly inhibit the differentiation of OBL precursors in culture.[133–135] More importantly, anti-IL-3 antibody has been shown to abrogate the ability of MM BM plasma to block OBL development. In addition, IL-3 also appears to act via $CD45^+/CD11b^+$ monocytes/macrophage to indirectly inhibit OBL development.[133,135] More work remains to be done to elucidate the exact mechanism of IL-3 action and its potential as a therapeutic target.

Increased OBL apoptosis may contribute to the reduced OBL numbers evident in MM BM samples. MMC express TRAIL and Fas-L, and OBL express death receptors 4/5 and Fas.[136] In addition, coculture of OBL with MMC results in enhanced OBL apoptosis, which is abrogated by neutralizing anti-FAS-L antibodies or OPG, a decoy receptor for TRAIL as well as RANKL.[137,138]

Summary and Conclusion

Skeletal integrity requires continuous skeletal remodeling, the resorption of damaged bone balanced by the deposition of new. This process is coordinated via a signaling network among OBL, OC, osteocytes, and the BM stroma. MM disrupts this process, arresting OBL development by inhibiting canonical Wnt signaling, suppressing Runx2/Cbfa1 expression, blocking intra-OBL signaling, and inducing OBL apoptosis. This not only prevents bone repair but also changes the RANKL/OPG balance in favor of increased osteoclastogenesis. OC development is further stimulated by multiple cytokines and chemokines, and by direct MMC–OC contact. In turn, OC and OC-mediated bone resorption support MMC growth and survival, resulting in a vicious cycle of tumor progression and bone destruction.

Despite this common presentation, the sheer number of molecular signals that have been implicated in MM bone disease suggests a heterogeneous process composed of multiple signals working both in parallel and series to each other. Currently, we do not know which of these signals is necessary, which is redundant, and how they are integrated to trigger bone destruction. However, this complex interplay may prove a limitation of therapies that target only one pathway, such as anti-DKK1, anti-MIP-1α, or anti-RANKL. Additional questions surrounding the mechanisms described above include (1) how MM can antagonize Wnt signaling, yet use Wnts as growth factors, (2) the impact of MM on ITAM-associated immunoglobulin-like receptors, (3) the impact of MM on Eph-ephrin signaling, and (4) the existence of a master signal for Runx2/Cbfa1, Wnts, and Notch that coordinates MM survival and bone destruction. Clearly, more work is required to clarify this pathophysiology.

References

1. Bataille R, Harousseau JL. MM. *N Engl J Med* 1997; 336:1657–1664.
2. Durie BG, Salmon SE. Cellular kinetics, staging, and immunoglobulin synthesis in MM. *Annu Rev Med* 1975; 26:283–288.
3. Robbiani D, Chesi M, Bergsagel PL. Bone lesions in molecular subtypes of MM. *N Engl J Med* 2004; 351:197–198.
4. Greipp PR, San Miguel J, Durie BG, et al. International staging system for multiple myeloma. *J Clin Oncol* 2005; 23(15):3412–3420.
5. Lane JM, Hong R, Koob J, et al. Kyphoplasty enhances function and structural alignment in multiple myeloma. *Clin Orthop Relat Res* 2004; 426:49–53.
6. Pearse R. Wnt antagonism in MM: A potential cause of uncoupled bone remodeling. *Clin Cancer Res* 2006; 12 (20 Suppl):6274s–6278s.
7. Roodman GD. Regulation of osteoclast differentiation. *Ann N Y Acad Sci* 2006; 1068:100–109.
8. Hadkidakis D, Androulakis I. Bone remodeling. *Ann N Y Acad Sci* 2006; 1092:385–396.
9. Niida S, Kaku M, Amano H, et al. Vascular endothelial growth factor can substitute for macrophage colony-stimulating factor in the support of osteoclastic bone resorption. *J Exp Med* 1999; 190:293–298.
10. Dai XM, Ryan GR, Hapel AJ, et al. Targeted disruption of the mouse colony-stimulating factor 1 receptor gene results in osteopetrosis, mononuclear phagocyte deficiency, increased primitive progenitor cell frequencies, and reproductive defects. *Blood* 2002; 99(1):111–120.
11. Han JH, Choi SJ, Kurihara N. Macrophage inflammatory protein-1 alpha is an osteoclastogenic factor in MM that is independent of receptor activator of nuclear factor kappa B ligand. *Blood* 2001; 97:3349–3353.
12. Tolar J, Teitelbaum SL, Orchard PJ. Osteopetrosis. *N Engl J Med* 2004; 351:2839–2849.
13. Hsu H, Lacey DL, Dunstan CR, et al. Tumor necrosis factor receptor family member RANK mediates osteoclast differentiation and activation induced by osteoprotegerin ligand. *Proc Natl Acad Sci* 1999; 96:3540–3545.
14. Boyle WJ, Simonet WS, Lacey DL. Osteoclast differentiation and activation. *Nature* 2003; 423(6937):337–342.
15. Lacey DL, Timms E, Tan HL, et al. Osteoprotegerin ligand is a cytokine that regulates osteoclast differentiation and activation. *Cell* 1998; 93:165–176.
16. Heider U, Hofbauer LC, Zacriski I, et al. Novel aspects of osteoclast activation and OBL inhibition in MM bone. *Biochem Biophys Res Commun* 2005; 338:687–693.
17. Roodman GD. Mechanisms of disease: mechanisms of bone metastasis. *N Engl J Med* 2004; 350:1655–1664.

18. Roodman GD, et al. Interleukin 6. A potential autocrine/paracrine factor in Paget's disease of bone. *J Clin Invest* 1992; 89:46–52.
19. Teitelbaum SL. Bone resorption by osteoclasts. *Science* 2000; 289:1504–1508.
20. Odgren PR, Kim N, MacKay CA, et al. The role of RANKL (TRANCE/TNFSF11), a tumor necrosis factor family member, in skeletal development: effects of gene knockout and transgenic rescue. *Connect Tissue Res* 2003; 44 Suppl 1:264–271.
21. Wong BR, Josien R, Lee SY, et al. The TRAF family of signal transducers mediates NF-kappaB activation by the TRANCE receptor. *J Biol Chem* 1998; 273(43):28355–28359.
22. Xing L, et al. NF-kappaB p50 and p52 expression is not required for RANK-expressing osteoclast progenitor formation but is essential for RANK- and cytokine-mediated osteoclastogenesis. *J Bone Miner Res* 2002; 17:1200–1210.
23. Asagiri M, Takayanagi H. The molecular understanding of osteoclast differentiation. *Bone* 2007; 40(2):251–264.
24. Mansky KC, Sankar U, Han J, et al. Microphthalmia transcription factor is a target of the p38 MAPK pathway in response to receptor activator of NF-kappa B ligand signaling. *J Biol Chem* 2002; 277(13):11077–11083.
25. Dougall WC, Glaccum M, Charrier K, et al. RANK is essential for osteoclast and lymph node development. *Genes Dev* 1999; 13(18):2412–2424.
26. Teitelbaum SL. Bone resorption by osteoclasts. *Science* 2000; 289:1504–1508.
27. Terpos E, Politou M, Rahemtulla A. New insights into the pathophysiology and management of bone disease in MM. *Br J Haematol* 2003; 123:758–769.
28. Kong YY, Yoshida H, Sarosi I, et al. OPGL is a key regulator of osteoclastogenesis, lymphocyte development, and lymph-node organogenesis. *Nature* 1999; 397: 315–323.
29. Bucay N, Sarosi I, Dunstan CR. Osteoprotegerin-deficient mice develop early-onset osteoporosis and arterial calcification. *Genes Dev* 1998; 12:1260–1268.
30. Robey PG, Young MF, Flanders KC, et al. Osteoblasts synthesize and respond to transforming growth factor-type beta (TGF-beta) in vitro. *J Cell Biol* 1987; 105(1):457–463.
31. Bonewald LF, Dallas SL. Role of active and latent transforming growth factor beta in bone formation. *J Cell Biochem* 1994; 55(3):350–357.
32. Janssens K, ten Dijke P, Janssens S, et al. Transforming growth factor-beta1 to the bone. *Endocr Rev* 2005; 26(6):743–774.
33. Takayanagi H, Ogasawara K, Hida S, et al. T-cell-mediated regulation of osteoclastogenesis by signaling cross-talk between RANKL and IFN-gamma. *Nature* 2000; 408(6812):600–605.
34. Zhou Z, Imme lD, Xi CX, et al. Regulation of osteoclast function and bone mass by RAGE. *J Exp Med* 2006; 203(4):1067–1080.
35. Kim N, Takami M, Rho J, et al. A novel member of the leukocyte receptor complex regulates osteoclast differentiation. *J Exp Med* 2002; 195(2):201–209.
36. Cella M, Buonsanti C, Strader C, et al. Impaired differentiation of osteoclasts in TREM-2-deficient individuals. *J Exp Med* 2003; 198(4):645–651.
37. Koga T, Inui M, Inoue K, et al. Costimulatory signals mediated by the ITAM motif cooperate with RANKL for bone homeostasis. *Nature* 2004; 428(6984):758–763.
38. Pearse RN, Sordillo EM, Yaccoby S, et al. MM disrupts the TRANCE/osteoprotegerin cytokine axis to trigger bone destruction and promote tumor progression. *Proc Natl Acad Sci* 2001; 98(20):11581–11586.
39. Lam J, Takeshita S, Barker JE, et al. TNF-alpha induces osteoclastogenesis by direct stimulation of macrophages exposed to permissive levels of RANK ligand. *J Clin Invest* 2000; 106(12):1481–1488.
40. Taichman RS, Emerson SG. The role of osteoblasts in the hematopoietic microenvironment. *Stem Cells* 1998; 16(1):7–15.
41. Zhang J, Niu C, Ye L, Huang H, et al. Identification of the haematopoietic stem cell niche and control of the niche size. *Nature* 2003; 425(6960):836–841.

42. Calvi LM, Adams GB, Weibrecht KW, et al. Osteoblastic cells regulate the haematopoietic stem cell niche. *Nature* 2003; 425(6960):841–846.

43. Ducy P, Zhang R, Geoffroy V, et al. Osf2/Cbfa1: a transcriptional activator of OBL differentiation. *Cell* 1997; 89:747–754.

44. Komori T, Yagi H, Nomura S, et al. Targeted disruption of Cbfa1 results in a complete lack of bone formation owing to maturational arrest of OBL. *Cell* 1997; 89:755–764.

45. Hu H, Hilton MJ, Tu X, et al. Sequential roles of Hedgehog and Wnt signaling in osteoblast development. *Development* 2005; 132(1):49–60.

46. Gong Y, Slee RB, Fukai N, et al. LDL receptor-related protein 5 (LRP5) affects bone accrual and eye development. *Cell* 2001; 107:513–523.

47. Boyden LM, Mao J, Belsky J, et al. High bone density due to a mutation in LDL-receptor-related protein 5. *N Engl J Med* 2002; 346:1513–1521.

48. Rawadi G, Vayssière B, Dunn F, et al. BMP-2 controls alkaline phosphatase expression and osteoblast mineralization by a Wnt autocrine loop. *J Bone Miner Res* 2003; 18(10):1842–1853.

49. Kato M, Patel MS, Levasseur R, et al. Cbfa1-independent decrease in osteoblast proliferation, osteopenia, and persistent embryonic eye vascularization in mice deficient in LRP5, a Wnt coreceptor. *J Cell Biol* 2002; 157(2):303–314.

50. Day TF, Guo X, Garrett-Beal L, et al. Wnt/beta-catenin signaling in mesenchymal progenitors controls osteoblast and chondrocyte differentiation during vertebrate skeletogenesis. *Dev Cell* 2005; 8(5):739–750.

51. Hill TP, Später D, Taketo MM, et al. Canonical Wnt/beta-catenin signaling prevents osteoblasts from differentiating into chondrocytes. *Dev Cell* 2005; 8(5):727–738.

52. Westendorf JJ, Kahler RA, Schroeder TM. Wnt signaling in OBL and bone diseases. *Gene* 2004; 341:19–39.

53. Franz-Odendaal TA, Hall BK, Witten PE. Buried alive: how osteoblasts become osteocytes. *Dev Dyn* 2006; 235(1):176–190.

54. Knothe Tate ML, Adamson JR, Tami AE, et al. The osteocyte. *Int J Biochem Cell Biol* 2004; 36(1):1–8.

55. Rodan GA, Martin TJ. Role of osteoblasts in hormonal control of bone resorption – a hypothesis. *Calcif Tissue Int* 1981; 33(4):349–351.

56. Zhao C, Irie N, Takada Y, et al. Bidirectional ephrinB2-EphB4 signaling controls bone homeostasis. *Cell Metab* 2006; 4(2):111–121.

57. Hayden JM, Mohan S, Baylink DJ. The insulin-like growth factor system and the coupling of formation to resorption. *Bone* 1995; 17(2 Suppl):93S–98S.

58. Pfeilschifter J, Mundy GR. Modulation of type beta transforming growth factor activity in bone cultures by osteotropic hormones. *Proc Natl Acad Sci USA*. 1987; 84(7):2024–2028.

59. Sheu TJ, Schwarz EM, Martinez DA, et al. A phage display technique identifies a novel regulator of cell differentiation. *J Biol Chem* 2003; 278(1):438–443.

60. Udagawa N, Takahashi N, Jimi E, et al. OBL/stromal cells stimulate osteoclast activation through expression of osteoclast differentiation factor/RANKL but not macrophage colony-stimulating factor: receptor activator of NF-kappa B ligand. *Bone* 1999; 25(5):517–523.

61. Glass D, Bialek P, Karsenty G, et al. Canonical Wnt signaling in differentiated OBL controls ostelast differentiation. *Dev Cell* 2005; 8:751–764.

62. Holmen SL, Zylstra CR, Mukherjee A, et al. Essential role of -catenin in postnatal bone acquisition. *J Biol Chem* 2005; 280:21162–21168.

63. Bataille R, Chappard D, Marcelli C, et al. OBL stimulation in MM lacking lytic bone lesions. *Br J Haematol* 1990; 76:484–487.

64. Abildgaard N, Brixen K, Eriksen EF, et al. Sequential analysis of biochemical markers of bone resorption and bone densitometry in MM. *Haematologica* 2004; 89(5):567–577.

65. Taube T, Beneton MN, McCloskey EV, et al. Abnormal bone remodeling in patients with myelomatosis and normal biochemical indices of bone resorption. *Eur J Haematol* 1992; 49:192–198.

66. Fonseca R, Trendle MC, Leong T, et al. Prognostic value of serum markers of bone metabolism in untreated MM patients. *Br J Haematol* 2000; 109:24–29.

67. Terpos E, Politou M, Rahemtulla A. The role of markers of bone remodeling in MM. *Blood Rev* 2005; 19(3):125–142.

68. Heider U, Hofbauer L, ZavrskiI, et al. Novel aspects of osteoclast activation and OBL inhibition in MM bone disease. *Biochem Biophys Res Commun* 2005; 338:1–7.

69. Sezer O, Heider U, Jakob C, et al. Immunohistochemistry reveals RANKL expression of MMC. *Blood* 2002; 99:4646–4647.

70. Lai FP, Cole-Sinclair M, Cheng WJ. MMC can directly contribute to the pool of RANKL in bone bypassing the classic stromal and osteoblast pathway of osteoclast stimulation. *Br J Haematol* 2004; 126:192–201.

71. Standal T, Seidel C, Hjertner O, et al. Osteoprotegerin is bound, internalized, and degraded by MMC. *Blood* 2002; 100:3002–3007.

72. Giuliani N, Bataille R, Mancini C, et al. Myeloma cells induce imbalance in the osteoprotegerin/osteoprotegerin ligand system in the human bone marrow environment. *Blood* 2001; 98(13):3527–3533.

73. Cook DC. The role of MIP-1 alpha in inflammation and hematopoeisis. *J Leukoc Biol* 1996; 59:61–66.

74. Choi S, Cruz JC, Craig F, et al. Macrophage inflammatory protein-1α (MIP-1α) is a potential osteoclast stimulatory factor in MM. *Blood* 2000; 96:671–675.

75. Hashimoto T, Abe M, Oshima T, et al. Ability of MMC to secrete macrophage inflammatory protein (MIP)-1alpha and MIP-1beta correlates with lytic bone lesions in patients with MM. *Br J Haematol* 2004; 125(1):38–41.

76. Abe M, Hiura J, Wilde K, et al. Role for macrophage inflammatory protein (MIP)-1 alpha and MIP-1 beta in the development of osteolytic lesions in MM. *Blood* 2002; 100:2195–2202.

77. Choi SJ, Oba Y, Gazitt Y, et al. Antisense inhibition of macrophage inflammatory protein 1-alpha blks bone destruction in a model of MM bone disease. *J Clin Invest* 2001; 108:1833–1841.

78. Han J, Choi S, Kurihara N, et al. Macrophage inflammatory protein-1 is an osteoclastogenic factor in MM that is independent of receptor activator of nuclear B ligand. *Blood* 2001; 97:3349–3353.

79. Lentzsch S, Gries M, Janz R, et al. Macrophage inflammatory protein-1 alpha triggers migration and signaling cascades mediating survival and proliferation in MM cells. *Blood* 2003; 101:3568–3573.

80. Menu E, De Leenheer E, De Raeve H. Role of CCR1 and CCR5 in homing and growth of MM and in the development of osteolytic lesions: a study in the 5TMM model. *Clin Exp Metastasis* 2006; 23(5–6):291–300.

81. Oba Y, Lee JW, Ehrlich LA, et al. MIP-1alpha utilizes both CCR1 and CCR5 to induce osteoclast formation and increase adhesion of MMC to marrow stromal cells. *Exp Hematol* 2005; 33(3):272–278.

82. Alsayed Y, Ngo H, Runnels J, et al. Mechanisms of regulation of CXCR4/SDF-1 (CXCL12)-dependent migration and homing in MM. *Blood* 2007; 109:2708–2717.

83. Zannettino AC, Farrugia AN, Kortesidis A, et al. Elevated serum levels of stromal-derived factor 1-alpha are associated with increased osteoclast activity and osteolytic bone disease in MM patients. *Cancer Res* 2005; 1700–1709.

84. Abe M, Hiura K, Matsumoto T, et al. Osteoclasts enhance MM cell growth and survival via cell-cell contact: a vicious cycle between bone destruction and MM expansion. *Blood* 2004; 104:2848–2491.

85. Michigami T, Shimizu N, Williams PJ, et al. Cell-cell contact between marrow stromal cells and MMC via VCAM-1 and alpha(4)beta(1)-integrin enhances production of osteoclast-stimulating activity. *Blood* 2000; 96:1953–1960.

86. Mori Y, Shimizu N, Dallas M, et al. Anti-(alpha)4 integrin antibody suppresses the development of MM and associated osteoclasic osteolysis. *Blood* 2004; 104(7):2149–2154.

87. Croucher PI, Shipman CM, Lippitt J, et al. Osteoprotegerin inhabits the development of osteolytic bone disease in multiple myeloma.. *Blood* 2001; 98(13):3534–3540.

88. Croucher PI, De Hendrik R, Perry MJ, et al. Zoledronic acid treatment of 5T2MM-bearing mice inhibits the development of myeloma bone disease: evidence for decreased osteolysis, tumor burden and angiogenesis, and increased survival. *J Bone Miner Res* 2003; 18(3):482–492.

89. Dhodapkar MV, Singh J, Mehta J, et al. Anti-myeloma activity of pamidronate in vivo. *Br J Haematol* 1998; 103(2):530–532.

90. Berenson JR, Lichtenstein A, Porter L, et al. Long-term pamidronate treatment of advanced multiple myeloma patients reduces skeletal events. Myeloma Aredia Study Group. *J Clin Oncol* 1998; 16(2):593–602.

91. Yaccoby S, Wezeman MJ, Henderson A, et al. Cancer and the microenvironment: myeloma-osteoclast interactions as a model. *Cancer Res* 2004; 64(6):2016–2023.

92. Tanaka Y, Abe M, Hiasa M, et al. Myeloma cell-osteoclast interaction enhances angiogenesis together with bone resorption: a role for vascular endothelial cell growth factor and osteopontin. *Clin Cancer Res* 2007; 13(3):816–823.

93. Moreaux J, Legouffe E, Jourdan E, et al. BAFF and APRIL protect myeloma cells from apoptosis induced by interleukin 6 deprivation and dexamethasone. *Blood* 2004; 103(8):3148–3157.

94. Abe M, Kido S, Hiasa M, et al. BAFF and APRIL as osteoclast-derived survival factors for myeloma cells: a rationale for TACI-Fc treatment in patients with multiple myeloma. *Leukemia* 2006; 20(7):1313–1315.

95. Moreaux J, Cremer FW, Reme T, et al. The level of TACI gene expression in myeloma cells is associated with a signature of microenvironment dependence versus a plasmablastic signature. *Blood* 2005; 106(3):1021–1030.

96. Yin L. Chondroitin synthase 1 is a key molecule in MM cell-osteoclast interactions. *J Biol Chem* 2005; 280(16):15666–15672.

97. Jundt F, Pröbsting KS, Anagnostopoulos I, et al. Jagged1-induced Notch signaling drives proliferation of multiple myeloma cells. *Blood* 2004; 103(9):3511–3515.

98. Nefedova Y, Cheng P, Alsina M, et al. Involvement of Notch-1 signaling in bone marrow stroma-mediated de novo drug resistance of myeloma and other malignant lymphoid cell lines. *Blood* 2004; 103(9):3503–3510.

99. Houde C, Li Y, Song L, et al. Overexpression of the NOTCH ligand JAG2 in malignant plasma cells from MM patients and cell lines. *Blood* 2004; 104:3697–3704.

100. Dallas SL, Rosser JL, Mundy GR, Bonewald LF. Proteolysis of latent transforming growth factor-beta (TGF-beta)-binding protein-1 by osteoclasts. A cellular mechanism for release of TGF-beta from bone matrix. *J Biol Chem* 2002; 277(24):21352–21360.

101. Hauschka PV, Chen TL, Mavrakos AE. Polypeptide growth factors in bone matrix. *Ciba Found Symp* 1988; 136:207–225.

102. Qiang YW, Yao L, Tosato G, Rudikoff S. Insulin-like growth factor I induces migration and invasion of human MMC. *Blood* 2004; 103:301–308.

103. Ferlin M, Noraz N, Hertogh C, et al. Insulin-like growth factor induces the survival and proliferation of MMC through an interleukin-6-independent transduction pathway. *Br J Haematol* 2000; 111(2):626–634.

104. Urashima M, Ogata A, Chauhan D, et al. Transforming growth factor-beta 1: differential effects on multiple myeloma versus normal B cells. *Blood* 1996; 87(5):1928–1938.

105. Hayashi T, Hideshima T, Nguyen AN, et al. Transforming growth factor beta receptor I kinase inhibitor down-regulates cytokine secretion and MM cell growth in the BM microenvironment. *Clin Cancer Res* 2004; 10(22):7540–7546.

106. Kehrl JH, Roberts AB, Wakefield LM, et al. Transforming growth factor beta is an important immunomodulatory protein for human B lymphocyte. *J Immunol* 1986; 137(12):3855–3860.

107. Kyrtsonis MC, Repa C, Dedoussis GV, et al. Serum transforming growth factor-beta 1 is related to the degree of immunoparesis in patients with multiple myeloma. *Med Oncol* 1998; 15(2):124–128.

108. Amoroso SR, Huang N, Roberts AB, et al. Consistent loss of functional transforming growth factor beta receptor expression in murine plasmacytomas. *Proc Natl Acad Sci USA* 1998; 95(1):189–194.

109. Bataille R, Chappard D, Marcelli C, et al. Recruitment of new osteoblasts and osteoclasts is the earliest critical event in the pathogenesis of human multiple myeloma. *J Clin Invest* 1991; 88(1):62–66.

110. Evans CE, Ward C, Rathour L, et al. MM affects both the growth and function of human OBL-like cells. *Clin Exp Metastasis* 1992; 10:33–38.

111. Giuliani N, Rizzoli V, Roodman G. MM bone disease: pathophysiology of OBL inhibition. *Blood* 2006; 108:3992–3996.

112. Tian E, Zhan F, Walker E, et al. The role of the Wnt-signaling antagonist DKK1 in the development of osteolytic lesions in MM. *N Engl J Med* 2003; 349:2483–2494.

113. Yaccoby S, Ling W, Zhan F, et al. Antibody-based inhibition of DKK1 suppresses tumor-induced bone resorption and MM growth in vivo. *Blood* 2007; 109:2106–2111.

114. Oshima T, Abe M, Matsumoto T. MMC suppress bone formation by secreting a soluble Wnt inhibitor, sFRP-2. *Blood* 2005; 106:3160–3165.

115. Glass D, Bialek P, Karsenty G, et al. Canonical Wnt signaling in differentiated OBL controls osteoblast differentiation. *Dev Cell* 2005; 8:751–764.

116. Yaccoby S, Wezeman MJ, Zangari M, et al. Inhibitory effects of osteoblasts and increased bone formation on myeloma in novel culture systems and a myelomatous mouse model. *Haematologica* 2006; 91(2):192–199.

117. Qiang Y, Walsh K, Rudikoff S. Wnts induce migration and invasion of MM plasma cells. *Blood* 2005; 106:1786–1793.

118. Nelson W, Russe R. Convergence of Wnt, beta-catenin, and cadherin pathways. *Science* 2004; 303:1483–1487.

119. Derkson PWB, Tjin E, Pals T. Illegitimate Wnt signaling promotes proliferation of MMC. *Proc Natl Acad Sci* 2004; 101:6122–6127.

120. Miller JR, Hking AM, Brown JD, Moon RT. Mechanism and function of signal transduction by the Wnt/beta-catenin and Wnt/Ca2+ pathways. *Oncogene* 1999; 18(55):7860–7872.

121. Staal FJ, Clevers HC. WNT signaling and haematopoiesis: a WNT-WNT situation. *Nat Rev Immunol* 2005; 5(1):21–30.

122. Dosen G, Tenstad E, Nygren MK, et al. Wnt expression and canonical Wnt signaling in human BM B lymphopoiesis. *BMC Immunol* 2006; 29:7–13.

123. Herbst A, Kolligs FT. Wnt signaling as a therapeutic target for cancer. *Methods Mol Biol* 2007; 361:63–91.

124. Karim R, Tse G, Putti T, et al. The significance of the Wnt pathway in the pathology of human cancers. *Pathology* 2004; 36(2):120–128.

125. Giuliani N, Colla S, Marandi F, et al. MMC blk RUNX2/CBFA1 activity in human BM OBL progenitors and inhibit OBL formation and differentiation. *Blood* 2005; 106:2472–2483.

126. Weitzmann MN, Roggia C, Tpraodp G, et al. Increased production of IL-7 uncouples bone formation from bone resorption during estrogen deficiency. *J Clin Invest* 2002; 110:1643–1650.

127. Gaur T, Lengner CJ, Hovhannisyan H, et al. Canonical Wnt signaling promotes osteogenesis by directly stimulating Runx2 gene expression. *J Biol Chem* 2005; 280:33132–33140.

128. Kahler RA, Westendorf JJ. Lymphoid enhancer factor-1 and beta-catenin inhibit Runx2-dependent transcriptional activation of the osteocalcin promoter. *J Biol Chem* 2003; 278(14):11937–11944.
129. Reinhold MI, Naski MC. Direct interactions of Runx2 and canonical Wnt signaling induce FGF18. *J Biol Chem* 2007; 282(6):3653–3663.
130. Haque T, Nakada S, Hamdy RC. A review of FGF18: Its expression, signaling pathways and possible functions during embryogenesis and post-natal development. *Histol Histopathol* 2007; 22(1):97–105.
131. Thirunavukkarasu K, Halliday DL, Miles RR, et al. The OBL-specific transcription factor Cbfa1 contributes to the expression of osteoprotegerin, a potent inhibitor of osteoclast differentiation and function. *J Biol Chem* 2000; 2675:25163–25172.
132. Ely SA, Knowles DM. Expression of CD56/neural cell adhesion molecule correlates with the presence of lytic bone lesions in multiple myeloma and distinguishes myeloma from monoclonal gammopathy of undetermined significance and lymphomas with plasmacytoid differentiation. *Am J Pathol* 2002; 160(4):1293–1299.
133. Ehrlich LA, Chung HY, Ghobrial I, et al. IL-3 is a potential inhibitor of OBL differentiation in MM. *Blood* 2005; 106:1407–1414.
134. Giuliani N, Morandi F, Tagliaferri S, et al. Interleukin-3 (IL-3) is overexpressed by T lymphocytes in MM patients. *Blood* 2006; 107:841–842.
135. Lee JW, Chung HY, Ehrilch LA, et al. IL-3 expression by MMC increases both osteoclast formation and growth of MMC. *Blood* 2004; 103:2308–2315.
136. Silvestris F, Cafforio P, Tucci M, et al. Upregulation of OBL apoptosis by malignant plasma cells: a role in MM bone disease. *Br J Haematol* 2003; 122:39–52.
137. Tinhofer I, Biedermann R, Krismer M, et al. A role of TRAIL in killing OBL by MMC. *FASEB J* 2006; 20:759–761.
138. Shipman CM, Croucher PI. Osteoprotegerin is a soluble decoy receptor for tumor necrosis factor-related apoptosis-inducing ligand/Apo2 ligand and can function as a paracrine survival factor for human myeloma cells. *Cancer Res* 2003; 63(5):912–916.

Chapter 28

Anemia and Erythropoeitic Growth Factors in Multiple Myeloma

Mark J Sloan and Noopur Raje

Introduction

Multiple myeloma (MM) is characterized by a clonal proliferation of plasma cells within the bone marrow compartment. Anemia is a common feature of MM and its presence often dictates the need for treatment. The proper management of anemia in MM can impact both the duration and the quality of life in myeloma patients. This chapter will focus on the prevalence, pathophysiology, and management of anemia associated with MM. Special attention will be paid to the use of erythropoietic growth factors in MM.

Prevalence and Severity of Anemia in Multiple Myeloma

Virtually no myeloma patient is exempt from the complication of anemia; of 1027 patients diagnosed with MM at the Mayo Clinic between 1985 and 1998, 73% were anemic at diagnosis and 97% had a hemoglobin (Hb) level of 12 g/dL or lower at some point in the course of their disease.[1] A 7% minority of patients had an Hb level of <8 g/dL at presentation. A similar prevalence was documented in the European Cancer Anaemia Survey.[2] Only 47% of the anemic patients with myeloma or lymphoma in this study received treatment for their anemia; transfusion and erythropoietin stimulating agents (ESAs) were used in approximately equal proportion.

Anemia is accepted as evidence of end organ damage and is one of the CRAB (Calcium, Renal, Anemia, Bone) criteria for myeloma diagnosis under the International Myeloma Working Group diagnostic criteria.[3] Its presence is a poor prognostic factor and is associated with shorter survival.[4] Approximately 10% of patients with MM are diagnosed in the absence of lytic bone lesions or symptoms.[5] Prevailing opinion holds that these patients with smoldering or indolent MM do not require specific antimyeloma therapy,[6] though treatment for anemia may be indicated depending on its severity and symptomatology.

Pathophysiology of Anemia in Multiple Myeloma

The basis for anemia in MM is multifactorial and complex. The panoply of reasons for anemia of chronic disease adds to features particular to MM to create a unique form of cancer-associated anemia. Marrow involvement by malignant plasma cells is an obvious but not exclusive etiology. All the hallmarks of anemia of chronic disease are present in MM patients including inappropriately low erythropoietin levels, bone marrow resistance to erythropoietin, iron dysregulation, and shortened red cell survival.

Because erythropoietin is synthesized in the juxtaglomerular cells of the kidney,[7] erythropoietin secretion is linked to renal function. Primary erythropoietin deficiency and anemia usually occur when the glomerular filtration rate drops below 60 mL/min.[8] Renal failure of this magnitude is present in over one quarter of patients with MM.[9] Myeloma patients without renal impairment or significant anemia have normal erythropoietin levels; the normal diurnal variation of erythropoietin secretion is also preserved, with peak levels in the afternoon. In contrast, patients with poor renal function have an absolute erythropoietin deficiency and lack the normal circadian rhythm of erythropoietin secretion.[10]

Blunted erythropoietin secretion in response to anemia has been proven in anemia of chronic disease[11] and cancer,[12] and explicitly (albeit inconsistently) in MM.[13,14] Inadequate erythropoietin secretion may occur even in the absence of renal impairment. Cancer patients have lost the reciprocal relationship between Hb level and erythropoietin,[12] creating even more discordant erythropoietin levels in severely anemic patients.

Erythropoietin production is regulated at the level of gene transcription; it is vulnerable to interference on a number of levels.[15] Inflammatory cytokines, notably IL-1 and TNF-α, impede the hypoxic upregulation of erythropoietin mRNA.[16] The mechanism for decreased erythropoietin production in MM may in part be related to this cytokine-driven suppression of erythropoietin transcription. The mechanism may, however, be more complicated because these cytokines are not consistently increased in this disease.[17]

Resistance to erythropoietin and impaired erythropoiesis can be found in patients even without primary bone marrow pathology. This is well illustrated by the dose escalation of erythropoietin required for treating anemia in patients with inflammation. For instance, the therapeutic erythropoietin dose in dialysis patients with high C-reactive protein levels was 80% higher than for dialysis patients without inflammation.[18] Variable resistance of bone marrow to erythropoietin has been documented in MM and is not necessarily reflective of the extent of marrow infiltration.[19] This effect is also cytokine mediated. Interferon-γ and TNF-α impair the proliferation and differentiation of erythroid progenitor cells through a variety of mechanisms, including induction of apoptosis and downregulation of the erythropoietin receptor.[20–23]

Diversion of available iron to the reticuloendothelial system at the expense of optimal erythropoiesis is an idiosyncrasy of anemia of chronic disease. The pathophysiology of iron dysregulation has been greatly illuminated by the discovery and characterization of the hepcidin molecule.[24,25] Hepcidin binds to the iron exporter ferroportin, causing its internalization and degradation.[25] This prevents the efflux of iron from macrophages, and thereby limits the iron supply available to the bone marrow for erythropoiesis. Interleukin-6 appears to be the most important stimulant of hepcidin synthesis, though others have been described.[26] The central role of these molecules is demonstrated in experiments where inflammation-induced hypoferremia is blocked in hepcidin or IL-6-deficient mice.[27,28] The effect of cytokines on hepcidin and erythropoietin synthesis is the molecular underpinning of the anemia of chronic disease, and the principal extramedullary cause of anemia in MM.[29]

Radioisotope studies were able to document shortened red cell survival in 75% of MM patients. The red cells of these patients were deemed "prematurely senescent" because they were susceptible to random destruction after only 40–60 days.[30] Evidence for shortened red cell survival due to extrinsic causes is found in transfusion studies; the red cells of normal subjects transfused into patients with anemia of inflammation had shortened survival times.[31]

Pernicious anemia is associated with MM.[32,33] A retrospective review of 664 patients at the Cleveland Clinic found that 14% of patients with plasma cell dyscrasias had vitamin B12 deficiency. The percentage was even higher in patients with immunoglobulin A (IgA) as the monoclonal protein.[34] The characteristic macrocytosis of B12 deficiency is usually missing in these patients. Low vitamin B12 levels should be identified and corrected to optimize anemia and minimize neuropathy associated with treatment.

In addition to these systemic reasons for anemia in MM, expansion of the malignant clone at the expense of erythropoietic progenitors significantly impairs erythropoiesis. Anemia does not necessarily correlate with the extent of marrow infiltration, but rather is related to the aggressiveness of the neoplasm. Hb level is inversely correlated with the percentage of marrow plasma cells and the percentage of plasma cells in S-phase.[35] In patients with an Hb level of <11 g/dL, the proportion of myeloma cells in S-phase was a more important determinant of anemia than were overall markers of disease burden. Fas ligand expression is increased on the malignant plasma cell in stage III myeloma; this is thought to induce apoptosis in erythroid precursors and exacerbate anemia.[36] Plasma cell expression of tumor necrosis factor-related apoptosis-inducing ligand (TRAIL) is also linked to ineffective erythropoiesis.[37]

Antimyeloma treatment improves anemia in the majority of cases although certain agents may exacerbate anemia as a potential toxicity. Of the commonly used regimens, those containing alkylating agents are the most myelosuppressive and may result in chemotherapy-induced anemia. Novel agents generally do not suppress erythropoiesis. Bortezemib produced anemia in 21% of patients,[38] lenalidomide in under 10%.[39]

It is again emphasized that anemia due to marrow infiltration of plasma cells should improve with antimyeloma therapy. Exogenous erythropoietin corrects only the minority of underlying reasons for anemia.

Anemia's Impact on Survival and Quality of Life in Cancer Patients

Anemia is associated with shorter survival times for many different malignancies, including MM.[4] While it is possible that the anemia itself contributes to decreased survival, it more likely serves as a surrogate marker for other adverse factors, such as tumor burden or aggressiveness. It is therefore not surprising that correction of anemia through ESAs or other means does not show a consistent survival benefit.

A substantial body of evidence exists to suggest that anemia contributes to functional impairment in cancer patients.[40] Treatment with erythropoietin improved patient-reported functional capacity and quality of life in three placebo-controlled trials[41–43] and several open-label community studies.[44–47] These improvements correlated with Hb levels and were mostly independent of tumor response. A randomized but uncontrolled study measured the quality-of-life advantage for prompt treatment of anemia (at an Hb level of <12 g/dL) versus withholding therapy until the Hb level was <9 g/dL in patients with hematologic malignancies (HM). This showed a significant but modest benefit in self-reported quality-of-life measures for the more aggressive strategy.[48] Efforts to quantify the relationship between changes in Hb level and quality of life for anemic cancer patients suggest that the maximal incremental gain in quality of life occurs when the Hb level is between 11 and 13 g/dL.[49] Others have viewed this data with skepticism, emphasizing that the small quality-of-life difference observed in these studies do not persist after multivariate analysis.[50]

Treatment of Anemia in Multiple Myeloma

Androgens were historically used to treat anemia; these were abandoned in favor of transfusion because of complications and poor response rates.[51] Transfusion works quickly and reliably, but carries with it the incumbent risks of infection and transfusion reactions. Very conservative transfusion thresholds (Hb level < 7 g/dL) have been validated in trials of critically ill adults[52] and children.[53] While similar data for cancer patients does not exist, the parsimonious use of transfusion is clearly good medicine. The decision to transfuse should be guided by symptoms rather than an arbitrary numerical trigger.

Erythropoietic growth factors are commonly used for the treatment of anemia in myeloma and other malignancies. It was hoped that they would offer the ability to reduce transfusions, improve quality of life, and possibly improve survival, without the risks and inconveniences of transfusion. Enthusiasm has been tempered by concern for increased thromboembolic events and risk of tumor progression. These concerns have caused the relative benefits of these medications to be called into question, as will be discussed below.[54]

Growth Factor Biology

Recombinant erythropoietin is available in several different forms. The two ESAs commercially available in the United States are erythropoietin alfa (sold as Epogen® or Procrit®) and darbepoetin alfa (sold as Aranesp®). A number of additional preparations are available in other countries, and several are under development. Both erythropoietin and darbepoetin are 165 amino acids long and manufactured by recombinant DNA technology from Chinese hamster ovary cells. While erythropoietin alfa reflects the sequence of endogenous erythropoietin, darbepoetin has been modified at five amino acids. These modifications result in the addition of two additional N-linked carbohydrates to the three carbohydrates already present on the native molecule. Sialic acids are attached to the carbohydrates and are necessary for in vivo activity. The additional carbohydrate prolongs the half-life of darbepoetin but reduces its affinity for the EPO receptor.[55] Darbepoetin's total biological activity is three- to fourfold greater than that of erythropoietin.

Treatment of Anemia in Multiple Myeloma with Erythropoiesis Stimulating Agents

Since 1990, over ten trials have studied the efficacy of erythropoietin and its derivatives for treatment of anemia associated with MM. Most of these are summarized in Table 1. They span a heterogeneous patient population and have different study designs and treatment strategies. The majority of trials were performed using erythropoietin alfa given daily or three times weekly. Response rates, as defined by a 2 g/dL increase in Hb level, range from 35% to 85% but are consistently in the 60–70% range. Most of these studies were well controlled; comparison with the control arms demonstrates that the responses seen are due to the study medication rather than evolution of the underlying disease. Importantly, few or none of these studies were designed or powered to detect differences in survival.

A 2006 meta-analysis for the Cochrane Reviews database concludes that ESAs raise the Hb level and reduce the need for transfusion. For studies composed of patients with HM, the weighted mean increase in Hb level was 1.73 g/dL. Fewer HM patients on ESAs needed transfusion (RR 0.72, 95% CI 0.64–0.80) and the number of red cells transfused was reduced.[56]

Potential of ESAs as Antitumor Agent in Multiple Myeloma

Conflicting and inconclusive data exist about the impact of ESAs as an anti-tumor agent in MM. These data come from animal models, case reports, and retrospective analyses.

In a murine model, Mittelman and colleagues allege that erythropoietin induces tumor regression by promoting an effective antitumor immune response.[57] In their experiments, mice bearing MOPC-315 MM tumors were treated with daily recombinant erythropoietin. This resulted in complete tumor regression in 30–60% of mice. These mice were able to reject a rechallenge with their tumor in a specific fashion. Both CD4[+] and CD8[+]T cells were involved in this response. Evidence to support the immunomodulatory proper-ties of erythropoietin in humans is less extraordinary. A nonrandomized study of patients with advanced MM treated with erythropoietin showed that several immunologic markers including CD4:CD8 ratios and IL-6 levels were signifi-cantly different from untreated patients.[58] A subgroup analysis from another study suggests that certain myeloma patients receiving erythropoietin may have improved B cell function.[59] The reproducibility and clinical relevance of these efforts is not clear.

Occasional responses to erythropoietin monotherapy are seen in MM[60] and speculation about the antimyeloma effects has arisen from clinical observations.[61] A retrospective study reports that recombinant erythropoietin is associated with increased overall survival in patients with MM; this effect was evident only after extensive adjustment for age, disease burden, and other parameters.[62]

Concern for Thromboembolic and Other Adverse Events

In the Cochrane Reviews database, hypertension was seen at a significantly higher rate in treated patients than in controls (RR 1.24, 95% CI 1.00–1.54).[63]

Table 1 Results of the use of erythropoeitic growth factors in multiple myeloma (MM).

Reference	Lead author	Trial type	Treatment population (MM/NHL)	Drug used	Starting dose	Mean starting Hb (g/dL) or Hct/3	Mean starting epo (U/L)	Response >2 g/ dL Hb increase in treatment arm (%)	Control (n/N)
NEJM 91	Ludwig	Single arm	13 MM	Epo	150 U/kg QMWF	10.03 ± 0.61	34 (range 22–82)	11/13 (85)	
Arch Intern Med 1995	Garton	Randomized, double blind, placebo-controlled	25 MM	Epo	150 U/kg	8.67		11/20 (55)	3/10 (30%)
Blood, 1995.	Cazzola	Randomized, unblinded, not placebo controlled	84 MM 62NHL	Epo	1000 U qid to 10,000 U qid	9.4	30 (range 11–70)	35/57 [a] (61) at 5000 U or 10000 U dose	2/29 (7%)
Blood 1996	Osterborg	Randomized, unblinded, not placebo controlled	65 MM 56 NHL	Epo	10,000 U QD or 2000 U – 10,000 U qid stepwise	8.0	55 (range 5–4,044)	13/22 (70)	8/49 (16%)
JCO 2001	Littlewood	Randomized, double blind, placebo controlled	37 MM 214 other (including solid tumors)	Epo	150 U/kg– 300 U/kg	9.9		85/113[a] (75)	9/54 (17%)
Eur J Haematol 1997.	Musto	Single arm	37 MM	Epo	10000 U QMWF			13/35 (35)[a]	
Br J Haematol 2003	Hedenus	Randomized, double bline, placebo controlled	89 MM 85 Lymphoma	Darbe- poetin	2.25 mcg/kg Qwk	9.59	68.99 (2– 1522)	113/171[a] (65)	31/170 (18%)
Br J Haematol 2001	Dammacco	Randomized, double blind, placebo controlled	69 MM	Epo	150 U/kg QMWF	9.3	116 (18– 5220)	38/66 (58)	6/66 (9%)
J Clin Oncol 2002	Osterborg	Randomized, double blind, placebo controlled	58 MM 112 NHL/ CLL	Epo	150 U/kg QMWF	9.2	38	44/58 (76)	46/173 (27%)
Ann Hematol 1995	Silvestris	Randomized, unblinded, NOT placebo controlled	30 MM	Epo	150 U/kg			23/30 (78)	
JCO 1998	Demetri	Single arm	515 Hematologic	Epo	10000 TIW	9.2	62	313/515 (61)	

MM multiple myeloma, *RR* relative risk, *CLL* chronic lymphocytic leukemia, *Hb* hemoglobin, *NHL* non hodgkins lymphoma.
[a]Alternative response definition of "abolition of transfusion," combined relative risk for multiple myeloma and lymphoma patients.

It is estimated that approximately one third of patients on erythropoietin have a rise in blood pressure or require an increase in antihypertensive medication.[64] While increased seizure risk has been postulated, this has not been substantiated in large trials of oncology patients. No significant difference in overall survival was observed (OR 1.12, 95% CI 0.98–1.36).

In the Cochrane database, the rate of thrombotic events was significantly higher in ESA-treated cancer patients than in controls (RR 1.67, 95% CI 1.35–2.06). This finding has been significant across several other meta-analyses,[65] and led to the revision of the package insert for erythropoietin and darbepoetin identifying the increased risk of venous thromboembolism. These studies do not separate thrombotic events by malignancy type, so it cannot yet be stated unequivocally that the risk of thrombosis in myeloma is disproportionately increased by ESAs.

A trial of thalidomide and darbepoetin in myelodysplastic syndrome was stopped early for a high number of thromboembolic events.[66] Concern was heightened even further with the report that patients receiving lenalidomide and dexamethasone have an increased risk of venous thrombosis and that erythropoetic agents may increase this risk.[67] This was not substantiated in a review of 199 patients treated with erythropoietin and thalidomide.[68] Another retrospective review of patients treated with erythropoietin and anthracycline-based chemotherapy with thalidomide did not indicate an association between erythropoietin use and thrombosis.[69]

Recent data from the non-oncology setting has further clarified the risk of maintaining higher Hb levels. In the Correction of Hemoglobin and Outcomes in Renal Insufficiency (CHOIR) trial, randomization to an Hb level target of 13.5 g/dL resulted in an increased risk of death over a lower Hb level target (11.3 g/dL).[70] This was largely the result of increased heart failure, perhaps from hypertension, and not from stroke, myocardial infarction, or thrombovascular events. A separate normalization of Hb level in patients with chronic kidney disease and anemia study showed that patients maintained at an Hb level of 13–15 g/dL had better general health and physical function than did patients maintained at 10.5–11.5 g/dL. While there was no significant difference in thrombovascular events, hypertensive episodes were more common in the higher Hb group and hemodialysis was more frequently required.

Long-term follow-up of the lymphoid cancers anemia study[43] has been submitted to the FDA but not yet fully published.[54] Half of the population in this study had myeloma. The long-term follow-up demonstrates inferior overall survival in the darbepoetin-treated patients (HR 1.37, 95% CI 1.02, 1.83) and a higher rate of thrombotic events. In this study, darbepoetin was withheld only for an Hb level of >15 g/dL (men) or 14 g/dL (women). Information on effects on tumor progression is not available.

Antibody-mediated pure red cell aplasia after exposure to erythropoietin was first reported in 1998; several hundred confirmed cases followed. The majority of these patients had received a subcutaneous formulation of epoetin alfa sold outside the United States. This particular formulation (Eprex) contained polysorbate as a stabilizer in place of human serum albumin. The number of antibody-mediated pure red cell aplasia cases reduced dramatically in 2003, when nephrologists switched patients receiving this formulation to intravenous (IV) administration.

Given the unique thrombotic susceptibility of many MM patients on treatment, there is a legitimate concern that thrombotic risk is amplified by exogenous erythropoietin. Data supports the assertion that thrombosis risk can be moderated by avoiding Hb levels in excess of 13 g/dL. The AHRQ meta-analysis, for instance, shows that thrombotic risk is significantly worse at a target Hb level of 14 g/dL but not at 13 g/dL or less.[71] The same analysis also shows that overall survival is not clearly worse until a target Hb level stop of 16 g/dL. In sum, extra care must be taken to avoid uncontrolled erythrocytosis in myeloma patients, and erythropoietin should be not be used to maintain Hb levels at a point higher than is needed in order to avoid transfusion. This should help minimize thrombotic and cardiovascular risk.

Potential for Impaired Tumor Control Due to ESAs

An even larger and more nebulous shadow looms over the ESAs. Most of the recent controversy surrounding the use of erythropoietic agents has focused on the potential for inferior tumor control. Trials designed to achieve normal Hb levels (12–14 g/dL) in cancer patients have demonstrated impaired disease control in the case of head and neck cancer[72] and inferior survival in patients with metastatic breast cancer.[73] Concerning data is also emerging for HM and MM. Transformation from MM to plasma cell leukemia has been attributed to erythropoietin.[74] Erythropoietin has been shown to stimulate growth of a human myeloma cell line in a dose-dependent manner.[75] A recent well-designed study of darbepoetin alfa for the treatment of anemia in patients with active cancer not receiving chemotherapy or radiotherapy included 71 MM patients.[76] For these patients, overall survival favored placebo, with a hazard ratio of 3.38 (1.19–9.61). Neither a rapid rate of rise in Hb level nor the achievement of Hb level > 12 g/dL was found to correlate with poor outcome. In the entire patient population the increased deaths while on study were attributed to cancer rather than thromboembolic events.

While this challenges the assumption that these drugs can be given safely if the rise in Hb level is monitored closely, it must be viewed in the context of multiple trials and meta-analyses that have demonstrated no overall survival difference in patients with myeloma or HM.[63] The Centers for Medicare and Medicaid Services (CMS) has proposed limiting coverage for patients with myeloma to those with an Hb level of <9 g/dL in addition to placing limits on the dose and duration of these agents. It bases its proposition on the reported presence of erythropoietin receptors on malignant plasma cells. These are not well substantiated. Even if the presence of erythropoietin receptors on plasma cells is verified, proving their functionality will require additional work, as will defining erythropoietin's effect on angiogenesis.[77] That the acceleration of tumor growth through direct or indirect stimulation of the malignant clone is biologically plausible is the source of considerable trepidation for clinicians and policy makers.

All of these concerns generated by ESA use prompted the Oncologic Drugs Advisory Commmittee (ODAC) of the US Food and Drug Administration (FDA) to release a brief in May 2007, suggesting that although an increased risk of venous thromboembolism was noted with the use of ESAs, the risk of tumor progression along with impact on survival remains to be determined. This briefing also cautions physicians and urges them to use the ESAs after weighing the risks and benefits.

Dosing Strategies

Several trials examined dosing strategies for both erythropoietin and darbe-poietin. Darbepoetin has a longer half-life (40 h vs 8 h for epoetin alfa) but less binding affinity for the EPO receptor as the result of additional sialic acids. While subcutaneous dosing is thought to be more effective in hemodialysis patients,[78] a randomized trial of IV versus subcutaneous darbepoetin for chemotherapy-induced anemia did not show a significant difference between the routes.[79] Fixed-dose and weight-based dosing have similar efficacy when given three times a week (150 IU/kg vs 10,000 IU for epoetin, 4.5 mcg/kg vs 325 mcg for darbepoetin).[80,81] Less frequent dosing is generally equivalent. Once weekly dosing with 40,000 U of epoetin performed similarly to historical controls receiving 10,000 U three times weekly[46,82] After three weekly doses of 40,000 U of epoetin, a dose of 120,000 U every three weeks can be safely administered with a mild diminution in level increment. Data also support using darbepoetin at 100 mcg Qweek, 200 mcg Q2weeks, or 300 mcg Q3weeks.[83]

Iron Supplementation

Effective erythropoiesis cannot take place without adequate iron stores. Ferritin should generally be kept above 100 ng/dL and transferrin saturations > 20% in patients initiating ESA therapy. In many trials, a significant proportion of patients do not achieve a meaningful rise in Hb level after ESA administration, despite having normal or elevated ferritin levels and transferrin saturations. This has been attributed to "functional iron deficiency," where the movement of usable iron from the reticuloendothelial system to the bone marrow is impaired. This effect appears to be mediated by hepcidin.[84] A similar situation occurs in the dialysis population, where IV iron is known to improve Hb response to erythropoietin. Two randomized trials demonstrate that IV iron improves the Hb response and quality of life in patients with chemotherapy-related anemia receiving erythropoietin.[85,86] Oral iron was much less effective. This has also been specifically proven in patients with HM.[87] A reasonable approach is to begin IV iron if the expected rise of 1 g/dL in Hb level is not seen in 4 weeks after standard dosing of ESAs. Intravenous iron can also be used to hasten the rise in Hb level when a rapid response is desired or when the minimum erythropoietin dose is preferred.

Prediction of Response to Erythropoietin

A large number of exploratory analyses have examined predictive factors for Hb response. These explore baseline erythropoietin levels, serum ferritin, renal function, and cell counts in an effort to determine who would benefit from erythropoietin. Unfortunately, none of these factors or algorithms has been validated with sufficiently high predictive values to be useful, and an empiric trial of erythropoietin cannot be circumvented in an individual patient.

Conclusions and Future Directions

Anemia is a central feature of MM and correlates with prognosis. The pathogenesis of anemia in MM has its origin in erythropoietin deficiency and resistance,

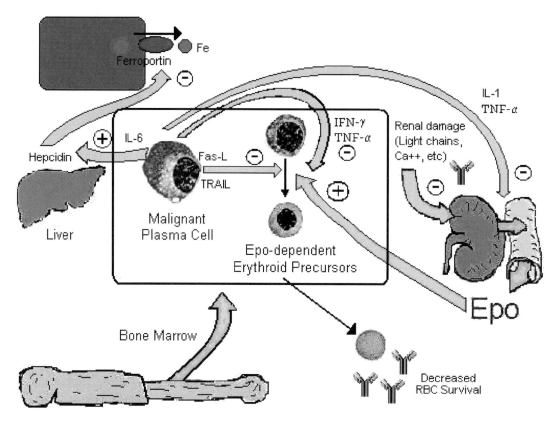

Fig. 1 Pathophysiology of anemia in multiple myeloma (*MM*): As demonstrated in the figure, the pathophysiology of anemia in MM is multifactorial resulting from marrow infiltration, ineffective erythropoiesis, and iron dysregulation (*see* Plate 10).

as well as in iron dysregulation and the interaction of the plasma cell with erythroid progenitors. Therapy of the underlying MM improves anemia in the majority of cases. Treatment with ESAs can also ameliorate anemia in the majority of patients and modestly improve quality of life. Hypertension and increased thromboembolic events accompany ESA treatment. These agents must be studied in more detail to determine their effects on tumor progression and overall survival. Until these data are available, ESAs should be used within the product label after evaluating the risks and benefits of such therapy (Fig1.).

References

1. Kyle, R.A., et al., *Review of 1027 patients with newly diagnosed multiple myeloma.* Mayo Clin Proc, 2003. **78**(1): p.21–33.
2. Birgegard, G., P. Gascon, and H. Ludwig, *Evaluation of anaemia in patients with multiple myeloma and lymphoma: findings of the European CANCER ANAEMIA SURVEY.* Eur J Haematol, 2006. **77**(5): p.378–86.
3. *Criteria for the classification of monoclonal gammopathies, multiple myeloma and related disorders: a report of the International Myeloma Working Group.* Br J Haematol, 2003. **121**(5): p.749–57.
4. Caro, J.J., et al., *Anemia as an independent prognostic factor for survival in patients with cancer: a systemic, quantitative review.* Cancer, 2001. **91**(12): p.2214–21.

5. Rosinol, L., et al., *Smoldering multiple myeloma: natural history and recognition of an evolving type*. Br J Haematol, 2003. **123**(4): p.631–6.

6. Rajkumar, S.V., *MGUS and smoldering multiple myeloma: update on pathogenesis, natural history, and management*. Hematology Am Soc Hematol Educ Program, 2005: p.340–5.

7. Hirashima, K. and F. Takaku, *Experimental studies on erythropoietin. II. The relationship between juxtaglomerular cells and erythropoietin*. Blood, 1962. **20**: p.1–8.

8. Astor, B.C., et al., *Association of kidney function with anemia: the Third National Health and Nutrition Examination Survey (1988–1994)*. Arch Intern Med, 2002. **162**(12): p.1401–8.

9. Blade, J., et al., *Renal failure in multiple myeloma: presenting features and predictors of outcome in 94 patients from a single institution*. Arch Intern Med, 1998. **158**(17): p.1889–93.

10. Pasqualetti, P., A. Collacciani, and R. Casale, *Circadian rhythm of serum erythropoietin in multiple myeloma*. Am J Hematol, 1996. **53**(1): p.40–2.

11. Baer, A.N., et al., *Blunted erythropoietin response to anaemia in rheumatoid arthritis*. Br J Haematol, 1987. **66**(4): p.559–64.

12. Miller, C.B., et al., *Decreased erythropoietin response in patients with the anemia of cancer*. N Engl J Med, 1990. **322**(24): p.1689–92.

13. Beguin, Y., et al., *Erythropoiesis in multiple myeloma: defective red cell production due to inappropriate erythropoietin production*. Br J Haematol, 1992. **82**(4): p.648–53.

14. Majumdar, G., et al., *Serum erythropoietin and circulating BFU-E in patients with multiple myeloma and anaemia but without renal failure*. Leuk Lymphoma, 1993. **9**(1–2): p.173–6.

15. Bondurant, M.C. and M.J. Koury, *Anemia induces accumulation of erythropoietin mRNA in the kidney and liver*. Mol Cell Biol, 1986. **6**(7): p.2731–3.

16. Jelkmann, W., *Proinflammatory cytokines lowering erythropoietin production*. J Interferon Cytokine Res, 1998. **18**(8): p.555–9.

17. Pisa, P., et al., *Tumor necrosis factor-alpha and interferon-gamma in serum of multiple myeloma patients*. Anticancer Res, 1990. **10**(3): p.817–20.

18. Barany, P., J.C. Divino Filho, and J. Bergstrom, *High C-reactive protein is a strong predictor of resistance to erythropoietin in hemodialysis patients*. Am J Kidney Dis, 1997. **29**(4): p.565–8.

19. Aoki, I., et al., *Responsiveness of bone marrow erythroid progenitors (CFU-E and BFU-E) to recombinant human erythropoietin (rh-Ep) in vitro in multiple myeloma*. Br J Haematol, 1992. **81**(4): p.463–9.

20. Taniguchi, S., et al., *Interferon gamma downregulates stem cell factor and erythropoietin receptors but not insulin-like growth factor-I receptors in human erythroid colony-forming cells*. Blood, 1997. **90**(6): p.2244–52.

21. Maciejewski, J.P., et al., *Nitric oxide suppression of human hematopoiesis in vitro. Contribution to inhibitory action of interferon-gamma and tumor necrosis factor-alpha*. J Clin Invest, 1995. **96**(2): p.1085–92.

22. Sato, T., et al., *Hematopoietic inhibition by interferon-gamma is partially mediated through interferon regulatory factor-1*. Blood, 1995. **86**(9): p.3373–80.

23. Selleri, C., et al., *Interferon-gamma and tumor necrosis factor-alpha suppress both early and late stages of hematopoiesis and induce programmed cell death*. J Cell Physiol, 1995. **165**(3): p.538–46.

24. Pigeon, C., et al., *A new mouse liver-specific gene, encoding a protein homologous to human antimicrobial peptide hepcidin, is overexpressed during iron overload*. J Biol Chem, 2001. **276**(11): p.7811–9.

25. Nemeth, E., et al., *Hepcidin regulates cellular iron efflux by binding to ferroportin and inducing its internalization*. Science, 2004. **306**(5704): p.2090–3.

26. Truksa, J., et al., *Bone morphogenetic proteins 2, 4, and 9 stimulate murine hepcidin 1 expression independently of Hfe, transferrin receptor 2 (Tfr2), and IL-6*. Proc Natl Acad Sci USA, 2006. **103**(27): p.10289–93.

27. Nicolas, G., et al., *The gene encoding the iron regulatory peptide hepcidin is regulated by anemia, hypoxia, and inflammation.* J Clin Invest, 2002.**110**(7): p.1037–44.

28. Nemeth, E., et al., *IL-6 mediates hypoferremia of inflammation by inducing the synthesis of the iron regulatory hormone hepcidin.* J Clin Invest, 2004. **113**(9): p.1271–6.

29. Theurl, I., et al., *Dysregulated monocyte iron homeostasis and erythropoietin formation in patients with anemia of chronic disease.* Blood, 2006. **107**(10): p.4142–8.

30. Cline, M.J. and N.I. Berlin, *Studies of the anemia of multiple myeloma.* Am J Med, 1962. **33**: p.510–25.

31. Cartwright, G.E., *The anemia of chronic disorders.* Semin Hematol, 1966. **3**(4): p.351–75.

32. Larsson, S.O., *Myeloma and pernicious anaemia.* Acta Med Scand, 1962. **172**: p.195–205.

33. Hsing, A.W., et al., *Pernicious anemia and subsequent cancer. A population-based cohort study.* Cancer, 1993. **71**(3): p.745–50.

34. Baz, R., et al., *Prevalence of vitamin B12 deficiency in patients with plasma cell dyscrasias: a retrospective review.* Cancer, 2004. **101**(4): p.790–5.

35. Fossa, A., et al., *Relation between S-phase fraction of myeloma cells and anemia in patients with multiple myeloma.* Exp Hematol, 1999. **27**(11): p.1621–6.

36. Silvestris, F., et al., *Fas-L up-regulation by highly malignant myeloma plasma cells: role in the pathogenesis of anemia and disease progression.* Blood, 2001. **97**(5): p.1155–64.

37. Silvestris, F., et al., *Negative regulation of erythroblast maturation by Fas-L(+)/ TRAIL(+) highly malignant plasma cells: a major pathogenetic mechanism of anemia in multiple myeloma.* Blood, 2002. **99**(4): p.1305–13.

38. Richardson, P.G., et al., *A phase 2 study of bortezomib in relapsed, refractory myeloma.* N Engl J Med, 2003. **348**(26): p.2609–17.

39. Rajkumar, S.V., et al., *Combination therapy with lenalidomide plus dexamethasone (Rev/Dex) for newly diagnosed myeloma.* Blood, 2005. **106**(13): p.4050–3.

40. Cella, D., *The Functional Assessment of Cancer Therapy-Anemia (FACT-An) Scale: a new tool for the assessment of outcomes in cancer anemia and fatigue.* Semin Hematol, 1997. **34**(3 Suppl 2): p.13–9.

41. Littlewood, T.J., et al., *Effects of epoetin alfa on hematologic parameters and quality of life in cancer patients receiving nonplatinum chemotherapy: results of a randomized, double-blind, placebo-controlled trial.* J Clin Oncol, 2001. **19**(11): p.2865–74.

42. Osterborg, A., et al., *Randomized, double-blind, placebo-controlled trial of recombinant human erythropoietin, epoetin Beta, in hematologic malignancies.* J Clin Oncol, 2002. **20**(10): p.2486–94.

43. Hedenus, M., et al., *Efficacy and safety of darbepoetin alfa in anaemic patients with lymphoproliferative malignancies: a randomized, double-blind, placebo-controlled study.* Br J Haematol, 2003. **122**(3): p.394–403.

44. Glaspy, J., et al., *Impact of therapy with epoetin alfa on clinical outcomes in patients with nonmyeloid malignancies during cancer chemotherapy in community oncology practice. Procrit Study Group.* J Clin Oncol, 1997. 15(3): p.1218–34.

45. Demetri, G.D., et al., *Quality-of-life benefit in chemotherapy patients treated with epoetin alfa is independent of disease response or tumor type: results from a prospective community oncology study. Procrit Study Group.* J Clin Oncol, 1998. **16**(10): p.3412–25.

46. Gabrilove, J.L., et al., *Clinical evaluation of once-weekly dosing of epoetin alfa in chemotherapy patients: improvements in hemoglobin and quality of life are similar to three-times-weekly dosing.* J Clin Oncol, 2001. 19(11): p.2875–82.

47. Boccia, R., et al., *The effectiveness of darbepoetin alfa administered every 3 weeks on hematologic outcomes and quality of life in older patients with chemotherapy-induced anemia.* Oncologist, 2007. **12**(5): p.584–93.

48. Straus, D.J., et al., *Quality-of-life and health benefits of early treatment of mild anemia: a randomized trial of epoetin alfa in patients receiving chemotherapy for hematologic malignancies.* Cancer, 2006. **107**(8): p.1909–17.

49. Crawford, J., et al., *Relationship between changes in hemoglobin level and quality of life during chemotherapy in anemic cancer patients receiving epoetin alfa therapy.* Cancer, 2002. **95**(4): p.888–95.

50. Wisloff, F., et al., *Quality of life may be affected more by disease parameters and response to therapy than by haemoglobin changes.* Eur J Haematol, 2005. **75**(4): p.293–8.

51. Bergsagel, D.E., et al., *Treatment of anemia associated with multiple myeloma.* N Engl J Med, 1991. **324**(1): p.59–60.

52. Hebert, P.C., et al., *A multicenter, randomized, controlled clinical trial of transfusion requirements in critical care. Transfusion Requirements in Critical Care Investigators, Canadian Critical Care Trials Group.* N Engl J Med, 1999. **340**(6): p.409–17.

53. Lacroix, J., et al., *Transfusion strategies for patients in pediatric intensive care units.* N Engl J Med, 2007. **356**(16): p.1609–19.

54. Khuri, F., *Weighing the hazards of erythropoiesis stimulation in patients with cancer.* N Engl J Med, 2007. **356**(24): p.2445–8.

55. Elliott, S., et al., *Control of rHuEPO biological activity: the role of carbohydrate.* Exp Hematol, 2004. **32**(12): p.1146–55.

56. Bohlius, J., et al., *Erythropoietin or darbepoetin for patients with cancer.* Cochrane Database Syst Rev, 2006. **3**: p.CD003407.

57. Mittelman, M., et al., *Erythropoietin induces tumor regression and antitumor immune responses in murine myeloma models.* Proc Natl Acad Sci USA, 2001. **98**(9): p.5181–6.

58. Prutchi-Sagiv, S., et al., *Erythropoietin treatment in advanced multiple myeloma is associated with improved immunological functions: could it be beneficial in early disease?* Br J Haematol, 2006. **135**(5): p.660–72.

59. Silvestris, F., et al., *Long-term therapy with recombinant human erythropoietin (rHu-EPO) in progressing multiple myeloma.* Ann Hematol, 1995. **70**(6): p.313–8.

60. Barrios, M. and C. Alliot, *IgA multiple myeloma responding to erythropoietin monotherapy.* Am J Hematol, 2005. **80**(2): p.165–6.

61. Mittelman, M., et al., *Erythropoietin has an anti-myeloma effect – a hypothesis based on a clinical observation supported by animal studies.* Eur J Haematol, 2004. **72**(3): p.155–65.

62. Baz, R., et al., *Recombinant human erythropoietin is associated with increased overall survival in patients with multiple myeloma.* Acta Haematol, 2007. **117**(3): p.162–7.

63. Bohlius, J., et al., *Recombinant human erythropoietins and cancer patients: updated meta-analysis of 57 studies including 9353 patients.* J Natl Cancer Inst, 2006. **98**(10): p.708–14.

64. Lee, M.S., J.S. Lee, and J.Y. Lee, *Prevention of erythropoietin-associated hypertension.* Hypertension, 2007.

65. Gleason, K., et al., *Recombinant erythropoietin (Epo)darbepoetin (Darb) associated venous thromboembolism (VTE) in the oncology setting: findings from the Research on Adverse Drug Events and Reports (RADAR) project.* Journal of Clinical Oncology, 2007 ASCO Annual Meeting Proceedings Part I., 2007. **25**(18S): p.2552.

66. Steurer, M., et al., *Thromboembolic events in patients with myelodysplastic syndrome receiving thalidomide in combination with darbepoietin-alpha.* Br J Haematol, 2003. **121**(1): p.101–3.

67. Knight, R., R.J. DeLap, and J.B. Zeldis, *Lenalidomide and venous thrombosis in multiple myeloma.* N Engl J Med, 2006. **354**(19): p.2079–80.

68. Galli, M., et al., *Recombinant human erythropoietin and the risk of thrombosis in patients receiving thalidomide for multiple myeloma.* Haematologica, 2004. **89**(9): p.1141–2.

69. Baz, R., et al., *An analysis of erythropoietin (Epo) and venous thromboembolic events (VTE) in multiple myeloma (MM) patients (pts) treated with anthracycline-based chemotherapy and the immunomodulator agent thalidomide.* Journal of Clinical Oncology, 2007 ASCO Annual Meeting Proceedings Part I., 2007. **25**(18S): p.8107.

70. Singh, A.K., et al., *Correction of anemia with epoetin alfa in chronic kidney disease.* N Engl J Med, 2006. **355**(20): p.2085–98.

71. Seidenfeld, J., et al., *Comparative effectiveness of epoetin and darbepoetin for managing anemia in patients undergoing cancer treatment. Comparative effectiveness review no. 3. (Prepared by Blue Cross and Blue Shield Association Technology Evaluation Center Evidence-based Practive Center under Contract No. 290-02-0026).* Agency for Healthcare Research and Quality, 2006 (available at: www.effectivehealthcare.ahrq.gov/reports/final.cfm).

72. Henke, M., et al., *Erythropoietin to treat head and neck cancer patients with anaemia undergoing radiotherapy: randomised, double-blind, placebo-controlled trial.* Lancet, 2003. **362**(9392): p.1255–60.

73. Leyland-Jones, B., et al., *Maintaining normal hemoglobin levels with epoetin alfa in mainly nonanemic patients with metastatic breast cancer receiving first-line chemotherapy: a survival study.* J Clin Oncol, 2005. **23**(25): p.5960–72.

74. Olujohungbe, A.,S. Handa, and J. Holmes, *Does erythropoietin accelerate malignant transformation in multiple myeloma?* Postgrad Med J, 1997. **73**(857): p.163–4.

75. Okuno, Y., et al., *Establishment and characterization of four myeloma cell lines which are responsive to interleukin-6 for their growth.* Leukemia, 1991. **5**(7): p.585–91.

76. Glaspy, J., *Results from a Phase III, randomized, double-blind, placebo-controlled study of darbepoetin alfa (DA) for th treatment of anemia in patients not receiving chemotherapy or radiotherapy.* Presented April 16, 2007 at the American Association for Cancer Research Meeting, 2007.

77. Longmore, G.D., *Do cancer cells express functional erythropoietin receptors?* N Engl J Med, 2007. **356**(24): p.2447.

78. Kaufman, J.S., et al., *Subcutaneous compared with intravenous epoetin in patients receiving hemodialysis. Department of Veterans Affairs Cooperative Study Group on Erythropoietin in Hemodialysis Patients.* N Engl J Med, 1998. **339**(9): p.578–83.

79. Justice, G., et al., *A randomized, multicenter study of subcutaneous and intravenous darbepoetin alfa for the treatment of chemotherapy-induced anemia.* Ann Oncol, 2005. **16**(7): p.1192–8.

80. Granetto, C., et al., *Comparing the efficacy and safety of fixed versus weight-based dosing of epoetin alpha in anemic cancer patients receiving platinum-based chemotherapy.* Oncol Rep, 2003. **10**(5): p.1289–96.

81. Hesketh, P.J., et al., *A randomized controlled trial of darbepoetin alfa administered as a fixed or weight-based dose using a front-loading schedule in patients with anemia who have nonmyeloid malignancies.* Cancer, 2004. **100**(4): p.859–68.

82. Cheung, W., N. Minton, and K. Gunawardena, *Pharmacokinetics and pharmacodynamics of epoetin alfa once weekly and three times weekly.* Eur J Clin Pharmacol, 2001. **57**(5): p.411–8.

83. Canon, J.L., et al., *Randomized, double-blind, active-controlled trial of every-3-week darbepoetin alfa for the treatment of chemotherapy-induced anemia.* J Natl Cancer Inst, 2006. **98**(4): p.273–84.

84. Rivera, S., et al., *Hepcidin excess induces the sequestration of iron and exacerbates tumor-associated anemia.* Blood, 2005. **105**(4): p.1797–802.

85. Auerbach, M., et al., *Intravenous iron optimizes the response to recombinant human erythropoietin in cancer patients with chemotherapy-related anemia: a multicenter, open-label, randomized trial.* J Clin Oncol, 2004. **22**(7): p.1301–7.

86. Henry, D.H., et al., *Intravenous ferric gluconate significantly improves response to epoetin alfa versus oral iron or no iron in anemic patients with cancer receiving chemotherapy.* Oncologist, 2007. **12**(2): p.231–42.

87. Hedenus, M., et al., *Addition of intravenous iron to epoetin beta increases hemoglobin response and decreases epoetin dose requirement in anemic patients with lymphoproliferative malignancies: a randomized multicenter study.* Leukemia, 2007. **21**(4): p.627–32.

Chapter 29

Percutaneous Vertebroplasty and Balloon Kyphoplasty for the Treatment of Acute Painful Pathologic and Nonpathologic Fractures

Sandra Narayanan and Frank C. Tong

Introduction

Percutaneous vertebroplasty, a procedure first performed in France in 1984[1] and in the United States in 1994,[2] is generally used for three primary indications: osteoporotic vertebral compression fractures, malignant vertebral tumors, and painful and/or aggressive vertebral hemangiomas.[3] The goal in all three scenarios is pain relief with the potential for early mobility while providing structural support of the destructive spine lesion.

Persons with destructive malignant lesions of the spine such as multiple myeloma are ideal candidates for vertebroplasty, as progressive and disproportionate bone resorption is responsible for the principal morbidity of this devastating illness. Fifty-five to seventy percent of fractures in multiple myeloma occur in the spine, most commonly in the lower thoracic or lumbar vertebrae.[4] A threefold increased fracture risk (mostly pathologic fractures) is noted in patients with monoclonal gammopathy of undetermined significance (MGUS)[5]; this risk sharply increases at the time of myeloma diagnosis.[6] Fractures in these patients may result from direct myelomatous involvement of the vertebra or may be due to the generalized osteopenia characteristic of this disease.[7] Myeloma-associated lytic lesions are different from osteolysis from other malignant or metastatic processes in that the former do not heal, even after years of disease remission,[8] likely from a total loss of local osteoblastic activity. Although chemotherapy and bisphosphonates form the basis of myeloma therapy, minimally invasive procedures such as percutaneous vertebroplasty or balloon kyphoplasty can produce long-term structural and functional support.

Percutaneous balloon kyphoplasty was initially developed in the late 1990s as a modification of the vertebroplasty procedure. Although much more costly (up to 10-fold more expensive[9]) than vertebroplasty, it is an alternative method of improving vertebral body height, kyphosis, and vertebral alignment with the goal of reducing the risk of cement extravasation frequently noted with vertebroplasty.[10–12] A series of 18 myeloma patients undergoing 55 kyphoplasty procedures and a series of 52 myeloma patients undergoing kyphoplasty have confirmed the safety and efficacy of this procedure in this specialized population.[13,14]

From: *Contemporary Hematology Myeloma Therapy*
Edited by: S. Lonial © Humana Press, Totowa, NJ

Indications

Indications for percutaneous vertebroplasty include patients with acute to subacute (usually <3 months old) painful vertebral compression fractures from osteo-porosis, osteolysis or invasion of benign (e.g., aggressive/painful hemangioma) or malignant tumors, and osteonecrosis (also known as Kummel's disease). Another process benefiting from vertebroplasty is the intravertebral vacuum cleft, which is felt to represent fracture nonunion and pseudoarthrosis and is exquisitely painful. Compression fractures associated with these clefts often demonstrate dynamic movement of osseous fragments with postural changes. The resultant severe back pain is particularly exacerbated by prolonged sitting or standing.[15-17]

Vertebroplasty and kyphoplasty are second-line approaches considered when the patient has failed standard medical therapy; this is defined by inadequate pain relief with prescribed analgesics and other conservative medical treatment (e.g., bed rest and back braces) after at least 4 weeks or adequate pain relief but with unacceptable adverse effects such as excessive sedation, confusion, or constipation.[18] However, some operators will intervene more acutely. The efficacy of prophylactic vertebroplasty in an osteoporotic patient is not known; this is currently not an acceptable indication, except in asymptomatic patients with osteolytic vertebral body lesions who are considered at high risk of vertebral collapse, spinal dislocation (e.g., when there is metastatic involvement of the facet joints), or impending thoracic insufficiency from severe kyphosis.[19]

Absolute contraindications to any vertebral augmentation procedure include asymptomatic vertebral compression fractures (with the above notable exceptions), ongoing local or systemic infection, uncorrectable coagulopathy, hypersensitivity to bone cement (although most patients with this condition are unaware of it due to lack of prior exposure to bone cement), or improving pain on medical therapy. Fractures of the posterior elements (without vertebral body fracture) are another absolute contraindication, as vertebroplasty does not target the former and would not be expected to improve the associated symptoms.

Relative contraindications include retropulsed osseous fragment or intracanalicular tumor extension with greater than one-third spinal canal compromise, as well as radicular symptoms in excess of vertebral pain that may suggest tumor extension or a compressive lesion (e.g., spinal stenosis) unrelated to the vertebral fracture. Burst fractures are another relative contraindication to vertebroplasty, as they have a high incidence of cement leakage and an increased risk of further canal compromise due to mass effect on fracture fragments by cement deposition. Malignant osteolytic lesions with posterior cortical destruction or with an epidural component are another relative contraindication,[20] as patients with an incompetent posterior vertebral body wall are at a higher risk for complications of cement extravasation.[21] Loss of greater than two-thirds of the vertebral body height increases the technical difficulty of vertebroplasty but is not a true contraindication. In patients with severe vertebral body height loss, however, vertebroplasty is more often technically feasible than kyphoplasty.

A hypersensitivity to iodinated contrast is not an absolute contraindication to a vertebral augmentation procedure, as the latter can be performed without venography. When a history of mild hypersensitivity (e.g., cutaneous reactions) to iodinated contrast is elicited, the patient can be given appropriate premedication. The protocol at the authors' institution is methylprednisolone 32 mg PO (intravenous) × 2 doses (given 12 and 2 h preprocedure), and Benadryl 25–50 mg IV × 2 doses (given 30 min prior to and 2 h after the procedure). In patients with severe allergic reactions such as anaphylaxis, the above regimen does not reliably prevent an adverse reaction, and beginning the procedure with the patient under general anesthesia is strongly recommended.

Indications for treatment of vertebral fractures associated with metastatic lesions to the spine are much the same as those for osteoporotic fractures but with the additional consideration that the former may be a palliative procedure that improves the quality of life. In cases where cord compression is present, a combination of fluoroscopy-guided vertebroplasty or kyphoplasty and laminectomy with decompression can be performed (Figs. 1–3).

A noncontrast computed tomography (CT) demonstrating a new or progressive vertebral compression fracture is ideal to visualize areas of cortical disruption, thereby predicting areas at risk for cement leakage. It may also demonstrate other potential etiologies of back pain, such as a neoplastic lesion, in patients with nonspecific histories. If there is doubt as to the acuity of the

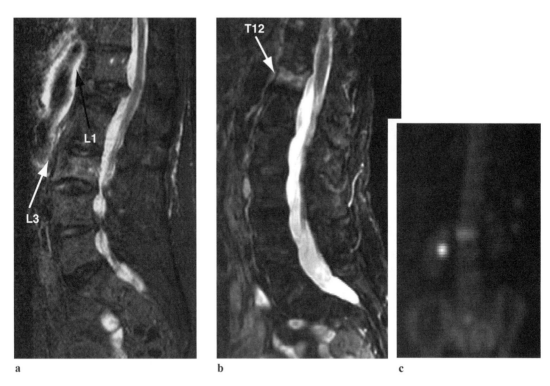

a   b   c

Fig. 1 Imaging findings of fracture acuity. MRI of the lumbar spine in two different patients with increased (abnormal) signal on the STIR sequence at L3 (white arrow, **a**) and at T12 (arrowhead, **b**). The L1 vertebral compression fracture (black arrow, **a**) is not a candidate for vertebroplasty, due to lack of abnormal STIR signal indicating fracture chronicity, severe loss of vertebral body height (nearly vertebra plana), and posterior retropulsion into the spinal canal. (**c**) Increased radionuclide uptake at L2 on a bone scan in a third patient with a vertebral compression fracture.

Indications	Absolute contraindications	Relative contraindications
•Painful vertebral body compression fracture refractory to medications	•Fracture of posterior elements without vertebral body fracture	•Posterior retropulsion with >1/3 spinal canal compromise or associated myelopathy
•Acute/subacute onset (as confirmed by history, abnormal STIR signal on MRI, and/or increased radionuclide uptake on bone scan/SPECT at level of fracture	•Asymptomatic or minimally symptomatic	•Burst fractures or lesion with incompetent posterior vertebral body wall
	•Local or systemic infection	•>2/3 loss of vertebral body height
•Reproducible midline pain over fracture	•Uncorrectable coagulopathy	•No abnormal STIR signal on MRI
	•Hypersensitivity to bone cement	•Normal bone scan
		•Radicular or musculoskeletal pain or pain off midline

Fig. 2 Indications and contraindications to vertebroplasty/kyphoplasty.

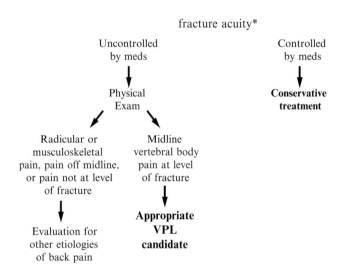

Fig. 3 Treatment algorithm for patients with back pain and imaging evidence of fracture acuity.

fracture, noncontrast magnetic resonance imaging (MRI) with short *tau* inversion recovery (STIR) sequence is useful to assess for bone marrow edema. Technetium-99 methylene diphosphonate (MDP) bone scan with SPECT (single photon emission CT) is another adjunctive test that may reveal occult vertebral fractures or metastatic lesions by demonstrating increased uptake from osteoblastic activity. This test may be falsely negative in the first several days (and up to 2 weeks) after the fracture, particularly in elderly patients, who have a slower healing response.

Patients can be referred for vertebral augmentation procedures either as outpatients or as inpatients. At our institution, many of the vertebroplasty consults are for patients hospitalized for fracture-related pain refractory to medications. A detailed assessment and the vertebroplasty, if indicated, is performed during the hospitalization, ideally as soon as possible. A careful history should be taken regarding the location, quality, intensity, and duration of the pain and triggering/relieving factors. The pain should be in the midline and focal over the fractured vertebral body and exacerbated by overlying pressure. Pain that is paraspinal in location suggests a musculoskeletal etiology, and pain that is radiating laterally or inferiorly (down the buttock/lower extremity) is likely radicular. Both of these types of pain are essentially contraindications to vertebroplasty, which would not be expected to alleviate the symptoms. The presence of a sensory level, paraparesis, and/or bowel/bladder incontinence suggests spinal cord compression, and vertebroplasty is strongly discouraged in this situation. On physical examination, firm pressure or tapping over the fractured level should reliably elicit pain; if there is no tenderness to palpation, the need for vertebroplasty should be reassessed. Baseline labs should include a coagulation profile and complete blood cell count. The goal INR should be ≤1.4, and the platelet count should be ≥50,000.

Materials

The cement most commonly used in both vertebroplasty and balloon kyphoplasty is polymethyl methacrylate (PMMA),[22] a rapidly setting bone cement, although the Food and Drug Administration (FDA) did not approve PMMA for this use until April 2004. Advantages of using PMMA include its bioinert character, ease of handling, good biomechanical strength, lack of thrombogenicity,[23] and cost-effectiveness. Disadvantages include excessive stiffness, short polymerization time (4–10 min) with nonlinear increases in viscosity,[24] lack of osteoconductive potential (i.e., potential to promote bone apposition along its surface), high polymerization temperature (up to 113°C),[25] and potential monomer toxicity.

The cement used for vertebroplasty at the authors' institution consists of a liquid PMMA monomer and a powdered PMMA polymer marketed under the trade name Cranioplastic™ (Codman, Boston, Massachusetts). Although increased quantity of liquid monomer can enhance cement penetration through cancellous bone, in vitro studies have demonstrated up to 24% weakening of cured cement when monomer is used in higher or lower ratios than recommended by the manufacturer, which is 0.57 mL/kg.[26] Both liquid and solid components are mixed with sterile barium sulfate powder, which comprises ~30% of the cement volume; this is to ensure that the cement is sufficiently radiopaque and does not cure prematurely or compromise the overall structural integrity of the cement.[27] While the combination of barium sulfate and tungsten results in increased visibility as opposed to either alone, the latter is not yet approved by the FDA in the United States for this indication. Both tungsten and barium sulfate have a tendency to clump and must be powdered and mixed thoroughly with the powdered PMMA.

In immunocompromised patients, powdered tobramycin can be mixed with the powdered PMMA prior to addition of the liquid polymer. This leaches out of the cured cement and provides local antibiotic coverage. In one series where patients underwent cranioplasty, vertebral body replacement, or spinal fusion with PMMA, there was a reduction in infection rate from 5% to 1% when

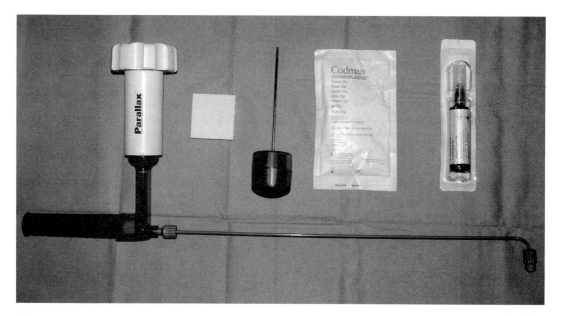

Fig. 4 Vertebroplasty materials. From left to right: cement injector, cement, access needle, powdered polymer, and liquid monomer (Cranioplastic™, Codman, Boston, Massachusetts) (*see* Plate 11).

tobramycin-impregnated PMMA was used.[28] Although addition of antibiotics to PMMA can adversely affect the mechanical properties of the cured cement, this effect is observed only with antibiotic quantities of >2 g per standard packet of polymer powder.[29,30] Recent changes in tobramycin formulation have been anecdotally noted to decrease cement stability, and tobramycin is no longer mixed with vertebroplasty cement at our institution. Intravenous antibiotics, usually cefazolin 1 g (or vancomycin 1 g/clindamycin 600 mg if allergic to penicillin), are routinely administered at the start of the procedure. The ideal consistency of cement is like that of pancake batter; a more liquid consistency increases the risk of cement leakage into epidural veins, and a more viscous consistency may cause premature cement hardening in the needle or vertebral body, causing inadequate cement penetration (Fig. 4).

Technique

Vertebroplasty

After obtaining informed written consent, the patient is placed prone on the angiography table and prepped and draped in a sterile fashion. A pillow is sometimes placed underneath the abdomen for patient comfort. Neuroleptic anesthesia, usually with midazolam and fentanyl, is administered intravenously, and the blood pressure, heart rate, and pulse oximetry are monitored throughout the procedure. The target vertebral body is localized under fluoroscopic guidance and sterilely marked over one of the pedicles. In the past, this procedure has been done under CT as well or, rarely, under a combination of fluoroscopy and CT, but fluoroscopy alone is the preferred modality.

High-quality fluoroscopy is of key importance to visualize the stylet tip in two planes, as well as to more quickly discern potential nontarget migration of cement material. The anteroposterior (AP) tube is angled to maximize the oval appearance of the pedicle and ensure precise needle placement.[2] Standard bipediculate technique may be helpful in filling the contralateral hemivertebra but prolongs the procedure and may potentially carry a higher risk of venous or epidural PMMA embolization, as the existing cement from the first injection obscures further injection on the lateral view. An angled AP oblique view can be used in this situation.

The most common technique for vertebroplasty is the transpedicular approach, which can be uni- or bipediculate, with the goal of cement deposition in both sides of the vertebral body. A modified unipediculate approach using a more oblique angle of entry (lateral to the superior articulating facet) to center the needle tip in the contralateral ventral vertebral body has been reported to produce filling across midline in 96% of cases. Initial cement filling is contralateral to the needle entry site, and as the needle is retracted 2–3 mm with each injection, filling is noted in the ipsilateral vertebral body.[31] When a transpedicular approach is impossible due to posterior fusion hardware or pedicular lysis from a metastatic lesion, a parapedicular approach is used.[30] In patients with osteolytic tumors posterior to the vertebral body, transpedicular access is favored over parapedicular access.[21]

Local anesthesia with 0.25% bupivacaine is administered superficially in the skin over the center of the pedicle oval and deeply (at the periosteum). After a small skin incision is made with a scalpel blade, a 10–15 cm-length beveled 11-gauge access needle is centered over the pedicle oval and advanced inferolateral to the superior articulating facet with the stylet in place until the tip abuts the bone. Beveled needles are preferred at our institution because of the ease with which rotating the bevel can change the course of the needle. Lateral fluoroscopy is useful to ensure that the needle is centered in craniocaudad dimension within the pedicle. Slow rotatory hand pressure or a small orthopedic mallet can be used at this point to gently push or "tap" the needle into the final position, which is ideally in the anterior one-third to one-fourth of the vertebral body. The trocar tip should be just superior to or just inferior to the equatorial plane (where the basivertebral plexus is located) to minimize the risk of venous cement leakage. The needle should be nearly parallel to the superior and inferior endplates of the vertebral body. Alternatively, a descending course through the pedicle can be used.

Venography is recommended for less experienced operators and can be performed prior to PMMA injection to exclude needle placement within a major venous outlet such as the basivertebral venous plexus, to delineate the venous drainage pattern, and to ensure integrity of the posterior vertebral wall. If early venous filling is significant, the needle can be repositioned or the cement made more viscous to reduce the risk of cement leakage. If a bone biopsy is indicated, especially for those patients with malignant vertebral tumors, a 14-gauge biopsy needle can be passed coaxially through the access needle to obtain a tissue sample prior to the vertebroplasty.

Injection of cement is best demonstrated in the lateral view, as tiny "pebbles" of barium sulfate are seen traveling in the trocar prior to entering the vertebral body. The injection is performed slowly with 1–3 mL Luer-Lock syringes (Medallion; Merit Medical System, South Jordan, Utah) with continuous lateral (and occasionally also with AP) fluoroscopic guidance. Careful attention toward averting a breach of the anterior or posterior surfaces of the vertebral body by radiopaque material and prevention of PMMA embolization in the ventral or dorsal epidural veins is important. If this occurs, the injection is temporarily halted to let the partially embolized cement harden and therefore prevent further passage of cement along the same route. If a second injection of cement continues to embolize in a similar manner, the needle tip can be advanced or withdrawn. Epidural cement extravasation is best detected on the lateral view, whereas paravertebral cement leakage is best seen on the AP view.

As the vertebral body fills, injection pressure will necessarily increase. The procedure is finished when hemi- or holovertebral filling is achieved, no further material can be injected, PMMA approaches the posterior one-fifth of the vertebral body (indicating impending cement leakage), cement extravasation into the disc, spinal canal, or neural foramen occurs, or there is persistent venous embolization of cement despite needle repositioning. The amount of cement injected is variable, and up to 10–12 mL of cement can be deposited in a vertebral body. Multiple levels can be treated at the same time, as tolerated by the patient, although we recommend treating no more than three levels per session to minimize patient discomfort. Removal of the trocar is done without the stylet to prevent injection of dead-space cement in an already PMMA-saturated vertebral body.

Postprocedural protocol includes placing the patient in a supine position for 1 h during cement curing. The patient may then sit up but is monitored for an additional 1 h prior to discharge. Inpatients are generally monitored for 24 h but can be discharged afterwards if stable and if their pain is adequately controlled (Fig. 5).

Kyphoplasty

The technique for kyphoplasty is similar to that of percutaneous vertebroplasty, with a few notable exceptions. It is generally performed under general anesthesia, as balloon inflation is quite painful. A bipediculate approach is often used in order to elevate both superior endplates *en masse*.[11] In the thoracic spine, an extrapedicular approach is sometimes used; the needle is placed between the rib head and lateral aspect of the pedicle. A guide pin is first placed into the pedicle and vertebral body, and a stylet and working cannula are then placed over the guide pin into the posterior one-third of the vertebral body. A hand-driven drill enlarges the channel and is passed to within 3–4 mm posterior to the ventral cortical margin of the vertebral body. Following this, an inflatable bone tamp attached to a manometer is inserted into the vertebral body. A balloon filled with ~60% iodinated contrast is inflated within the collapsed vertebra, compacting surrounding bone, elevating the fractured vertebral body, and creating a sterile cavity for the injection of viscous, partially cured PMMA cement. The initial starting pressure is ~50 pounds per square inch (psi), and the maximal achievable pressure is 220 psi. After the balloon is removed, a bone filler device is inserted and the cement is injected into the cavity. Chilled PMMA is often preferred to cement that has been kept at room temperature, as the former cures at a

slower rate, allowing more working time.[12] The ideal vertebroplasty cement
has a longer liquid phase with a short set time, whereas the ideal kyphoplasty
filler material has a shorter liquid phase and a longer partially cured cement
time (Figs. 6 and 7).[32]

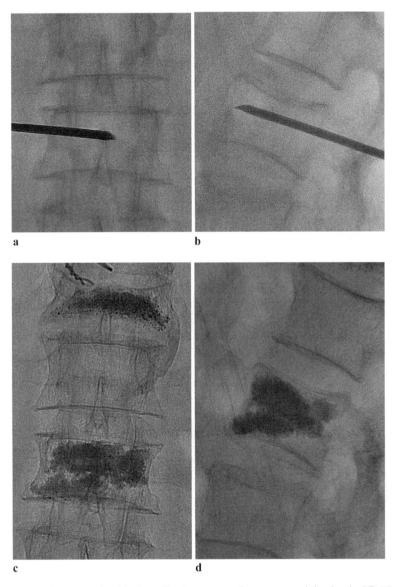

Fig. 5 AP fluoroscopy demonstrating ideal needle placement prior to cement injection in AP (**a**) and lateral (**b**)
views. The needle tip is just past the midline in the AP view. Final cement filling in AP (**c**) and lateral (**d**) views.
Cement fills the ventral vertebral body adjacent to both superior and inferior endplates, as well as the dorsal
superior vertebral body. (**d**)

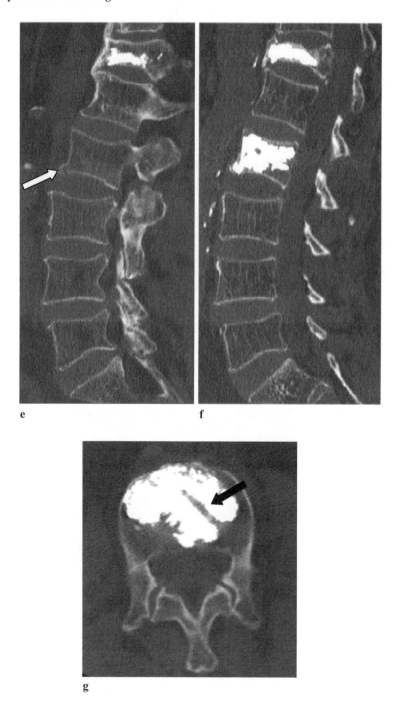

Fig. 5 (continued) This patient has had a prior T12 vertebroplasty. Preprocedure CT reveals a ventral inferior endplate fracture of L2 (white arrow, **e**). Postprocedure CT shows cement filling the region of fracture without evidence of cement extravasation outside the vertebral body (**f,g**). A needle tract can be seen in the left side of the vertebral body (black arrow, **g**).

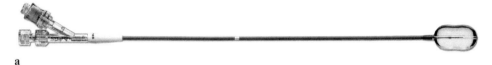

a

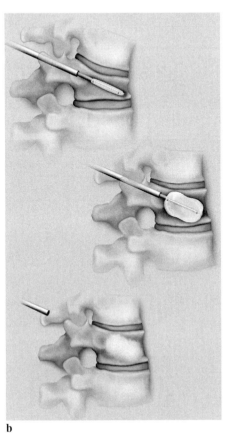

b

Fig. 6 Kyphoplasty materials and technique. (**a**) Inflatable balloon tamp. (**b**) Transpedicular insertion, inflation, and removal of balloon tamp. (Images courtesy of Kyphon Inc.) (*see* Plate 12).

Results

An effective and safe vertebroplasty (both structurally and functionally) depends on multiple factors: operator experience, adequate and timely preparation of PMMA, approach (bipediculate vs modified unipediculate), hemi- versus holovertebral filling, and presence of PMMA leakage in nontarget locations, possibly resulting in pain, further fractures, neurological sequelae, and hypoxia or hemodynamic instability. Although it is unclear why vertebroplasty produces pain relief in patients with vertebral fractures, theories include mechanical stabilization of microfractures, chemical toxicity, and thermal injury to nerve endings by an exothermic reaction of the deposited PMMA.[31],[32] Additionally, there may be an antitumoral effect of methylmethacrylate, which has a known cytotoxic effect when incompletely polymerized[33] and may be responsible

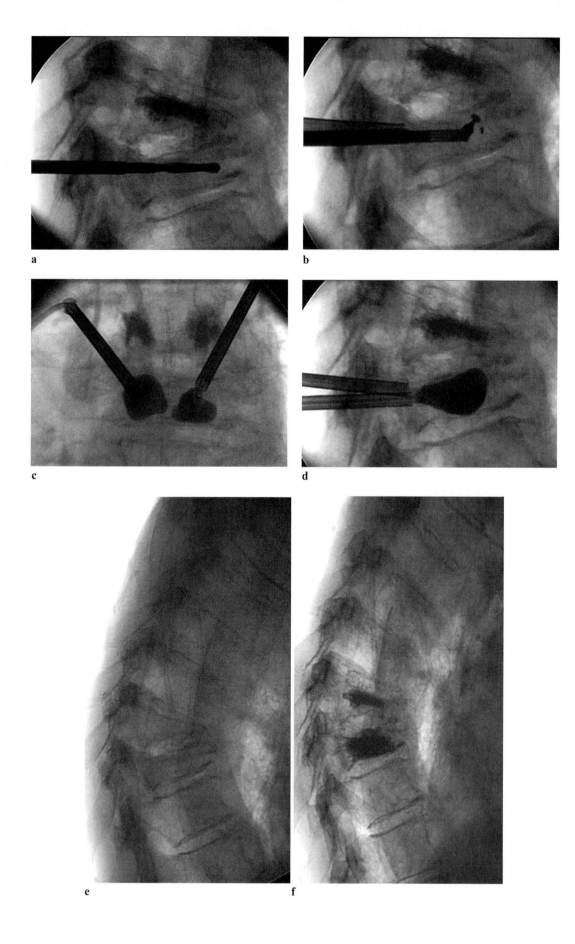

a

b

c

d

e

f

for the low rate of local metastatic recurrence observed after vertebroplasty. No direct relationship has been established between percentage of lesion filling and pain relief in patients with either osteoporotic or malignant osteolytic vertebral compression fractures,[21,34] although we have observed improved pain relief with retreatment and addition of cement to previously vertebroplastied levels. While it has been suggested that 2 mL of bone cement is sufficient to normalize the ultimate strength of osteoporotic vertebrae in cadavers,[35] the practice at our institution is to instill as much cement as the fractured vertebral body will safely tolerate.

Pain relief following vertebroplasty is frequently immediate, with the majority of patients experiencing marked pain relief in the first 3–5 days following the procedure. A small percentage of patients may actually have increased pain following vertebroplasty, likely due to local irritation from needle placement. In a recent prospective study of percutaneous vertebroplasty in patients with osteoporotic vertebral compression fractures, visual analog scale (VAS) scores for pain at the treated level dropped from 8.8 (preprocedure) to 2.5–3.3.[36] Eighty-six percent and greater than ninety-five percent of the patients were satisfied with the outcome on short- and long-term follow-up visits, respectively. Significant or complete pain relief is achieved in over 90% of patients with vertebral hemangiomas or osteoporotic vertebral compression fractures.[19] Nearly 100% of patients with spinal metastases who underwent vertebroplasty had marked pain relief postprocedure; this dropped to 73% at 6 months and 65% at 1 year.[20] There is a suggestion of a placebo effect for pain relief following vertebroplasty.[37] The Investigational Vertebroplasty Efficacy and Safety Trial (INVEST) is an ongoing, National Institute of Health (NIH)-sponsored trial to randomize patients with osteoporotic vertebral compression fractures to vertebroplasty at up to two levels versus a control (sham) intervention procedure. The goal of the study is to assess the true effect of vertebroplasty apart from the placebo effect.

Few studies emphasize the potential for height restoration and correction of kyphosis following vertebroplasty.[9,17,38,39] Several recent reports have described successful height restoration of vertebral compression fractures with postural reduction,[40–43] which can lead to an immediate increase in vertebral body height; this is termed "dynamic mobility." Maintaining a hyperextended supine position with a pillow under the back at the level of the fracture for a prolonged period, usually overnight, can further reduce the fracture; this is known as "latent mobility."[44] As osteoporotic fractures frequently involve the anterior column and the anterior longitudinal ligament is usually intact,[45] a ligamentotaxis, or molding effect, can be shown to re-expand the collapsed vertebra. Mobility is generally but not exclusively associated with intravertebral clefts, occurs more commonly at the thoracolumbar junction (T11-L1), and is associated with more severe fractures.[16,17,44,46,47] In one study, 93% of osteoporotic compression fractures were re-expanded with prolonged postural reduction, enabling vertebroplasty to be safely performed in many cases with

---

Fig. 7 (**a**) Insertion of drill bit into ventral vertebral body. (**b**) Placement of balloon tamp. AP (**c**) and lateral (**d**) fluoroscopy of bipediculate balloon tamp inflation to elevate the superior endplate *en masse*. Pre- (**e**) and post- (**f**) kyphoplasty fluoroscopy images demonstrate moderate improvement in vertebral body height and kyphosis. (Images courtesy of Dr. David Miller, Mayo Clinic, Jacksonville, Florida).

greater than two-thirds loss of height preprocedure that otherwise would have been excluded from vertebroplasty.[48] In another study, the mean dynamic mobility (as measured by anterior vertebral body height) was +4.7 mm, and the mean latent mobility was +2.7 mm.[44] Injection of bone cement preserves the positional changes in vertebral body height and may further improve the height of the fractured vertebra; this is particularly true for fractures associated with unstable fluid-filled cavities.[9]

Preoperative dynamic mobility is a good indicator of height restoration potential and postprocedure reduction in kyphotic angle following vertebroplasty.[17,38,46] This may be true for kyphoplasty as well, as the majority of kyphoplasties have been performed on acute fractures. The presence of associated bone marrow edema increases the likelihood of the fracture being mobile.[49] The relationship between age of the fracture and amount of height/deformity correction is unclear.[10,50,51] Lack of standardized reporting of methods of determining height and kyphosis correction make comparison between studies somewhat challenging. For example, depending on where the measurement is made, it is possible to have an increase in height without a reduction in angle of kyphosis[52] or reduction in kyphotic angle without an increase in height.[49]

If performed within 3 months from the time of fracture (i.e., onset of pain), kyphoplasty improves the wedge angle (angle between superior and inferior endplates of a fractured vertebra[38]) by over 50%. If performed after 3 months from onset of fracture, there is some, although less noticeable, improvement in vertebral body height.[11] A review of 69 clinical studies of kyphoplasty and vertebroplasty procedures demonstrated an appreciable restoration of height in 66% and 61% of cases, respectively. Mean kyphotic angle restoration was 6.6° for both interventions.[49] This is similar to the results of Dublin et al.,[9] who reported a mean improvement of 6° in Cobb angle , improvement of 3.5° in wedge angle, and an improvement of 47.6% in pretreatment height with vertebroplasty. Only 15% of patients had no improvement in either kyphosis or vertebral body height. Preservation of pain relief, restoration of height, and correction of kyphosis has been demonstrated in osteoporotic[53] and pathologic fractures from multiple myeloma[54] at least 1 year postvertebroplasty.

Complications

Nontarget PMMA Embolization

In a systematic review of vertebroplasty and kyphoplasty procedures by Hulme et al., cement leaks occurred in 41% and 9% of treated vertebrae, respectively.[49] Attention to fractures of the endplates or anterior and posterior vertebral body margins is essential, as cement leaking through these regions can penetrate the adjacent disc and then into the spinal canal, epidural veins, or epidural soft tissue. Intradiscal cement leakage as seen under fluoroscopy is usually globular but may also outline the adjacent endplate. While intradiscal cement leakage does not interfere with pain relief, it does predispose to adjacent vertebral body fractures (58% of vertebral bodies vs 12% of vertebral bodies without adjacent cement extravasation).[55]

Posterior epidural passage of cement, either via a breached posterior wall of the vertebral body or via the disc, can cause mass effect on the thecal sac. Intradural cement leakage has been rarely reported.[56] Cement leakage in the cervical spine may be associated with transient dysphagia and a higher risk for other neurological complications as compared to thoracic or lumbar verte-broplasty. A general rule for prevention of this complication is to ensure that the needle tip crosses the posterior cortex of the vertebral body on the lateral view prior to crossing the medial border of the pedicle on the AP view. This will also avoid tearing the thecal sac during needle placement.

Cement extravasation is usually asymptomatic (96% of vertebroplasty and 89% of kyphoplasty cases), although leakage into certain locations such as neural foramina frequently produces radicular symptoms. The rates of radiculopathy and spinal cord compression in patients with vertebroplasty for osteoporotic compression fractures are 4% and 0.5%, respectively.[57] Nerve root compression or irritation occurs at higher rates with parapedicular/pos-terolateral approaches that cross the neural foramen. Embolization of PMMA material into paraspinal veins occurs in up to 30% of patients undergoing vertebroplasty for osteoporotic compression fractures.[58] It is often asympto-matic,[59] but as reported in an intraoperative vertebroplasty of a patient with a patent foramen ovale, it can result in pulmonary hypertension and paradoxical intracranial embolization of cement.[60]

The risk of asymptomatic and symptomatic neurological complications from percutaneous vertebroplasty in pathologic fractures is much higher (5–10%) than in osteoporotic fractures, as the former are typically more difficult to treat (from a technical perspective) and often have irregular PMMA filling patterns. Epidural cement leakage is due to breach of the posterior vertebral body wall by fracture, decreased ability to accommodate cement due to tumor cells occu-pying the medullary cavity, and the hypervascularity associated with certain malignant tumors.[19,27,61] Cement extravasation is as high as 37%[21]–72.5%[62] in metastatic vertebral compression fractures and 30%[2]–65%[62] in osteoporotic fractures. The locations of PMMA leaks as detected by CT in post-vertebro-plasty patients with either spinal metastases or multiple myeloma were most commonly the paravertebral tissue and epidural space, followed by neural foramen, disc, and lumbar venous plexus.[21]

A correlation with cement pulmonary embolism as detected on chest radio-graphy has been made with the presence of paravertebral venous cement leak ($p < 0.001$) but not with the number of levels treated. In this series, all patients with cement pulmonary embolism had multiple myeloma, and three out of four cases occurred in vertebroplasty patients (the fourth being a kyphoplasty patient).[63] PMMA pulmonary emboli occur 1%[18]–4.6%[63] of the time and may cause clinically significant and, rarely, catastrophic complications.[64,65] This can be minimized with safe technique and good fluoroscopy.

Although the authors do not suggest ordering routine postprocedure chest imaging on asymptomatic patients, if there is any evidence of dyspnea, hypoxia, chest pain, or hemodynamic instability, an emergent chest CT and pulmonary CT angiogram should be obtained to evaluate for cement pulmonary embolism. Typical findings include multiple radiopaque objects in a tubular branching pattern corresponding to the pulmonary segmental arterial distribution, usually at or near the levels treated. A large amount of cement extravasation into para-vertebral and epidural veins as seen under fluoroscopy is a relative indication for obtaining chest imaging in an asymptomatic patient.

Cement embolization occurs at a much lower rate with kyphoplasty, as the material used in this procedure is thicker and is poured into a low-pressure

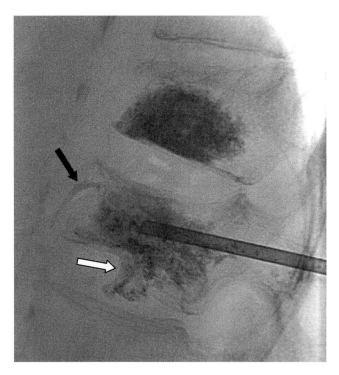

Fig. 8 Lateral fluoroscopic image demonstrating cement extravasation into a ventral epidural vein (black arrow) and into the adjacent disc (white arrow).

balloon-tamped cavity in a more controlled fashion. In vertebroplasty, PMMA deposition is in cancellous bone matrix, which is a risk in itself for cement leakage, and the usage of a more liquid form of PMMA signifies a greater quantity of "free" monomer that may potentially enter the paravertebral veins Fig. 8.[32]

Adjacent Vertebral Body or Rib Fractures

Fractures adjacent to vertebroplastied levels are common in patients with generalized osteopenia. Although the exact mechanism for these fractures is unclear, biomechanical models show that rigid cement vertebral augmentation increases loading in adjacent structures by up to 17%.[66] As normal endplate disc bulge into the treated vertebra is inhibited by cement, this increases pressure within the adjacent disc, thereby increasing loading of an adjacent untreated vertebra.[67] Several series have documented a higher incidence of adjacent vertebral fractures (as high as 67% of all new fractures) in the first 2 years after vertebroplasty[68,69]; most of these occurred within the first 30 days following the procedure.[69] Trout et al. reported that fractures at adjacent levels also occur sooner (mean of 55 days) after vertebroplasty than do those at nonadjacent levels (mean of 127 days).[70] Iatrogenic pedicle fractures have rarely been noted during needle placement and are more common with vertebra plana. A potential treatment for this condition is pediculoplasty.[71]

Osteopenic patients undergoing thoracic vertebroplasties are at highest risk for adjacent rib fractures, which are thought to occur because of forces transmitted to the rib cage during needle placement in a prone patient. Usage of a small orthopedic hammer to tap the needle into final position and avoidance of excessive torque when advancing the needle may decrease the incidence of iatrogenic rib fracture.[27] Factors increasing the risk of adjacent vertebral fractures following one-level vertebroplasty include intradiscal leak of cement[19,55] and the presence of intravertebral clefts from bony necrosis due to pseudoarthrosis or avascular necrosis of the vertebral body.[72,73]

Infection

Several case reports have documented the rare complication of infection presenting either early (within a few days) or late (up to 6 months) after vertebroplasty. Most of these cases were associated with an infectious illness during the periprocedural period, suggesting hematogenous dissemination of infection as a possible cause of spondylitis or osteomyelitis. Typical radiographic findings of osseous destruction/lysis and focal osteopenia may not always be present. It is thought that the presence of mature intravertebral clefts lined with cartilage may not be filled by PMMA during vertebroplasty. The clefts can potentially serve as a site for persistent infection in the event of transient periprocedural bacteremia, as their poor vascularity make them relatively inaccessible to systemic antibiotics.[74]

Other

A unique but rare complication of kyphoplasty is rupture of the inflatable balloon tamp, which can occur because of puncture by sharp osseous fragments or because of high inflation pressure when abutting bone with a higher density. This is not dangerous, although the patient may be exposed to a small volume of radiopaque contrast material. Some studies report a transient exacerbation of pain, low-grade fever, or hypoxia following a vertebral augmentation procedure.[61] There is also a small risk of epidural hematoma with both vertebral augmentation procedures, particularly with postprocedural heparin administration. Noncement pulmonary emboli are rare but can be secondary to bone marrow or fat particles displaced from the vertebral body into the venous circulation.

Conclusion

Percutaneous vertebroplasty and balloon kyphoplasty are safe and minimally invasive procedures that provide significant and enduring analgesic effects, increased mobility, and improved quality of life. They are indicated for painful and destabilizing osteoporotic and malignant compression fractures and aggressive vertebral body hemangiomas failing conservative medical management, and can be successfully combined with antiresorptive medications, radiation, chemotherapy, and posterior laminectomy. In addition, because of the high incidence of instrumentation failure in osteopenic patients and the lack of surgical candidacy of patients with widespread metastatic disease to the spine, vertebral augmentation procedures may be the only significant treatment option.

At present, both vertebroplasty and balloon kyphoplasty are often utilized with similar efficacy in treating vertebral compression fractures. Although no randomized, controlled, double-blinded trials of vertebroplasty versus kyphoplasty in osteoporotic or pathologic fractures have yet been done, this is one of the future directions for this rapidly developing field. A large national randomized study is currently ongoing to compare kyphoplasty and vertebro-plasty in the treatment of osteoporotic vertebral body fractures (KAVIAR, Kyphoplasty and Vertebroplasty in the Augmentation and Restoration of Vertebal Body Compression Fractures) and will likely help clarify each meth-od's relative strengths and weaknesses.

References

1. Galibert P, Déramond H, Rosat P, Le Gars D. Preliminary note on the treatment of vertebral angioma by percutaneous acrylic vertebroplasty. *Neurochirurgie* 1987;33(2):166–168.
2. Jensen ME, Evans AJ, Mathis JM, Kallmes DF, Cloft HG, Dion JE. Percutaneous polymethylmethacrylate vertebroplasty in the treatment of osteoporotic verte-bral body compression fractures: technical aspects .*AJNR Am J Neuroradiol* 1997;18(10):1897–1904.
3. Déramond H, Depriester C, Toussaint P, Galibert P. Percutaneous Vertebroplasty. *Semin Musculoskelet Radiol* 1997;1(2):285–296.
4. Lecouvet FE, Vande Berg BC, Maldague BE, Michaux L, Laterre E,Michaux JL, Ferrant A, Malghem J. Vertebral compression fractures in multiple myeloma. Part I. distribution and appearance at MR imaging. *Radiology* 1997;204(1):195–199.
5. Melton LJ 3rd, Rajkumar SV, Khosla S, Achenbach SJ, Oberg AL, Kyle RA. Fracture risk in monoclonal gammopathy of undetermined significance. *J Bone Miner Res* 2004;19(1):25–30.
6. Melton LJ 3rd, Kyle RA, Achenbach SJ, Oberg AL, Rajkumar SV. Fracture risk with multiple myeloma: a population-based study. *J Bone Miner Res* 2005;20(3):487–493. Epub 2004 Nov 29.
7. Angtuaco EJ, Justus M, Sethi R, Analysis of compression fractures in patients with newly diagnosed multiple myeloma on comprehensive therapy (abstr). *Radiology* 2001;221(P):138.
8. Epstein J, Walker R. Myeloma and bone disease: "the dangerous tango". *Clin Adv Hematol Oncol* 2006;4(4):300–306.
9. Dublin AB, Hartman J, Latchaw RE, Hald JK, Reid MH. The vertebral body frac-ture in osteoporosis: restoration of height using percutaneous vertebroplasty. *AJNR Am J Neuroradiol* 2005;26(3):489–492.
10. Lieberman IH, Dudeney S, Reinhardt MK, Bell G . Initial outcome and efficacy of "kyphoplasty" in the treatment of painful osteoporotic vertebral compression fractures. *Spine* 2001;26(14):1631–1638.
11. Garfin SR, Yuan HA, Reiley MA. New technologies in spine: kyphoplasty and vertebroplasty for the treatment of painful osteoporotic compression fractures. *Spine* 2001;26(14):1511–1515.
12. Theodorou DJ, Theodorou SJ, Duncan TD, Garfin SR, Wong WH. Percutaneous balloon kyphoplasty for the correction of spinal deformity in painful vertebral body compression fractures. *Clin Imaging* 2002;26(1):1–5.
13. Dudeney S, Lieberman IH, Reinhardt MK, Hussein M. Kyphoplasty in the treat-ment of osteolytic vertebral compression fractures as a result of multiple myeloma. *J Clin Oncol* 2002;20(9):2382–2387.
14. Lieberman I, Reinhardt MK. Vertebroplasty and kyphoplasty for osteolytic verte-bral collapse. *Clin Orthop Relat Res* 2003;(415 Suppl):S176-S186.
15. Heran MK, Legiehn GM, Munk PL Current concepts and techniques in percutaneous vertebroplasty.. *Orthop Clin N Am* 2006;37(3):409–434.
16. McKiernan F, Faciszewski T. Intravertebral clefts in osteoporotic vertebral compression fractures. *Arthritis Rheum* 2003;48(5):1414–1419.
17. McKiernan F, Jensen R, Faciszewski T. The dynamic mobility of vertebral compression fractures. *J Bone Miner Res* 2003;18(1):24–29.

18. McGraw JK, Cardella J, Barr JD, Mathis JM, Sanchez O, Schwartzberg MS, Swan TL, Sacks D. Society of Interventional Radiology quality improvement guidelines for percutaneous vertebroplasty. *J Vasc Interv Radiol* 2003;14(7):827–831.

19. Déramond H, Depriester C, Galibert P, Le Gars D. Percutaneous vertebroplasty with polymethylmethacrylate: technique, indications, and results. *Radiol Clin North Am* 1998;36(3):533–546.

20. Weill A, Chiras J, Simon JM, Rose M, Sola-Martinez T, Enkaoua E. Spinal metastases: indications for and results of percutaneous injection of acrylic surgical cement. *Radiology* 1996;199(1):241–247.

21. Cotten A, Dewatre F, Cortet B, Assaker R, Leblond D, Duquesnoy B, Chastanet P, Clarisse J. Percutaneous vertebroplasty for osteolytic metastases and myeloma: effects of the percentage of lesion filling and the leakage of methyl methacrylate at clinical follow-up. *Radiology* 1996;200(2):525–530.

22. Jasper LE, Déramond H, Mathis JM, Belkoff SM. Material properties of various cements for use with vertebroplasty. *J Mater Sci Mater Med* 2002;13(1):1–5.

23. Blinc A, Bozic M, Vengust R, Stegnar M. Methyl-methacrylate bone cement surface does not promote platelet aggregation of plasma coagulation in vitro. *Thromb Res* 2004;114(3):179–184.

24. Baroud G, Yahia FB. A finite element rheological model for polymethylmethacrylate flow: analysis of the cement delivery in vertebroplasty. *Proc Inst Mech Eng [H]* 2004;218(5):331–338.

25. Belkoff SM, Molloy S. Temperature measurement during polymerization of polymethylmethacrylate cement used for vertebroplasty. *Spine* 2003;28(14):1555–1559.

26. Jasper LE, Déramond H, Mathis JM, Belkoff SM. The effect of monomer-to-powder ratio on the material properties of cranioplastic. *Bone* 1999;25(2 suppl):27S-29S.

27. Resnick DK, Garfin SR. Vertebroplasty and Kyphoplasty. Thieme Medical Publishers, Inc., 2005.

28. Shapiro SA. Cranioplasty, vertebral body replacement, and spinal fusion with tobramycin-impregnated methylmethacrylate. *Neurosurgery* 1991;28(6): 789–791.

29. Lautenschlager EP, Jacobs JJ, Marshall GW, Meyer PR Jr. Mechanical properties of bone cements containing large doses of antibiotic powders. *J Biomed Mater Res* 1976;10(6):929–938.

30. Lautenschlager EP, Marshall GW, Marks KE, Schwartz J, Nelson CL. Mechanical strength of acrylic bone cements impregnated with antibiotics. *J Biomed Mater Res* 1976;10(6):837–845.

31. Kim AK, Jensen ME, Dion JE, Schweickert PA, Kaufmann TJ, Kallmes DF. Unilateral transpedicular percutaneous vertebroplasty: initial experience. *Radiology* 2002;222(3):737–741.

32. Lieberman IH, Togawa D, Kayanja MM. Vertebroplasty and kyphoplasty: filler materials. *Spine J* 2005;5(6 Suppl):305S-316S.

33. Jefferiss CD, Lee AJ, Ling RS. Thermal aspects of self-curing polymethylmethacrylate. *J Bone Joint Surg Br* 1975;57(4):511–518.

34. Mousavi P, Roth S, Finkelstein J, Cheung G, Whyne C. Volumetric quantification of cement leakage following percutaneous vertebroplasty in metastatic and osteoporotic vertebrae. *J Neurosurg* 2003;99(1 Suppl):56–69.

35. Belkoff SM, Mathis JM, Jasper LE. Ex vivo biomechanical comparison of hydroxyapatite and polymethylmethacrylate cements for use with vertebroplasty. *AJNR Am J Neuroradiol* 2002;23(10):1647–1651.

36. Voormolen MH, Lohle PN, Lampmann LE, van den Wildenberg W, Juttmann JR, Diekerhof CH, de Waal Malefijt J. Prospective clinical follow-up after percutaneous vertebroplasty in patients with painful osteoporotic vertebral compression fractures. *J Vasc Interv Radiol* 2006;17(8):1313–1320.

37. Kallmes DF, Jensen ME. Percutaneous vertebroplasty. *Radiology* 2003;229(1):27–36.

38. Teng MM, Wei CJ, Wei LC, Luo CB, Lirng JF, Chang FC, Liu CL, Chang CY. Kyphosis correction and height restoration effects of percutaneous vertebroplasty. *AJNR Am J Neuroradiol* 2003;24(9):1893–1900.

39. Hiwatashi A, Moritani T, Numaguchi Y, Westesson PL. Increase in vertebral body height after vertebroplasty. *AJNR Am J Neuroradiol* 2003;24(2):185–189.

40. Bedbrook GM. Treatment of thoracolumbar dislocation and fractures with paraplegia. *Clin Orthop Relat Res* 1975;112:27–43.

41. Kim YS, Kim KW, Park HC, Chung SS, Lee KC. Postural reduction for the compression fracture of the thoracolumbar spines. *J Korean Neurosurg Soc* 1988;17(6):1421–1431. (Korean)

42. Krompinger WJ, Fredrickson BE, Mino DE, Yuan HA. Conservative treatment of fractures of the thoracic and lumbar spine. *Orthop Clin North Am* 1986;17(1):161–170.

43. Youn SH, Kim KS, Zhang HY, Kim YS. Postural reduction in compression fracture of spines. *J Korean Neurosurg Soc* 1996;25(7):1473–1479. (Korean)

44. McKiernan F, Faciszewski T, Jensen R. Latent mobility of osteoporotic vertebral compression fractures. *J Vasc Interv Radiol* 2006;17(9):1479–1487.

45. Bedbrook GM. Stability of spinal fractures and fracture dislocations. *Paraplegia* 1971;9(1):23–32.

46. Carlier RY, Gordji H, Mompoint DM, Vernhet M, Feydy A, Vallée C. Osteoporotic vertebral collapse: percutaneous vertebroplasty and local kyphosis correction. *Radiology* 2004;233(3):891–898. Epub 2004 Oct 14.

47. Mirovsky Y, Anekstein Y, Shalmon E, PeerA. Vacuum clefts of the vertebral bodies. *AJNR Am J Neuroradiol* 2005;26(7):1634–1640.

48. Chin DK, Kim YS, Cho YE, Shin JJ. Efficacy of postural reduction in osteoporotic vertebral compression fractures followed by percutaneous vertebroplasty. *Neurosurgery* 2006;58(4):695–700.

49. Hulme PA, Krebs J, Ferguson SJ, Berlemann U. Vertebroplasty and kyphoplasty: a systematic review of 69 clinical studies. *Spine* 2006;31(17):1983–2001.

50. Phillips FM, Ho E, Campbell-Hupp M, McNally T, Todd Wetzel F, Gupta P. Early radiographic and clinical results of balloon kyphoplasty for the treatment of osteoporotic vertebral compression fractures. *Spine* 2003;28(19):2260–2265; discussion2265–2267.

51. Berlemann U, Franz T, Orler R, Heini PF. Kyphoplasty for treatment of osteoporotic vertebral fractures: a prospective non-randomized study. *Eur Spine J* 2004;13(6):496–501.

52. Kasperk C, Hillmeier J, Noldge G, Grafe IA, Dafonseca K, Raupp D, Bardenheuer H, Libicher M, Liegibel UM, Sommer U, Hilscher U, Pyerin W, Vetter M, Meinzer HP, Meeder PJ, Taylor RS, NawrothP. Treatment of painful vertebral fractures by kyphoplasty in patients with primary osteoporosis: a prospective nonrandomized controlled study. J Bone Miner Res 2005;20(4):604–612. Epub 2005 Apr 5.

53. Pflugmacher R, Kandziora F, Schröder R, Schleicher P, Scholz M, Schnake K, Haas N, Khodadadyan-Klostermann C. [Vertebroplasty and kyphoplasty in osteoporotic fractures of vertebral bodies – a prospective 1-year follow-up analysis]. *Rofo* 2005;177(12):1670–1676. (Ger)

54. Pflugmacher R, Schleicher P, Schröder RJ, Melcher I, Klostermann CK. Maintained pain reduction in five patients with multiple myeloma 12 months after treatment of the involved cervical vertebrae with vertebroplasty. *Acta Radiol* 2006;47(8):823–829.

55. Lin EP, Ekholm S, Hiwatashi A, Westesson PL. Vertebroplasty: cement leakage into the disc increases the risk of new fracture of adjacent vertebral body. *AJNR Am J Neuroradiol* 2004;25(2):175–180.

56. Chen YJ, Tan TS, Chen WH, Chen CC, Lee TS. Intradural cement leakage: a devastatingly rare complication of vertebroplasty. *Spine* 2006;31(12):E379-E382.

57. Chiras J, Depriester C, Weill A, Sola-Martinez MT, Déramond H. [Percutaneous vertebral surgery. Technics and indications.] *J Neuroradiol* 1997;24:45–59. (Fr)

58. Yeom JS, Kim WJ, Choy WS, Lee CK, Chang BS, Kang JW. Leakage of cement in percutaneous transpedicular vertebroplasty for painful osteoporotic compression fractures. *J Bone Joint Surg Br* 2003;85(1):83–89.

59. MacTaggart JN, Pipinos II, Johanning JM, Lynch TG. Acrylic cement pulmonary embolus masquerading as an embolized central venous catheter fragment. *J Vasc Surg* 2006;43(1):180–183.

60. Scroop R ,Eskridge J, Britz GW. Paradoxical cerebral arterial embolization of cement during intraoperative vertebroplasty: case report. *AJNR Am J Neuroradiol* 2002;23(5):868–870.

61. Cotten A, Boutry N, Cortet B, Assaker R, Demondion X, Leblond D, Chastanet P, Duquesnoy B, Déramond H. Percutaneous vertebroplasty: state of the art. *Radiographics* 1998;18(2):311–320; discussion320–323.

62. Laredo JD, Hamze B. Complications of percutaneous vertebroplasty and their prevention. *Semin Ultrasound CT MR* 2005;26(2):65–80.

63. Choe DH, Marom EM, Ahrar K, Truong MT, Madewell JE. Pulmonary embolism of polymethyl methacrylate during percutaneous vertebroplasty and kyphoplasty. *AJR Am J Roentgenol* 2004;183(4):1097–1102.

64. Padovani B, Kasriel O, Brunner P, Peretti-Viton P. Pulmonary embolism caused by acrylic cement: a rare complication of percutaneous vertebroplasty. *AJNR Am J Neuroradiol* 1999;20(3):375–377.

65. Tozzi P, Abdelmoumene Y, Corno AF, Gersbach PA, Hoogewoud HM, von SegesserL K. Management of pulmonary embolism during acrylic vertebroplasty. *Ann Thorac Surg* 2002;74(5):1706–1708.

66. Baroud G, Vant C, Wilcox R. Long-term effects of vertebroplasty: adjacent vertebral fractures. *J Long Term Eff Med Implants* 2006;16(4):265–280.

67. Ananthakrishnan D, Lotz JC, Berven S, Puttlitz C. Changes in spinal loading due to vertebral augmentation: vertebroplasty versus kyphoplasty. In: Annual Meeting of the American Academy of Orthopaedic Surgeons. 2003. p.472(New Orleans).

68. Grados F, Depriester C, Cayrolle G, Hardy N, Déramond H, Fardellone P. Long-term observations of vertebral osteoporotic fractures treated by percutaneous vertebroplasty. *Rheumatology* (Oxford) 2000;39:1410–1414.

69. Uppin AA, Hirsch JA, Centenera LV, Pfiefer BA, Pazianos AG, Choi IS. Occurrence of new vertebral body fracture after percutaneous vertebroplasty in patients with osteoporosis. *Radiology* 2003;226(1):119–124.

70. Trout AT, Kallmes DF, Kaufmann TJ. New fractures after vertebroplasty: adjacent fractures occur significantly sooner. *AJNR Am J Neuroradiol* 2006;27(1):217–223.

71. Eyheremendy EP, De Luca SE, Sanabria E. Percutaneous pediculoplasty in osteoporotic compression fractures. *J Vasc Interv Radiol* 2004;15(8):869–874.

72. Trout AT, Kallmes DF, Lane JI, Layton KF, Marx WF. Subsequent vertebral fractures after vertebroplasty: association with intraosseus clefts. *AJNR Am J Neuroradiol* 2006;27(7):1586–1591.

73. Trout AT, Kallmes DF. Does vertebroplasty cause incident vertebral fractures? A review of available data. *AJNR Am J Neuroradiol* 2006;27(7):1397–1403.

74. Vats HS, McKiernan FE. Infected vertebroplasty: case report and review of literature. *Spine* 2006;31(22):E859–E862.

Chapter 30

The Role of Anatomic and Functional Imaging in Myeloma

Brian G.M. Durie

Introduction

Multiple myeloma is a heterogeneous disease which can present with or without overt symptomatology.[1] The heterogeneity relates both to the intrinsic biology of the myeloma cells and bone marrow microenvironment and to systemic host responses to the myeloma.[2] The patient's age, health status, and the time of presentation to the healthcare system all impact outcome.

In an effort to standardize the treatment approaches, it is essential to characterize the disease as clearly as possible at the time of diagnosis. The Durie/Salmon myeloma staging system was introduced in 1975 to permit easy clinical staging, which correlated with measured myeloma cell mass.[3] This system has been widely used over the past 30 years. Despite the fact that classification based on the number and extent of bone lesions found on X-ray is observer dependent, the system has proved to be remarkably reliable.[4,5] Nonetheless, the availability of much more sensitive imaging techniques has mandated the integration of computed tomography (CT), magnetic resonance imaging (MRI), and FDG-PET scanning into routine anatomic and functional staging.[6–9]

Limitations of Anatomic Staging Using Standard Radiographs

Multiple myeloma can produce both localized lytic lesions and diffuse osteopenia evident on standard radiographs. Fracture of weakened areas is common. Early myeloma may not reveal observable changes on X-ray. Other imaging techniques show evidence of active myeloma in ~20% of patients with negative X-rays.[8,9] In addition, osteopenia may or may not be due to myeloma and can require further characterization. In some cases, it may be difficult to determine if bone collapse or fracture is a true pathologic process secondary to myeloma.

The ideal baseline diagnostic evaluation to overcome the limitations of standard radiography is summarized in Table 1. The diagnosis and disease stage are

From: *Contemporary Hematology Myeloma Therapy*
Edited by: S. Lonial © Humana Press, Totowa, NJ

Table 1 Ideal baseline diagnostic evaluation for staging and prognosis.

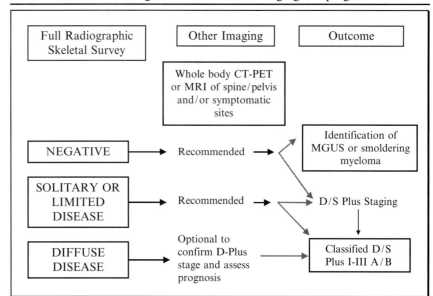

Recommendations:
- Whole body CT-PET is ideal. Whole body FDG-PET combined with localized CT is also excellent.
- MRI with spin echo (T1 and T2 weighted [-wt]), gradient-echo T2-wt, short T1 inversion recover (STIR), and Gadolinium-enhanced spine echo sequences (with and without fat supression); encompassing the whole spine and pelvis is a reasonable alternative and is the basis for the new DS-Plus Staging. MRI of symptomatic sites and/or areas of special concern is helpful, but does not constitute baseline staging.

Gadolinium can be used to enhance myeloma lesions. However, attention is drawn to the risk of nephrogenic systemic fibrosis, a serious late adverse reaction to Gadolinium which can occur in patients with renal insufficiency (30, 31, 32). Gadolinium must be used with due caution in patients with myeloma and renal insufficiency.

usually clear-cut for patients with multiple lytic lesions and/or severe osteopenia with fractures. The diagnostic and staging challenges emerge in patients with earlier disease. The goal is to provide systematic guidance for detection of early bone destruction or loss with screening of the whole body or the major areas of potential involvement in the axial skeleton. The problem is both technical and financial in that extensive imaging is costly. There is thus a strong requirement to show the clinical impact of the new imaging approaches. Obvious advantages of more precise anatomic and functional staging include the following:

- Correct staging using current imaging technology
- Avoidance of unnecessary treatment for patients with MGUS and/or smoldering myeloma[1]
- Early treatments for patients with impending overt bone disease
- Identification of poorer risk subgroups
- Accurate staging for patients with oligosecretory or nonsecretory myeloma
- Specific advantages of Durie/Salmon PLUS staging are summarized in Table 2.

Table 2 Advantages of Durie/Salmon PLUS staging.

Advantages of Durie/Salmon PLUS staging
• Direct confirmation of active myeloma for stage I patients with negative X-rays
• Cell mass assessment and staging for patients with hyposecretory or nonsecretory disease
• Identification of poor-risk patients with >27 focal lesions and/or extramedullary disease
• Overall, direct assessment of the patient versus assignment of risk based on statistical probability related to cytogenetic or other factors. This facilitates immediate clinical decision making.

Role of Computed Tomography

CT is the ideal tool for detection of early bone destruction.[4,6] Use of CT has enhanced the diagnosis of localized bone problems for many years. With the more recent availability of wide field and whole body techniques,[7,8] larger screening and assessment are possible (see Table 1). The combined use with FDG-PET is discussed below.[9] Incorporation of FDG-PET helps overcome the difficulty in determining the age or activity status of lesions identified on CT. Since myeloma lesions frequently do not heal, despite eradication of myeloma in a particular area, CT scan typically shows persistent bone lesions throughout the course of the disease. Both MRI and FDG-PET reflect the myeloma activity over time. However, CT alone cannot assess continued activity of myeloma in areas of prior bone destruction.

The Role of Magnetic Resonance Imaging

The use of MRI has added enormously to the ability to identify and monitor marrow infiltration with myeloma.[10–13] MRI is especially helpful for the evaluation of the axial skeleton. Infiltration at the site(s) of osteopenia or questionable lytic disease is diagnostically important. However, it is important to note that the MRI predominately reflects marrow infiltration, which may or may not be associated with bone destruction. Abnormal MRIs occur in patients with early smoldering disease. An abnormal MRI does not necessarily equate with a need for immediate therapy. Conversely, in patients with documented active myeloma, the number of lesions on MRI correlates very well with the outcome of treatment and overall survival.[14]

Advantages of MRI include gadolinium enhancement of areas of myeloma, which can thus be distinguished from other morphologic displacements, and the different settings (e.g., STIR, sagittal T1-weighted inversion recovery) which allow discrimination of fatty tissue (e.g., following radiation therapy), vascular abnormalities, and degenerative changes (However: see footnote Table 1 regarding use of Gadolinium). Disadvantages include the time and expense required to scan large portions of the body. The commonest and recommended approach is to scan the spine and pelvis for screening purposes. Other areas can be encompassed if symptomatic. Larger field screening of limb girdle areas and extremities can be utilized with detailed follow-up for areas of concern. An additional disadvantage of the MRI is for serial monitoring (Fig. 1). It

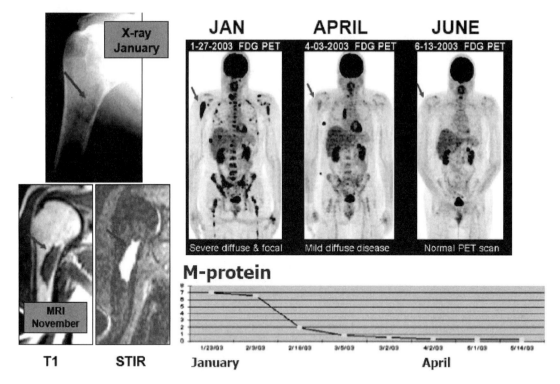

Fig. 1 Serial PET shows early response.

takes 9–12 months for lesions evident on MRI to resolve and be clearly indicative of response.[11,14] Thus although very accurate, MRI is cumbersome for routine screening and not ideal for serial whole body monitoring.

Whole Body FDG-PET

This relatively new technique has several advantages for whole body screening.[7,9,14–16] Firstly, it is possible to scan the whole body in a reasonable time frame. Since 18F-fluro-deoxy glucose is taken up and retained by areas of active myeloma, one can assess both the location and the activity of myeloma lesions. By considering the level of FDG uptake (SUV, standardized uptake values, which take into account the injected FDG dose and body weight) one can generally distinguish between active myeloma and other pathologies. One must be alert for areas of infection or abscesses since such lesions can have substantial FDG uptake.[17] However, fever, pain, and other clinical abnormalities are usually obvious clues to the presence of sepsis. Nonetheless, this is an important caution or caveat, and other diagnostic evaluations including biopsy may be required to confirm the correct pathology.

The currently available data indicate the utility of whole body FDG-PET in several settings:

- **MGUS is FDG negative.**[9,14,15] MGUS and low-level smoldering myeloma are consistently negative on scan. Conversely, only very low-level myeloma is not detectable on FDG-PET. Technetium-99 sesta MIBI imaging may be especially helpful in this setting to detect indolent disease.[18–22] Whole body technetium-99msesta MIBI has been used as an alternative to FDG-PET with one study showing rather similar results.[18] Interesting and important nuances include the enhanced uptake of technetium-99m sesta MIBI by drug-resistant myeloma cells versus enhanced uptake of FDG by metabolically active myeloma cells.[9,19]

- **Active myeloma is FGD positive.**s[9,14,15] Untreated myeloma patients manifest both focal and diffuse abnormalities on FDG-PET (Fig. 2). Patients with and without high-risk extramedullary disease are also identified. FDG-PET identifies active myeloma and allows enumeration of sites of focal disease for classification within the new Durie/Salmon PLUS myeloma staging system.
- **Systemic intramedullary and extramedullary disease can be monitored with FDG-PET.**[9,14,15] FDG-PET uptake decreases rapidly with effective therapy. Uptake can decrease within hours and within a few days to 3–4 weeks reduced uptake reflects ongoing response. Conversely, as noted above,[11,14] there is a substantial time lag of 9–12 months in the reversal of MRI abnormalities with successful therapy.
- **Persistent FDG-PET positivity correlates with likely earlier relapse.**[9] In the posttransplant setting a persistent positive scan is a poor prognostic factor and correlates with likely relapse in ~6 months. Importantly, this can occur when bone marrow and M-component markers are negative.
- **CT-PET is the ideal screening technology.**[7] Since FDG-PET uptake indicates active myeloma and CT shows bone destruction, combined whole body CT-PET is an excellent method to evaluate myeloma.[7,9,14,15]

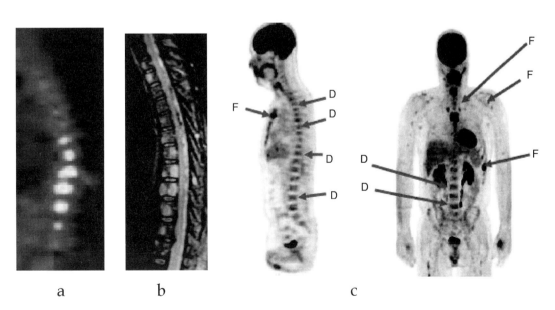

a   b   c

Fig.2 Staging with FDG-PET and CT. (**a** and **b**) FL on PET and MRI. (**a**) FDG PET scan of thoracic spine. (**b**). MRI-STIR weighted of thoracic spine. (**c**) Multiple myeloma FDG PET: severe diffuse (**d**) and focal (**f**) disease (*see* Plate 13).

The Need for a Multifaceted Approach to Staging and Prognostic Factor Classification

Myeloma is heterogeneous at both the cellular and clinical levels.[23–25] Therefore, no single system can encompass all patients. Some patients are hypo or non-secretory. For such patients high tumor burden is accompanied by low serum B2 microglobulin. ISS staging can therefore be misleading. Very indolent myeloma is not FDG avid and may not be detected with FDG-PET.[9] However, such disease is usually detected by MRI[26] and/or MIBI imaging.[18,22] Early disease has low serum B2 microglobulin, but can be associated with abnormal cytogenetic findings identifying a poor prognosis subset.[23,24] The clinician and clinical researcher must be alert to these nuances of heterogeneity. An advantage of the Durie/Salmon PLUS staging system[27] is that it can form the basis for ancillary or complementary prognostic factor classification. For example, cytogenetic abnormalities can identify low- and high-myeloma cell mass patients with drug-resistant and/or especially high-risk features.[14,23,24] High levels of soluble receptor activator of NFkB ligand/osteoprotegerin ratio predict particularly poor survival and have been proposed as useful for prognostic subclassification.[25] Using anatomic/functional and prognostic factor staging systems in a complementary fashion is ideal (Table 3).

Current and Future Role of Imaging in Myeloma

It is essential to integrate new imaging technology into myeloma staging in a systematic fashion. The anatomic/functional staging is a direct approach which serves as a basis for immediate clinical assessment and as a basis for clinical decision-making. A single focal lesion can be irradiated. Multiple lesions require a systemic approach. Both MRI and FDG-PET are included and can be used in a flexible fashion as feasible. Whole body FDG-PET (or CT-PET) is more efficient for whole body screening. MRI is especially helpful for evaluation of axial disease and also helpful for more indolent disease likely to be less FDG avid. Another alternative is technetium-99m sesta MIBI imaging for evaluation of more indolent disease.[20,21,22]

It is conceptually useful to plan immediate therapy and/or clinical trials based on combined information about myeloma tumor burden and risk fac-

Table 3 Comparison of staging systems.

	Median survival (months)			
	Original Durie/ Salmon myeloma staging systema	Durie/ Salmon PLUSb		International staging system (ISS) a
STAGE I				
A	69	72	I	62
B	22	20		
STAGE II				
A	58	61	II	44
B	34	28		
STAGE III				
A	45	40	III	29
B	24	19		

aSee Greipp et al.[5]
bSee Durie et al.[9]

tors. The A/B framework for the Durie/Salmon PLUS system is amenable to the addition of genetic-, proteomic-, and cytokine-based prognostic stratification.[25] It has already been shown that integration of PET information positively impacts clinical care overall.[28] Refinement of patient classification will occur over time. In a recent analysis of MRI the presence or absence of more than seven MRI lesions is a major discriminator.[29] New data further affirm the role of CT-PET in myeloma and related diseases. Results from the National Oncologic PET Registry (NOPR) in the U.S. indicated that physicians often change their intended management on the basis of PET scan results across the full spectrum of potential uses[33]. In addition a recent French study illustrates the role of the whole body CT-PET in patients with solitary plasmacytomata[34]. CT-PET detected additional lesions in 10 patients whereas MRI missed a total of 18 lesions. CT-PET was recommended as the best current tool in this setting. Another benefit of whole body CT-PET is that it provides sensitive screening for both sites of infection and/or occult malignancy[17, 35].

It is reasonable to anticipate that refined individual decision making can be derived from a complementary combination of anatomic/functional staging and prognostic factor classification. Novel therapies will target cell mass and prognostic factor subsets to allow evolution of personalized approaches to myeloma care.

References

1. Durie BGM, Kyle RA, et al. Myeloma management guidelines: a consensus report from the Scientific Advisors of the International Myeloma Foundation. Hematol J. 2003; 4: 379–98.
2. Durie BGM, Jacobson J, et al. Magnitude of response with myeloma frontline therapy does not predict outcome: importance of time to progression in Southwest Oncology Group chemotherapy trials. J Clin Oncol. 2004; 22(10): 1857–63.
3. Durie BGM, Salmon SE. A clinical staging system for multiple myeloma. Cancer 1975; 36: 842–854.
4. Gahrton G, Durie BGM, et al. Multiple Myeloma and Related Disorders, The role of imaging in myeloma. Arnold 2004; 10: 155–63.
5. Greipp PR, Durie BGM, et al. International sStaging sSystem for multiple myeloma. J Clin Oncol. 2005; 23(15): 3412–20.
6. Kyle RA, Schreiman JS, et al. Computer tomography in diagnosis and management of multiple myeloma and its variants. Arch Intern Med. 1985; 145: 1451–2.
7. Antoch G, Vogt FM, Freudenberg LS, et al. Whole-body dual-modality PET/CT and whole-body MRI for tumor staging in oncology. JAMA 2003; 290: 3199–206.
8. Modic MT, Obuchowski N. Whole-body CT screening for cancer and coronary disease: does it pass the test? Cleveland Clin J Med 2004; 71(1): 47–56.
9. Durie BGM, Waxman AD, et al. Whole Body F-FDG PET identifies high-risk myeloma. J Nucl Med. 2002; 43: 1457–63.
10. Bauer A, Stabler A, et al. Magnetic resonance imaging as a supplement for the clinical staging system of Durie and Salmon? Cancer. 2002; 95(6): 1334–5.
11. Walker R, Jones-Jackson L, et al. Diagnostic imaging of multiple myeloma- – FDG PET and MRI complementary for tracking short vs long term tumor response [abstract #758]. Blood. 2004; 104(11): 217a.
12. Kusumoto S, Jinnai I, Itoh K, et al. Magnetic resonance imaging patterns in patients with multiple myeloma. Br J of Haematol. 1997; 99: 649–655.
13. Mariette X, Zagdanski AM, Guermazi A, et al. Prognostic value of vertebral sessions detected by magnetic resonance imaging in patients with stage I multiple myeloma. Br J of Haematol. 1999; 104: 723–729.
14. Walker R, Barlogie B, et al. Prospective evaluation of 460 patients from total therapy II – —identification of characteristics on baseline MRI examinations of

prognostic significance – —importance of focal lesions (FL) in multiple myeloma (MM). Hematol J. 2003; 4: S171. Abstract 188.

15. Schirmeister H, Bommer M, et al. Initial results in the assessment of multiple myeloma using 18 F-FDG PET. Eur J Nucl Med. 2002; 29: 361–6.

16. Walker RC, Barlogie B, Shaughnessy J. DKK1 in myeloma: correlation with FDG-PET. New Engl J Med. 2004; 350(14): 1465–6.

17. Miceli M, Atoui R, Walker R, et al. Diagnosis of deep septic thrombophlebitis in cancer patients by fluorine-18 flurodeoxyglucose positron emission tomography scanning: a preliminary report. J Clin Oncol. 2004; 22(10): 1949–56.

18. Mileshkin L, Blum R, Seymour JF, et al. A comparison of fluorine-18 fluoro-deoxyglucose PET and technetium-99m sestamibi in assessing patients with multiple myeloma. Europ J Haematol. 2004; 72(1): 32–7.

19. Fonti R, Vecchio S, Zannetti A, et al. Functional imaging of multidrug resistant phenotype by 99mTcMIBI scan in patients with multiple myeloma. 2004; 19(2): 165–70.

20. Durie BGM, et al. Technetium-99m-MIBI scanning in multiple myeloma (MM): comparison with PET (FDG) imaging. Blood 1996; 88: 10. Abstract 1559.

21. Tirovola EB, Biassoni L, Britton KE, et al. The use of 99mTc-MIBI scanning in multiple myeloma. Br J Cancer. 1996; 74: 1815–20.

22. Durie BGM, Waxman AD, D'Agnolo A. A whole-body Tc-99m-MIBI scanning in the evaluation of multiple myeloma (MM). J Nucl Med. 1998; 39: 138.

23. Jaksic W, Trudel S, Chang H, et al. Clinical outcomes in t(4;14) multiple myeloma: a chemotherapy-sensitive disease characterized by rapid relapse and alkylating agent resistance. J Clin Oncol. 2005; 23(28): 7069–73.

24. Dewald GW, Therneau T, et al. Relationship of patient survival and chromosome anomalies detected in metaphase and/or interphase cells at diagnosis of myeloma. Blood. 2005; 106(10): 3553–8.

25. Terpos E, Szydlo R, Apperley JF, et al. Soluble receptor activator of nuclear factor kB ligand-osteoprotegerin ratio predicts survival in multiple myeloma: proposal for a novel prognostic index. Blood. 2003; 102(3): 1064–9.

26. Chim CS, Ooi GC, et al. Unusual presentations of hematologic malignancies: role of MRI and FDG-PET in evaluation of solitary plasmacytoma. J Clinic Oncol. 2004; 22(7): 1328–30.

27. Durie BGM. The roll of anatomic and functional staging in myeloma: Description description of Durie/Salmon plus staging system. European J of Cancer. 2006; 42:1539–43.

28. Hillner BE, et al. Clinical decisions associated with positron emission tomography in a prospective cohort of patients with suspected or known cancer at one United States center. J Clinic Oncol. 2004; 22(20):4147–56.

29. Walker R, Barlogie B, et al. Magnetic resonance imaging in multiple myeloma: Diagnostic diagnostic and clinical implications. J Clinic Oncol. 25(9):1121–28.

30. Thomsen HS. Nephrogenic systemic fibrosis: A serious late adverse reaction to gadodiamide. Eur Radiol. 2006; 16:2619–2621.

31. Moran GR, Pekar J, Bartolini M, et al. An Investigation of the toxicity of gadolinium based MRI contrast agents. Proc Intl Soc Mag Reson Med. 2002. 10.

32. Swaminathan S, Horn T, Pellowski, et al. Nephrogenic systemic fibrosis, gadolinium, and iron mobilization. N Engl J Med. 2007; 357(7): 720–722.

33. Hillner BE, Siegel BA, Liu D, et al. Impact of positron emission tomography/computed tomography and positron emission tomography (PET) alone on expected management of patients with cancer: Initial results from the national oncologic PET registry. J Clin Onco. 2008; 26(13). (Published ahead of print.)

34. Salaun P-Y, Gastinne T, Frampas E, et al. FDG-positron-emission tomography for staging and therapeutic assessment in patients with plasmacytoma. Haematologica. 2008; 93(8):1269–1271.

35. Patel RR, Subramaniam RM, Mandrekar JN. Occult malignancy in patients with suspected paraneoplastic neurologic syndromes: value of positron emission tomography in diagnosis. Mayo Clin Proc. 2008; 83(8):917–922.

Chapter 31

Management of Multiple Myeloma Patients with Renal Dysfunction

Sikander Ailawadhi and Asher Chanan-Khan

Introduction

Multiple myeloma (MM) is a systemic disorder with ability to affect multiple organ systems including the renal system. Renal dysfunction is an important complication in patients with MM that can result in a limitation of therapeutic options and is associated with a compromised survival.[1] Among newly diagnosed MM patients, ~50% are noted to have a decrease in creatinine clearance (Cr Cl) while 10% of the patients will require dialysis due to severe renal impairment.[2] The incidence of renal failure in MM patients differs among various reported series depending on the criteria used to define renal failure as well as the patient population studied. Among the MM patients who present with renal dysfunction on initial presentation, at least 20% can be classified as having renal failure defined by an increase ≥ 2.0 mg/dL (177 micromole/L) in serum creatinine concentrations.[3] In a series of 66 MM patients at Roswell Park Cancer Institute we used the National Kidney Foundation's Kidney Disease Outcomes Quality Initiative (NKF KDOQI) categories and observed that 54% patients had grade 3 or higher renal dysfunction (GFR, glomerular filtration rate < 60 ml/min/1.73 m[2)] at initial presentation of the disease (Fig. 1).[4] A high tumor burden in MM patients has been reported to be associated with an increased predisposition to develop renal failure and this can develop as an acute or a chronic process.[1] Both the presence of renal dysfunction and the response of renal disease to therapy appear to have a prognostic significance in these patients.[1] Bladé et al. have reported that improvement in renal function with antimyeloma therapy resulted in improved median overall survival compared to those patients with persistent or irreversible renal failure (28 vs 4 months, respectively).[3] Recent years have witnessed a significant advancement in myeloma therapeutics resulting in approval of several new drugs by the Food and Drug Administration (FDA). Importantly, there continues to be a void in understanding of the use of some of these agents in patients with renal dysfunction. Prospective clinical trials focusing on this patient population are lacking and there continues to be a need to understand how novel therapies could be safely incorporated into the management of patients with MM with renal dysfunction.

From: *Contemporary Hematology Myeloma Therapy*
Edited by: S. Lonial © Humana Press, Totowa, NJ

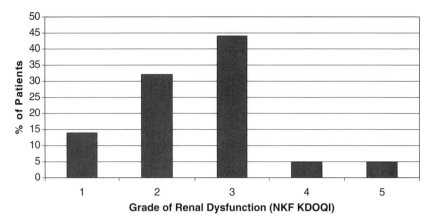

Fig. 1 Degree of renal dysfunction in a single institution series of MM patients as per the National Kidney Foundation's Kidney Disease Outcomes Quality Initiative (*NKF KDOQI*) categories (*see* Plate 14).

Pathophysiology and Types of Renal Disease in Multiple Myeloma

Plasma cells synthesize light chains and heavy chains separately which are then combined in the endoplasmic reticulum to form the immunoglobulin (Ig) molecules.[5] A mismatch in this synthesis leads to escape of free light chains in the circulation and can be detected and quantified by serum free light chain assays.[6] Although these free light chains are filtered through the glomerulus, they are readily reabsorbed in the proximal tubule. The reabsorption of light chains in the proximal tubule is a saturable process,[7] and thus excess protein load that remains unabsorbed present to the distal renal tubule and appear in the urine as Bence Jones proteins.[8]

The pathogenesis of renal failure in MM is usually multifactorial.[1,9–14] Some of the common etiologies of renal dysfunction in myeloma patients are summarized in Table 1. Among these the most common cause is hypercalcemia and dehydration reported in up to 58% of the patients who present with acute renal failure (ARF).[15] Furthermore, it is important to note that the median age of diagnosis of MM is 71 years, and many of these patients have concurrent illnesses that may require treatment with potentially nephrotoxic medications. Some of the more specific causes of renal dysfunction in MM patients are described below. Apart from these conditions that can result in kidney disease but are Ig-unrelated, renal dysfunction inherent to MM can have a variety of pathogeneses as described below (Table 1).

Myeloma Cast Nephropathy

Myeloma cast nephropathy is one of the most common diagnoses among MM patients who present with renal dysfunction and accounts for up to 60% of the cases determined by autopsy or renal biopsy.[16–18] Myeloma cast nephropathy occurs most often in patients with high rates of production and excretion of

Table 1 Pathogenesis of renal dysfunction in multiple myeloma.

Immunoglobulin-related causes of renal failure in multiple myeloma
Urinary light chain excretion
• Myeloma cast nephropathy (Myeloma kidney)
Tissue deposition of immunoglobulins
• AL Amyloidosis (light chains)
• Light chain deposition disease (LCDD)
• Heavy chain deposition disease (HCDD)
Tubular dysfunction
• Fanconi syndrome
Immunoglobulin-unrelated causes of renal failure in multiple myeloma
Hypercalcemia
Volume depletion (dehydration)
Hyperuricemia
Hyperviscosity
Medications
Angiotensin-converting enzyme inhibitors
Angiotensin receptor blockers
Loop diuretics
Antimicrobials (amphotericin B, acyclovir)
Intravenous radiocontrast media

LCDD Light chain deposition disease, *HCDD* Heavy chain deposition disease

free light chains. The normal rate of light chain excretion is <30 mg/day. Overproduction of light chains, as occurs in MM, can result in an increased light chain excretion ranging from 100 mg to more than 20 g per day. The light chains bind and form complexes with Tam-Horsfall mucoprotein (THMP), which is a protein normally synthesized by the renal tubular cells in the thick ascending limb of the loop of Henle.[19,20] These complexes are central to the pathogenesis of myeloma cast nephropathy.

On light microscopy, these complexes appear as large refractile tubular casts surrounded by multinucleated giant cells located in the distal and collecting tubules. They are strongly eosinophilic, non-argyrophilic, and stain positively with Periodic acid-Schiff stain.[21,22] These complexes are themselves toxic to the tubules and can also form obstructing tubular casts particularly in patients with intravascular volume depletion.[11] Volume depletion is a significant risk factor, both by slowing flow within the tubules and by increasing the light chain concentration, thereby promoting the formation of large aggregates of the light chain-mucoprotein complexes. Also, loop diuretics (by increasing luminal sodium chloride) and radiocontrast media (through interaction with light chains) can accelerate intratubular obstruction and renal failure in MM patients.[19,23–25]

Another contributing factor to THMP binding and predisposition to cast nephropathy may be the isoelectric point (pI) of the light chain.[19,24,26] Tubular fluid pH in the distal nephron is 5.1 and when the Bence Jones proteins have a pI above this value, they possess a net positive charge, a characteristic that may promote binding via charge interaction to anionic THMP (pI = 3.2).[11,24,27] Urinary alkalinization might therefore be beneficial by reducing binding of the light chain to THMP, by causing the light chains to become less cationic, and by changing the charge on a single histidine residue in the binding site of Tamm-Horsfall mucoprotein.[24,27,28] Acute reversible renal failure seems to be associated with low pI light chains and chronic irreversible renal failure with high pI light chains.[29]

Yet another determinant of the ability of light chains to cause renal disease may be their tendency to form high molecular weight aggregates that are more likely to form casts.[30] Data from myeloma animal models also suggests that the degree of renal dysfunction in myeloma kidney may be related to the type of light chains secreted, with different light chains having a variable nephrotoxic potential.[11,19,26–28,31,32] This may also be determined by the affinity of a specific light chain type to bind the THMP.[19,28] As an example, infusion of light chains from individual patients into mice produces the same form of renal disease (cast nephropathy, amyloid deposition, or lack of disease) as was seen in the patient.[11,32] Addition of furosemide to this model aggravated nephrotoxicity by increasing direct binding to THMP and coprecipitation of THMP with Bence Jones proteins in vitro.[11]

Amyloidosis

Amyloid kidney refers to the extracellular tissue deposition of fibrils composed of low molecular weight subunits (molecular weight range of 5–25 kD) of a variety of plasma proteins. These have an antiparallel beta-pleated sheet configuration (noted on X-ray diffraction), and can be identified on biopsy specimens both by their characteristic appearance on electron microscopy and by their ability to bind Congo red (leading to green birefringence under polarized light) and thioflavine T (producing an intense yellow-green fluorescence)[33] (Fig. 2a–2c). On light microscopy, the deposits are extracellular, eosinophilic, and metachromatic.

Primary amyloidosis (also called AL amyloidosis) refers to the subtype in which the precursor proteins are monoclonal Ig light chains produced by an underlying clonal plasma cell proliferative disorder. In ~10% of cases the disorder overlaps with overt MM. There are several forms of amyloidosis with distinct clinical patterns based on the nature of the precursor protein. Of these, AL amyloidosis is most commonly associated with IgD myeloma[34] and light-chain disease.[35] The fibrils in primary amyloidosis are derived from the variable region of lambda light chains in ~75% of cases and from kappa light chains in the rest.[36,37] In vitro studies suggest that the amino acid composition and the net charge of the protein may be an important determinant of amyloidogenic potential.[38]

Light Chain Deposition Disease

Light chain deposition disease (LCDD) is similar pathogenetically to primary amyloidosis, but the light chain fragments do not have the necessary biochemical characteristics to form amyloid fibrils.[39,40] It is therefore a non-amyloid monoclonal Ig light chain deposition caused by an underlying clonal plasma cell proliferative disorder. Tissue deposits in LCDD are usually composed of kappa light chains, are granular not fibrillar, and do not stain with Congo red or thioflavine-T.[41] As opposed to the deposits in primary amyloidosis, the deposits in LCDD are typically formed by the constant region of the Ig chains.

Fig. 2a Congo red staining of amyloid in kidney glomeruli under light microscopy. (Courtesy Dr Edit Weber) (*see* Plate 15).

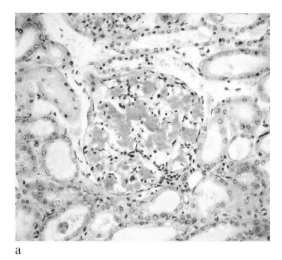

a

Fig. 2b Green birefringence of Congo red staining in renal amyloid deposits under polarized light. (Courtesy Dr Edit Weber) (*see* Plate 16).

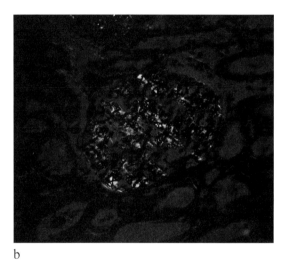

b

Fig. 2c Electron microscopy with fibrillar deposits of amyloid in renal glomerular basement membranes. (Courtesy Dr Edit Weber)

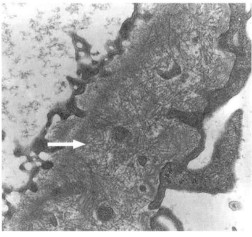

c

As a result, immunofluorescence microscopy is typically strongly positive for the monoclonal light chain.[42]

Renal involvement in LCDD is often associated with deposits in the tubular basement membranes and Bowman's capsule that may cause tubulointerstitial fibrosis.[39] These deposits may be seen in the glomeruli less commonly. The variation in pathology also affects clinical presentation. Patients with predominant glomerular deposition may present with nephrotic syndrome (similar to primary amyloidosis),[40] while those with predominant tubular deposition may present with renal insufficiency and relatively mild proteinuria.[39]

Fanconi Syndrome

An acquired Fanconi syndrome can be caused by light chain deposition in proximal renal tubules and the resulting tubular dysfunction. This causes a generalized dysfunction of tubular transport, leading to urinary excretion, and hence, wasting of amino acids, glucose, phosphate, potassium, bicarbonate, uric acid, and low molecular weight proteins. Symptoms of Fanconi syndrome may appear prior to the development of overt myeloma or amyloidosis.[43–45] Tissue specimens of bone marrow and renal tubular cells reveal crystalline cytoplasmic inclusion bodies in the lymphoplasmacytic elements in such cases. These inclusion bodies are rectangular, rhomboid, or rounded, with slight basophilic staining, as reported in several case reports.[46–48]

Heavy Chain Disease

Heavy chain disease (HCD) is caused by a monoclonal gammopathy involving the truncated heavy chains with no associated excess light chains. Involvement of all three Ig classes has been described, with α-HCD, γ-HCD, and μ-HCD occurring in that order of frequency. HCD proteins usually consist of the fragment crystallizable (Fc) region with a normal C-terminal end. Renal biopsy in these patients usually shows nodular sclerosing glomerulopathy,[49–51] though rapidly progressing glomerulonephritis has also been described.[52] Long-term follow-up in these patients demonstrate progressive renal failure in nearly all patients with HCD.

Diagnosis

The most common laboratory findings suggestive of renal dysfunction in MM are asymptomatic proteinuria and/or an elevation in serum creatinine or blood urea nitrogen (Table 2). Notably, random urine dipstick test can detect only albuminuria but not Bence Jones proteinuria.[53] Evaluation of urinary proteins by electrophoresis as well as assessment of renal function by 24-h Cr Cl are preferred investigations to assess myeloma-associated renal dysfunction. Urine protein electrophoresis will demonstrate presence of a monoclonal protein while immunofixation can identify monoclonal protein subtype (Fig. 3a and 3b). Tissue diagnosis of myeloma kidney, LCDD, or amyloidosis should be confirmed by a renal biopsy when possible, although recovery of renal dysfunction with MM-specific therapy can be an indication of the presumptive diagnosis. LCDD and amyloidosis usually do not coexist with myeloma kidney.[39,54] These disorders should be suspected with clinical signs of nephrotic syndrome, including heavy proteinuria, hypoalbuminemia, and edema. Up to

Table 2 Diagnosis of renal dysfunction in multiple myeloma.

Diagnosis of renal dysfunction in multiple myeloma
Serum chemistries
    Blood urea nitrogen
    Creatinine
Random urine sample
    Urine dipstick test
    Protein electrophoresis
24-h urine sample
    Creatinine-clearance
    Protein electrophoresis
    Immunofixation electrophoresis
Renal ultrasound
Renal biopsy

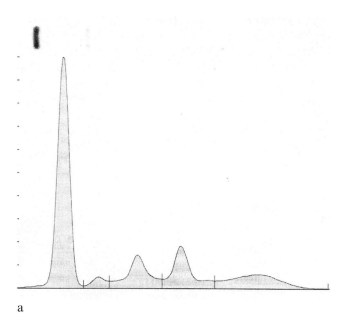

a

Fig. 3a Normal protein electrophoresis.

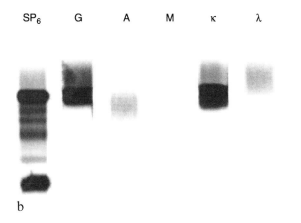

b

Fig. 3b Protein immunofixation electrophoresis showing Immunoglobulin G (*IgG*) kappa positivity (*see* Plate 17).

25% patients with LCDD may have nephrotic-range proteinuria at presentation.[55] Renal ultrasonography may show enlarged kidney size in amyloidosis. Fanconi syndrome should be suspected in patients with normoglycemia and the presence of hypokalemia, hypophosphatemia, hypouricemia, normal anion gap metabolic acidosis, and glycosuria.

Increased light chain excretion and renal failure may rarely be seen in conditions other than MM. These include monoclonal gammopathy in lymphoma,[56] Waldenstrom's macroglobulinemia,[57] and polyclonal gammopathy due to proximal tubular damage induced by rifampin.[58] HCD may not be detected as a monoclonal spike on protein electrophoresis alone due to the larger molecular weight of the paraprotein and thus, diagnosis should include serum immunoelectrophoresis, immunofixation, and immunoselection.[59]

Clinical Features

Myeloma cast nephropathy is usually associated with renal insufficiency and varying degrees of proteinuria, but nephrotic-range proteinuria is uncommon. Renal insufficiency is progressive in nature, though ARF can occur in the event of dyselectrolytemia, hypovolemia, or iatrogenic causes.[1,9–12]

Tubulointerstitial damage, fibrosis, and severe cast formation as seen on renal biopsy in myeloma kidney are associated with a poorer outcome and a lack of recovery of renal function.[15,16,60,61] Sex, tumor load, the severity of renal failure, and light-chain pI have not been shown to correlate with prognosis in patients with renal dysfunction and MM,[62] while recovery of renal function with chemotherapy, disease stage, and creatinine at 1 month have been suggested as important prognostic factors predicting survival.[63] Patients with amyloidosis or LCDD may not have significantly reduced kidney function at disease presentation, although renal failure may occur if amyloidosis or LCDD is not recognized and treated early in the disease course. Renal vein thrombosis may rarely be diagnosed in patients with nephrotic syndrome, although its contribution to renal failure in MM is not well described.

Treatment Options in Myeloma Patients with Renal Dysfunction

Acute Renal Insufficiency

In the event of ARF due to a potential offending agent, the primary goal should be to eliminate the causative factor. Hydration, alkaline diuresis (to facilitate elimination of nephrotoxic agents), and avoiding exposure to radiographic contrast media can potentially reverse an acute renal process.[15,63–65] Treatment and response may be followed with serial protein electrophoreses (Fig. 4a and 4b).

Plasma exchange is a means for rapidly reducing the paraprotein level and potentially improving or reversing ARF secondary to MM.[66,67] Although it is a temporizing measure by itself, it may have a role in combination with hydration, forced alkaline diuresis, dialysis, and chemotherapy for the treatment of myeloma-associated ARF.[66–68] Several studies have reported the use of plasmapheresis as a beneficial modality for ARF in MM.[15,61,69] Johnson et al.

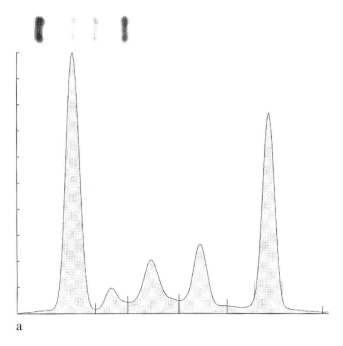

Fig. 4a Protein electrophoresis showing abnormal monoclonal spike (on extreme right).

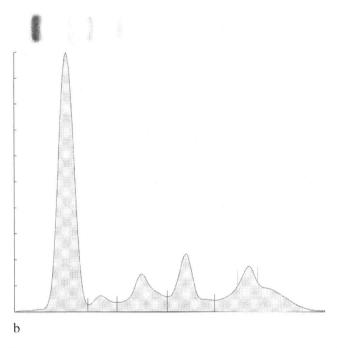

Fig. 4b Protein electrophoresis showing resolution of abnormal monoclonal spike after treatment. (Same patient as Fig. 4a).

reported 21 myeloma patients with ARF, who were treated with forced diuresis and chemotherapy, with or without plasmapheresis.[61] The only patients to recover renal function with treatment belonged to the group who received plasmapheresis. A retrospective review of 50 cases showed that renal function improved in 61% patients among those who received plasma exchange, as against 27% in patients who did not.[15] A regimen of five to seven plasma exchanges over 7–10 days concurrently with specific antimyeloma therapy is usually recommended. Quantification assays for monoclonal paraprotein should be repeated within 1–2 days after completing the initial course of plasmapheresis to assess the need for continued treatment.

Chronic Renal Insufficiency

Renal replacement therapy (RRT) is required in ~10% patients with MM due to end-stage renal disease.[2] This could be in the form of continuous ambulatory peritoneal dialysis (CAPD) or hemodialysis (HD). Although there are advantages and disadvantages of each of these processes, CAPD clears light chains better than HD. This, however, has not been reported to influence recovery of renal function[69–71] and no significant difference in survival outcome has been reported among patients on HD versus CAPD.[72] Also, there does not seem to be any increase in the risk of peritonitis among MM patients when compared to those without myeloma.[73] The overall survival of patients begun on RRT is comparable to that of other myeloma patients.[74] The response rate to chemotherapy in patients who survive beyond the first 2 months from initiation of RRT seems to be similar to that of patients with normal renal function.[75] Thus, it is more important to initiate specific therapy for myeloma at the earliest, as, essentially, the control of MM is more important in prolonging survival than just the reversal of renal dysfunction.

Renal transplantation has been reported in some cases with preexisting myeloma and others who developed MM shortly after an allograft.[74,76–81] This experience is limited. Nevertheless, prolonged survival and graft function have been reported following renal transplantation in these patients. Although there are no established criteria for patient selection it is suggested that the patients be in complete remission for at least 1 year prior to being considered for a renal transplant.

Conventional Chemotherapy

Response rates of myeloma patients with renal failure to conventional chemotherapeutic strategies have been reported by several authors and are in the range of 40–50%.[3,64,72,82–84] Bladé et al. have reported an increase in mortality early on in patients with MM and renal failure, when compared to patients without renal failure (30% vs 7%).[3] This may be a reason for the lower response rate to conventional chemotherapy in these patients. Interestingly, if patients who die within the first 2 months are excluded from the overall analysis, response to therapy is similar in all patients regardless of their pretreatment renal function.[3] This suggests that renal failure per se may not be contributory to chemotherapy resistance. Melphalan is an important therapeutic agent in myeloma therapy and requires dose adjustment for renal dysfunction. Thus, melphalan-based regimens may be suboptimal for treatment of patients with renal dysfunction. On the contrary anthracycline-based regimens with doxorubicin plus vincristine and dexamethasone (VAD)[85] or methylprednisolone (VAMP)[86] could be more effective in these patients as no dose reductions are warranted in these regimens.

High-Dose Therapy/Stem Cell Transplantation

Several authors have reported their experience with high-dose therapy/stem cell transplant (HDT/SCT) in patients with MM and renal failure.[87–90] While most of these have been case reports and small case series, the experience helps to understand possible patient outcome and therapeutic options. San Miguel et al. reported a comparison in the outcomes of patients with MM with or without renal failure, who underwent HDT/SCT.[91] The treatment-related mortality (TRM) was reported higher in the group with renal failure (29% vs 4%), although there was no significant difference in overall survival or overall event-free survival between the two groups. Poor performance status (ECOG > 2), higher serum creatinine level (>5 mg/dl), and a low hemoglobin level (<9.5 mg/dl) were factors significantly associated with the TRM.[91] Badros et al. studied different conditioning regimens for patients undergoing HDT/SCT with a comparison between melphalan at doses 200 mg/m^2 (MEL-200) and 140 mg/m^2 (MEL-140).[92] This study looked only at elderly population (>70 years). A total of 81 patients with nonreversible renal failure were enrolled and it was noted that the incidence of complications was significantly higher in the MEL-200 group, especially in dialysis-dependent patients. Interestingly though, there was no difference in outcome between the two groups. Older age, refractory disease, and low serum albumin were associated with a significantly shorter overall survival.[92] Thus, current data suggests that while HDT/SCT in MM patients with renal failure is feasible, it should be individualized to patients with a higher likelihood of a better outcome such as those who are young in age or with good performance status and chemosensitive disease.

Novel Agents and Myeloma Patients with Renal Dysfunction

Immunomodulating Agents

Treatment of MM has seen remarkable evolution due to the approval of several newer agents (Table 3). Among these immunomodulating agents, thalidomide and lenalidomide have clearly made a major impact.

Table 3 Novel agents for the treatment of multiple myeloma (MM): Standard dosage and recommendations for dose adjustment in patients with renal dysfunction.

Drug	Usual dosage	Dose adjustment with renal failure	Reference
Thalidomide	200 mg PO	None	96
Pegylated Liposomal Doxorubicin	30 mg/m^2 IV	Nonc	
Bortezomib	1.3 mg/m^2 IV	None	98,99
Lenalidomide	25 mg PO	Not defined	97

PO per os (by mouth), *IV* intravenous

Thalidomide has been studied in patients with renal failure in several small clinical trials. The efficacy and toxicity profile of thalidomide with or without dexamethasone was reported by Tosi et al. in 20 patients with stage III relapsed/refractory MM and renal failure, defined as serum creatinine >130 mmol/L.[93] An overall response rate (ORR) of 75% was reported, with 45% patients achieving partial remission. Median duration of response was 7 months and 4 patients were refractory to treatment. Recovery to a normal renal function was observed in 12 (80%) of 15 responsive patients. Toxicity profile of thalidomide with or without dexamethasone was comparable with that observed in patients with a normal renal function. This is contrary to the observation by other investigators who have reported higher incidence of severe neuropathy, constipation, lethargy, and bradycardia with thalidomide among patients who had serum creatinine of 3 mg/dl.[94] Hyperkalaemia is a specific and serious potential complication of thalidomide in patients with renal failure and usually occurs during the first few weeks of treatment but may occur later during the treatment with thalidomide.[95] The mechanisms underlying this adverse event remain unclear. Eriksson et al. studied the pharmacokinetics of thalidomide in renal failure patients and reported that the drug concentration profiles in patients with renal failure were very similar to those reported by others for patients with normal renal function.[96] Although dialysis increases thalidomide clearance, the dose or schedule of thalidomide does not need to be changed in patients with decreased renal function.

Lenalidomide is a more potent analog of thalidomide recently approved for myeloma treatment. It has been investigated in various combination regimens. Since lenalidomide is primarily excreted unchanged in the urine, it is expected to have an enhanced toxicity in myeloma patients with impaired renal function.[97] For this reason patients with renal insufficiency were excluded from the clinical trials with lenalidomide, and those who developed renal insufficiency during the clinical trials had the drug held. Since there is lack of adequate clinical experience with lenalidomide in renally impaired patients with myeloma, it is reasonable to avoid its use in this patient population. Ongoing clinical trials are investigating appropriate dose and schedule in myeloma patients with renal dysfunction. These studies will be beneficial in identifying appropriate use of this agent in the context of renal impairment.

Bortezomib

Another novel agent used in MM is the proteasome inhibitor, bortezomib. Initial clinical experience of bortezomib use in patients with renal dysfunction was reported by Jagannath et al.[98] They noted that the response rates, toxicity profiles, and treatment discontinuation rates were similar in patients with or without renal dysfunction (Cr Cl < 30 ml/min). In a retrospective review we investigated the efficacy and toxicity of bortezomib-based regimens in patients with advanced MM and chronic renal failure requiring HD.[99] In twenty-four patients the ORR was 75%, with 30% achieving a CR or near-CR. Three patients became independent of dialysis following bortezomib-based treatment. Interestingly, no increase in treatment-related toxicities was reported.[99] Bortezomib is now approved by the FDA for the treatment of myeloma patients with renal insufficiency with or without dialysis support.

The impact of high-dose dexamethasone-containing regimens with or without thalidomide and bortezomib on the reversal of renal failure was evaluated in 41 consecutive newly diagnosed patients with MM by Kastritis et al.[100] Renal function was reversed in 73% of all patients within a median of 1.9 months. In patients treated with dexamethasone and novel agents (thalidomide and/or bortezomib) the reversibility rate was 80% within a median of 0.8 months. Severe renal failure and significant Bence Jones proteinuria were associated with a lower probability of reversal of renal function. Patients who responded to the treatment achieved reversal of renal function more often than those who did not (85% vs 56%, $p = 0.046$) (Table 3).

Supportive Therapy

A common clinical manifestation of MM is the lytic bone disease. Bone resorption in MM is accelerated because of an increase in the number and activity of osteoclasts at the interface of these lytic lesions.[101] Bisphosphonates are used to treat bony disease in MM as they inhibit osteoclastic activity among other mechanisms of action.[102–106] Clinical practice guidelines for the use of bisphosphonates in patients with MM have been published by the American Society of Clinical Oncology (ASCO).[107] Alterations in dose, infusion schedule, or dosing interval are unnecessary in patients with preexisting renal disease and a serum creatinine < 3.0 mg/dL. Dose adjustment is recommended for zoledronic acid in patients with Cr Cl between 30 and 60 ml/min.[108] No adjustments are recommended for pamidronate in patients with Cr Cl > 30 ml/min.[109] In patients with more severe renal failure, or those undergoing HD, there are no specific guidelines and treatment should be individualized based on the risks and benefits.

Acknowledgments: Dr. Edit Weber, Department of Pathology, Buffalo General Hospital, Buffalo, NY.

References

1. CG W. Acute myeloma kidney. Kidney Int. 1995;48:1347–1361.
2. Torra R BJ, Cases A. Patients with multiple myeloma requiring long-term dialysis: presenting features, response to therapy, and outcome in a series of 20 cases. Br J Haematol. 1995;91:854–859.
3. Bladé J F-LP, Bosch F, et al. Renal failure in multiple myeloma: presenting features and predictors of outcome in 94 patients from a single institution. Arch Intern Med. 1998;158:1889–1893.
4. K/DOQI clinical practice guidelines for chronic kidney disease: evaluation, classification, and stratification; 2000.
5. Bergman LW KW. Co-translational modification of nascent immunoglobulin heavy and light chains. J Supramol Struct. 1979;11:9–24.
6. Endelman GM GJ. The nature of Bence-Jones proteins'' chemical similarities to polypeptide chains of myeloma globulins and normal gamma-globulins. J Exp Med. 1962;116:207–227.
7. Baylis C F-SJ, Ross B. Glomerular and tubular handling of differently charged human immunoglobulin light chains by the rat kidney. Clin Sci. 1988;74:639–644.
8. Sanders PW HG. Monoclonal immunoglobulin light chain-related renal diseases. Semin Nephrol. 1993;13:324–341.
9. Uchida M KK, Okubo M. Renal dysfunction in multiple myeloma. Intern Med. 1995;34:364–370.

10. Rota S MB, Baudouin B, et al. Multiple myeloma and severe renal failure: a clinicopathologic study of outcome and prognosis in 34 patients. Medicine (Baltimore). 1987;66:126–137.

11. Sanders PW BB. Pathobiology of cast nephropathy from human Bence Jones proteins. J Clin Invest. 1992;89:630–639.

12. Cohen DJ SW, Osserman EF, et al. Acute renal failure in patients with multiple myeloma. Am J Med. 1984;76:247–256.

13. Hoitsma AJ WJ, Koene RA. Drug-induced neprotoxicity. Aetiology, clinical features and management. Drug Saf. 1991;6:131–147.

14. Rashed A AB, Abu Romesh SH. Acyclovir-induced acute tubulo-interstitial nephritis. Nephron. 1990;56:436–438.

15. Pozzi C PS, Donini U, et al. Prognostic factors and effectiveness of treatment in acute renal failure due to multiple myeloma: a review of 50 cases. Clin Nephrol. 1987;27:1–9.

16. Pasquali S ZP, Casanova S, et al. Renal histological lesions and clinical syndromes in multiple myeloma. Renal Immunopathology Group. Clin Nephrol. 1987;27:222–228.

17. B I. Renal complications in multiple myeloma. Acta Morphol Hung. 1989;37:235–243.

18. Montseny JJ KD, Meyrier A, et al. Long-term outcome according to renal histological lesions in 118 patients with monoclonal gammopathies. Nephrol Dial Transplant. 1998;13:1438–1445.

19. PW S. Pathogenesis and treatment of myeloma kidney. J Lab Clin Med. 1994;124:484–488.

20. Leboulleux M LB, Mougenot B, et al. Protease resistance and binding of Ig light chains in myeloma-associated tubulopathies. Kidney Int. 1995;48:72–79.

21. Sanders PW HG, Kirk KA, et al. Spectrum of glomerular and tubulointerstitial renal lesions associated with monotypical immunoglobulin light chain deposition. Lab Invest. 1991;64:527–537.

22. Pirani CL SF, D''Agati V, et al. Renal lesions in plasma cell dyscrasias: ultrastructural observations. Am J Kidney Dis. 1987;10:208–221.

23. Smolens P BJ, Kreisberg R Hypercalcemia can potentiate the nephrotoxicity of Bence Jones proteins. J Lab Clin Med. 1987;110:460–465.

24. Holland MD GJ, Sanders PW, et al. Effect of urinary pH and diatrizoate on Bence Jones protein nephrotoxicity in the rat. Kidney Int. 1985;27:46–50.

25. Morgan C Jr HW. Intravenous urography in multiple myeloma. N Engl J Med. 1966;275:77.

26. Sanders PW BB, Bishop JB, et al. Mechanisms of intranephronal proteinaceous cast formation by low molecular weight proteins. J Clin Invest. 1990;85:570–576.

27. Sanders PW HG, Chen A, et al. Differential nephrotoxicity of low molecular weight proteins including Bence Jones proteins in the perfused rat nephron in vivo. J Clin Invest. 1988;82:2086–2096.

28. Huang ZQ SP. Localization of a single binding site for immunoglobulin light chains on human Tamm-Horsfall glycoprotein. J Clin Invest. 1997;99:732–736.

29. Melcion C MB, Baudouin B, et al. Renal failure in myeloma: relationship with isoelectric point of immunoglobulin light chains. Clin Nephrol. 1984;22:138–143.

30. Myatt EA WF, Weiss DT, et al. Pathogenic potential of human monoclonal immunoglobulin light chains: relationship of in vitro aggregation to in vivo organ deposition. Proc Natl Acad Sci USA. 1994;91:3034–3038.

31. Decourt C RA, Bridoux F, et al. Mutational analysis in murine models for myeloma-associated Fanconi''s syndrome or cast myeloma nephropathy. Blood. 1999;94:3559–3566.

32. Solomon A WD, Kattine AA. Nephrotoxic potential of Bence Jones proteins. N Engl J Med. 1991;324:1845–1851.

33. Kisilevsky R YI. Pathogenesis of amyloidosis. Baillieres Clin Rheumatol. 1994;8:613–626.

34. Jancelewicz Z TK, Sugai S, et al. IgD multiple myeloma. Arch Intern Med. 1975;135:87–93.

35. Stone MJ FE. The clinical spectrum of light chain myeloma. A study of 35 patients with special reference to the occurrence of amyloidosis. Am J Med. 1975;58:601–619.

36. Bellotti V MG, Bucciarelli E, et al. Relevance of class, molecular weight and isoelectric point in predicting human light chain amyloidogenicity. Br J Haematol. 1990;74:65–69.

37. Perfetti V CS, Palladini G, et al. Analysis of V(lambda)-J(lambda) expression in plasma cells from primary (AL) amyloidosis and normal bone marrow identifies 3r (lambdaIII) as a new amyloid-associated germline gene segment. Blood. 2002;100:948–953.

38. Hurle MR HL, Li L, et al. A role for destabilizing amino acid replacements in light-chain amyloidosis. Proc Natl Acad Sci USA. 1994;91:5446–5450.

39. Buxbaum JN CJ, Hellman GC, et al. Monoclonal immunoglobulin deposition disease: light chain and light and heavy chain deposition diseases and their relation to light chain amyloidosis. Clinical features, immunopathology, and molecular analysis. Ann Intern Med. 1990;112:455–464.

40. Lin J MG, Valeri AM, et al. Renal monoclonal immunoglobulin deposition disease: the disease spectrum. J Am Soc Nephrol. 2001;12:1482–1492.

41. Pozzi C DAM, Fogazzi GB, et al. Light chain deposition disease with renal involvement: clinical characteristics and prognostic factors. Am J Kidney Dis. 2003;42:1154–1163.

42. Noel LH DD, Ganeval D, et al. Renal granular monoclonal light chain deposits: morphological aspects in 11 cases. Clin Nephrol. 1984;21:263–269.

43. Dragsted PJ HN. The association of the Fanconi syndrome with malignant disease. Danish Med Bull. 1956;3:177–179.

44. Headley RN KJ, Cooper MR, et al. Multiple myeloma presenting as adult Fanconi syndrome. Clin Chem. 1972;18:293–295.

45. Lee DB DJ, Rosen VJ, et al. The adult Fanconi syndrome: observations on etiology, morphology, renal function and mineral metabolism in three patients. Medicine (Baltimore). 1972;51:107–138.

46. Aucouturier P BM, Khamlichi AA, et al. Monoclonal Ig L chain and L chain V domain fragment crystallization in myeloma-associated Fanconi''s syndrome. J Immunol. 1993;150:3561–3568.

47. Orfila C LJ, Modesto A, et al. Fanconi''s syndrome, kappa light-chain myeloma, non-amyloid fibrils and cytoplasmic crystals in renal tubular epithelium. Am J Nephrol. 1991;11:345–349.

48. Troung LD, Mawad J CP, et al. Cytoplasmic crystals in multiple myeloma-associated Fanconi''s syndrome. A morphological study including immunoelectron microscopy. Arch Pathol Lab Med. 1989;113:781–785.

49. Kambham N MG, Appel GB, et al. Heavy chain deposition disease: the disease spectrum. Am J Kidney Dis. 1999;33:954–962.

50. Aucouturier P KA, Touchard G et al. Heavy-chain deposition disease. N Engl J Med. 1993;329:1389–1393.

51. Liapis H PI, Nakopoulou L. Nodular glomerulosclerosis secondary to mu heavy chain deposits. Human Pathol. 2000;31:122–125.

52. Vedder AC WJ, Krediet RT. Intracapillary proliferative glomerulonephritis due to heavy chain deposition disease. Nephrol Dial Transplant. 2004;19:1302–1304.

53. Geneval D CM, Noel L-H, et al. Kidney involvement in multiple myeloma and related disorders. Contrib Nephrol. 1982;33:210–222.

54. Hill GS M-ML, Mery JP, et al. Renal lesions in multiple myeloma: their relationship to associated protein abnormalities. Am J Kidney Dis. 1983;2:423–438.

55. Choukroun G VB, Grunfeld J-P. Multiple myeloma. Part I: Renal renal involvement. Clin Issues Nephrol. 1995;70:11–17.

56. Burke JR Jr FR, Lasker N, et al. Malignant lymphoma with "''myeloma kidney''" acute renal failure. Am J Med. 1976;60:1055–1060.

57. Isaac J HG. Cast nephropathy in a case of Waldenstrom''s macroglobulinemia. Nephron. 2002;91:512–515.

58. Soffer O NV, Campbell WG Jr, et al. Light chain cast nephropathy and acute renal failure associated with rifampin therapy. Renal disease akin to myeloma kidney. Am J Med. 1987;82:1052–1056.

59. Doe WF DF, Seligmann M. Immunodiagnosis of alpha chain disease. Clin Exp Immunol. 1979;36:189–197.

60. Levi DF WR, Lindstrom FD. Immunofluorescent studies of the myeloma kidney with special reference to light chain disease. Am J Med. 1968;44:922–933.

61. Johnson WJ KR, Pineda AA, et al. Treatment of renal failure associated with multiple myeloma: plasmapheresis, hemodialysis, and chemotherapy. Arch Intern Med. 1990;150:863–869.

62. Pasquali S CS, Zucchelli P, et al. Long-term survival in patients with acute and severe renal failure due to multiple myeloma. Clin Nephrol. 1990;34:247–254.

63. Geneval D RC, Guerin V, et al. Treatment of multipe myeloma with renal involvement. Adv Nephrol. 1992;21:347–370.

64. Misiani R TG, Mingardi G, et al. Management of myeloma kidney: an anti-light-chain approach. Am J Kidney Dis. 1987;10:28–33.

65. Iggo N WC, Davies ER. The development of cast nephropathy in multiple myeloma. QJM. 1997;90.

66. Feest TG BP, Cohen SL. Successful treatment of myeloma kidney by diuresis and plasmapheresis. BMJ. 1976;i:503–507.

67. Misiani R RG, Bertani T, et al. Plasmapheresis in the treatment of acute renal failure in multiple myeloma. Am J Med. 1979;66:684–688.

68. Locatelli F PC, Pedrini L, et al. Steroid pulses and plasmapheresis in the treatment of acute renal failure in multiple myeloma. Proc EDTA. 1980;17:690–694.

69. Zucchelli P PS, Cagnoli L, et al. Controlled plasma exchange trial in acute renal failure due to multiple myeloma. Kidney Int. 1988;33:1175–1180.

70. Rosansky SJ RF. Use of peritoneal dialysis in the treatment of patients with renal failure and paraproteinemia. Am J Nephrol. 1985;5:361–365.

71. Solling K SJ. Clearance of Bence-Jones proteins during peritoneal dialysis or plasmapheresis in myelomatosis associated with renal failure. Contrib Nephrol. 1988;68:259–262.

72. Iggo N PA, Severn A, et al. Chronic dialysis in patients with multiple myeloma and renal failure: a worthwile treatment. QJM. 1989;73:903–910.

73. Shetty A OD. Myeloma patients do well on CAPD too! Br J Haematol. 1997;96:654–657.

74. Cosio FG PT, Shapiro FL, et al. Severe renal failure in multiple myeloma. Clin Nephrol. 1981;15:206–210.

75. DE B. The role of chemotherapy in the treatment of multiple myeloma. Bailliere''s Clin Haematol. 1995;8:783–794.

76. Walker F BR. Renal transplantation in light-chain multiple myeloma. Am J Nephrol. 1983;3:34–37.

77. Humphrey RL WJ, Zachary JB, et al. Renal transplantation in multiple myeloma. Ann Intern Med. 1975;83:651–653.

78. Sammett D DF, abbi R, et al. Renal transplantation in multiple myeloma: case report and review of literature. Transplantation. 1996;62:1577–1580.

79. Passweg J BH, Tichelli A, et al. Transient multiple myeloma after intense immunosuppression in a renal transplant patient. Nephrol Dial Transplant. 1993;8:1393–1394.

80. Gerlag PGG KR, Berden JHM. Renal transplantation in light chain nephropathy: case report and review of the literature. Clin Nephrol. 1986;25:101–104.

81. Scully RE GJ, McNeely BU. Case records of the Massachusetts General Hospital: case 1–1981. N Engl J Med. 1981;304:33–43.

82. Knudsen LM HM, Hippe E. Renal failure in multiple myeloma: reversibility and impact on prognosis. Eur J Haematol. 2000;65:175–181.

83. Korzets A TF, Russell G, et al. The role of continuous ambulatory peritoneal dialysis in end-stage renal failure due to multiple myeloma. Am J Kidney Dis. 1990;6:216–223.

84. Medical Research Council Working Party on Leukemia in Adults. Analysis and management of renal failure in the fourth myelomatosis trial. Br Med J. 1984;288:1411–1416.

85. Barlogie B SL, Alexanian R. Effective treatment of advanced multiple myeloma refractory to alkylating agents. N Engl J Med. 1984;310:1353–1356.

86. Aitchison RG RI, Morgan AG, et al. Vincristine, adriamycin and high dose steroids in myeloma complicated by renal failure. Br J Cancer. 1990;61:765–766.

87. Ballester OF TR, Janssen WE, et al. High-dose chemotherapy and autologous peripheral blood stem cell transplantation in patients with multiple myeloma and renal failure. Bone Marrow Transplant. 1997;20:653–656.

88. Rebibou JM CD, Cassanovas RO, et al. Peripheral blood stem cell transplantation in a myeloma patient with end-stage renal failure. Bone Marrow Transplant. 1997;20:63–65.

89. Reiter E KP, Keil F, et al. Effects of high-dose melphalan and peripheral blood stem cell transplantation on renal function in patients with multiple myeloma and renal insufficiency: a case report and review of the literature. Ann Hematol. 1999;78:189–191.

90. Tosi F ZE, Ronconi S, et al. Safety of autologous hematopoietic stem cell transplantation in patients with multiple myeloma and chronic renal failure. Leukemia. 2000;14:1310–1313.

91. San Miguel JF LJ, Gar ia-Sanz R, et al. Are myeloma patients with renal failure candidates for autologous stem cell transplantation? Hematologica. 2000;1:28–36.

92. Badros A BB, Siegel E, et al. Autologous stem cell transplantation in elderly multiple myeloma patients over the age of 70 years. Br J Haematol. 2001;114:600–607.

93. Tosi P ZE, Cellini C, et al. Thalidomide alone or in combination with dexamethasone in patients with advanced, relapsed or refractory multiple myeloma and renal failure. Eur J Haematol. 2004;73:98–103.

94. Pineda-Roman M TG. High-dose therapy in patients with plasma cell dyscrasias and renal dysfunction. Contrib Nephrol. 2007;153:182–194.

95. Harris E BJ, Samson D, et al. Use of thalidomide in patients with myeloma and renal failure may be associated with unexplained hyperkalaemia. Br J Haematol. 2003;122:160–161.

96. Eriksson T HP, Turesson I, et al. Pharmacokinetics of thalidomide in patients with impaired renal function and while on and off dialysis. J Pharm Pharmacol. 2003;55:1701–1706.

97. Revlimid® (lenalidomide);: package Package insert.: Celgene Corporation; 2006.

98. Jagannath S BB, Berenson JR, et al. Bortezomib in recurrent and/or refractory multiple myeloma; initial clinical experience in patients with impaired renal function. Cancer. 2005;103:1195–1200.

99. Chanan-Khan AA KJ, Mehta J, et al. Activity and safety of bortezomib in multiple myeloma patients with advanced renal failure: a multicenter retrospective study. Blood. 2007;109:2604–2606.

100. Kastritis E AA, Roussou M, et al. Reversibility of renal failure in newly diagnosed multiple myeloma patients treated with high dose dexamethasone-containing regimens and the impact of novel agents. Hematologica. 2007;92:546–549.

101. Croucher PI AJ. Bone disease in multiple myeloma. Br J Haematol. 1998;103:902–910.

102. Rodan GA FH. Bisphosphonates: mechanisms of action. J Clin Invest. 1996;97:2692–2696.

103. Sato M GW, Endo N, et al. Bisphosphonate action. Alendronate localization in rat bone and effects on osteoclast ultrastructure. J Clin Invest. 1991;88:2095–2105.
104. H F. Bisphosphonates: mechanisms of action. Endocr Rev. 1998;19:80–100.
105. Owens JM FK, Chambers TJ. Osteoclast activation: potent inhibition by the bisphosphonate alendronate through a nonresorptive mechanism. J Cell Physiol. 1997;172:79–86.
106. Reszka AA H-NJ, Masarachia PJ, et al. Bisphosphonates act directly on the osteoclast to induce caspase cleavage of mst1 kinase during apoptosis. A link between inhibition of the mevalonate pathway and regulation of an apoptosis-promoting kinase. J Biol Chem. 1999;274:34967–34973.
107. Berenson JR HB, Kyle RA, et al. American Society of Clinical Oncology clinical practice guidelines: the role of bisphosphonates in multiple myeloma. J Clin Oncol. 2002;20:3719–3736.
108. Zometa (zoledronic acid): Prescribing information.: Novartis Pharmaceuticals Corporation; 2007.
109. Aredia (pamidronate): Prescribing information.: Novartis Pharmaceuticals Corporation; 2007.

Section 7

Other Plasma Cell Disorders

Chapter 32

Waldenstrom's Macroglobulinemia

Lijo Simpson and Morie Gertz

Waldenstroms macroglobulinemia (WM) was first described by Jan Waldenstrom in 1944. He described two patients with oronasal bleeding, lymphadenopathy, normochromic anemia, increased erythrocyte sedimentation rate (ESR), thrombocytopenia, hypoalbuminemia, low serum fibrinogen, and increased number of lymphoid cells in bone marrow.[1] Waldenstrom went on to point out: "The cellular basis of macroglobulinemia is the proliferation of one clone of cells that produces one definitive macroglobulin molecule. These cells may appear in different histological patterns. The most common is diffuse infiltration of the bone marrow but many patients also have enlargement of lymph glands ("lymphoma"). In some instances the spleen is also invaded and rare patients have a lymphoma picture in the lungs and even in the brain. The characteristic finding is that these cells contain immunoglobulin M (IgM) with the same light-chain type, either κ (kappa) or λ (lambda), as the increased IgM in the serum."[2]

Much has changed in our understanding of this disease since then. Some groups postulated that WM was a clinical syndrome (IgM paraproteinemia) characterized by the presence of monoclonal IgM secretion which can be generated by different types of plasma cell disorders (MGUS, monoclonal gammopathy of undetermined significance) or low-grade lymphoproliferative diseases, namely, lymphoplasmacytic lymphoma (LPL), small lymphocytic lymphoma (SLL), or marginal zone lymphoma (MZL), while others defined it as a distinct clinicopathological syndrome. This has resulted in some confusion in the minds of treating physicians.

The median age at diagnosis of WM is 63 years. WM is currently incurable, and most patients die of disease progression, with a median survival of 5 years.[3] However, many patients live over 10 years with good quality of life. WM has an overall incidence of ~3.4 per million persons per year among males and 1.7 per million persons per year among women. This translates to ~1,500 new cases annually in the United States. In a study looking at the incidence of WM across 11 population-based cancer registries that participate in the Surveillance, Epidemiology, and End Results (SEER) Program of the National Cancer Institute there were 551 cases of WM diagnosed among whites (326 males and 225 females), 31 among blacks (16 males and 15 females),

From: *Contemporary Hematology Myeloma Therapy*
Edited by: S. Lonial © Humana Press, Totowa, NJ

22 among other races (14 males and 8 females), and 20 among those with unknown race (11 males and 9 females).[4] Thus, white males represented 52% of all cases, white females represented 36%, blacks represented 5%, other races represented 4%, and those whose race was unspecified represented 3%. Interestingly, the incidence rate among white males (3.6 per million persons per year) was more than twice that reported in the other three major race/gender groups. This seems to parallel the pattern observed in hairy cell leukemia. The cause of this is unknown.

Etiology and Predisposing Factors

The role of environmental factors in WM is unclear. In a case-control study of WM among 65 cases, diagnosed in the greater Baltimore area, compared with 213 hospital controls without cancer, cases were slightly better educated, but there were no other differences in sociodemographic factors, history of prior medical conditions, medication use, cigarette smoking, alcohol consumption, specific occupational exposures, employment in any particular industries or occupations, or familial cancer history. Cases were more likely to have first-degree relatives with a history of pneumonia, diphtheria, rheumatic fever, and diabetes mellitus. An evaluation of immunologic profiles of first-degree relatives of cases revealed that relatives of two cases had asymptomatic IgM (>750 mg/dL) monoclonal gammopathy and close to 40% of the 109 evaluated had diverse immunologic abnormalities.[5] One case series suggested a link between WM and shoe repairers.[6] But other studies have not shown any occupational link.[7]

Familial Waldenstroms Macroglobulinemia

There has been some indirect evidence of a genetic predisposition toward WM. A report outlined the occurrence of WM in monozygotic twins.[8] The two monoclonal IgMs differed by their light-chain type and their idiotype. While there may have been a genetic predisposition to cancer in these twins, the gene recombination leading to idiotypic specificity and light-chain assortment occurred independently. Similar findings were reported in another family with four brothers with WM.[9] The four patients had IgMs differing in the light-chain components.

The four brothers did not share a common human leukocyte antigen (HLA) A, B, DR haplotype, and a genetic linkage to the HLA complex could not be found. Five of their 12 relatives had high serum immunoglobulin concentration (four IgG, three IgA, and two IgM) with no evidence of monoclonality.

A recent review of the literature of familial WM outlined 12 families containing 31 cases of WM.[10] The number of patients in this review was small, but the familial cases differ from sporadic WM being diagnosed around a decade earlier and more common in males than sporadic cases.[10]

Presenting symptoms and signs were generally similar to those found in sporadic WM. The most common symptoms were bleeding diathesis, malaise, and/or weakness followed by weight loss. Examination was significant for hepatosplenomegaly, lymphadenopathy, and retinal dysproteinemic findings. Anemia was common and peripheral lymphocytosis was often noted. Nearly all patients had an elevated erythrocyte sedimentation rate, and Bence-Jones proteinuria was reported in half. When other immunoglobulins were evaluated, most patients (84.2%) had some abnormality, usually deficiencies of IgG alone (31.2%) or in association with IgA (50.0%). When sought, 41.2% of patient relatives had evidence of autoantibodies, but definite clinical autoimmune disease was rare. For instance, the prevalence of IgM monoclonal gammopathy (IgM MG) in first-degree relatives of WM cases was reportedly as high as 6.3%. The implications of these findings are unclear. Sixteen cases (69.6%) were κ restricted while seven cases (30.4%) were λ light-chain restricted. The light-chain typing was discordant in five of eight families.

Conventional cytogenetic studies in familial WM have been inconsistent. Unfortunately, none of the reported families have yet had cytogenetic analysis using more sensitive molecular techniques.

Another large recent review of familial WM showed that 18.7% of patients with WM who were diagnosed had at least one first degree relative with either WM (5.1%), or other hematologic disorders such as non-Hodgkin's lymphoma (3.5%), multiple myeloma (MM) (3.1%), chronic lymphocytic leukemia (CLL) (2.7%), MGUS (1.9%), acute lymphoblastic leukemia (ALL) (1.2%), and Hodgkin's disease (1.2%). This is the most comprehensive data that gives us an estimate of the incidence of familial WM and indicates a relation with multiple hematologic malignancies in affected families. This study also indicated that patients from families with a history of WM had higher bone marrow involvement at the time of diagnosis and therefore a higher disease burden compared with de novo patients. A subset of patients in this study had conventional GTG karyotyping and fluorescent in situ hybridization (FISH) studies performed. The only recurrent structural chromosomal abnormality was deletions in the 6q21–q22 regions. These were found only in patients without a family history of WM. Using FISH assay the authors observed loss of hybridization for RP11-91C23 and RP11-171J20 in 37/77 (48%) and 31/77 (40%) of all WM patients, respectively, with a total of 53/77 (69%) showing loss of at least one of the probes. There was no statistically significant difference between patients with and without a family history of WM.[11]

Classification

Historically, the term WM was loosely applied to denote a clinicopathologic syndrome of lymphoma associated with an IgM paraprotein. LPL associated with WM, or "true" WM, was separated from other lymphomas by an arbitrary serum IgM level. Although this approach was practical from the clinical standpoint, it was problematic for the pathologist trying to classify different types of B-cell lymphoma associated with IgM paraprotein. Several terms introduced by different classification systems over the last several decades added to the confusion because terms used to label "lymphomas with lymphoplasmacytic differentiation" are not necessarily interchangeable in different classification systems.

These terms included plasmacytoid lymphoma in the Rappaport classification, plasmacytic–lymphocytic lymphoma in the Lukes-Collins classification, SLL with plasmacytoid differentiation (Working Formulation), lymphoplasmacytic lymphocytoid immunocytoma (Kiel classification), lymphoplasmacytoid lymphoma/immunocytoma (REAL, Revised European/American Lymphoma classification), and LPL in the World Health Organization (WHO) classification.[12]

The WHO classification attempted to bring together the diagnosis of WM and LPL. It defined LPL/WM as a clinicopathologic entity characterized by a monoclonal expansion of predominantly small B-lymphocytes with variable plasmacytoid differentiation that are usually negative for CD5, CD10, and CD23 and associated with IgM paraprotein. The WHO classification does not define a specific cut off for serum IgM paraprotein but observed that a paraprotein level of >3 g/dL occurs in most patients with LPL/WM.

To further define the diagnostic criteria of WM and to establish guidelines for clinical management, the Second International Workshop on WM was held in Greece in 2002. This is the most accepted definition of WM.

Definition

The consensus panel from the Second International Workshop on WM recommended that the diagnosis of WM required the demonstration of bone marrow infiltration by LPL. This is defined as a tumor of small lymphocytes showing evidence of plasmacytoid/plasma cell differentiation without any of the clinical, morphological, or immunophenotypic features of other lymphoproliferative disorders. This is as defined by the WHO and REAL classifications.[13]

The diagnostic criteria of WM are outlined in Table 1. The panel defined WM as a distinct clinicopathologic entity confined to cases of LPL and recommended against use of the term in patients with other types of B-cell lymphoma. Also, cases of LPL associated with IgG or IgA or other B-cell lymphomas with IgM paraprotein are not considered WM. Some members of the panel also believe that LPL/WM has a distinctive immunophenotype, that is, CD19[+], CD5[-], CD10[-], and CD23[-], as described below.

The committee also recommended that there was no threshold for IgM to establish a diagnosis of WM provided the other criteria are met.

Immunophenotype

IgM paraproteins can occur in a variety of low-grade B-cell lymphoproliferative disorders making a diagnosis of WM difficult. Immunophenotyping provides an important tool in excluding other B-cell lymphoproliferative disorders (Table 2). The immunophenotypic profile of WM has been explored in numerous studies; however, the results have been inconsistent due to the small number of patients involved, different techniques used (immunohistochemistry

Table 1 Diagnostic criteria for Waldenstroms macroglobulinemia.

1. IgM gammopathy of any concentration
2. Bone marrow infiltration by small lymphocytes showing plasmacytoid/plasma cell differentiation
3. Intertrabecular pattern of bone marrow infiltration
4. Surface IgM[+], CD5[+], CD10[-], CD19[+], CD20[+], CD22[+], CD23[-], CD25[+], CD27[+], FMC7[+], CD103[-], CD138[-] immunophenotype

Adapted from Owen RG, Treon SP, Al-Katib A, Fonseca R, Greipp PR, McMaster ML, Morra E, Pangalis GA, San Miguel JF, Branagan AR, Dimopoulos MA. Clinicopathological definition of Waldenstrom's macroglobulinemia: consensus panel recommendations from the Second International Workshop on Waldenstrom's Macroglobulinemia. Semin. Oncol. 2003 Apr;30(2):110–5.

vs flow cytometry), and criteria used to define positive results. The WHO definition of WM is positive for monotypic surface immunoglobulin light chain, IgM, CD19, and CD20, and is negative for CD5, CD10, and CD23.[14]

However, these observations have not been supported by all. Owen et al. reviewed their immunophenotyping experience.[15] Ninety-eight cases of LPL/WM were analyzed by flow cytometry. The WHO immunophenotype was seen in 90% of cases with CD19, CD20, and CD22 expression noted in 100%, 100%, and 98.2% of cases, respectively. However, CD5, CD10, and CD23 expression was also found in 5.4%, 4.5%, and 0.9% of cases, respectively. San Miguel et al. in their review[16] noted that there was constant expression of CD19, CD20, and CD22 with CD5 and CD23 being detected in 20% and 29% of WM patients, respectively. Another review of 75 patients with WM[17] indicated that the neoplastic cells, in all cases, expressed monoclonal immunoglobulin light chains and CD19, and every case assessed was positive for CD20 ($n = 68$) and CD52 ($n = 60$). The results for other antigens assessed in decreasing frequency of positivity were as follows: surface IgM (26/28 [93%]), CD79b (11/13 [85%]), CD11c (13/16 [81%]), CD25 (5/7 [71%]), CD23 (17/28 [61%]), CD38 (24/50 [48%]), FMC7 (11/29 [38%]), CD22 (4/12 [33%]), CD5 (3/65 [5%]), and CD10 (1/38 [3%]). The immunophenotype was similar in involved lymph nodes and bone marrow in examined cases. Interestingly, all patients tested for CD52 expressed this antigen. This has also been confirmed independently,[18] indicating a potential use of alemtuzumab (anti-CD52) in this condition. There therefore is considerable heterogeneity in the immunophenotyping of WM and the overall clinical and bone marrow picture should be taken into account.

The clinical significance and impact on survival of CD5, CD10, or CD23 expression in LPL/WM is unclear. One study has indicated that CD23 and CD5 positivity correlates with higher disease burden (71% of positive cases had IgM > 30 g/L vs 43% of CD23 negative cases; 91% of CD5+ cases had

Table 2 Use of peripheral blood immunophenotyping and fluoresent in situ hybridization to distinguish B-cell lymphoproliferative disorders.

	CD5	CD19	CD20	CD23	CD10	CD103	CD11c/c22	Surface Ig
Chronic lymphocytic leukemia	Present	Present	Present (dim)	Present	Absent	Absent	Absent	Present (dim)
Mantle cell lymphoma	Present	Present	Present (bright)	Dim to absent	Absent	Absent	Absent	Present (bright)
Follicular lymphoma	Absent	Absent	Present	Present or absent	Present or absent	Absent	Absent	Present
Nodal and splenic marginal zone lymphoma	Absent	Present	Present (bright)	Absent	Absent	Absent	Absent	Present
Hairy cell leukemia	Absent	Present (bright)	Present (bright)	Absent	Absent	Present	Present (bright)	Present
Lymphoplasmacytic lymphoma	Present or absent	Present	Present	Present or absent	Absent	Absent	Absent	Present (dim)

Adapted from Tait et al.[35]

IgM > 20 g/L vs 71% of CD5⁻ cases). FMC7-positive patients had lower mast cell count and bone marrow infiltration. Other studies have not confirmed this, showing that in CD23⁺ patients there was no statistically significant difference in patient age, serum monoclonal IgM level, total serum IgM level, and extent of bone marrow involvement (Tables 1 and 2).[17]

Cytogenetics

Early studies indicated that the t(9; 14) (p13; q32) translocation is present in 50% of cases of LPL/WM as well as other plasmacytic lymphomas.[19,20] This translocation juxtaposes the PAX-5 gene encoding for B-cell-specific activator protein (BSAP), an essential B-cell transcription factor, with the joining region of IgH, resulting in deregulated expression of BSAP. The t(9; 14) (p13; q32) translocation results in the upregulation of PAX-5. The resulting increase in BSAP causes an increase in B-cell proliferation and is believed to be important in disease pathogenesis. However, this finding has not been confirmed in subsequent studies in WM and this association has held more strongly with LPL without any IgM paraproteinemia. Thus, WM, a type of LPL with IgM paraproteinemia, and LPL with no paraproteinemia differ not only in phenotype but also in the presence of the t(9; 14) (p13; q32) translocation.

Metaphase cytogenetic studies in WM are hampered by the slow rate of proliferation of WM cells with difficulty obtaining meaningful metaphases for analysis. This results in low rate of detection of chromosomal abnormalities with conventional cytogenetics. Mansoor et al.[21] looked at conventional G band karyotype analysis of 37 patients with WHO-defined LPL/WM. Among all 37 cases, 25 (68%) had a diploid karyotype and 12 (32%) were abnormal. Eight (67%) of these 12 cases had complex cytogenetic abnormalities. In 12 cases with an abnormal karyotype, 4 (33%) were pseudodiploid, 5 (42%) were hyperdiploid, and 3 (25%) were hypodiploid. Trisomy 5 and monosomy 8 each were identified in 3 cases (25%) and this was the commonest numeric chromosomal abnormality. Trisomy 3 and loss of chromosome Y were each seen in 2 cases (17% each). Monosomy of chromosome 4, 7, 13, 19, 21, or 22 was identified in one case each. Using FISH study, deletion of chromosome 6q, encompassing q13–q22, was the most common structural change, seen in 6 cases (50%). Deletions 3q21 and 13q12 were each seen in 2 (17%) cases. Structural abnormalities of 12p occurred in 2 cases (17%), both add (12) (p11–13). One case each had del(1)(q32) and add(17)(p13). Cytogenetic abnormalities were detected in 3 (17%) of 18 lymphoplasmacytoid, 2 (20%) of 10 lymphoplasmacytic, and 7 (78%) of 9 polymorphous cases. When the lymphoplasmacytoid and lymphoplasmacytic groups were combined for statistical analysis, polymorphous tumors were significantly more likely to be aneuploid (7/9 [78%] vs 5/28 [18%]) and carry a poorer prognosis than were lymphoplasmacytoid and lymphoplasmacytic tumors. Thus, the bone marrow morphology predicted karyotype abnormalities and stratified a subpopulation with a poorer prognosis.[21]

In a similar study by Schop et al.,[22] 35 patients with WM had karyotyping performed. Twenty-two (63%) patients had normal metaphases. Abnormal metaphases were obtained in 13 (37%) patients. For the 13 patients with abnormal karyotype, 4 (31%) had recurrent abnormalities of chromosome 13, with del(13)(q14) in 3 and monosomy 13 in 1; 2 (15%) had del(6)(q13q21)(q13q25);

1 (8%) had an addition at chromosome 6q27 (add(6)(q27)); 2 (15%) had abnormalities of chromosome 17q25 and 1 (8%) had chromosome 17 monosomy; 2 had del(5q)(13q35); and 4 had diverse abnormalities in chromosome 8. Using more sensitive FISH strategies, deletions of 6q21 were observed in 42% of patients. In addition, there were no t(9;14)(p13;q32) translocations observed.

Other rarer mutations have been reported. Liu et al.[23] reported a single case of WM with deletion of 20q as the sole initial cytogenetic abnormality. Ten cases with plasma cell dyscrasias and del(20q) were also reviewed. None of the cases in whom del(20q) was present developed MDS/AML but three patients with this mutation appearing after chemotherapy developed MDS/AML. This suggests that the significance of del(20q) differs depending on whether it appears at diagnosis or after chemotherapy.

Another large study of cytogenetics in WM by Ocio et al.[24] studied 102 patients. Patients were stratified according to the ISS in three categories: stage I: albumin $\geq$ 35 g/L and β2M < 3.5 mg/L; stage II: albumin < 35 g/L and β2M < 3.5 mg/L or β2M 3.5–5.5 mg/L; and stage III: β2M > 5.5 mg/L. Of the 102 patients included in the study, deletion in the 6q21 region was present in 40 (39%) by FISH. Only in 4 of 39 patients with 6q deletion detected by FISH was the abnormality also detected by conventional cytogenetics. Patients with 6q deletion displayed features which, in previous studies, have been associated with worse prognosis in WM. Patients with 6q deletion had significantly higher levels of β2M (β2M $\geq$ 4.0 mg/L: 52% vs 14%, $P = 0.001$), anemia (hemoglobin [Hb] < 110 g/L in 66% vs 40%, $P = 0.01$), and hypoalbuminemia (albumin < 40 g/L in 90% vs 54% of cases, respectively, $P = 0.001$). The amount of paraprotein has also been described in some reports as having prognostic influence in WM. In this study, IgM levels were higher than 20 g/L in 90% of patients with loss of 6q when compared with 72% of patients without the deletion ($P = 0.03$). The frequency of 6q– increased with the stage of the International Staging System, which revealed a trend toward statistical significance. Only 24% of patients in stage 1 displayed the abnormality when compared with 42% and 67% of patients included in stage 2 and 3, respectively ($P = 0.05$). Patients who had deletion of 6q more frequently required treatment; 87% of patients with 6q– required treatment while only 67% of patients without the abnormality were treated during follow-up ($P = 0.02$). In this subset of patients, those with 6q deletion displayed a shorter treatment-free survival (median of 55.2 months), when compared with not reached after a follow-up of 100 months for patients without the deletion ($P = 0.03$). There was no survival advantage demonstrated in this study.

Data was recently published on gene expression profiling in WM and contrasted with related lymphocyte malignancies.[25] WM had a homogeneous transcription profile, clustering with CLL and normal B cells. In contrast, the expression profile of WM is very different from that of MM and normal plasma cells. Only a small set of genes has a unique expression profile in WM. Among the upregulated genes, IL-6 is the most significant. It has been demonstrated that IL-6 levels are elevated in WM and that IL-6 is required for plasmacytic differentiation of the clonal B cells in WM. The functional and biologic importance of IL-6 in WM therefore requires further study and may provide therapeutic targets. Serum IL-6 levels have been reported to reflect disease severity and high tumor burden in MM patients and to correlate with several other laboratory parameters, such as bone marrow plasmacytosis, serum LDH, and β2M.[26] It has also been shown that clonal blood B cells from patients with WM spontaneously differentiate in vitro to plasma cells through an IL-6 pathway. These findings suggest that IL-6 may be a marker reflecting tumor burden and response to treatment in WM.[27]

Of the various genes that have been localized to 6q21, BLIMP-1 is postulated to be of importance in WM. BLIMP-1, a tumor suppressor gene, has the ability to drive activated B cells to become antibody-secreting cells with a plasma cell phenotype. Blimp-1 proteins use five zinc-finger motifs for sequence-specific binding to DNA. Blimp-1 is a transcriptional repressor and exerts much of its effect by repression of c-Myc, MHC2TA, and PAX-5.[28] It facilitates the transition from the mature B-cell stage to the plasma cell stage. Partial or whole losses in this gene could result in a predisposition for B-cell malignancies such as WM.

Another area of interest in WM is the B-lymphocyte stimulator (BLyS), a B-cell-activating factor of the tumor necrosis factor family member expressed by monocytes, macrophages, dendritic cells, and neutrophils. BLyS has been shown to be critical for the maintenance of normal B-cell development and homeostasis. It stimulates B-cell proliferation and immunoglobulin secretion. Three receptors have been identified as receptors for BLyS: B-cell maturation antigen (BCMA), transmembrane activator and calcium-modulator and cyclophilin ligand interactor (TACI), and B-cell activating factor of the tumor necrosis factor family receptor (BAFF-R). BCMA and BAFF-R are predominantly expressed on B lymphocytes, while TACI can be found on B cells as well as on activated T cells. BAFF-R has been identified as the main BLyS receptor responsible for peripheral B-cell homeostasis and specifically binds BLyS.[28] BCMA and TACI can also bind the related molecule, a proliferation-inducing ligand (APRIL). In WM, IgG and IgA hypogammaglobulinemia are more prevalent among cases with mutations in the TACI-signaling process.[29] In a study by Elsawa et al.,[30] lymphoplasmacytic cell infiltrates in the bone marrow of patients with WM stained positive for BLyS expression, and serum BLyS levels in patients with WM were significantly higher than in healthy controls. Because of the role of BLyS in WM, strategies to inhibit BLyS potentially may have therapeutic efficacy.

Abnormal expression of hyaluronan synthases (HASs) has been reported as a possible pathogenetic factor in WM.[31] Hyaluronan has a role in malignant cell migration and metastasis. Of the three HAS isoenzymes detected in humans, Adamia et al.[32] postulated that overexpressed HAS1 and HAS3 form a hyaluronan matrix around WM cells, thereby preventing their elimination by the immune system and promoting spread of the disease. A later report stated that a single nucleotide polymorphism in the HAS1 gene resulted in an enhanced risk of WM development.[32] These findings are important considering that serum hyaluronan levels have been shown to have prognostic value in MM.

Cell of Origin

The cell of origin of LPL/WM has been debated. Several studies have shown a lack of IgH translocations in WM. This indicates that WM is derived from IgM + postgerminal center memory B-cells. Also, IGH sequence analysis in WM has demonstrated evidence of somatic hypermutation without intraclonal diversity and isotype switching in most cases. Zeta-chain-associated protein kinase 70 (ZAP–70), a marker predicting unmutated status of the neoplastic cells in SLL/CLL, is usually not expressed in LPL/WM.[33] These phenotypic and sequence data suggest that WM is derived from a B cell that has completed somatic hypermutation and has exited the germinal center.

Differential Diagnosis

The differential diagnosis of LPL/WM includes small lymphocytic leukemia (SLL) CLL, mantle cell lymphoma (MCL), follicular lymphoma (FL), MM, and various types of MZL.

In the bone marrow, the neoplastic cells of LPL/WM show a spectrum of cytologic features including small lymphocytes, plasmacytoid lymphocytes, and plasma cells. The plasma cells are usually mature (Marchalko type) and may contain cytoplasmic globules (Russell bodies) and intranuclear pseudoinclusions (Dutcher bodies). Mast cells may be increased, but this is a nonspecific finding. The infiltrate may be nodular (interstitial or paratrabecular), interstitial, mixed, or diffuse.

The consensus panel proposed that the diagnosis of LPL/WM should be based on detection of bone marrow involvement by the disease. Specifically, an intertrabecular pattern of infiltration is considered to be helpful supporting evidence. There is no defined minimal infiltrate required for the diagnosis. In the literature, the minimal requirement for the percentage of lymphocytes has ranged from 10% to 30%. Similar to the levels of serum IgM paraprotein, the extent of bone marrow infiltrate does not appear to correlate with clinical symptoms. The extent of bone marrow infiltration in smoldering or asymptomatic LPL/WM overlaps with that of overt LPL/WM.

Cases of SLL/CLL can exhibit plasmacytoid differentiation and morphologically mimic LPL/WM. These neoplasms also can be associated with serum IgM paraprotein. In Kyle et al.'s series,[34] 5% of patients with IgM paraproteinemia had CLL. Immunophenotypically, SLL/CLLs express dim monotypic surface immunoglobulin and CD20. They are virtually always positive for CD5, and commonly are CD19+ and CD23+.[35] Cytogenetic abnormalities may be found in ~80% of patients with CLL. Frequently identified abnormalities include 13q– (65% of patients), trisomy 12 (20% of patients), 11q– (10% of patients), and 17 p– (5% of patients). ZAP-70 may be positive in IgH unmutated cases. These mutations are uncommon in WM.

MCL is usually composed of monomorphous atypical small to medium-sized lymphoid B cells with scant cytoplasm, slightly to markedly irregular indented nuclei, moderately dispersed chromatin, and inconspicuous nucleoli. MCL cells show a characteristic phenotype: CD19+, CD20+, CD22+, CD23–, CD24+, CD79a+, moderate to strong surface IgM or IgD expression or both, CD43+, FMC7+, HLA-DR+, BCL2+, CD5+, CD10–, and nuclear cyclin D1 (CCND1, BCL1, PRAD1)+.[36] MCL rarely exhibits plasmacytoid differentiation, but they can be morphologically confused with the lymphoplasmacytoid variant of LPL/WM. Thus, most cases of LPL/WM can be distinguished from MCL by histopathology, immunophenotyping, and the presence of t(11;14)(q13;q32) and cyclin D1 overexpression.

Cases of FL also need to be considered in the differential diagnosis with LPL/WM. Although a paratrabecular infiltrate in the bone marrow is typical of FL, this pattern is also reported in a small subset of LPL/WM cases. Cytologically, the neoplastic cells in FL are small, cleaved, with minimal cytoplasm, unlike the round and often plasmacytoid cells of LPL/WM. Immunophenotypically, most cases of FL are positive for CD10, CD19, CD20, and BCL6; CD10 expression is rare in LPL/WM. Detection of the t(14;18)(q32;q21) or BCL3 gene rearrangement supports the diagnosis of FL.[12]

Most cases of plasma cell myeloma are easily distinguished from LPL/WM. Plasma cell myeloma is composed of sheets of atypical plasma cells showing large prominent nucleoli. By contrast, the neoplastic cells of LPL/WM are smaller lymphoid cells without prominent nucleoli. However, the small cell variant of plasma cell myeloma can be confused with the lymphoplasmacytic variant of LPL/WM because of its lymphoid appearance and frequent expression of the B cell marker CD20. In difficult cases, clinical data are helpful. Lytic bone lesions, renal failure, and IgG or IgA serum paraprotein are common in plasma cell myeloma and are not seen in LPL/WM according to the consensus panel definition. In MM, immunoperoxidase staining detects either κ or λ light chains, but not both, in the cytoplasm of bone marrow plasma cells, thereby confirming that the plasma cell proliferation is monoclonal. Also the malignant plasma cells in MM usually stain for CD38, CD56 (neural cell adhesion molecule), and CD138 and are usually negative for surface immunoglobulin and the pan-B-cell antigen CD19. Although morphologically WM is often characterized by plasmacytoid cells, very few CD138+ cells (1–5%) are detectable in either blood or in BM and almost all patients are CD20 positive. In addition, karyotyping and cytogenetics in myeloma reveal characteristic mutations such as del17p−, t(4;14), t(14;16), del13, hypodiploidy, hyperdiploidy and t(11;14), t(6,14). These mutations are rare in WM.[37]

Most extranodal marginal zone B-cell lymphoma of mucosa-associated lymphoid tissue (MALT) type (MALT-type lymphoma, MALT lymphoma) are easily distinguished from LPL/WM. Presence of serum IgM paraprotein is uncommon in patients with MALT lymphoma, and involvement of an extranodal site is uncommon in LPL/WM. The extranodal MALT lymphomas involve stomach, lung, orbit, conjunctiva, skin, and salivary gland while WM typically does not involve these areas. Histologically, MALT lymphoma is characterized in most cases by monocytoid B-cells, lymphoepithelial lesions, and reactive follicles. In the small subset of LPL/WM cases that involve an extranodal site, these histologic findings are less frequent. Epidemiologic studies support a strong association between MALT-type gastric lymphomas and chronic *Helicobacter pylori* infection. In a case control study conducted by Parsonnet et al., patients with gastric lymphoma were significantly more likely than matched controls to have evidence of previous *H. pylori* infection (matched odds ratio, 6.3; 95% confidence interval (CI), 2.0–19.9).[38] This association is not found with WM. Immunophenotypically, the tumor cells express surface membrane immunoglobulin (IgM > IgG > IgA) and lack IgD; 50% have monotypic cytoplasmic immunoglobulin, indicating plasmacytoid differentiation. They express B-cell-associated antigens (CD19, CD20, CD22, and CD79a) and complement receptors (CD21 and CD35), and are usually negative for CD5, CD10, and CD23. Immunophenotypically, therefore, they are similar to WM. Trisomy 3 (60%) and t(11;18) involving AP12–MALT1 (25–40%) are the most commonly reported cytogenetic abnormalities. Other translocations characteristic of MALT lymphoma include the t(11;18)(q21;q21), the t(14;18)(q32;q21) involving IgH–MALT1, and t(1;14)(p22;32). These translocations

Color Plates

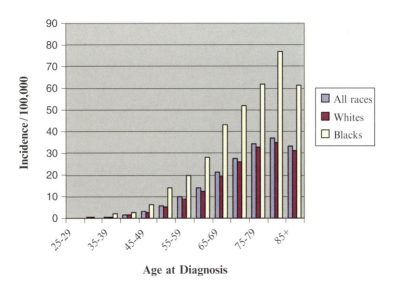

Plate 1 Incidence of multiple myeloma according to age (SEER Data, 2000–2004).

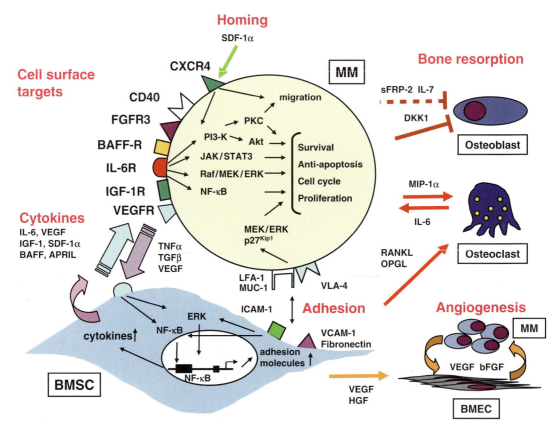

Plate 2 Interaction of multiple myeloma (MM) cells with their bone marrow microenvironment. The adhesion of MM cells to bone marrow stromal cells (BMSCs) triggers cytokine-mediated tumor cell growth, survival, drug resistance, and migration. In both MM cells and BMSCs, adhesion mediates activation of NF-KB, thereby further upregulating adhesion molecules including intercellular adhesion molecule (ICAM-1) and vascular cell adhesion molecule-1 (VCAM-1). Binding of MM cells to BMSCs upregulates cytokine secretion from both BMSCs and tumor cells. These cytokines activate via their cell surface receptors major signaling pathways, such as extracellular signal-regulated kinase (ERK), Janus kinase (JAK) 2/signal tranducers and activators of transcription (STAT)-3, phosphatidylinositol-3 kinase (P13-K)/Akt, and nuclear factor-id3 (NF-κB). Their downstream targets include cytokines, such as interleukin-6 (IL-6), insulin-like growth factor-1 (IGF-l), and vascular endothelial growth factor (VEGF), antiapoptotic proteins, and cell cycle modulators. Homing of MM cells to their BM milieu is mediated by stromal-derived factor-la (SDF-la) and its receptor CXCR4 on MM cells. Osteoclastogenesis is stimulated by receptor activator of NF-κB ligand (RANKL) and osteoprotegerin ligand (OPGL) from BMSCs, as well as macrophage inflammatory protein 1α (MIP-1α) from MM cells. In addition, MM cells inhibit osteoblastogenesis via the secretion of IL-7 and Dickkopf 1 (DKK1), thereby further enhancing osteolysis. Secretion of factors like VEGF and basic fibroblast growth factor (bFGF) stimulates angiogenesis.

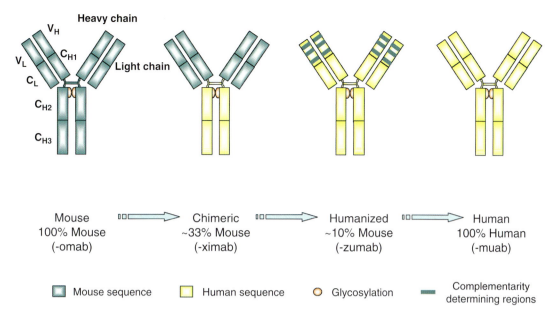

Plate 3 A schematic representation of the process involved in engineering murine mAbs to reduce their immunogenecity. A chimeric antibody (*Ab*) splices the variable light (V$_L$) and variable heavy (V$_H$) portions of the murine IgG to a human IgG. A humanized Ab splices only the complementarity determining region (*CDR*) portions from the murine monoclonal antibody (*mAb*), along with some of the adjacent "framework" regions to help maintain the conformational structure of the *CDRs*.

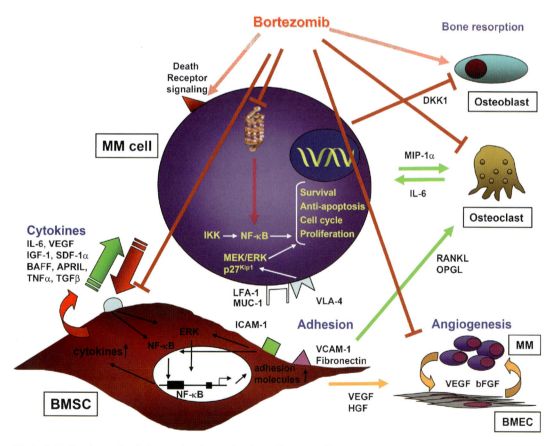

Plate 4 Molecular and cellular mechanisms of action of bortezomib.

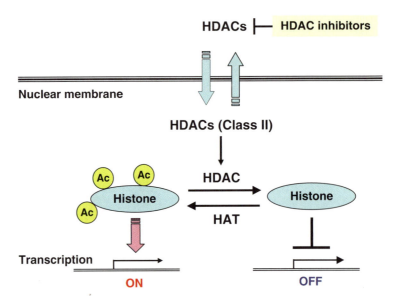

Plate 5 Among histone deacetylases (HDACs), only class II HDACs can shuttle between cytoplasm and nucleus. HDAC inhibitors block HDACs activity, thereby accumulating acetylated histones, which facilitates transcriptional activity.

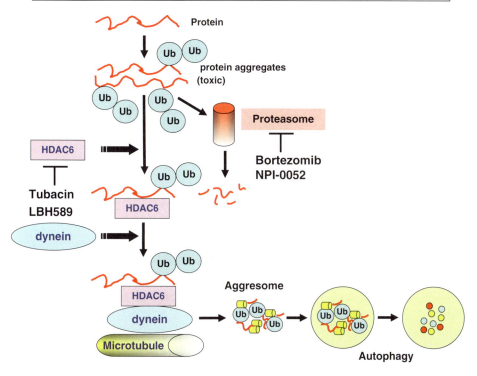

Synergistic anti-tumor activity by HDAC6 inhibitors plus proteasome inhibitors

Protein

protein aggregates
(toxic)

Proteasome

Bortezomib
NPI-0052

HDAC6

Tubacin
LBH589

dynein

HDAC6

HDAC6
dynein
Microtubule

Aggresome

Autophagy

Hideshima et al, PNAS 2005;102: 8567.
Hideshima et al, Clin Cancer Res;2005;11: 8530
Catley et al, Blood 2006;108: 3441.

Plate 6 Possible ubiquitinated protein catabolism in tumor cells and rationale for combination treatment of HDAC6 inhibitors with proteasome inhibitors. Misfolded proteins become polyubiquitinated and normally degraded by proteasomes. However, misfolded proteins can escape degradation due to abnormal or pathological conditions and form toxic aggregates. These misfolded and aggregated proteins are recognized and bound by HDAC6 through the presence of polyubiquitin chains. This allows for the loading of polyubiquitinated misfolded protein cargo onto the dynein motor complex by HDAC6. The polyubiquitinated cargo-HDAC6-dynein motor complex then travels to the aggresome, where the misfolded and aggregated proteins are processed and degraded, clearing the cell of cytotoxic protein aggregates. Inhibition of both proteasomal and aggresomal protein degradation pathway by bortezomib/NPI0052 and tubacin/LBH589, respectively, induces endoplasmic reticulum stress, followed by synergistic cytotoxicity. *HDAC* histone deacetylase.

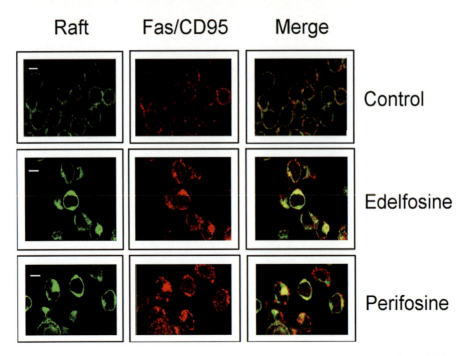

Plate 7 Edelfosine and perifosine induce coclustering of membrane rafts and Fas/CD95 in multiple myeloma (MM) cells. MM cell line MM144 was either untreated (Control) or treated with 10 μM edelfosine or perifosine for 12 h, and then stained with fluorescein isothiocyanate (FITC)-cholera toxin B subunit to identify membrane rafts (green fluorescence), due to its binding to ganglioside GM1 mainly found in lipid rafts, and with an anti-Fas/CD95 monoclonal antibody, followed by CY3-conjugated antimouse immunoglobulin antibody (red fluorescence). Areas of colocalization between membrane rafts and Fas/CD95 in the merge panels are yellow. Fas/CD95 was homogenously distributed in the cell membrane prior to alkyl-lysophospholipid treatment and formed clusters after stimulation. The FITC-cholera toxin B subunit staining shows profound reorganization of membrane rafts leading to aggregates that contain clustered Fas/CD95, as evidenced in the merge picture. Bar, 10 μm. From Gajate and Mollinedo.[36] © American Society of Hematology, used with permission.

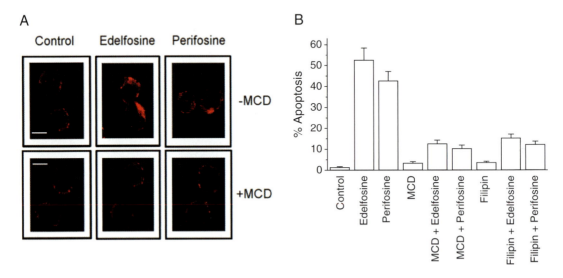

Plate 8 Disruption of membrane rafts inhibits alkyl-lysophospholipid-induced Fas/CD95 clustering and apoptosis. MM144 cells were untreated (Control) or pretreated with methyl-β-cyclodextrin (MCD) or filipin to disrupt lipid rafts, and then incubated with 10 μM edelfosine or perifosine for 12 h and analyzed for Fas/CD95 clustering by confocal microscopy (**a**), or for 24 h and examined for the percentage of apoptotic cells by flow cytometry (**b**). Bar, 10 μm. From Gajate and Mollinedo.[36] © American Society of Hematology, used with permission.

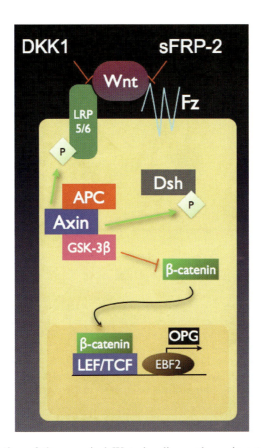

Plate 9 Regulation of the canonical Wnt signaling pathway in osteoblasts (OBL) (adapted from Pearse[6]). APC/Axin/glycogen synthase 3-beta (GSK-3β) form a complex which phosphorylates β-catenin. Phosphorylated beta-catenin is then degraded by the proteosome (not shown above). Binding of Wnt glycoproteins to the frizzled (*Fz*)/lipoprotein-related protein (*LRP*) receptor complex triggers the phosphorylation of Disheveled (*Dsh*) and LRP. Phosphorylated Dsh and LRP recruit and bind Axin, which disrupts the APC/Axin/GSK-3β complex, thereby preventing the degradation of β–catenin. As a result, β-catenin is allowed to translocate to the nucleus, where it is associated with lymphoid enhancer-binding factor (*LEF*)/T-cell transcription factor (*TCF*) to facilitate transcription of their target genes. In mature OBL, β-catenin complexes with TCF1 and TCF4 to facilitate the transcription of osteoprotegerin (*OPG*), in cooperation with early B cell factor 2 (*EBF*2). Inhibition of Wnt signaling in OBL leads to reduced expression of OPG, which results in heightened osteoclastogenesis, and increased bone resorption. Myeloma inhibits Wnt signaling through the secretion of Wnt antagonists, Dickkopf1 (*DKK*1), and secreted frizzled-related proteins2 (*sFRP*-2) (DKK1 binds to the Wnt coreceptors, LRP5/6, to block activation of the receptor complex; sFRP-2 is a decoy receptor for Wnts). Secretion of DKK1 and sFRP-2 may therefore contribute to the dysregulation of RANKL/OPG expression seen in multiple myeloma (*MM*1).

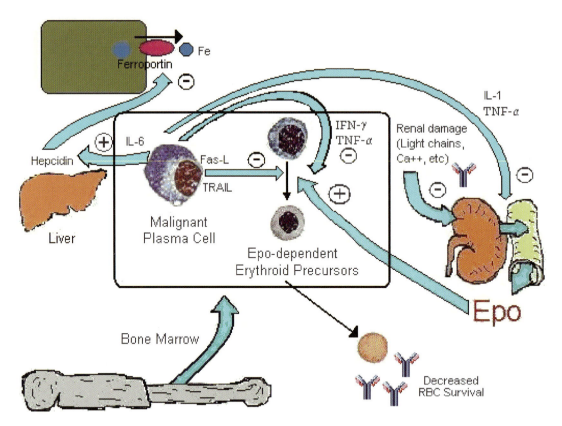

Plate 10 Pathophysiology of anemia in multiple myeloma (*MM*): As demonstrated in the figure, the pathophysiology of anemia in MM is multifactorial resulting from marrow infiltration, ineffective erythropoiesis, and iron dysregulation.

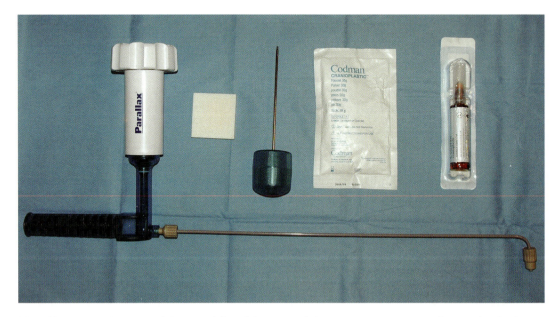

Plate 11 Vertebroplasty materials. From left to right: cement injector, cement, access needle, powdered polymer, and liquid monomer (Cranioplastic™, Codman, Boston, Massachusetts).

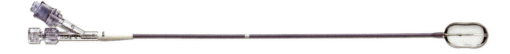

a

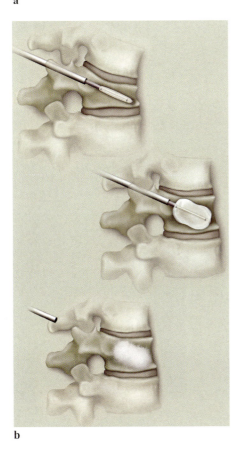

b

Plate 12 Kyphoplasty materials and technique. (**a**) Inflatable balloon tamp. (**b**) Transpedicular insertion, inflation, and removal of balloon tamp. (Images courtesy of Kyphon Inc.)

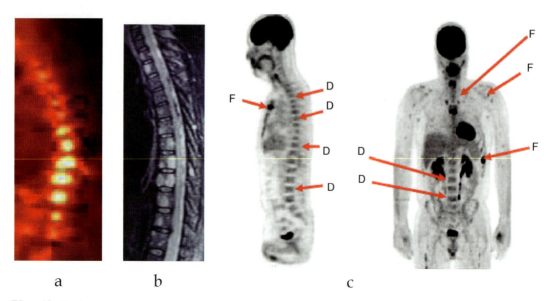

a   b   c

Plate 13 Staging with FDG-PET and CT. (**a** and **b**) FL on PET and MRI. (**a**) FDG PET scan of thoracic spine. (**b**). MRI-STIR weighted of thoracic spine. (**c**) Multiple myeloma FDG PET: severe diffuse (**d**) and focal (**f**) disease (*See Color Plates*).

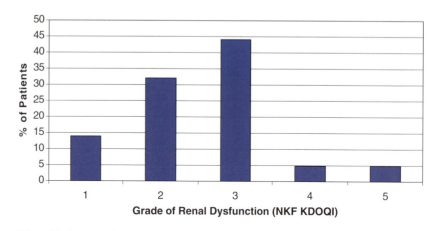

Plate 14 Degree of renal dysfunction in a single institution series of MM patients as per the National Kidney Foundation's Kidney Disease Outcomes Quality Initiative (*NKF KDOQI*) categories

Plate 15 Congo red staining of amyloid in kidney glomeruli under light microscopy. (Courtesy Dr Edit Weber)

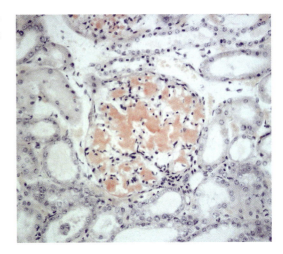

Plate 16 Green birefringence of Congo red staining in renal amyloid deposits under polarized light. (Courtesy Dr Edit Weber)

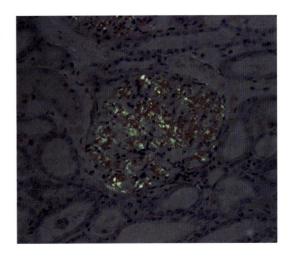

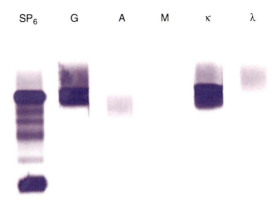

Plate 17 Protein immunofixation electrophoresis showing Immunoglobulin G (*IgG*) kappa positivity.

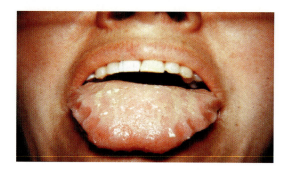

Plate 18 Macroglossia.

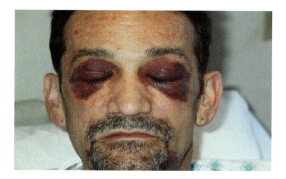

Plate 19 Periorbital purpura, raccoon eyes.

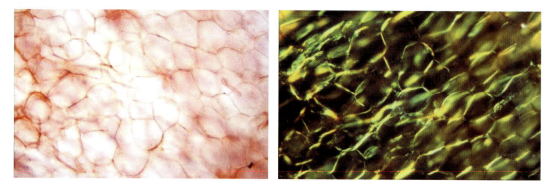

Plate 20 Fat pad aspiration, Congo red stain under polarizing microscope.

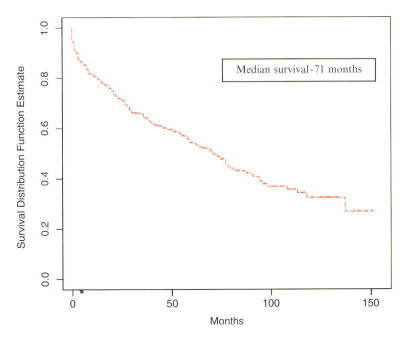

Plate 21 Kaplan-Meier survival curve of 382 patients with AL amyloidosis treated with high-dose melphalan/stem cell transplantation, Boston University Medical Center (BUMC), 1994–2006.

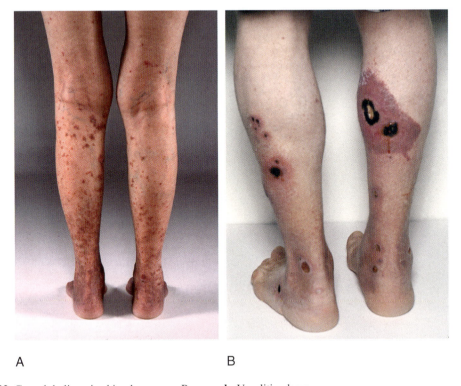

A   B

Plate 22 Cryoglobulinemic skin changes. **a**. Purpura. **b**. Vaculitic ulcers.

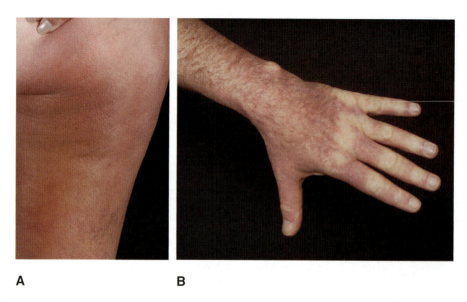

A **B**

Plate 23 Scleromyxedema skin changes. **a**. Small waxy papules. **b**. Stiffening of the skin and decreased range of motion in the hands.

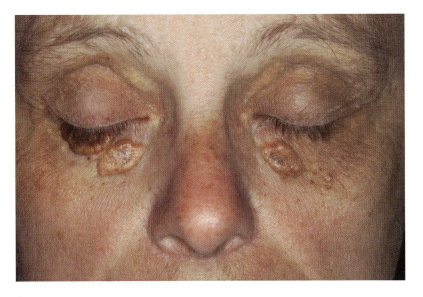

A

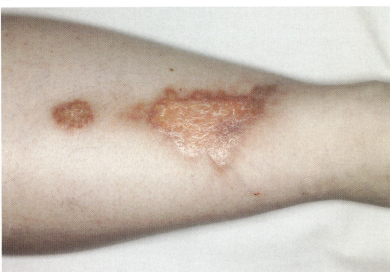

B

Plate 24 Xanthogranuloma necrobiotica skin changes. **a**. Periorbital lesions. **b**. Cutaneous involvement.

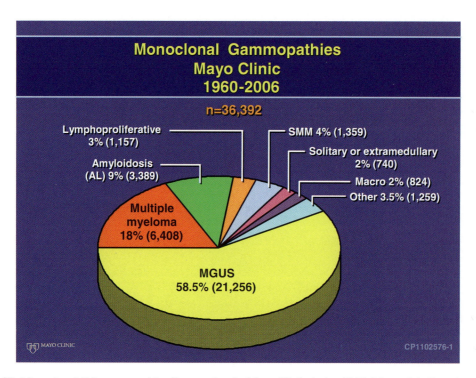

Plate 25 Monoclonal (*M*) gammopathies diagnosed at the Mayo Clinic during 2006. Macroglobulinemia; *MGUS* monoclonal gammopathy of undetermined significance, *SMM* smoldering multiple myeloma.

have been detected in 13.5%, 10.8%, and 1.6% of MALT lymphomas, respectively, and have not yet been reported in cases of LPL/WM.

The distinction between LPL/WM and IgM-secreting splenic MZL can be difficult. Bone marrow involvement is constant in splenic MZL, and serum IgM paraprotein is present in ~45% of patients. A deletion of 7q and occasionally del(10)(q22–q24) are chromosomal aberrations commonly associated with splenic MZL.[12] In most patients with nodal and splenic MZL, the IgM serum levels generally do not exceed 3 g/dL. Ocio and colleagues[39] compared the pattern of markers expressed by LPL/WM with that of splenic MZL. They emphasized that cases of LPL/WM were more likely to express κ, with an overall frequency of κ to λ of 4:5:1 versus 1:2:1 in splenic MZL cases. The combination of CD25+ and CD22+ dim best discriminates LPL/WM (88%) from splenic MZL (21%) (P < 0.001).

Clinical Features

The clinical manifestations of WM are variable. Most patients present with fatigue, shortness of breath, complications of anemia, chronic epistaxis, gingival oozing, weight loss, night sweats, and chronic infections. Lymphadenopathy occurs in 15–20% of LPL/WM patients at the time of presentation and usually is not as prominent as is seen in patients with other types of non-Hodgkin lymphoma. Splenomegaly occurs in 10–20% of patients. Other symptoms could be classified based on the mechanisms underlying the symptoms.

Manifestations Related to Direct Tumor Infiltration
WM by definition always involves the bone marrow causing anemia, leukopenia, and thrombocytopenia. One third of patients present with lymphadenopathy, splenomegaly, or hepatomegaly caused by tumor infiltration of these organs.[40] Patients with WM have been reported with infiltration of virtually every organ.[41–43] Rarely, in 3–5% of patients with WM, a lymphoplasmacytic infiltration of the lung occurs with diffuse pulmonary infiltrates, nodules, masses, or pleural effusion.[44] Orbital involvement can be caused by lesions involving the retro-orbital lymphoid tissue and lacrimal glands. Conjunctival and vitreal involvement (malignant vitreitis) have been described.[45] The Bing-Neel syndrome consists of confusion, memory loss, disorientation, motor dysfunction, and eventually coma. This syndrome is a result of long-standing hyperviscosity that alters vascular permeability and allows for perivascular infiltrations of lymphoplasmacytoid cells.[46] Schnitzler syndrome is the term for IgM monoclonal gammopathy associated with urticarial skin lesions, fever, and arthralgia.[47] Involvement of the gastrointestinal (GI) tract has also been described[48] as has the involvement of the skull base. Lytic bone lesions, however, are extremely rare, occurring in <5% of cases. These patients have typical features of WM and should be treated as such.[49]

Manifestation Related to Circulating IgM
The monoclonal IgM in WM has several unique properties such as its physical size and high carbohydrate content. IgM proteins when present in sufficiently high quantities form aggregates and bind water through their carbohydrate component, resulting in an increased oncotic pressure, an increase in the resistance to blood flow, and impaired transit through the microcirculation. They are confined to the intravascular compartment due to large size. Also the

monoclonal IgM may interact with red blood cells, increasing the viscosity of blood cells and reducing their deformability.[50] This causes an increase in the viscosity of serum. If left unchecked this may result in the hyperviscosity syndrome, a hallmark of WM. Today, it is observed in <15% of patients at diagnosis.[51] Symptoms of hyperviscosity usually appear when the normal serum viscosity of 1.4–1.8 cP reaches 4–5 cP (corresponding to a serum IgM level of at least 3 g/dL) and include chronic bleeding from the nose, gums, and GI tract. In addition, patients complain of headache, tinnitus, vertigo, impaired hearing, or ataxia. There may be blurring and loss of vision with funduscopy showing distended sausage-shaped retinal veins, flame-shaped hemorrhages, and papilledema. If untreated, edema, high output cardiac failure, somnolence, stupor, and coma may occur. The hyperviscosity syndrome is uncommon today due in part to earlier diagnosis and/or prophylactic plasmapheresis given to patients at high risk.

Monoclonal IgM can interact with circulating proteins, including several coagulation factors, and may cause prolonged clotting times. The macroglobulin can coat platelets, impair their adhesion and aggregation, and result in a prolonged bleeding time.[52]

Manifestations Related to IgM Deposition in tissues

Macroglobulinemia cutis is a condition characterized by deposition of amorphous IgM deposits in the dermis (storage papules) without evidence of malignant infiltration. These appear as firm, flesh-colored skin papules and nodules in the skin. In most patients with cutaneous involvement with WM, the skin involvement occurred after the diagnosis of WM, often many years following the diagnosis. The lesions involve the trunk commonly and less commonly the ear lobes, face, and lower extremities. The lesions appear as infiltrated, red brown papules and plaques. There are usually no symptoms attributable to the cutaneous disease.[53] The implications of cutaneous disease on the natural history and prognosis of WM are unknown.

Manifestations Related to Amyloidogenic Properties of IgM

There have been case reports of secondary amyloidosis in WM. In secondary amyloidosis, fibrils are derived from the acute-phase reactant serum amyloid A (SAA) protein, by dysregulated proteolytic cleavage, with subsequent deposition in tissues. Such rare patients may present with nephrotic syndrome and GI involvement.[54]

Deposition of monoclonal light chain as fibrillar amyloid deposits (primary amyloidosis) has been reported in WM. At our institution we identified 50 patients with a serum IgM monoclonal protein and biopsy-proven amyloidosis. The amyloidosis developed in 2% of patients with monoclonal IgM of whom 10 (20%) had WM. Compared with other patients with primary systemic amyloidosis, there was a higher incidence of amyloid cardiomyopathy in this group. There was also a higher incidence of pulmonary and pleural amyloidosis compared with amyloidosis unassociated with IgM monoclonal proteins.[55] The median age of the patients was 68 years, and λ light chain was detected in 68% of the patients.

Virtually every patient with amyloid could be diagnosed by biopsy of the subcutaneous fat, rectum, or bone marrow. Most patients received conventional chemotherapy based on melphalan or chlorambucil with median overall survival (OS) time of 24.6 months. Organ dysfunction as a result of amyloidosis was the cause of death more often than the underlying WM. The commonest cause of death was cardiac amyloid, in 53% of patients, followed by pulmonary failure, in 12%. Macroglobulinemia was the cause of death in 7% of patients. The presence or absence of cardiac amyloid had the greatest impact on survival. Of the 22 patients with cardiomyopathy at diagnosis, the median survival was 11.1 months, with only 2 of the 22 surviving longer than 5 years and none of the patients alive at 6 years. Of the 28 patients without cardiomyopathy at diagnosis, the median survival was 27 months, with 8 of the 28 being 5-year survivors.

Manifestations Related to Autoantibody Activity of IgM

Peripheral neuropathy occurs commonly in patients with WM. The incidence is hard to estimate but varies between 15 and 30%.[3] It usually presents as a slowly progressive distal symmetric sensorimotor polyneuropathy. It can also present with cranial nerve palsies or mononeuropathies.[56] Sensory abnormalities predominate early in the disease process with motor weakness appearing later on in the disease course. Tremor may also be present.[57] Electrophysiologic studies show a demyelinating neuropathy, although cases of distal axonal neuropathy and neuropathy with axonal and demyelinating features also are reported. Anti-MAG antibodies are present in 50% of patients who have neuropathy.[57] Prolongation of P100 latency on visual evoked response may be present in patients who have neuropathy and IgM paraprotein that reacts with MAG, suggesting a subclinical central involvement. Morphologic studies of the sural nerve show reduction in the number of myelinated nerve fibers and findings of demyelination and remyelination on teased nerve fiber preparation. In addition, small collections of atypical lymphocytes may be present in the perineurium or endoneurium. Immunofluorescence studies show binding of monoclonal IgM to the myelin sheaths or the endoneurium and ultrastructural studies show widening of myelin lamellae.[57]

Once neuropathic symptoms begin, typical first-line chemotherapeutic regimens are to be used as outlined below under treatment. A combination of plasmapheresis and chlorambucil may be effective in treatment of peripheral neuropathy.[58] Otherwise, the standard treatment options may be used.[50]

WM has rarely been associated with type-II cryoglobulinemia. This occurs because of antibody activity of monoclonal IgM against polyclonal IgG. This is an immune complex disease characterized by symptoms including Raynaud's phenomenon, livedo reticularis, cutaneous ulcers, skin necrosis, urticaria, visceral dysfunction, or other manifestations of vasculitis affecting small vessels of skin, kidneys, liver, and peripheral nerves. In our review of a prospectively maintained dysproteinemia database, we found 66 cases of type-II cryoglobulinemia, two patients had WM indicating the rarity of this condition. Both patients had coexisting hepatitis C infection.[59]

Furthermore, occasional patients with WM have been reported in whom monoclonal IgM may behave as an antibody against basement membrane of glomeruli, skin, and retina. As a consequence glomerulonephritis, paraneoplastic pemphigus, and retinitis may occur.[60,61] Renal disease in WM is caused by deposition of IgM along the glomerular basement membrane, lymphocyte infiltration of the interstitium, cryoglobulinemia, or amyloidosis. There are two case reports of WM associated with nephrotic syndrome. Renal involvement in WM presents as a usually mild nonselective proteinuria and microscopic hematuria. Massive proteinuria and a nephrotic syndrome may develop and is in most cases caused by amyloidosis. Bence-Jones proteinuria is present in 80–90% of the patients, but the quantity is much smaller than in MM. Acute renal failure is rare in WM. It can occur after the use of intravenous (IV) contrast, however. The nephropathy can reoccur in renal allografts.[62] In most patients, however, renal failure is chronic.

Smoldering Waldenstrom's Macroglobulinemia

Approximately 25–30% of LPL/WM patients are asymptomatic at diagnosis and are referred to as "smoldering WM." These patients have a detectable IgM monoclonal paraprotein and evidence of bone marrow infiltration with LPL cells; however, they do not have any symptoms (as outlined above) referable to tumor infiltration or the circulating IgM. The serum level of IgM is not a good marker to distinguish between the smouldering and symptomatic WM as the median and range of serum monoclonal IgM levels in asymptomatic patients overlap with those of overt WM (1.8 [0.1–70] g/dL in symptomatic patients vs 2.2 [0.2–3.6] g/dL in overt disease), according to one study reporting that IgM levels do not predict clinical status.[12] Therefore, the consensus panel definition does not include any minimum level of IgM paraproteinemia

Large-cell transformation occurs in LPL/WM, and similar to Richter transformation in CLL/SLL, the high-grade tumor may or may not arise from the same clone. The onset of large-cell transformation is usually accompanied by new onset or increasing size of lymphadenopathy, organomegaly, worsening cytopenia, and rarely hypercalcemia. Serum IgM levels may paradoxically decrease at the time of transformation, a result of dedifferentiation of the neoplastic cells. Large-cell transformation is associated with poor prognosis. Classic Hodgkin lymphoma may also occur in LPL/WM patients, similar to patients with SLL/CLL.

Approach to a Patient with Suspected WM

A thorough history, physical examination including funduscopic examination (to exclude retinal vein engorgement with hemorrhage exudates, and papilledema), and determination of a serum viscosity level (if available) should be undertaken at initial examination and on follow-up examinations as needed for evaluation of hyperviscosity. A history of oronasal bleeding, blurred vision, headache, dizziness, vertigo, ataxia, encephalopathy, or altered consciousness would suggest hyperviscosity. Most patients with a serum viscosity <4 cp will not have symptoms of hyperviscosity (normal = 1.8 cp). Those patients who demonstrated signs or symptoms suggestive of symptomatic hyperviscosity should be considered for immediate plasmapheresis, and initiation of chemotherapy as soon as possible. The tests required to aid in the diagnosis and treatment of WM are summarized in Table 3. The use of densitometry should not be adopted to determine IgM levels for serial evaluations since nephelometry remains unreliable and shows large intralaboratory as well as interlaboratory variation. Estimation of peak size on elecrophoresis is to be preferred.

Prognostic Markers and Criteria to Initiate Therapy in Waldenstrom's Macroglobulinemia

Patients with asymptomatic or smoldering macroglobulinemia should be diagnosed and recognized early. No treatment is required as they may remain stable for many years. Treatment of this cohort has not been proven to improve outcomes.[63]

Table 3 Diagnostic testing for waldenström macroglobulinemia.

1. Serum protein electrophoresis.
2. Immunofixation – to characterize the type of light and heavy chains.
3. 24-h urine collection for protein electrophoresis.
4. Serum β2-microglobulin – for prognostic evaluation.
5. Bone marrow aspiration and biopsy.
6. Cytogenetic studies.
7. Computed tomography of the abdomen and pelvis – to detect organomegaly and lymphadenopathy.
8. Blood or serum viscosity – if signs and symptoms of hyperviscosity syndrome are present or IgM >5,000

Adapted from Vijay and Gertz[3]

The median survival of patients with WM averages 5 years, but at least 20% of patients survive for more than 10 years, and 10–20% die of unrelated causes.[40] Given the long natural history of this disease it is important to be cautious in the selection of therapies. The panel convened during the Second International Workshop on WM in Athens considered that initiation of therapy was appropriate for patients who demonstrated an Hb level of <10 g/dL and/or platelet count of <100 × 109/L that were attributable to disease, bulky adenopathy, or organomegaly, or any other disease-related complaints that were serious enough to warrant therapy including recurrent fever, night sweats, weight loss, fatigue, or symptomatic manifestations associated with WM including hyperviscosity, symptomatic neuropathies, nephropathy, amyloidosis, symptomatic cryoglobulinemia, or evidence of disease transformation. In the absence of the above, close observation was recommended.

Factors Identifying Patients Likely to Require Treatment in the Short Term
The Second International Workshop on WM felt that there was insufficient data to affirm the use of any prognostic marker in the initiation and selection of therapy. Also, initiation of therapy should not be based on consideration of IgM levels per se, since these may not correlate with clinical manifestations and prognosis of WM. However, initiation of therapy is reasonable for those patients who demonstrate rising IgM levels with progressive signs or symptoms of disease.

With such variability in clinical course, determining which patient needs treatment can prove difficult. In the Italian study done by Gobbi et al.,[64] the criteria that discriminated two prognostically different populations were age (≤ or ≥70), weight loss (a minimum of 3 kg during the last 6 months), Hb level (≤ or ≤9 g/dL), and cryoglobulinemia. These criteria were valid by multivariate analysis. The group that had one or less adverse criteria had a median survival of 84 months compared to 48 months in the group that had more than one adverse criterion. In the study by Morel et al.,[65] statistically significant adverse prognostic factors for survival were age 65 years or older, male gender, albumin level lower than 40 g/L, Hb level lower than 12 g/dL, platelet count less than150 × 10(9)/L, white blood cell count less than 4 × 10(9)/L, a high number of cytopenias, and hepatomegaly. Taking age (age 65 years or older, 1 point; younger than 65 years,

0 points), albumin (<40 g/L, 1 point; 40 g/L or more, 0 points), and total number of cytopenias (no cytopenia, 0 points; 1 cytopenia, 1 point; 2 or 3 cytopenias, 2 points) into account, the patients can be divided into three groups with low (score 0 or 1), intermediate (score 2), or high (score 3 or 4) risk, associated with 5-year survival rates at 87%, 62%, and 25%, respectively.

We analyzed 337 patients with symptomatic WM from our database who were diagnosed between 1960 and 2001. The median survival from the time of diagnosis was 6.4 years. The median disease-specific survival was 11.2 years. Univariate analysis for OS identified the following adverse prognostic factors: age > 65 years ($P < 0.001$), organomegaly ($P < 0.001$), elevated β2-microglobulin (<0.001), anemia (Hb < 10.0 g/dL) ($P = 0.01$), leucopenia (<4.0 × 109/L) ($P = 0.03$), thrombocytopenia (<150 × 109/L) ($P = 0.01$), serum albumin < 40 g/L ($P = 0.001$), and quantitative IgM < 0.4 g/L ($P = 0.04$). On multivariate analysis, age > 65 years and organomegaly were associated with poor prognosis. A prognostic model was built based on these two variables. Patients at high risk (1–2 risk factors, median survival 4.2 years) experienced worse survival than patients at low risk (0 risk factors, median survival 10.6 years), $P < 0.001$. β2-microglobulin levels of 4 mg/L or higher were associated with a threefold increase in the risk of death when added to the prognostic model.[66] It seems reasonable to consider treatment in the patients with poor prognostic criteria at the outset. However, this approach has not been validated in a prospective model yet.

Response Criteria for Treatment of WM
During the Second International Workshop on WM, a consensus panel proposed guidelines for standardized response criteria.[67]

Complete Response: Complete response (CR) is defined as complete disappearance of serum and urine monoclonal protein by immunofixation, resolution of lymphadenopathy and organomegaly, and no signs or symptoms that are directly attributable to WM (unexplained recurrent fevers ≥38.4°C, drenching night sweats, 10% weight loss, hyperviscosity, or symptomatic cryoglobulinemia). These findings must be confirmed 6 weeks later. The bone marrow examination should not show malignant cells.

Partial Response: Partial response (PR) is defined as a >50% reduction in serum monoclonal IgM on protein electrophoresis and a >50% reduction in bulky lymphadenopathy and organomegaly on computed tomography. There should be no new symptoms, signs, or other evidence of disease relapse.

Relapse from CR is defined as reappearance of serum monoclonal protein as determined by immunofixation confirmed by a second measurement or reappearance of clinically significant symptoms and signs attributable to WM or development of any other clinically significant disease-related complication.

Progressive Disease: Progressive disease is defined as >25% increase in serum monoclonal IgM protein levels from the lowest attained response value as determined by serum electrophoresis and confirmed by measurement 3 weeks later. For monoclonal protein nadirs <20 g/L, an absolute increase of 5 g/L is required to determine progressive disease. Progressive disease may also be documented if there is worsening of anemia, thrombocytopenia, leukopenia, lymphocytosis, lymphadenopathy, organomegaly, or any other symptom such as unexplained fever, night sweats, weight loss, neuropathy, nephropathy, symptomatic cryoglobulinemia, or amyloidosis directly attributable to WM.

Treatment of WM

Various treatment strategies for WM are available depending on the disease presentation, aggressiveness of symptoms, goals of treatment, and patient and physician preferences. The optimal treatment strategy is unclear due to the lack of phase III trials comparing different options. Standardized response criteria were only recently published so comparison between studies is not always feasible.

Plasmapheresis

In some patients with WM, the predominant symptoms are caused by elevated serum viscosity. Because 70–80% of monoclonal IgM protein is contained within the intravascular space, plasmapheresis is an effective means of rapidly reducing the amount of circulating IgM.[68] Continuous-flow centrifugation systems, which are fully automated, are usually used. Usually a 1–1.5 times plasma volume exchange is performed, which will lower plasma IgM levels by around 70%.[69] Higher exchange volumes have not been shown to be more helpful because the incremental decrease in plasma proteins will be minimal in subsequent plasma exchanges. Higher volumes also increase the time required to perform the process. The typical replacement fluid is 5% human albumin and 0.9% saline. If the patients have had a recent hemostatic challenge (within 48 h of the procedure) or will be challenged we provide three units of FFP at the very end of the plasmapheresis. In case of monoclonal IgM protein, a single plasmapheresis session can result in significant clinical improvement and serum viscosity reduction by 50% or more.[70] In severe cases, daily or every other day single plasma volume exchanges are used initially until symptoms are relieved. Definitive cytoreductive therapy should follow the plasmapheresis once the patient is clinically better from the plasmapheresis. Drug therapy should be withheld until after plasma exchange so that protein-bound drugs are not removed from the circulation by this procedure[50] The rare patient will need long-term plasma exchange if hyperviscosity persists or if the patient is resistant to treatment.

Splenectomy

There have been several case reports of patients with refractory macroglobulinemia and massive splenomegaly who responded to splenectomy. In one series of two patients with macroglobulinemia and massive splenomegaly, palliative splenectomy produced a CR and both patients are alive at 12 and 13 years, respectively, after splenectomy.[71] Another treatment option described in a case report was splenic irradiation. However, this produced a PR and was followed by a splenectomy with the patient being in remission for 6 years after splenectomy.[72] The proposed mechanism of response was removal of a large number of tumor cells. However, it is unclear whether some of the patients who benefited from splenectomy might have had splenic MZL as these case series were much older.

Chemotherapy

Alkylating Agents: The historical primary therapy for patients with WM has been the administration of oral alkylating agents, such as chlorambucil, melphalan, or cyclophosphamide. The agent most commonly used has been oral chlorambucil.

There have been very few phase III studies in this disease. In one study done at our institution, patients were randomized to receive chlorambucil 0.1 mg/kg/day or chlorambucil 0.3 mg/kg/day orally for 7 days, repeated every 6 weeks. Seventy-nine percent of patients given continuous therapy had an objective improvement by either reduction in serum M-protein or increase in Hb. Sixty-eight percent of patients given chlorambucil intermittently had an objective response. The size of the liver decreased by ≥ 2 cm in 55% of patients, and the size of the spleen decreased ≥ 2 cm in 67%. Lymphadenopathy decreased in 71%. However, acute leukemia or refractory anemia developed in four patients. The median duration of survival was 5.4 years, and there were no statistically significant differences between the regimens. CRs are rare with this regimen. The rate of decrease in monoclonal protein level was slow and treatment for 6 months is advised prior to abandoning the drug as ineffective.[73] Another combination of alkylator agents was reported by Annibali et al.[74] They used melphalan (6 mg/m^2 p. o.), cyclophosphamide (125 mg/m^2 p.o.), and prednisone (40 mg/m^2 p.o.) given on days 1 through 7 every 4–6 weeks for a maximum of 12 courses; patients with responsive or stable disease (SD) then received chlorambucil (3 mg/m^2 p.o. per day) and prednisone (6 mg/m^2 p.o. per day) until progression. Following induction therapy, 55 of 71 evaluable patients (77%) responded and another 10% had SD. Median duration of response and OS were 5.3 and 5.5 years, respectively. Toxicity was limited to transient nausea and vomiting and mild neutropenia. One patient developed AML and one patient developed MDS. The authors stressed the cost-effectiveness compared with other therapies of equivalent benefit.

The addition of corticosteroids does not seem to increase response rate or survival, although they may be useful in patients who present or develop autoimmune hemolytic anemia, mixed cryoglobulinemia, or cold agglutinin disease.[50]

Nucleoside Analogs: Fludarabine and 2-chlorodeoxyadenosine (cladribine) are purine nucleoside analogs that have been effective for a variety of low-grade lymphoid malignancies. A trial performed by the Southwest Oncology Group (SWOG) treated 182 patients with symptomatic or progressive WM with four to eight cycles of therapy with fludarabine (30 mg/m2 of body surface area (BSA) daily for 5 days every 28 days).[75] The overall rate of response to fludarabine therapy was 36% (with 2% complete remissions, 1% unconfirmed CR). Patients who were 70 years old or older had a substantially lower likelihood of response than did younger patients. On multivariate analysis, a serum β2M level of 3 mg/L or higher, Hb level below 120 g/L, and serum IgM level below 40 g/L (4 g/dL) were significant adverse prognostic factors for survival. In an update to this study,[76] the authors found that event-free and OSs were significantly longer in the presence of lower levels of serum β2m. Neither the occurrence of response (CR or PR) using current criteria nor the time to response was associated with superior overall or event-free survival. Serum β2m is the dominant prognostic indicator in WM, and this factor alone therefore can provide valuable disease risk assessment. Also, the authors found that response to therapy using current criteria is not a reliable predictor for survival in this disease. At least 50% reduction in serum monoclonal protein levels was documented in 40% of patients, including CR in 3%. The median time to response was 2.8 months (range, 0.7–22.5 months). The median event-free and OS times were 43 and 84 months, respectively.[76]

The authors published prognostic criteria dividing patients into four stages and risk groups each with unique 5-year OS and progression-free survival (PFS). Stage A or low-risk patients had β2M < 3 mg/L + Hb ≥ 120 g/L and had a 5 year OS of 87% and 5 year PFS of 83%. Stage B or medium-risk patients had β2M < 3 mg/L + Hb < 120 g/L and had a 5 year OS of 63% and 5 year PFS of 55%. Stage C or medium-risk patients had β2M ≥ 3 mg/L and IgM β 40 g/L and had a 5 year OS of 53% and 5 year PFS of 33%. Stage D or high-risk patients had β2M ≥ 3 mg/L and IgM < 40 g/L and had a 5 year OS of 21% and 5 year PFS of 12%. These criteria could be used to help determine which patients would potentially benefit from early treatment; however, this has not been validated in a prospective fashion.

In a study looking at the efficacy of fludarabine in WM in the relapsed setting, 92 patients with WM resistant to first-line therapy (42 patients) or with first relapse (50 patients) after alkylating-agent therapy were randomly assigned to receive fludarabine (25 mg/m2 of BSA on days 1–5) or cyclophosphamide, doxorubicin (Adriamycin), and prednisone (CAP; 750 mg/m2 cyclophosphamide and 25 mg/m2 doxorubicin on day 1 and 40 mg/m2 prednisone on days 1–5).[77] There was no difference between the two arms with regards to hematologic toxicity or infections. As expected, mucositis and alopecia occurred significantly more often in patients treated with CAP. After six cycles of treatment, PRs were obtained in 14 patients (30%) treated with fludarabine and 5 patients (11%) treated with CAP and the difference was statistically significant. There were no CRs in either treatment group. The responses were more durable in patients treated with fludarabine compared to CAP (19 months vs 3 months). There was no statistical difference in the median OS in the two study arms. This was due to the use of effective salvage agents in the patients who relapsed. Four cases of secondary acute myeloid leukemia/myelodysplastic syndrome (AML/MDS) and three cases of disease transformation into diffuse large-cell lymphoma (Richter syndrome) occurred in the fludarabine group, and two cases of secondary AML/MDS and two cases of disease transformation into diffuse large-cell lymphoma occurred in the CAP group. Fludarabine was thus more active than CAP in salvage therapy of WM in terms of response rate and durability of response.

Fludaribine has also been explored in other studies in combination with alkylating agents and with monoclonal antibodies. In a study from Australia,[78] four different combinations with fludarabine were studied. These included FC (fludarabine 25 mg/m2 for 3 days plus cyclophosphamide 250 mg/m2 for 3 days; n = 9), FM (fludarabine 25 mg/m2 for 3 days plus mitoxantrone 10 mg/m2 for 1 day; n = 3), FCR (FC plus rituximab 375 mg/m2; n = 5), or fludarabine/rituximab (n = 1). Four patients had previously untreated disease, and 14 had pretreated disease. Patients received a median of four cycles (range, 1–6 cycles), with grade 3 or higher neutropenia and infection complicating 25% and 4% of cycles, respectively. Objective responses (all partial) were attained in 13 patients (76%). Response rates did not significantly differ by regimen, previous treatment, age, performance status, β2-microglobulin level, Hb level, time from diagnosis, previous fludarabine exposure, or alkylator refractoriness. Median remission duration was 38 months; no previously untreated patient had died at a median of 37 months of follow-up, and the actuarial 5-year survival rate was 55% for pretreated patients. No cases of secondary myelodysplasia or leukemia were encountered.

Single-agent cladribine was given to 26 consecutive, previously untreated and symptomatic patients with WM.[79] Patients received two courses as outpatients through a central catheter for 7 days using a continuous infusion strategy. Responding patients were followed without further therapy and were scheduled to receive two additional treatments with 2CdA on disease relapse. The overall response rate (ORR)was 85% (22 of 26 patients, 95% , 65–96%) including three patients who achieved a CR and 19 patients who had a PR. Treatment was well tolerated, with no acute hematologic toxicity. One patient died 16 months after retreatment of disseminated HSV infection. A marked and sustained reduction in CD4+ lymphocytes occurred in all patients and may have contributed to a fatal infection with disseminated herpes simplex in one patient. With a median follow-up of 13 months, five patients had relapsed, four patients were retreated, and all retreated patients responded to 2CdA.

In another smaller study,[80] ten symptomatic patients without prior therapy received 2CdA daily at 0.12 mg/kg body weight in a 2-h IV infusion over 5 consecutive days repeated every 28 days for four cycles. Patients achieving a remission received interferon alfa-2 15μg subcutaneously 3 times a week for 1 year. This was a prospective multicenter study. All ten patients responded to 2CdA (100%; 95% CI, 68–100%), with one complete (CR) and eight partial responders (PR): one patient had only one 2-CdA cycle and showed a minor improvement (MR). Tolerability of the regimen was good with infections occurring in two patients (WHO grade 1 and 2 only). After a median observation period of 57 weeks, three patients had shown progression, including one who died of lymphoma. Several other studies of cladribine in the patients with untreated WM show similar high response rates.[81,82,83] The median time to a 50% reduction in monoclonal protein was 1.2 months, and the median PFS was 18 months in one study. However, other studies have reported longer times to response (median, 5.8 months).[50]

Pentostatin has been studied in WM albeit in smaller studies. A small phase-II study looked at the combination regimen of PC with and without R (pentostatin/cyclophosphamide with or without rituximab) in 14 patients with WM and three patients with LPL without monoclonal serum IgM, followed by a maintenance regimen with rituximab (375 mg/m² every 3 months) for patients exhibiting a CR or a PR after 4–6 cycles.[84] Nine patients never received treatment, and eight had been previously treated with 1–3 regimens. The first nine patients received PC therapy (pentostatin 4 mg/m² plus cyclophosphamide 600 mg/m²), and eight patients received the same combination with rituximab 375 mg/m² on day 1. Cycles were repeated every 3 weeks. The ORR was 64.7%, with 2 CRs (11.7%) and 9 PRs (52.9%). In patients who received rituximab ($n = 13$) simultaneously or subsequently, the ORR was 76.9%. Grade 3 hematologic toxicity occurred after 9 of 49 cycles (18.3%), and grade 4 toxicity occurred after two cycles (4%). In many patients after completion of chemotherapy, IgM levels continued to decline.

Stem Cell Transplantation for WM

In spite of therapeutic advances made in the treatment of WM it still remains incurable. High-dose therapy followed by autologous SCT (ASCT) has shown activity in several malignancies that share similarities with WM, such as MM, FL, and CLL. However, the published experience is limited. The Center for International Blood and Marrow Transplant Research (CIBMTR) provided the largest review on this topic recently.[85] They reviewed 57 patients who underwent stem cell transplantation (SCT) (35 allogeneic and 22 autologous) for WM. Complete data was available for 36 patients who underwent transplantation and was the subject of the analysis. The data was from 24 transplant centers in seven countries. Overall, 53% of the patients ($n = 19$) had received three or more prior therapies with 68% receiving nucleoside analogs. Twenty-six patients underwent allogeneic SCT, and ten patients underwent ASCT. It is possible that more patients underwent allogeneic transplantation due to heavier pretreatment making autologous transplantation not feasible due to failure of adequate stem cell collection. The median follow-up of the survivors was 65 months (range, 24–103 months). Fifty-two percent of the patients were resistant to their most recent salvage chemotherapy, with only 33% of the patients being in at least a PR at the time of transplantation. Twenty-five percent of patients were progressing or relapsing despite salvage chemotherapy at the time of transplant. There were no statistically significant differences in any parameters between the two SCT groups. Median follow-up of survivors was 65 months (range, 24–103 months). Seventy percent of patients in the ASCT group received peripheral blood stem cells and the other 30% received bone marrow as the stem cell source. Fifty percent of patients in the allogeneic SCT group received a bone marrow graft, 46% received a peripheral blood stem cell graft, and 4% received both. A TBI-containing conditioning regimen was utilized in 50% of the patients. More patients in the allogeneic SCT group received TBI conditioning than in the ASCT group. A nonmyeloablative conditioning regimen was given to 19% of the patients ($n = 5$) who received allogeneic SCT. Nine patients (25%) achieved complete remission (CR) at 100 days posttransplantation, 12 (33%) were in PR, 4 (11%) were in less than PR, 1 (3%) had progressive disease, and 10 (28%) were not evaluable/had died at 100 days. The response rates to transplantation were similar regardless of the disease status at time of transplantation. Overall NRM was 32% (95% CI, 18%–49%) for the entire group. NRM was 40% for the allogeneic SCT group and 11% for the ASCT group at both 1 year and 3 years. The overall risk of progression was 15% at 1 year, with 16% for the allogeneic SCT group and 11% for the ASCT group, and 28% at 3 years, with 29% for the allogeneic SCT group and 24% for the ASCT group. PFS was 53% at 1 year, with 44% for the allogeneic group and 78% for the autologous group, and 40% at 3 years, with 31% for the allogeneic group and 65% for the autologous group. OS was 64% at 1 year, with 58% for the allogeneic group and 80% for the autologous group, and 52% at 3 years, with 46% for the allogeneic group and 70% for the autologous group. At a median follow-up of 65 months, 15 of the 36 patients (42%) were alive, 9 from the allogeneic SCT group (35%) and 6 (60%) from the ASCT group. Despite the absence of further NRM beyond year 1, relapses continued to occur, indicating absence of a strong graft versus tumor effect in the allogeneic transplantation group.

Others have also reviewed their experience.[86–90] A variety of preparative regimens have been used. Some patients received high-dose chemotherapy alone, such as melphalan or the combination of carmustine, etoposide, cytarabine, and melphalan (BEAM), whereas others were treated with total-body irradiation (TBI) combined with melphalan, cyclophosphamide, or etoposide. The median age of these patients was ~55 years. All studies indicate a treatment-related mortality of <5% with autologous transplantation. Almost all patients had an objective response, indicating the inherent chemosensitive nature of this disease. Overall it appears that ASCT for advanced WM is feasible and safe with good response rates. It is well known that prior exposure to nucleoside analogs impairs stem cell collection and candidates who are potential stem cell transplant candidates need to be identified and have stem cells harvested and stored early in the course of their disease.

Allogeneic SCT on the contrary seems to carry a much higher risk of NRM and higher TRM. Therefore, this cannot be recommended outside of a trial setting. Innovative transplantation strategies with nonmyeloablative conditioning may be required. In a study available in abstract form,[91] a nonmyeloablative conditioning regimen involving low-dose TBI at 2 Gy with fludarabine 90 mg/m^2 and postgrafting immunosuppression with mycophenolate mofetil and cyclosporine was administered to nine WM patients with a median age of 54 years who had failed a median of four prior regimens. Six patients received stem-cell transplantations from HLA-matched siblings, and three patients received stem-cell transplantations from HLA-matched unrelated donors. Among the eight patients evaluated for response, there were four CRs and two PRs. There was no transplantation-related mortality. However, follow-up data is required and until available this modality should be limited to the research setting.

Monoclonal Antibody Therapy

Rituximab: WM almost always widely expresses CD20. Therefore, anti-CD20 or rituximab is a rational treatment for this disease. Several small studies have suggested a benefit from the anti-CD20 monoclonal antibody rituximab (Rituxan) in patients with WM. In an initial retrospective study by Treon et al.,[92] 30 patients with WM who received treatment with single-agent rituximab was reported. The median number of prior treatments for these patients was 1 (range 0–6), and 14 patients (47%) received a nucleoside analog before rituximab therapy. Overall, treatment was well tolerated with a median of four treatment cycles with rituxan. Median IgM levels for all patients declined from 2,403 mg/dL (range 720–7639 mg/dL) to 1,525 mg/dL (range 177–5,063 mg/dL) after rituximab therapy ($P = 0.001$), with 8 of 30 (27%) and 18 of 30 (60%) patients demonstrating >50% and >25% decline in IgM, respectively. Seventeen patients had a pre- and posttreatment bone marrow performed and the lymphoplasmacytic cell involvement declined from 60% (range 5–90%) to 15% (range 0–80%). Overall responses after treatment with rituximab were as follows: 8 (27%) and 10 (33%) of the patients achieved a partial (PR) and a minor (MR) response, respectively, and an additional 9 (30%) of the patients demonstrated SD. No patients attained a CR.

A phase-II prospective study reported from Europe confirmed these results.[93] Twenty-seven consecutive patients with WM were treated with rituximab (375 mg/m^2) for 4 weeks. Twelve patients were previously treated, with two patients being primary refractory, and eight patients having a chemotherapy-resistant relapse, and two patients were relapsing while being observed without treatment. Seven patients had received at least three previous regimens. Twelve patients (44%) achieved a PR after treatment with rituximab. Median time to response was 3.3 months. Responses occurred in 6 (40%) of 15 previously untreated patients and in 6 (50%) of 12 pretreated patients. Patients with a serum IgM <40 g/L had a significantly higher response rate. The median time to progression for all patients was 16 months, and with a median follow-up of 15.7 months, 9 of 12 responding patients remain free of progression. Treatment with rituximab was well tolerated, with approximately one fourth of patients experiencing some mild (WHO grade 1and 2) infusion-related toxicity. One patient out of three had significant improvement of neuropathy with treatment. The other two patients had SD with unchanged neuropathy. Another patient had resolution of autoimmune hemolytic anemia with the treatment.

A response to rituximab is not uniformly observed in all patients in spite of the uniform expression of CD20 on these cells. One of the mechanisms involved in Rituximab activity is ADCC (antibody-dependent cellular cytotoxicity). In ADCC, the antibody binds to tumor cells and then is engaged by effector cells via their receptors for immunoglobulin G (FcγRs). A role for Fcγ receptor has been suggested by a recent study that a polymorphism of FcγRIIIa was associated with tumor response in FL patients treated with rituximab as first-line therapy. In this study,[94] the FcγRIIIa 158 valine/valine and the Fc γRIIa 131 histidine/histidine genotypes were found to be independently associated with the response rate and freedom from progression in patients treated with rituximab. In a study of receptor polymorphisms in WM, the response trend was higher for patients with FcγRIIIA-48L/H (38.5%) versus -48L/R (25.0%) and LL (22.0%), and was significantly higher for patients with FcγRIIIA-158V/V (40.0%) and -V/F (35%) versus -158F/F (9.0%; $P = 0.030$). Responses for patients with FcγRIIIA-48L/L were higher when at least one valine was present at FcγRIIIA-158 ($P = 0.057$), thereby supporting a primary role for FcγRIIIA-158 polymorphisms in predicting rituximab responses. Therefore, when valine was absent from Fcγ IIIA–158, the response rate to rituximab was only 9%. When at least one valine was present, the response rate ranged between 35% and 40%.[95] Studies have also been done using an extended schedule of rituximab consisting of four weekly courses at 375 mg/m2/week, which are repeated later by another 4-week course. This demonstrates response rates similar to standard-dose rituximab (around 44% PR rate) with a prolonged time to progression at 13–29 months. Responses rates were higher in patients with lower circulating monoclonal IgM (<6000 mg/dL in two studies and <4000 mg/dL in another study).[9698]

Time to response after rituximab is slow and exceeds 3 months on the average.[50] In many patients, a transient increase in serum IgM may be noted immediately after initiation of treatment. Such an increase does not herald treatment failure, and most patients will return to their baseline serum IgM level by 12 weeks.[99,100] In one of these studies, of the 54 patients for whom the IgM measurements were available, 29 (54%) experienced an increase in IgM levels between baseline and the first scheduled post baseline time point. At 2 months, 59% continued to have elevated IgM levels, and at 4 months, elevated IgM levels persisted in 27%. In responding patients, the IgM decreased within 4 months of the initiation of therapy. This may have therapeutic consequences, in that patients with baseline serum IgM levels of more than 50 g/dL or serum viscosity of more than 3.5 cp may be particularly at risk for a hyperviscosity-related event, and in such patients, plasmapheresis should be considered in advance of rituximab therapy. Because of the decreased likelihood of response in patients with higher IgM levels as well as the possibility that serum IgM and viscosity levels may abruptly increase, rituximab monotherapy should be used with caution for the treatment of patients at risk for hyperviscosity symptoms.

There may also be an increase in cryoglobulin levels after initiation of rituximab therapy.[101]

Because rituximab is an active and nonmyelosuppressive agent, its combination with chemotherapy has a sound rationale, Treon et al. reported on its combination with CHOP chemotherapy (cyclophosphamide, doxorubicin, vincristine, prednisone, and rituximab). They reported three CRs unconfirmed, eight PRs, one MR. At a median follow-up of 9 months, 10 of the 11 patients who had a major response remained in remission.[102]

Treon et al.[103] administered a combination of rituximab and fludarabine to 32 previously untreated patients. An objective response was noted in 80% of patients with a median follow-up of 17 months and 92% of patients remain without progression.

Alemtuzumab: With the use of three-color flow cytometry, Owen et al. demonstrated CD52 expression in the B-cells of 47 cases of WM, with a median of 99% of cells (range, 81–100%) expressing the antigen. Antigen density was very similar to that seen in CLL.[104] Owen et al. presented data on the use of alemtuzumab in previously treated patients with WM.[105] This was a phase-II study with seven heavily pretreated with WM. This group included five men and two women with a median age of 62 years. Patients were previously treated with purine analog (seven patients), alkylating agents [6], anthracycline-containing regimens[5], and rituximab [4]. Five of the seven patients were refractory to their previous regimen while two patients were treated in untested relapse. Alemtuzumab was given by IV infusion at a dose of 30 mg for 3 days/week for a maximum of 12 weeks. Patients received a median of 10 weeks of therapy (range, 2–12 weeks) and all received prophylaxis against Pneumocystis carinii pneumonia and herpes infection. Weekly PCR was used to monitor for CMV reactivation. Responses were documented in five of the seven patients, with PRs in four patients and a CR in one patient. A further patient had SD whereas the remaining patient was considered to have failed when treatment was discontinued at 2 weeks following bacterial sepsis. Of the four patients who had previously received rituximab, responses were documented in two patients (both PR) while SD was documented in another. The median duration of response was 13 months from the completion of therapy (range, 1–37 months). Infective complications were common composed of CMV reactivation requiring ganciclovir in three patients and bacterial infections necessitating hospital admission in three patients. Herpes simplex reactivation, aspergillosis, and tuberculosis all occurred in one patient each. Of the responding patients, four have died, two from infective complications (aspergillosis and tuberculosis), one from progressive disease, and one from an unrelated cause while still in a PR. One responding patient remains in a PR at 37 months posttreatment. This treatment modality while effective had significant infectious morbidity associated with it. It is also unclear if the infectious risks are magnified in patients in whom purine analogs were used previously with their own immunosuppressive complications. Further studies with this agent are warranted.

New Agents

Thalidomide: In the initial phase-II study of single-agent thalidomide, the drug was administered at a starting dose of 200 mg orally at bedtime, with dose escalation in 200-mg increments every 14 days, as tolerated, to a maximum dose of 600 mg. Five (25%) of 20 patients achieved a PR. The time to response was short, ranging between 0.8 and 2.8 months, and the median duration of response was 11 months. Responses occurred in three of ten previously untreated and in two of ten pretreated patients. None of the patients treated during refractory relapse or with disease duration exceeding 2 years responded to thalidomide. Because of side effects, most patients could not tolerate more than 400 mg of thalidomide daily. The common toxicities of thalidomide were noted with constipation, somnolence, fatigue, and mood changes. The daily dose of thalidomide was escalated to 600 mg in only five patients (25%), and in seven patients (35%), this agent was discontinued within 2 months because of intolerance.[106] Two subsequent studies assessed the activity of the combination of clarithromycin, low-dose thalidomide, and dexamethasone in patients with WM. In one study,[107] twelve patients with WM underwent treatment with BLT-D, utilizing clarithomycin 500 mg orally twice daily, thalidomide 50 mg orally escalated to 200 mg daily, and dexamethasone 40 mg orally once weekly. All patients received prophylaxis with omeprazole and enteric-coated aspirin. All patients had been previously treated with at least one purine analog or alkylating agent. With a minimum of 6 weeks of treatment, ten had a significant response (83%) consisting of three near complete, three major, four partial, and two MRs. Toxicities were GI (primarily constipation), neurological (100%); endocrine (42%), and thrombotic (8%). All were WHO grade 1 or 2 toxicities. However, neurological toxicity was particularly severe with this regimen. In another study of this regimen,[108] the response rate was 25%, all PRs. Thalidomide is nonmyelosuppressive, immunomodulatory, and antiangiogenic and may be a reasonable choice for patients with pancytopenia in whom first-line therapies have failed or if they are not candidates for alkylating agents, nucleoside analogs, or rituximab therapy.

Studies are ongoing with thalidomide derivatives such as CC-5013 (lenalidomide) and CC-4047 in WM.

Bortezomib: Bortezomib (PS-341) is a reversible proteasome inhibitor that has been approved in the treatment of relapsed MM. Several preclinical studies of this agent in WM have shown evidence of activity in terms of inducing growth arrest and apoptosis of the WM–Wayne State University (WM–WSU) cell-line model. The proposed mechanism of action of this drug is through suppression of nuclear factor–κB activity and decreased expression of kinases required for growth and survival

In a phase-II study reported by Chen et al.,[109] 27 patients with WM previously treated with up to two prior chemotherapy regimens received bortezomib at a dose of 1.3 mg/m2/day on days 1, 4, 8, and 11 in a 21-day cycle. Patients were planned to be treated until PD or until two cycles after CR. Of the 27 patients enrolled, the overall objective response rate was 26% (95% CI, 11–46%). Twenty-one patients (78%) had at least a 25% decrease in their monoclonal protein. The median PFS was 16.3 months and duration of response was 10 months for patients with PR and 14.3 months with SD. Common toxicities observed with bortezomib was fatigue, nausea, neuropathy, myalgias, infections (non-neutropenic), diarrhea, and constipation. Twenty patients (74%) developed new or worsening neuropathy while on study. Neuropathy led to dose reductions in four patients and discontinuation of study drug in five patients. Drug-related toxicity led to discontinuation of bortezomib in 12 patients (44%). Another phase-II study[110] of ten heavily pretreated patients with bortezomib revealed a 60% PR rate with an expected duration of response exceeding 11 months. This agent therefore has activity in WM: however, more studies are needed to elucidate its place in the sequence of treatments for WM.

Other agents that are being studied in WM include oblimersen sodium. Oblimersen sodium, G3139 (oblimersen sodium; Genasense, Genta, Inc., Berkeley Heights, NJ), is an antisense phosphorothioate oligonucleotide compound designed specifically to bind to the first six codons of the human Bcl-2 mRNA sequence. This binding results in degradation of bcl-2 mRNA and subsequent decrease in Bcl-2 protein translation and intracellular concentration.[111] The Bcl-2 protein, which is located in the inner mitochondrial membrane, is a key inhibitor of apoptosis and confers resistance to treatment with traditional cytotoxic chemotherapy, radiotherapy, and monoclonal antibodies. Preclinical models appear promising.

Other agents that have been observed to be effective include sildenafil, a phosphodiesterase inhibitor, used conventionally to treat erectile dysfunction. Reduction in serum monoclonal protein was unexpectedly noted in five WM patients. One patient had a CR while four patients had a reduction in the IgM paraprotein.[112] In a prospective study[113] of 30 patients with WM not meeting criteria for treatment, use of sildenafil citrate induced a response in 63% of patients, with 17% of patients demonstrating an MR ($\geq$25% decrease in IgM). This drug therefore warrants further study.

One patient was found to have normalization of blood counts and a more than 50% decrease in his M spike with the initiation of testosterone supplementation.[114] Other therapeutic options currently being evaluated for WM include I-131 tositumomab.[115] Use of I-131 tositumomab in a patient with WM that had transformed into a diffuse large B-cell lymphoma resulted in a CR with disappearance of IgM. Other agents that are being studied in WM include Akt inhibitors such as perifosine, triciribine, protein kinase C inhibitors (such as AZD6244 and enzastaurin), and combinations of these novel agents with established drugs. Atacicept is a protein that binds to APRIL and BLyS receptors, thereby enhancing cytotoxicity. In a phase-I study of atacicept, out of four heavily pretreated patients with WM three patients had SD and one patient had minimal response with >25% decrease in serum IgM.

Conclusions

The treatment of WM has undergone tremendous changes in the last decade. Several new classes of drugs are available for treatment now. It is conceivable that with these treatments the median survival of patients will increase. Given the slow progression of the disease in many cases it is imperative not to overtreat patients and thus expose them to toxic or infectious side effects.

References

1. Waldenstrom J. Incipient myelomatosis or "essential" hyperglobulinema with fibrinogenopenia. A new syndrome? Acta Med Scand. 1944;117:216–22.
2. Waldenström J. Macroglobulinemia. A review. Haematologica 1986;71:437–40.
3. Vijay A, Gertz MA. Waldenstrom Macroglobulinemia. Blood. 2007 Feb 15; [Epub ahead of print].
4. Groves FD, Travis LB, Devesa SS, Ries LA, Fraumeni JF Jr. Waldenstroms macroglobulinemia: incidence patterns in the United States, 1988–1994. Cancer. 1998;82(6):1078–81.
5. Linet MS, Humphrey RL, Mehl ES, Brown LM, Pottern LM, Bias WB, McCaffrey L. A case-control and family study of Waldenstroms macroglobulinemia. Leukemia. 1993;7(9):1363–9.

6. Williamson LM, Greaves M, Waters JR, Harling CC. Waldenstroms macroglobuli-naemia: three cases in shoe repairers. BMJ. 1989;298:498–9.

7. Travis LB, Li CY, Zhang ZN, Li DG, Yin SN, Chow WH, et al. Hematopoietic malignancies and related disorders among benzene-exposed workers in China. Leuk Lymphoma. 1994;14:91–102.

8. Fine JM, Muller JY, Rochu D, Marneux M, Gorin NC, Fine A, Lambin P. Waldenstroms macroglobulinemia in monozygotic twins. Acta Med Scand. 1986;220(4):369–73.

9. Renier G, Ifrah N, Chevailler A, Saint-Andre JP, Boasson M, Hurez D. Four broth-ers with Waldenstrom's macroglobulinemia. Cancer. 1989;64(7):1554–9.

10. McMaster ML. Familial Waldenstrom's macroglobulinemia. Semin Oncol 2003;30(2):146–52.

11. Treon SP, Hunter ZR, Aggarwal A, Ewen EP, Masota S, Lee C, Ditzel Santos1 D, Hatjiharissi E, Xu L, Leleu X, Tournilhac O, Patterson1 CJ, Manning R, Branagan AR, Morton CC. Characterization of familial Waldenström's macroglobulinemia. Ann Oncol. 2006;17(3):488–94.

12. Lin P, Medeiros LJ. Lymphoplasmacytic lymphoma/Waldenstroms macroglob-ulinemia: an evolving concept. Adv Anat Pathol. 2005;12(5):246–55.

13. Harris NL, Jaffe ES, Stein H, et al. A revised European–American classification of lymphoid neoplasms: a proposal from the International Lymphoma Study Group. Blood. 1994;84:1361–92.

14. Jaffe ES, Harris NL, Stein H, Vardiman JW, editors. World Health Organization classification of tumours: pathology and genetics of tumours of hematopoietic and lymphoid tissues. Lyon: IARC Press, 2001:132–4.

15. Owen RG, Barrans SL, Richards SJ, O'Connor SJ, Child JA, Parapia LA, Morgan GJ, Jack AS. Waldenstrom macroglobulinemia. Development of diagnostic criteria and identification of prognostic factors. Am J Clin Pathol. 2001;116(3):420–8.

16. San Miguel JF, Vidriales MB, Ocio E, et al. Immunophenotypic analysis of Waldenstrom's macroglobulinemia. Semin Oncol. 2003;30:187–95.

17. Konoplev S, Medeiros LJ, Bueso-Ramos CE, Jorgensen JL, Lin P. Immunophenotypic profile of lymphoplasmacytic lymphoma/Waldenstrom macroglobulinemia. Am J Clin Pathol. 2005;124(3):414–20.

18. Owen RG, Hillmen P, Rawstron AC, et al. CD52 expression in Waldenström's mac-roglobulinemia: implications for alemtuzumab therapy and response assessment. Clin Lymphoma. 2005;5:278–81.

19. Offit K, Parsa NZ, Filippa D, et al. t(9;14)(p13;q32) denotes a subset of low-grade non-Hodgkin's lymphoma with plasmacytoid differentiation. Blood. 1992;80:2594–9.

20. Iida S, Rao PH, Ueda R, et al. Chromosomal rearrangement of the PAX-5 locus in lymphoplasmacytic lymphoma with t(9;14)(p13;q32). Leuk Lymphoma. 1999;34:25–33.

21. Mansoor A, Medeiros LJ, Weber DM, Alexanian R, Hayes K, Jones D, Lai R, Glassman A, Bueso-Ramos CE. Cytogenetic findings in lymphoplasmacytic lym-phoma/Waldenstroms macroglobulinemia. Chromosomal abnormalities are associ-ated with the polymorphous subtype and an aggressive clinical course. Am J Clin Pathol. 2001;116(4):543–9.

22. Schop RF, Kuehl WM, Van Wier SA, Ahmann GJ, Price-Troska T, Bailey RJ, Jalal SM, Qi Y, Kyle RA, Greipp PR, Fonseca R. Waldenstrom macroglobulinemia neoplastic cells lack immunoglobulin heavy chain locus translocations but have frequent 6q deletions. Blood. 2002;100(8):2996–3001.

23. Liu YC, Miyazawa K, Sashida G, Kodama A, Ohyashiki K. Deletion (20q) as the sole abnormality in Waldenström macroglobulinemia suggests distinct pathogen-esis of 20q11 anomaly. Cancer Genet Cytogenet. 2006;169:69–72.

24. Ocio EM, Schop RF, Gonzalez B, Van Wier SA, Hernandez-Rivas JM, Gutierrez NC, Garcia-Sanz R, Moro MJ, Aguilera C, Hernandez J, Xu R, Greipp PR, Dispenzieri A, Jalal SM, Lacy MQ, Gonzalez-Paz N, Gertz MA, San Miguel JF,

Fonseca R. 6q deletion in Waldenstrom macroglobulinemia is associated with features of adverse prognosis. Br J Haematol. 2007;136(1):80–6.

25. Chang WJ, Schop RF, Price-Troska T, Ghobrial I, Kay N, Jelinek DF, Gertz MA, Dispenzieri A, Lacy M, Kyle RA, Greipp PR, Tschumper RC, Fonseca R, Bergsagel PL. Gene-expression profiling of Waldenstrom macroglobulinemia reveals a phenotype more similar to chronic lymphocytic leukemia than multiple myeloma. Blood. 2006;108(8):2755–63. Epub 2006 Jun 27.

26. Klein B, Zhang XG, Lu ZY, Bataille R. Interleukin 6 in human multiple myeloma. Blood. 1995;85:863–72.

27. Hatzimichael EC, Christou L, Bai M, Kolios G, Kefala L, Bourantas KL. Serum levels of IL-6 and its soluble receptor (sIL-6R) in Waldenström's macroglobulinemia. Eur J Haematol. 2001;66:1–6.

28. Calame KL. Plasma cells: finding new light at the end of B cell development. Nat Immunol. 2001;2:1103–8.

29. Hunter Z, Leleu X, Hatjiharissi E, Santos D, Xu L, Ho A, et al. IgA and IgG hypogammaglobulinemia are associated with mutations in the APRIL/BLYS receptor TACI in Waldenström's. Blood. (ASH Annual Meeting Abstracts) 2006;108:Abstract 228.

30. Elsawa SF, Novak AJ, Grote DM, Ziesmer SC, Witzig TE, Kyle RA, et al. B-lymphocyte stimulator (BLyS) stimulates immunoglobulin production and malignant B-cell growth in Waldenström macroglobulinemia. Blood. 2006;107:2882–8. Epub 2005 Nov 22.

31. Adamia S, Crainie M, Kriangkum J, Mant MJ, Belch AR, Pilarski LM. Abnormal expression of hyaluronan synthases in patients with Waldenström's macroglobulinemia. Semin Oncol. 2003;30:165–8.

32. Adamia S, Treon SP, Reiman T, Tournilhac O, McQuarrie C, Mant MJ, et al. Potential impact of a single nucleotide polymorphism in the hyaluronan synthase 1 gene in Waldenström's macroglobulinemia. Clin Lymphoma. 2005;5:253–6.

33. Kriangkum J, Taylor BJ, Reiman T, et al. Origins of Waldenstroms macroglobulinemia: does it arise from an unusual B–cell precursor? Clin Lymphoma. 2005;5:217–9.

34. Kyle RA, Garton JP. The spectrum of IgM monoclonal gammopathy in 430 cases. Mayo Clin Proc. 1987;62(8):719–31.

35. Shanafelt TD, Byrd JC, Call TG, Zent CS, Kay NE. Narrative review: initial management of newly diagnosed, early-stage chronic lymphocytic leukemia. Ann Intern Med. 2006;145:435–47.

36. Bertoni F, Zucca E, Cavalli F. Mantle cell lymphoma. Curr Opin Hematol. 2004;11(6):411–8.

37. Dispenzieri A, Rajkumar SV, Gertz MA, Fonseca R, Lacy MQ, Bergsagel PL, Kyle RA, Greipp PR, Witzig TE, Reeder CB, Lust JA, Russell SJ, Hayman SR, Roy V, Kumar S, Zeldenrust SR, Dalton RJ, Stewart AK. Treatment of newly diagnosed multiple myeloma based on Mayo Stratification of Myeloma and Risk-adapted Therapy (mSMART): consensus statement. Mayo Clin Proc. 2007;82(3):323–41.

38. Parsonnet J, Hansen S, Rodriguez L, Gelb AB, Warnke RA, Jellum E, Orentreich N, Vogelman JH, Friedman GD. Helicobacter pylori infection and gastric lymphoma. N Engl J Med. 1994;330(18):1267–71.

39. Ocio EM, Hernandez JM, Mateo G, Sanchez ML, Gonzalez B, Vidriales B, Gutierrez NC, Orfao A, San Miguel JF. Immunophenotypic and cytogenetic comparison of Waldenstroms macroglobulinemia with splenic marginal zone lymphoma. Clin Lymphoma. 2005;5(4):241–5.

40. Dimopoulos MA, Panayiotidis P, Moulopoulos LA, et al. Waldenstroms macroglobulinemia: clinical features, complications, and management. J Clin Oncol. 2000;18:214–26.

41. Dimopoulos MA, Alexanian R. Waldenstroms macroglobulinemia. Blood. 83:1452–9.

42. Fudenberg HH, Virella G. Multiple myeloma and Waldenstroms macroglobulinemia: unusual presentations. Semin Hematol. 1980;17(1):63–79. Review

43. Lin P, Buesco–Ramos C, Wilson CS, et al. Waldenstrom macroglobulinemia involving extramedullary sites. Am J Surg Pathol. 2003;27:1104–13.
44. Fadil A, Taylor DE. The lung and Waldenstroms macroglobulinemia. South Med J. 1998;91:681–5.
45. Oveliama J, Friedman AH. Ocular manifestations of multiple myeloma, Waldenstroms macroglobulinemia and benign monoclonal gammopathy. Surv Ophthalmol. 1981;26:157–69.
46. Civit T, Coulbois S, Baylac F, et al. Waldenstroms macroglobulinemia and cerebral lymphoplasmacytic proliferation: Bing and Neel syndrome—Apropos of a new case. Neurochirurgie. 1997;43:245–9.
47. Schnitzler L, Schubert B, Boasson M, Gardais J, Tourmen A. Urticaire chronique, lésions osseuses, macroglobulinémie IgM: maladie de Waldenström? Bull Soc Fr Derm Syph. 1974;81:363–7.
48. Rosenthal JA, Curran WJ Jr, Schuster SJ. Waldenström's macroglobulinemia resulting from localized gastric lymphoplasmacytoid lymphoma. Am J Hematol. 1998;58:244–5.
49. Dimopoulos MA, Galani E, Matsouka C. Waldenstroms macroglobulinemia., Hematol Oncol Clin North Am. 1999;13(6):1351–66.
50. Dimopoulos MA, Kyle RA, Anagnostopoulos A, and Treon SP. Diagnosis and Management of Waldenstrom's Macroglobulinemia. J Clin Oncol. 2005;23(7):1564–77.
51. Gertz MA, Kyle RA. Hyperviscosity syndrome. J Intensive Care Med. 1995;10:128–41.
52. Farhangi M, Merlini G. The clinical implications of monoclonal immunoglobulins. Semin Oncol. 1986;13:366–79.
53. Libow LF, Mawhinney JP, Bessinger GT. Cutaneous Waldenstrom's macroglobulinemia: report of a case and overview of the spectrum of cutaneous disease. Am Acad Dermatol. 2001;45(6 Suppl):S202–6.
54. Gardyn J, Schwartz A, Gal R, Lewinski U, Kristt D, Cohen AM. Waldenstrom's macroglobulinemia associated with AA amyloidosis. Int J Hematol. 2001;74(1):76–8.
55. Gertz MA, Kyle RA, Noel P. Primary systemic amyloidosis: a rare complication of immunoglobulin M monoclonal gammopathies and Waldenstrom's macroglobulinemia. J Clin Oncol. 1993;11:914–20.
56. Baldini L, Nobile-Orazio E, Guffanti A, Barbieri S, Carpo M, Cro L, . Peripheral neuropathy in IgM monoclonal gammopathy and Waldenström's macroglobulinemia: a frequent complication in elderly males with low MAG-reactive serum monoclonal component. Am J Hematol. 1994;45:25–31.
57. Kwan JY. Paraproteinemic neuropathy. Neurol Clin. 2007;25(1):47–69.
58. Dalakas MC, Flaum MA, Rick M, : Treatment of polyneuropathy in Waldenstrom's macroglobulinemia: role of paraproteinemia and immunologic studies. Neurology. 1983;33:1406–10.
59. Bryce AH, Kyle RA, Dispenzieri A, Gertz MA. Natural history and therapy of 66 patients with mixed cryoglobulinemia. Am J Hematol. 2006;81(7):511–8.
60. Lindstrom FD, Hed J, Enestrom S. Renal pathology of Waldenstrom's macroglobulinemia with monoclonal antiglomerular antibodies and nephritic syndrome. Clin Exp Immunol. 1980;41:196–204.
61. Sen HN, Chan CC, Caruso RC, et al. Waldenstrom's macroglobulinemia–associated retinopathy. Ophthalmology. 2004;111:535–9.
62. Bradley JR, Thiru S, Bajallan N, Evans DB. Renal transplantation in Waldenstrom's macroglobulinaemia. Nephrol Dial Transplant. 1988;2:214–6.
63. Alexanian R, Weber D, Delasalle K, Cabanillas F, Dimopoulos M. Asymptomatic Waldenstrom's macroglobulinemia. Semin Oncol. 2003;30(2):206–10.
64. Gobbi PJ, Bettini R, Montecucco C, et al. Study of Prognosis in Waldenstrom's macroglobulinemia: a proposal for a simple binary classification with clinical and investigational utility. Blood. 1994;83:2939–45.
65. Morel P, Monconduit M, Jacomy D, et al. Prognostic factors in Waldenstrom's macroglobulinemia: a report on 232 patients with the description of a new scoring system and its validation on 253 other patients. Blood. 2000;96:852–8.

66. Ghobrial IM, Fonseca R, Gertz MA, Plevak MF, Larson DR, Therneau TM, Wolf RC, Hoffmann RJ, Lust JA, Witzig TE, Lacy MQ, Dispenzieri A, Vincent Rajkumar S, Zeldenrust SR, Greipp PR, Kyle RA. Prognostic model for disease-specific and overall mortality in newly diagnosed symptomatic patients with Waldenstrom macroglobulinaemia. Br J Haematol. 2006;133(2):158–64.

67. Weber D, Treon SP, Emmanouilides C, et al. Uniform response criteria in Waldenstrom's macroglobulinemia: Consensus Panel recommendation from the Second International Workshop on Waldenstrom's Macroglobulinemia. Semin Oncol. 2003;30:127–31.

68. Dimopoulos MA, Kyle RA, Anagnostopoulos A, Treon SP. Diagnosis and management of Waldenström's macroglobulinemia. J Clin Oncol. 2005;23(7):1564–77.

69. Kaplan AA. Therapeutic apheresis for the renal complications of multiple myeloma and the dysglobulinemias. Ther Apher. 2001;5:171–5.

70. Zarkovic M, Kwaan HC. Correction of hyperviscosity by apheresis. Semin Thromb Hemost. 2003;29:535–42.

71. Humphrey JS, Conley CL. Durable complete remission of macroglobulinemia after splenectomy: a report of two cases and review of the literature. Am J Hematol. 1995;48(4):262–6.

72. Takemori N, Hirai K, Onodera R, Kimura S, Katagiri M. Durable remission after splenectomy for Waldenstrom's macroglobulinemia with massive splenomegaly in leukemic phase. Leuk Lymphoma. 1997;26(3–4):387–93.

73. Kyle, RA, Greipp, PR, Gertz, MA, et al. Waldenstrom's macroglobulinaemia: a prospective study comparing daily with intermittent oral chlorambucil. Br J Haematol. 2000;108:737.

74. Annibali O, Petrucci MT, Martini V, Tirindelli MC, Levi A, Fossati C, Del Bianco P, Mandelli F, Foa R, Avvisati G. Treatment of 72 newly diagnosed Waldenstrom macroglobulinemia cases with oral melphalan, cyclophosphamide, and prednisone: results and cost analysis. Cancer. 2005;103(3):582–7.

75. Dhodapkar MV, Jacobson JL, Gertz MA, Rivkin SE, Roodman GD, Tuscano JM, Shurafa M, Kyle RA, Crowley JJ, Barlogie B. Prognostic factors and response to fludarabine therapy in patients with Waldenstrom macroglobulinemia: results of United States intergroup trial (Southwest Oncology Group S9003). Blood. 2001;98(1):41–8.

76. Dhodapkar MV, Jacobson JL, Gertz MA, Crowley JJ, Barlogie B. Prognostic factors and response to fludarabine therapy in Waldenstrom's macroglobulinemia: an update of a US intergroup trial (SW0G S9003). Semin Oncol. 2003;30(2):220–5.

77. Leblond V, Levy V, Maloisel F, Cazin B, Fermand JP, Harousseau JL, Remenieras L, Porcher R, Gardembas M, Marit G, Deconinck E, Desablens B, Guilhot F, Philippe G, Stamatoullas A, Guibon O; French Cooperative Group on Chronic Lymphocytic Leukemia and Macroglobulinemia. Multicenter, randomized comparative trial of fludarabine and the combination of cyclophosphamide-doxorubicin-prednisone in 92 patients with Waldenstrom macroglobulinemia in first relapse or with primary refractory disease. Blood. 2001;98(9):2640–4.

78. Tam CS, Wolf MM, Westerman D, Januszewicz EH, Prince HM, Seymour JF. Fludarabine combination therapy is highly effective in first-line and salvage treatment of patients with Waldenstrom's macroglobulinemia. Clin Lymphoma Myeloma. 2005;6(2):136–9.

79. Dimopoulos MA, Kantarjian H, Weber D, O'Brien S, Estey E, Delasalle K, Rose E, Cabanillas F, Keating M, Alexanian R. Primary therapy of Waldenstrom's (12):2694–8.

80. Fridrik MA, Jager G, Baldinger C, et al. First–line treatment of Waldenstrom's disease with cladribine. Ann Hematol. 1997;74:7–10.

81. Hellmann A, Lewandowski K, Zauche JM. Effect of a 2–hour infusion of 2–chlorodeoxyadenosine in the treatment of refractory or previously untreated Waldenstrom's macroglobulinemia. Eur J Haematol. 1999;63:35–41.

82. Delannoy A, Van de Neste E, Michaux JL, et al. Cladribine for Waldenstrom's macroglobulinemia. Br J Haematol. 1999;104:933–4.

83. Hampshire A, Saven A: update of bolus administration of cladribine in the treatment of Waldenstrom's macroglobulinemia. Blood. 2003;102:402a, (abstr).

84. Hensel M, Villalobos M, Kornacker M, Krasniqi F, Ho AD. Pentostatin/cyclophosphamide with or without rituximab: an effective regimen for patients with Waldenstrom's Macroglobulinemia /lymphoplasmacytic lymphoma. Clin Lymphoma Myeloma. 2005;6(2):131–5.

85. Anagnostopoulos A, Hari PN, Perez WS, Ballen K, Bashey A, Bredeson CN, Freytes CO, Gale RP, Gertz MA, Gibson J, Goldschmidt H, Lazarus HM, McCarthy PL, Reece DE, Vesole DH, Giralt SA. Autologous or allogeneic stem cell transplantation in patients with Waldenstrom's macroglobulinemia. Biol Blood Marrow Transplant. 2006;12(8):845–54.

86. Desikan R, Dhodapkar M, Siegel D, et al. High–dose therapy with autologous haemopoietic stem cell support for Waldenstrom's macroglobulinemia. Br J Haematol. 1999;105:993–6.

87. Anagnostopoulos A, Dimopoulos MA, Aleman A, et al. High-dose chemotherapy followed by stem-cell transplantation in patients with resistant Waldenstrom's macroglobulinemia. Bone Marrow Transplant. 2001;27:1027–9.

88. Toumilhac O, Leblond V, Tabrizi R, et al. Transplantation in Waldenstrom's macroglobulinemia: the French experience. Semin Oncol. 2003;30:291–6.

89. Dreger P, Stilgenbauers S, Seyfarth B, et al. Autologous and allogeneic stem cell transplantation for treatment of Waldenstrom's macroglobulinemia, 3rd International Workshop on Waldenstrom's Macroglobulinemia, Paris, France, October, 2004, p 70.

90. Fassas A, Dhodapkar M, Mc Coy J, et al. Management of Waldenstrom's macroglobulinemia in the pre–rituximab era: update on US Intergroup Trial 59003 and the Arkansas autotransplant experience, 3rd International Workshop on Waldenstrom's Macroglobulinemia, Paris, France, October, 2004, p 59.

91. Maloney DG, Sandmaier BM, Maris M, et al. Allogeneic hematopoietic cell transplantation for refractory Waldenstrom's macroglobulinemia: replacing high-dose cytotoxic therapy with graft-versus-tumor effect. Blood. 2003;102:472b, (abstr).

92. Treon SP, Hansen M, Branagan AR, Verselis S, Emmanouilides C, Kimby E, Frankel SR, Touroutoglou N, Turnbull B, Anderson KC, Maloney DG, Fox EA. Polymorphisms in FcgammaRIIIA (CD16) receptor expression are associated with clinical response to rituximab in Waldenstrom's macroglobulinemia. J Clin Oncol. 2005;23(3):474–81.

93. Dimopoulos MA, Zervas C, Zomas A, Kiamouris C, Viniou NA, Grigoraki V, Karkantaris C, Mitsouli C, Gika D, Christakis J, Anagnostopoulos N. Treatment of Waldenstroms macroglobulinemia with rituximab. J Clin Oncol. 2002;20(9):2327–33.

94. Weng WK, Levy R. Two immunoglobulin G Fc receptor polymorphisms independently predict response to rituximab in patients with follicular lymphoma. J Clin Oncol. 2003;21:3940–47.

95. Treon SP, Hansen M, Branagan AR, Verselis S, Emmanouilides C, Kimby E, Frankel SR, Touroutoglou N, Turnbull B, Anderson KC, Maloney DG, Fox EA. Polymorphisms in FcgammaRIIIA (CD16) receptor expression are associated with clinical response to rituximab in Waldenstrom's macroglobulinemia. J Clin Oncol. 2005;23(3):474–81.

96. Dimopoulos MA, Zervas C, Zomas A, et al. Treatment of Waldenström's macroglobulinemia with rituximab. J Clin Oncol. 2002;20:2327–33.

97. Dimopoulos MA, Zervas K, Zomas A, et al. Treatment of Waldenstrom's macroglobulinemia with rituximab: prognostic factors for responses and progression. Leuk Lymphoma. 2004;45:2057–61.

98. Treon P, Emmanoullides CA, Kimby E, et al: Extended rituximab therapy in Waldenstrom's macroglobulinemia. Ann Oncol. 2005;16:132–8.

99. Ghobrial IM, Fonseca R, Greipp PR, et al. The initial "flare" of IgM level after rituximab therapy in patients diagnosed with Waldenstrom Macroglobulinemia. An Eastern Cooperative Oncology Group Study. Blood. 2003;102:448a, (abstr).

100. Treon SP, Branagan AR, Hunter Z, et al. Paradoxical increases in serum IgM and viscosity levels following rituximab in Waldenstrom's macroglobulinemia. Ann Oncol. 2004;15:1481–3.

101. Ghobrial IM, Uslan DZ, Call TG, Witzig TE, Gertz MA. Initial increase in the cryoglobulin level after rituximab therapy for type II cryoglobulinemia secondary to Waldenstrom macroglobulinemia does not indicate failure of response. Am J Hematol. 2004;77(4):329–30.

102. Treon SP, Hunter Z, Barnagan AR. CHOP plus rituximab therapy in Waldenstrom's macroglobulinemia. Clin Lymphoma. 2005;5(4):273–7.

103. Treon SP, Branagan A, Wasi P, et al. Combination therapy with rituximab and fludarabine in Waldenstrom's macroglobulinemia. 3rd International Workshop on Waldenstrom's Macroglobulinemia, Paris, France, October 2004, p 27.

104. Owen RG, Hillmen P, Rawstron AC. CD52 expression in Waldenstrom's macroglobulinemia: implications for alemtuzumab therapy and response assessment. Clin Lymphoma. 2005;5(4):278–81.

105. Owen RG, Rawstron AC, Osterborg A, et al. Activity of alemtuzumab in relapsed/refractory Waldenstrom's macroglobulinemia. Blood. 2003;102:644a, (abstr).

106. Dimopoulos MA, Zomas A, Viniou NA, et al. Treatment of Waldenstrom's macroglobulinemia with thalidomide. J Clin Oncol. 2001;19:3596–601.

107. Coleman M, Leonard J, Lyona L, et al. Treatment of Waldenstrom's macroglobulinemia with clarithromycin, low–dose thalidomide and dexamethasone. Semin Oncol. 2003;30:270–4.

108. Dimopoulos MA, Tsatalas C, Zomas A, et al. Treatment of Waldenstrom's macroglobulinemia with single–agent thalidomide or with the combination of clarithromycin, thalidomide and dexamethasone. Semin Oncol. 2003;30:265–9.

109. Chen CI, Kouroukis CT, White D, Voralia M, Stadtmauer E, Stewart AK, Wright JJ, Powers J, Walsh W, Eisenhauer E; National Cancer Institute of Canada Clinical Trials Group. Bortezomib is active in patients with untreated or relapsed Waldenstrom's macroglobulinemia: a phase II study of the National Cancer Institute of Canada Clinical Trials Group. J Clin Oncol. 2007;25(12):1570–5. Epub 2007 Mar 12.

110. Dimopoulos MA, Anagnostopoulos A, Kyrtsonis MC, Castritis E, Bitsaktsis A, Pangalis GA. Treatment of relapsed or refractory Waldenstrom's macroglobulinemia with bortezomib. Haematologica. 2005;90(12):1655–8.

111. Frankel S. Oblimersen sodium (G 3139 Bcl–2 antisense oligonucleotide) therapy in Waldenstrom's macroglobulinemia. Semin Oncol. 2003;30:300–4.

112. Treon SP, Tourmihac O, Branagan AR, et al. Clinical responses to sildenafil in Waldenstrom's macroglobulinemia. Clin Lymphoma. 2004;5:205–7.

113. Patterson CJ, Soumerai J, Hunter Z, Leleu X, Ghobrial I, Treon SP. Sildenafil citrate suppresses disease progression in patients with Waldenström's macroglobulinemia [abstract]. J Clin Oncol. 2006;24(18 Suppl):435S.

114. Porrata LF, Markovic SN. Androgenic therapy for Waldenstrom's macroglobulinemia. Am J Hematol. 2006;81(11):892–3.

115. Tsai DE, Maillard I, Downs LH, Alavi A, Nasta SD, Glatstein E, Schuster SJ. Use of iodine 131I-tositumomab radioimmunotherapy in a patient with Waldenstrom's macroglobulinemia. Leuk Lymphoma. 2004;45(3):591–5.

Chapter 33

AL (Immunoglobulin Light-Chain) Amyloidosis

Vaishali Sanchorawala

Introduction

The amyloidoses are a group of diseases that have in common the extracellular deposition of pathologic, insoluble fibrils in various tissues and organs. The fibrils have a characteristic beta-pleated sheet configuration that produces apple-green birefringence under polarized light when stained with Congo red dye.[1] Many different proteins can misfold and form amyloid fibrils, and the types of amyloidosis are classified based on the amyloidogenic protein as well as by the distribution of amyloid deposits as either systemic or localized.[2] In the systemic amyloidoses, the amyloidogenic protein is produced at a site distant from the site of amyloid deposition. In contrast, in localized disease, the amyloidogenic protein is produced at the site of amyloid deposition (Table 1).

AL (primary) amyloidosis is the most common type of systemic amyloidosis. Although AL amyloidosis is typically viewed as a rare disease, its incidence is similar to that of Hodgkin's lymphoma or chronic myelogenous leukemia.[3] It is estimated to affect 5–12 persons per million per year, although autopsy studies suggest that the incidence might be higher.[4] The amyloiodogenic protein in AL amyloidosis is an immunoglobulin light chain or a fragment of a light chain produced by a clonal population of plasma cells in the bone marrow. The plasma cell burden in this disorder is low, typically 5–10%, although in ~10–15% of patients AL amyloidosis occurs in association with multiple myeloma.[5]

Several advances during the past decade have substantially impacted the approach to treatment and the prognosis of AL amyloidosis. This chapter will focus on diagnosis, assessment of organ involvement, and treatment of the disease. Treatments aimed at inducing hematologic remissions to improve patient survival and the function of affected organs, as well as aspects of symptomatic treatment that are relatively unique to this disease, will be presented.

Table 1 Types of amyloidosis.

Disease	Precursor protein	Amyloid protein
Systemic disease		
AL amyloidosis	Immunoglobulin light chain	AL
AA amyloidosis	Serum amyloid A (SAA)	AA
Familial amyloidosis	Transthyretin, apolipoprotein AI, apolipoprotein AII, fibrinogen A α, gelsolin, lysozyme	ATTR, AApoI, AApoII, AFibA, Alys, AGel
Senile amyloidosis	Transthyretin (wild-type)	ATTR
Dialysis-related amyloidosis	Beta-2-microglobulin	Aβ2M
Localized disease		
Localized AL	Immunoglobulin light chain	AL
Alzheimer's disease	Aβ protein precursor	Aβ
Creutzfeldt-Jakob disease	Prion protein	APrP
Type 2 diabetes mellitus	Islet amyloid polypeptide	AIAPP

Pathogenesis

A detailed elaboration of the pathogenesis of AL amyloidosis is beyond the scope of this chapter, but a few points warrant discussion (Fig. 1).[1,6] A key feature of all types of amyloidosis is abnormal folding of a protein that is normally soluble. In AL amyloidosis, the abnormal folding is the result of either a proteolytic event or an amino acid sequence that renders a light chain thermodynamically unstable and prone to self-aggregation. The aggregates form protofilaments that associate into amyloid fibrils. In all types of amyloidosis, glycosaminoglycan (GAG) moieties of proteoglycans and serum amyloid P protein interact with the amyloid fibrils or deposits, promoting fibril formation and stability in tissue. Organ dysfunction results from disruption of tissue architecture by amyloid deposits. However, increasing evidence is emerging indicating that amyloidogenic precursor proteins or precursor aggregates have direct cytotoxic effects that also contribute to disease manifestations.[7]

In AL amyloidosis, the clonal plasma cells express light chains of the lambda (λ) isotype more frequently than the kappa (κ), with a ratio of ~3:1, despite the greater proportion of κ-than λ-expressing plasma cells in a normal bone marrow. The immunoglobulin light-chain variable region (V_L) genes expressed by AL clones include several that are less frequently expressed in the normal repertoire, indicating that germ line-encoded features may contribute to the propensity of certain subtypes of light chains to form amyloid. Evidence of antigen selective pressure on amyloidogenic V_L genes as well as homogeneity of somatic mutations support the concept that the monoclonal transformation of most amyloidogenic plasma cells occurs after B-cell maturation and clonal selection in the lymphoid follicle.[8] Associations between immunoglobulin light-chain V_L germ line gene use and amyloid-related organ involvement have been described by several groups. This organ tropism may be related to the antigenic affinities of the clonal light chains.[9]

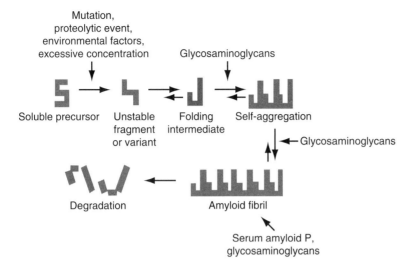

Fig. 1 Amyloid formation from precursor protein to tissue deposit (Adapted from Dember, Nephrology Forum, 2005).

Clinical Presentations

The organs most frequently affected in AL amyloidosis are the kidneys and the heart; however, virtually any tissue other than the brain can be involved.[10] Kidney involvement usually presents as nephrotic syndrome with progressive worsening of renal function. In a small proportion of patients (~10%), amyloid deposition occurs in the renal vasculature or tubulointerstitium, causing renal dysfunction without significant proteinuria.[6] Amyloid deposition in the heart results in rapidly progressive heart failure due to restrictive cardiomyopathy. The ventricular walls are concentrically thickened with normal or reduced cavity size. The ventricular ejection fraction can be normal or only slightly decreased, but impaired ventricular filling limits cardiac output. Low voltage on the electrocardiogram (ECG) is found in a high proportion of patients and is often associated with a pseudo-infract pattern.[11] Hepatomegaly is common and can occur as a result of either congestion from right heart failure or amyloid infiltration of the liver. Hepatomegaly from amyloid infiltration can be massive and on physical examination, the liver is typically "rock-hard" and nontender. Profound elevation of alkaline phosphatase with only mild elevation of transaminases is characteristic of hepatic amyloidosis since infiltration occurs in the sinusoids.[12] Autonomic nervous system involvement by AL amyloidosis can lead to orthostatic hypotension, early satiety due to delayed gastric emptying, erectile dysfunction, and intestinal motility issues. Painful, bilateral, symmetric, distal sensory neuropathy that progresses to motor neuropathy is the usual manifestation of peripheral nervous system involvement. Soft tissue involvement is characterized by macroglossia (Fig. 2a), carpal tunnel syndrome, skin nodules, arthropathy, alopecia, nail dystrophy, submandibular gland enlargement, periorbital purpura (Fig. 2b), and hoarseness of voice. Although present in a minority of patients, macroglossia is a hallmark feature of AL amyloidosis. Endocrinopathies such as hypothyroidism and hypoadrenalism are rare but are reported to occur with AL amyloidosis due to amyloid infiltration of the glands.[5]

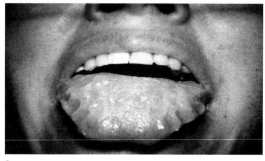

a

Fig. 2a Macroglossia (*see* Plate 18).

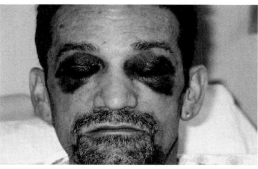

b

Fig. 2b Periorbital purpura, raccoon eyes (*see* Plate 19).

Diagnosis

The nonspecific and often vague nature of symptoms associated with AL amyloidosis frequently leads to delay in diagnosis such that organ dysfunction is advanced by the time treatment is initiated. The diagnosis of AL amyloidosis should be considered in patients with unexplained proteinuria, cardiomyopathy, neuropathy, or hepatomegaly, and in patients with multiple myeloma that has atypical manifestations.

The diagnosis of AL amyloidosis requires (1) demonstration of amyloid in tissue and (2) demonstration of a plasma cell dyscrasia. Tissue amyloid deposits demonstrate apple-green birefringence when stained with Congo red and viewed under polarizing microscopy (Fig. 3). Fine-needle aspiration of abdominal fat is a simple procedure that is positive for amyloid deposits in greater than 70% of patients with AL amyloidosis.[13,14] Other tissues that allow for relatively noninvasive biopsy procedures are the minor salivary glands, gingiva, rectum, and skin. However, obtaining tissue from an affected organ may be necessary to establish the diagnosis of amyloidosis.

Once a tissue diagnosis of amyloidosis has been established, confirmation of AL disease requires demonstration of a plasma cell dyscrasia by a bone marrow biopsy showing predominance of λ- or κ-producing plasma cells, or by the presence of a monoclonal light chain in the serum or urine. Immunofixation electrophoresis should be performed on the serum and urine

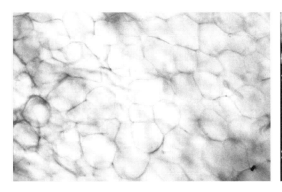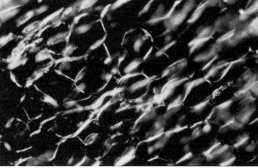

Fig. 3 Fat pad aspiration, Congo red stain under polarizing microscope (*see* Plate 20).

because, in contrast to multiple myeloma, the concentration of the monoclonal component is often too low to be detected by simple protein electrophoresis.

The recently introduced serum free light chain (FLC) assay, a nephelometric immunoassay, has a sensitivity for circulating free light chains that is reportedly more than tenfold that of immunofixation electrophoresis.[15,16] Because the FLC assay is quantitative, it has utility not only in diagnosis but also in following disease progression or response to treatment, as will be discussed later. Because free light chains undergo glomerular filtration, the ratio, rather than the absolute level, is the relevant measurement in individuals with renal impairment. A low κ:λ ratio (<0.26) strongly suggests the presence of a population of plasma cells producing clonal λ free light chains, whereas a high ratio (>1.65) suggests production of clonal κ free light chains.

The diagnostic utility of the FLC is not firmly established but is under evaluation. In a study of 110 patients with a diagnosis of AL amyloidosis, serum immunofixation was positive in 69%, urine immunofixation was positive in 83%, and the κ:λ ratio by the FLC assay was abnormal in 91%. The combination of an abnormal free κ:λ ratio and a positive serum immunofixation identified 99% of patients with AL amyloidosis.[17] Another study of 169 patients with AL amyloidosis found that an abnormal free κ:λ ratio had greater specificity and predictive value than absolute levels of free light chains in patients with κ clonal disease.[18]

Even if a monoclonal immunoglobulin light chain is identified in the serum or urine, a bone marrow biopsy is mandatory to assess the plasma cell burden[19] and exclude multiple myeloma and other less common disorders that can be associated with AL amyloidosis such as Waldenstrom's macroglobulinemia.[20] It is important to recognize that a monoclonal band present on serum immunofixation may be seen as an apparently incidental finding in 5–10% of patients over the age of 70 years (i.e., "monoclonal gammopathy of uncertain significance"). The serum free light chain assay is often normal in such cases.[21] Because of the high incidence of monoclonal gammopathy of undetermined significance (MGUS) in elderly individuals, further testing should be done to exclude familial or senile forms of amyloidosis if the clinical picture is at all atypical for AL disease. Such testing includes immunohistochemistry, immunofluorescence, or immunogold electron microscopy of amyloid deposits to identify the amyloidogenic protein,[22,23] or genetic testing to rule out familial forms of amyloidosis.[24,25]

Imaging Techniques for Assessment of Organ Involvement

Evaluation of the extent of amyloid deposition is desirable as it can help to prognosticate, formulate therapeutic options, and determine the response to treatment. Currently, physical examination and tissue biopsies are the most widely used methods to determine organ involvement. Scintigraphy using substances that bind to amyloid is a tool that also has utility in identifying affected organs. Technetium Tc 99m pyrophosphate binds avidly to many types of amyloid and has been used to identify cardiac amyloid.[26] However, quantitative assessment is not possible with this agent and strongly positive scintigraphic images usually occur only in patients with severe disease in whom echocardiography is generally diagnostic. Preliminary results suggest that technetium-labeled aprotinin may be more sensitive for imaging amyloid deposits than technetium Tc 99m pyrophosphate. Quantitative scintigraphy can also be performed with ^{123}I-labeled serum amyloid P component, a molecule that binds to all types of amyloid.[27] Multiple studies have suggested that both disease progression and response to treatment correlate with the degree of uptake of the serum amyloid P component, but this test is currently not widely available.

The echocardiographic features of cardiac amyloidosis have been well described and are reasonably distinctive in advanced disease. Early experience suggests that magnetic resonance (MR) imaging may provide an additional method for evaluation of cardiac involvement in amyloidosis, and may be particularly useful in distinguishing ventricular wall thickening due to amyloid infiltration from ventricular hypertrophy caused by hypertension. Several investigators have demonstrated abnormal delayed contrast enhancement and abnormal gadolinium distribution kinetics in patients with amyloid cardiomyopathy as compared to hypertensive control subjects.[28,29] It has been postulated that the delayed enhancement results from an increase in myocardial interstitial space due to amyloid infiltration. In addition to the delayed enhancement, additional work utilizing the inherent advantage of cardiac MR as a three-dimensional imaging technique has suggested that the ratio of left ventricular mass to left ventricular end-diastolic volume might be useful in differentiating cardiac amyloidosis from normal and hypertensive controls (Ruberg et al., unpublished data), particularly at an early stage of disease. Given these promising findings, cardiac MR imaging may soon play an important role in both the identification of amyloid cardiomyopathy and assessment of patients following therapy. The utility of MR in evaluating amyloid in other organs is not known.

Biomarkers of Prognosis and Treatment Response

The rate of disease progression is variable in AL amyloidosis and depends on the extent of organ involvement. The presence of clinically apparent cardiac involvement is an important determinant of outcome. The serum concentration of N-terminal pro-brain natriuretic peptide (NT-proBNP), either alone or in conjunction with levels of cardiac troponins, has been shown to be a sensitive marker of AL amyloidosis-associated cardiac dysfunction and a strong predictor of survival following aggressive treatment.[30,31] High circulating levels of free light chains have recently been shown to be associated with poor outcome, and greater reductions in levels following treatment of the underlying plasma cell dyscrasia are associated with both reduction in NT-proBNP and improved survival.[32],[33]

Treatment

The current therapeutic approach to systemic amyloidosis is based on the observations that organ dysfunction improves and survival increases if the synthesis of the amyloidogenic protein precursor is halted. Therefore, the aim of therapy in AL amyloidosis is to rapidly reduce the supply of amyloidogenic monoclonal light chains by suppressing the underlying plasma cell dyscrasia. Decisions about specific treatment regimens for individual patients must take into consideration the balance between anticipated treatment efficacy and tolerability.

Treatment Targets

Each of the steps in the pathogenesis of amyloidosis, from the production of the precursor protein to formation of amyloid deposits, is a potential target for treatment. Preclinical and clinical studies are being designed or are ongoing for several of these targets. Reducing the amyloidogenic precursor protein, that is, light chains produced by the clonal plasma cell dyscrasia, with chemotherapeutic agents has been used for the past several decades. Several interventions aimed at facilitating degradation of the amyloid deposits have been reported in AL amyloidosis.

Supportive Therapy

Regardless of the specific treatment directed against the plasma cell dyscrasia, supportive care to decrease symptoms and support organ function plays an important role in the management of this disease and requires the coordinated care by specialists in multiple disciplines. The mainstay of the treatment of amyloid cardiomyopathy is sodium restriction and the careful administration of diuretics. Achieving a balance between heart failure and intravascular volume depletion is particularly important especially in patients with autonomic nervous system involvement or nephrotic syndrome. Diuretic resistance is common in patients with severe nephrotic syndrome, and metolazone or spironolactone may be required in conjunction with loop diuretics. Patients with reduced stroke volume can benefit from afterload reduction with angiotensin-converting enzyme (ACE) inhibitors. However, these agents should be used cautiously, starting with a low dose and withdrawing if postural hypotension develops. Digoxin is not generally helpful, with the possible exception in patients with atrial fibrillation and rapid ventricular response. Calcium channel blockers can aggravate congestive heart failure in amyloid cardiomyopathy and should generally be avoided. Patients with recurrent syncope may require permanent pacemaker implantation, and ventricular arrhythmias are usually treated with amiodarone and, in some patients, implantable defibrillators.

Orthostatic hypotension can be severe and difficult to manage. Fitted waist-high elastic stockings and midodrine are helpful. Fludrocortisone is often not a good option because of associated fluid retention. Continuous norepinephrine infusion has been reported to be a successful treatment of severe hypotension refractory to conventional treatment. Supportive treatment of amyloid-associated kidney disease, as for other causes of nephrotic syndrome, includes salt restriction, diuretics, and treatment of hyperlipidemia. An impact of ACE inhibitors or angiotensin receptor blockers on proteinuria has not been established, but it is reasonable to use these agents if not precluded by hypotension. Both hemodialysis and peritoneal dialysis are used for amyloidosis-associated end-stage renal disease. Hemodynamic fragility and gastrointestinal (GI) symptoms such as early satiety should be considered in modality selection. Diarrhea is a common and incapacitating problem for patients with autonomic nervous system involvement. Octreotide decreases diarrhea in many patients, but chronic intestinal pseudo-obstruction is usually refractory to treatment. Adequate oral or intravenous feeding is mandatory in patients who are undernourished. Neuropathic pain is difficult to control. Gabapentin, although well tolerated, often fails to relieve pain. Other analgesics may be used as adjuvant agents. Duloxetine may be effective in controlling pain of neuropathy. Nonnephrotoxic analgesics may be used as adjuvant agents. Bleeding in AL amyloidosis is frequent and multifactorial.

Assessment of Treatment Response

Criteria for hematologic and organ responses for AL amyloidosis were unified and formalized in a recent consensus report.[34] Complete hematologic response is defined as absence of monoclonal protein in serum and urine by immunofixation electrophoresis, normal serum free light chain ratio, and bone marrow biopsy with less than 5% plasma cells with no clonal predominance by immunohistochemistry. Hematologic response is associated with a substantial survival advantage, improved quality of life, and improved organ function.[35–37] Improved organ function may be evident 3–6 months following treatment, although more delayed responses also occur. Reduction in proteinuria is gradual with continued improvement over 2 or more years. Importantly, a complete clonal hematologic response is not a prerequisite for clinical response and clinical improvement may still occur in patients with a partial clonal response. However, the rate of clinical response is higher in patients with a complete hematologic response than in those with a partial one. In one report, a reduction of greater than 90% in FLC was associated with a similar high likelihood of clinical improvement and prolonged survival, whether or not patients achieved a complete response after treatment.[38]

High-Dose Melphalan and Autologus Peripheral Blood Stem Cell Transplantation

High-dose melphalan (HDM) followed by autologous peripheral blood stem cell transplantation (SCT) is presently considered the most effective treatment of AL amyloidosis. The results of single and multicenter studies of HDM/SCT are summarized in Table 2. Encouraging hematologic and clinical responses have been reported in these studies, and although these are not controlled trials, the rates of complete hematologic response (25–67%) far exceed those observed with cyclic oral melphalan and prednisone, treatment that had been standard until the past several years. A case-matched control study has suggested the superiority of HDM/SCT compared to conventional chemotherapy regimens (oral melphalan and prednisone),[47] but the only randomized phase

Table 2 Results of single and multicenter studies of HDM/SCT in AL amyloidosis.

	No. of patients	TRM (%)	Hematologic CR (%)	Organ response (%)
Single center				
Gertz [39]	270	11	33	NR
Mollee [40]	20	35	28	Renal 46, cardiac 25, liver 50
Schonland [41]	41	7	50	40
Skinner [35]	277	13	40	44
Chow[42]	15	0	67	27
Multicenter				
Moreau [43]	21	43	25	83
Gertz [44]	28	14	NA	75
Goodman [45]	92	23	83 (CR + PR)	48
Vesole [46]	114	18	36	Renal 46, liver 58, cardiac 47

TRM treatment-related mortality, *CR* complete response, *PR* partial response, *HDM* high-dose melphalan, *SCT* stem cell transplantation.

III study by the French group in the literature failed to show a survival benefit for HDM/SCT. However, in this study, many of the patients randomized to the HDM/SCT arm were not actually transplanted, the toxicity on the transplant arm was excessive, and follow-up is short. Thus, the question of optimal therapy remains open, particularly as transplant techniques are refined, and nontransplant regimens are improved. However, it is clear that patients should be carefully selected for transplant, as advanced cardiac disease, more than two organ involvement, hypotension, and poor performance status are poor prognostic factors for the outcome of HDM/SCT.

Survival
The updated results demonstrate the median survival of 71 months (5.9 years) for 382 patients with AL amyloidosis treated with HDM/SCT at my institution from 1994 to 2006 (Fig. 4).

Eligibility Criteria for HDM/SCT
The eligibility criteria for HDM/SCT in AL amyloidosis vary among institutions and have evolved as experience has accrued, but all aim to make the treatment available to as many patients as possible while excluding those at greatest risk for severe morbidity and mortality. The Boston University Amyloid Program eligibility criteria include a confirmed tissue diagnosis of amyloidosis, clear evidence of a clonal plasma cell dyscrasia, age more than 18 years, performance status of 0–2 using the Southwest Oncology Group (SWOG) criteria, left ventricular ejection fraction greater than 40%, room air oxygen saturation greater than 95%, and supine systolic blood pressure greater than 90 mm Hg. Renal impairment including dialysis dependence is not an exclusion criteria.[35] The dose of melphalan can vary from 100 to 200 mg/m^2 depending on anticipated tolerability, using risk-adapted approaches.[48,49]

Stem Cell Mobilization and Collection
Several aspects of stem cell mobilization and collection pose particular challenges in patients with AL amyloidosis. As with other diseases, previous exposure to alkylating agents impairs hematopoietic stem cell collection; for melphalan, a prior cumulative dose exceeding 200 mg significantly reduces

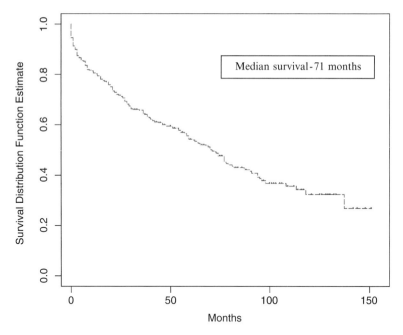

Fig. 4 Kaplan-Meier survival curve of 382 patients with AL amyloidosis treated with high-dose melphalan/stem cell transplantation, Boston University Medical Center (BUMC), 1994–2006 (*see* Plate 21).

the ability to mobilize stem cells. This is an important consideration if oral melphalan therapy is used before embarking on HDM/SCT, or if a second course of HDM is a possibility in the event of an incomplete hematologic response with the initial course. Patients with AL amyloidosis have more difficulty tolerating the stem cell mobilization and collection processes than do patients with other underlying diseases. Contrary to the typical experience in multiple myeloma, deaths have been reported during mobilization and leukapheresis in patients with AL amyloidosis with cardiac or multiorgan involvement. Overall, the major complication rate during mobilization or collection is ~15% in this disease.[35]

To minimize the risk of toxicity, it is recommended that granulocyte colony-stimulating factor (G-CSF) be used as a sole mobilizing agent since its use in combination with cyclophosphamide is associated with increased cardiac morbidity, the need for a greater number of aphereses sessions to obtain adequate numbers of stem cells, greater need of hospitalization, and increased toxicity overall. Contamination of the apheretic product with clonotypic immunoglobulin-positive plasma cells has been demonstrated, but CD34 selection is not presently recommended.[50]

Preparative Chemotherapy Regimen Before SCT
Because the burden of clonal plasma cells is modest in most patients with AL amyloidosis, induction with a cytoreducing regimen before HDM/SCT, as is done in multiple myeloma, seems unnecessary although possible benefits from VAD (vincristine, Adriamycin, and dexamethasone) treatment before SCT have been claimed. Evidence from a randomized trial indicates that the delay

associated with pretransplant cytoreduction using two cycles of oral melphalan and prednisone is likely to allow disease progression.[51] Total body irradiation (550 cGy) before SCT was investigated in a small feasibility study but is not used in current regimens because of cardiac toxicity and what appears to be greater overall morbidity and mortality. Tandem cycles of HDM in which adequate stem cells for two courses of chemotherapy are collected before the initial course of treatment have shown promising results.

Special Problems Associated with HDM/SCT in AL Amyloidosis

Several challenges with HDM/SCT are unique to patients with AL amyloidosis. Amyloid deposition in the GI tract predisposes to GI bleeding during periods of cytopenia; this can be exacerbated by amyloid-associated coagulopathies such as Factor X deficiency. Anasarca is common in patients with nephrotic syndrome particularly in association with G-CSF administration. Hypotension from cardiac disease or autonomic nervous system involvement, atrial and ventricular arrythmias in patients with amyloid cardiomyopathy, difficulties with emergent endotracheal intubation due to macroglossia, and spontaneous splenic and esophageal rupture are also problems that can arise during treatment in these patients.

HDM/SCT Following Heart Transplantation

In patients with end-stage heart failure, heart transplantation may be required as a life-saving procedure. Because of the high likelihood of amyloid recurrence in the transplanted organ, as well as progression in other organs, heart transplantation must be followed by anticlone therapy. Although the long-term survival is statistically inferior to that of patients with nonamyloid heart disease, the actuarial 5-year survival appears to be 50% with treatment of the underlying plasma cell dyscrasia. Thus, carefully selected patients, without other significant organ involvement, can benefit from heart transplantation followed by aggressive antiplasma cell treatment.[52]

Allogeneic Bone Marrow Transplantation

There is a small experience with allogeneic and syngeneic bone marrow transplantation for AL amyloidosis. A recent report by the European Cooperative Group for Blood and Marrow Transplantation describes 19 patients who underwent allogeneic transplantation.[53] The group is heterogeneous since it included 4 syngeneic, 8 reduced-intensity conditioning, and 7 full-dose allogeneic transplants, and 10 were T-cell-depleted grafts. Complete hematologic responses were seen in 10 of the 19 patients. However, the follow-up period was short, the treatment-related mortality was 40%, and only 4 patients were alive at 36 months. This report was compiled from registry data from 11 centers. The patient selection and the total number of patients evaluated at these centers as potential allogeneic transplant recipients are not known. Nonetheless, it represents the largest number of patients reported, and it is important for the scientific community to be aware of the feasibility of allogeneic transplant and its potential for graft versus tumor, as 5 of 7 patients with complete remission had chronic graft-versus-host disease. The data are of insufficient power to justify the use of this technique in clinical practice, and it should remain the subject of clinical trials.

Oral Melphalan-Based Regimens

The conventional treatment approach for AL amyloidosis, adopted from experience with multiple myeloma, is to administer low-dose oral melphalan in association with prednisone in a cyclical fashion. Two randomized clinical trials have demonstrated the efficacy of this regimen; however, the impact was modest increasing the median survival to only ~18 months.[54],[55] This form of treatment only rarely results in complete hematologic responses or reversal of amyloid-related organ dysfunction.

Many patients with advanced disease, particularly those with cardiac involvement, are unable to tolerate the fluid retention and worsening congestive heart failure associated with steroid treatment. The use of sole therapy with oral melphalan administered continuously rather than cyclically has been studied in patients with cardiac amyloidosis. In 30 such treated patients, 7 out of 13 patients evaluable after 3–4 months of treatment achieved a partial hematologic response and 3 achieved a complete hematologic response.[56] Six of the patients survived for more than 1 year. This regimen appeared to be effective in inducing hematologic responses in patients who received total doses of melphalan more than 300 mg.

High-Dose Dexamethasone-Based Regimens

A rapid response to therapy is essential in AL amyloidosis. In multiple myeloma, VAD (infusional vincristine, doxorubicin, and dexamethasone) may induce a quick clonal response. However, this regimen presents potential problems in patients with AL amyloidosis: Vincristine can exacerbate autonomic or peripheral neuropathy; doxorubicin can worsen cardiomyopathy; and the intensive high-dose dexamethasone can cause severe fluid retention in patients with renal and cardiac amyloidosis or trigger severe, often fatal, ventricular arrhythmias.[57] At the UK National Amyloidosis Center, 98 patients with AL amyloidosis were treated with a median of four cycles of standard VAD or CVAMP (cyclophosphamide, vincristine, Adriamycin, methyl-prednisolone). A hematologic response occurred in 54%, an organ response was evident in 42%, and the treatment-related mortality was only 7%. However, the responses were not durable with evidence of hematologic relapse in 21% of patients after a median time of 20 months (range 7–54).

Experience with multiple myeloma has indicated that dexamethasone accounted for most (80%) of the plasma cell reduction achieved with VAD and avoided the potential toxicity of vincristine and Adriamycin. Pulsed high-dose dexamethasone, as used in the VAD regimen, has been reported to benefit patients with AL amyloidosis with varying response rates. A recently completed SWOG trial with 87 eligible and analyzable patients found that 53% of patients had a hematologic response, and the hematologic response was complete in 24%. Organ function improved in 45%. The median progression-free survival was 27 months and overall survival was 31 months.[58]

The toxicity of dexamethasone used with the same schedule of the VAD regimen in patients with AL amyloidosis is substantial. A modified-dexamethasone, milder, less toxic schedule (40 mg/day for 4 days every 21 days) induced organ response in 35% of patients in a median time of 4 months, without significant toxicity.[59] The combination of melphalan and dexamethasone produced hematologic response in 67% in a median time of 4.5 months, with complete remission in 33% and functional improvement of the involved organs in 48%. Treatment-related mortality was low (4%). Median duration of response was 24 months (range 12–48).[60]

Thalidomide

Thalidomide is poorly tolerated in patients with AL amyloidosis, causing fatigue, progressive edema, cognitive difficulties, constipation, neuropathy, syncope due to bradycardia, thromboembolic complications, and worsening of renal function.[61],[62] Severe side effects impeded dose escalation above 200–300 mg/day and necessitated thalidomide withdrawal in 25–50% of the patients. Thalidomide was given in combination with intermediate dose dexamethasone in 31 patients with AL amyloidosis as a second-line therapy.[63] Hematologic and organ responses correlated with the dose of thalidomide. Overall hematologic response was observed in 15 patients (48%), of whom 6 (19%) attained a complete response, and organ response in 8 patients (26%). Median time to response was 3.6 months (range 2.5– 8.0 months). Hematologic response to treatment resulted in a significant survival benefit ($P = 0.01$). Treatment-related toxicity was frequent (65%), and symptomatic bradycardia was a common (26%) adverse reaction.

Overall, it appears that the combination of thalidomide and dexamethasone may be a valid option for refractory or relapsed patients. Because of the fragility of these patients, reduced doses of thalidomide should be used and careful monitoring for toxicity is necessary.

Thalidomide has also been combined with cyclophosphamide and steroids Cyclophosphamide Thalidomide Dexamethasone (CTD regimen) in a oral regimen and has shown to be effective in inducing hematologic responses in 74% (CR 21%, PR 53%) of patients with low treatment-related mortality of 4% and median overall survival of 41 months.[64]

Lenalidomide

In a small study of 34 patients with AL amyloidosis who either had persistent disease following HDM/SCT or were ineligible for HDM/SCT, lenalidomide with dexamethasone has been found to produce hematologic responses in 67% of patients with considerable organ responses.[65] Similar study from a different center showed a hematologic response in 41% of patients and organ response in 23% of patients.[66] Lenalidomide has a different toxicity profile than thalidomide. Adverse events of thromboembolic complications, myelosuppression, and immunosuppression are noted with lenalidomide, and neurotoxicity is generally not associated with lenalidomide. Of note, the median time to hematologic response in both the studies was 6 months.

Investigational Therapies

The proteasome inhibitor, bortezomib, is active in multiple myeloma. The ability of this drug, in combination with dexamethasone, to rapidly reduce the concentration of the circulating monoclonal protein in multiple myeloma makes this an attractive option also for AL amyloidosis, and a multicenter, international phase I/II trial is currently accruing patients.

An iodinated derivative of doxorubicin, 4-iodo-4-deoxydoxorubucin (IDOX), binds with high affinity to amyloid fibrils and promotes their disaggregation in vitro and in vivo in experimentally induced murine AA amyloidosis. Administration of IDOX to patients with AL amyloidosis showed promising results in a small, uncontrolled series, but its efficacy was unable to be demonstrated in a larger multicenter trial, possibly because the effect size was less than anticipated.[67,68] Strategies that combine IDOX with chemotherapy to suppress precursor production and promote amyloid resorption are a rational approach that warrants investigation.

Disruption of the interaction between serum amyloid P (SAP) and amyloid is another approach being investigated as a degradation-promoting treatment. Because SAP is present in all types of amyloid deposits, targeting the SAP–amyloid interaction could have broad application. SAP itself is highly resistant to proteolysis, and binding of SAP to amyloid fibrils protects them from proteolysis in vitro. SAP exists in a dynamic equilibrium between the circulation, where it is unbound, and tissue, where it is bound to amyloid. Pepys et al. hypothesized that removal of circulating SAP would drive SAP from tissue amyloid to the circulation and render the tissue amyloid less resistant to proteolysis. R-1-[6-[R-2-carboxy-pyrrolidin-1-yl]-6-oxo-hexanoyl]pyrrolidine-2-carboxylic acid (CPHPC), a palindromic compound that binds with high affinity to SAP, cross-links two SAP molecules together in a manner that occludes the binding surface of SAP.[69] CPHPC administration depleted SAP from the circulation and from amyloid deposits in murine models, and studies in humans demonstrated rapid SAP clearance from the circulation. However, the impact of CPHPC administration on amyloid deposits in either animal models or in humans is not known and is currently being studied in phase II trials.

Anti-tumor necrosis factor-α (TNF-α) therapy, in the form of etanercept, in 16 patients with advanced AL produced symptomatic improvement in most of them, and half had objective responses, notably in those with macroglossia.[70] However, this approach does not have any impact on the underlying plasma cell dyscrasia and therefore is of limited benefit.

Immunotherapy, both active and passive, is another approach that is actively being pursued. Dendritic cell-based idiotype vaccination has been shown to be well tolerated, but to have limited clinical impact. AL amyloid burden can be markedly reduced in mice by passive immunization with an anti-light chain murine monoclonal antibody specific for an amyloid-related epitope.[71] A humanized antibody is being produced for a phase I/II clinical trial in patients with AL disease.

Conclusions

Promising treatments are available for patients with AL amyloidosis. Prompt diagnosis of amyloidosis and appropriate referral has the potential to improve outcome for these patients. Maintaining AL amyloidosis in the differential diagnosis of patients being evaluated for a variety of syndromes, particularly with nephrotic range proteinuria, unexplained nonischemic cardiomyopathy, peripheral neuropathy, unexplained hepatomegaly, or atypical multiple myeloma, should improve diagnostic efficiency. Despite these improvements in the treatment and diagnosis of AL amyloidosis, continued basic and clinical research effort in this field is needed to help improve the outcome for these patients.

References

1. Merlini G, Bellotti V: Molecular mechanisms of amyloidosis. N Engl J Med 2003;349:583--596.
2. Westermark P, Benson MD, Buxbaum JN, Cohen AS, Frangione B, Ikeda S, Masters CL, Merlini G, Saraiva MJ, Sipe JD: Amyloid: toward terminology clarification. Report from the Nomenclature Committee of the International Society of Amyloidosis. Amyloid 2005;12:1--4.
3. Gertz MA, Lacy MQ, Dispenzieri A: Amyloidosis. Hematol Oncol Clin North America 1999;13:1211--1220.
4. Kyle RA, Linos A, Beard CM, Linke RP, Gertz MA, O''Fallon WM, Kurland LT: Incidence and natural history of primary systemic amyloidosis in Olmsted County, Minnesota, 1950 through 1989. Blood 1992;79:1817--1822.
5. Kyle RA, Gertz MA: Primary systemic amylodiosis: cClinical and laboratory features in 474 cases. Semin Hematol 1995;32:45--49.
6. Dember LM: Emerging treatment approaches for the systemic amyloidoses. Kidney Int 2005;68:1377--1390.
7. Brenner DA, Jain M, Pimentel DR, Wang B, Connors LH, Skinner M, Apstein CS, Liao R: Human amyloidogenic light chains directly impair cardiomyocyte function through an increase in cellular oxidant stress. Circ Res 2004;94:1008--1010.
8. Abraham RS, Ballman KV, Dispenzieri A, Grill DE, Manske MK, Price-Troska TL, Paz NG, Gertz MA, Fonseca R: Functional gene expression analysis of clonal plasma cells identifies a unique molecular profile for light chain amyloidosis. Blood 2005;105:794--803.
9. Comenzo RL, Zhang Y, Martinez C, Osman K, Herrera GA: The tropism of organ involvement in primary systemic amyloidosis: contributions of Ig V(L) germ line gene use and clonal plasma cell burden. Blood 2001;98:714--720.
10. Falk RH, Comenzo RL, Skinner M: The systemic amyloidoses. N Engl J Med 1997;337:898--909.
11. Falk RH: Diagnosis and management of the cardiac amyloidoses. Circulation 2005;112:2047--2060.
12. Park MA, Mueller PS, Kyle RA, Larson DR, Plevak MF, Gertz MA: Primary (AL) hepatic amyloidosis: clinical features and natural history in 98 patients. Medicine (Baltimore) 2003;82:291--298.
13. Libbey CA, Skinner M, Cohen AS: Use of abdominal fat tissue aspirate in the diagnosis of systemic amyloidosis. Arch Intern Med 1983;143:1549--1552.
14. Ansari-Lari MA, Ali SZ: Fine-needle aspiration of abdominal fat pad for amyloid detection: a clinically useful test? Diagn Cytopathol 2004;30:178--181.
15. Abraham RS, Katzmann JA, Clark RJ, Bradwell AR, Kyle RA, Gertz MA: Quantitative analysis of serum free light chains. A new marker for the diagnostic evaluation of primary systemic amyloidosis. Am J Clin Pathol 2003;119:274--278.
16. Katzmann JA, Clark RJ, Abraham RS, Bryant S, Lymp JF, Bradwell AR, Kyle RA: Serum reference intervals and diagnostic ranges for free kappa and free lambda immunoglobulin light chains: relative sensitivity for detection of monoclonal light chains. Clin Chem 2002;48:1437--1444.
17. Katzmann JA, Abraham RS, Dispenzieri A, Lust JA, Kyle RA: Diagnostic performance of quantitative kappa and lambda free light chain assays in clinical practice. Clin Chem 2005;51:878--881.
18. Akar H, Seldin DC, Magnani B, O''Hara C, Berk JL, Schoonmaker C, Cabral H, Dember LM, Sanchorawala V, Connors LH, Falk RH, Skinner M: Quantitative serum free light chain assay in the diagnostic evaluation of AL amyloidosis. Amyloid 2005;12:210--215.
19. Swan N, Skinner M, O'Hara O'Hara CJ: Bone marrow core biopsy specimens in AL (primary) amyloidosis. A morphologic and immunohistochemical study of 100 cases. Am J Clin Pathol 2003;120:610--616.

20. Sanchorawala V, Blanchard E, Seldin DC, O'Hara O'Hara C, Skinner M, Wright DG: AL amyloidosis associated with B-cell lymphoproliferative disorders: fFrequency and treatment outcomes. Am J Hematol 2006.

21. Kyle RA, Therneau TM, Rajkumar SV, Larson DR, Plevak MF, Melton LJ, 3rd: Long-term follow-up of 241 patients with monoclonal gammopathy of undetermined significance: the original Mayo Clinic series 25 years later. Mayo Clin Proc 2004;79:859--866.

22. Arbustini E, Verga L, Concardi M, Palladini G, Obici L, Merlini G: Electron and immuno-electron microscopy of abdominal fat identifies and characterizes amyloid fibrils in suspected cardiac amyloidosis. Amyloid 2002;9:108--114.

23. O''Hara CJ, Falk RH: The diagnosis and typing of cardiac amyloidosis. Amyloid 2003;10:127--129.

24. Lachmann HJ, Booth DR, Booth SE, Bybee A, Gilbertson JA, Gillmore JD, Pepys MB, Hawkins PN: Misdiagnosis of hereditary amyloidosis as AL (primary) amyloidosis. N Engl J Med 2002;346:1786--1791.

25. Comenzo RL, Zhou P, Fleisher M, Clark B, Teruya-Feldstein J: Seeking confidence in the diagnosis of systemic AL (Ig light-chain) amyloidosis: patients can have both monoclonal gammopathies and hereditary amyloid proteins. Blood 2006;107:3489--3491.

26. Falk RH, Lee VW, Rubinow A, Skinner M, Cohen AS: Cardiac technetium-99m pyrophosphate scintigraphy in familial amyloidosis. Am J Cardiol 1984;54:1150--1151.

27. Hawkins PN, Lavender JP, Pepys MB: Evaluation of systemic amyloidosis by scintigraphy with 123I-labeled serum amyloid P component. N Engl J Med 1990;323:508--513.

28. Maceira AM, Joshi J, Prasad SK, Moon JC, Perugini E, Harding I, Sheppard MN, Poole-Wilson PA, Hawkins PN, Pennell DJ: Cardiovascular magnetic resonance in cardiac amyloidosis. Circulation 2005;111:186--193.

29. Perugini E, Rapezzi C, Piva T, Leone O, Bacchi-Reggiani L, Riva L, Salvi F, Lovato L, Branzi A, Fattori R: Non-invasive evaluation of the myocardial substrate of cardiac amyloidosis by gadolinium cardiac magnetic resonance. Heart 2006;92:343--349.

30. Dispenzieri A, Gertz MA, Kyle RA, Lacy MQ, Burritt MF, Therneau TM, McConnell JP, Litzow MR, Gastineau DA, Tefferi A, Inwards DJ, Micallef IN, Ansell SM, Porrata LF, Elliott MA, Hogan WJ, Rajkumar SV, Fonseca R, Greipp PR, Witzig TE, Lust JA, Zeldenrust SR, Snow DS, Hayman SR, McGregor CG, Jaffe AS: Prognostication of survival using cardiac troponins and N-terminal pro-brain natriuretic peptide in patients with primary systemic amyloidosis undergoing peripheral blood stem cell transplantation. Blood 2004;104:1881--1887.

31. Palladini G, Campana C, Klersy C, Balduini A, Vadacca G, Perfetti V, Perlini S, Obici L, Ascari E, d''Eril GM, Moratti R, Merlini G: Serum N-terminal pro-brain natriuretic peptide is a sensitive marker of myocardial dysfunction in AL amyloidosis. Circulation 2003;107:2440--2445.

32. Palladini G, Lavatelli F, Russo P, Perlini S, Perfetti V, Bosoni T, Obici L, Bradwell AR, D'Eril D'Eril GM, Fogari R, Moratti R, Merlini G: Circulating amyloidogenic free light chains and serum N-terminal natriuretic peptide type B decrease simultaneously in association with improvement of survival in AL. Blood 2006;107:3854--3858.

33. Dispenzieri A, Lacy MQ, Katzmann JA, Rajkumar SV, Abraham RS, Hayman SR, Kumar SK, Clark R, Kyle RA, Litzow MR, Inwards DJ, Ansell SM, Micallef IM, Porrata LF, Elliott MA, Johnston PB, Greipp PR, Witzig TE, Zeldenrust SR, Russell SJ, Gastineau D, Gertz MA: Absolute values of immunoglobulin free light chains are prognostic in patients with primary systemic amyloidosis undergoing peripheral blood stem cell transplant. Blood 2006. 107:3378--3383.

34. Gertz MA, Comenzo R, Falk RH, Fermand JP, Hazenberg BP, Hawkins PN, Merlini G, Moreau P, Ronco P, Sanchorawala V, Sezer O, Solomon A, Grateau G: Definition of organ involvement and treatment response in immunoglobulin light chain amyloidosis (AL): a consensus opinion from the 10th International Symposium

on Amyloid and Amyloidosis, Tours, France, 18-–22 April 2004. Am J Hematol 2005;79:319-–328.

35. Skinner M, Sanchorawala V, Seldin DC, Dember LM, Falk RH, Berk JL, Anderson JJ, O'Hara O'Hara C, Finn KT, Libbey CA, Wiesman J, Quillen K, Swan N, Wright DG: High-dose melphalan and autologous stem-cell transplantation in patients with AL amyloidosis: an 8-year study. Ann Intern Med 2004;140:85-–93.

36. Seldin DC, Anderson JJ, Sanchorawala V, Malek K, Wright DG, Quillen K, Finn KT, Berk JL, Dember LM, Falk RH, Skinner M: Improvement in quality of life of patients with AL amyloidosis treated with high-dose melphalan and autologous stem cell transplantation. Blood 2004;104:1888-–1893.

37. Dember LM, Sanchorawala V, Seldin DC, Wright DG, LaValley M, Berk JL, Falk RH, Skinner M: Effect of dose-intensive intravenous melphalan and autologous blood stem-cell transplantation on al amyloidosis-associated renal disease. Ann Intern Med 2001;134:746-–753.

38. Sanchorawala V, Seldin DC, Magnani B, Skinner M, Wright DG: Serum free light-chain responses after high-dose intravenous melphalan and autologous stem cell transplantation for AL (primary) amyloidosis. Bone Marrow Transplant 2005;36:597-–600.

39. Gertz MA, Lacy MQ, Dispenzieri A, Hayman SR, Kumar S: Transplantation for amyloidosis. Curr Opin Oncol 2007;19:136-–141.

40. Mollee PN, Wechalekar AD, Pereira DL, Franke N, Reece D, Chen C, Stewart AK: Autologous stem cell transplantation in primary systemic amyloidosis: the impact of selection criteria on outcome. Bone Marrow Transplant 2004;33:271-–277.

41. Schonland SO, Perz JB, Hundemer M, Hegenbart U, Kristen AV, Hund E, Dengler TJ, Beimler J, Zeier M, Singer R, Linke RP, Ho AD, Goldschmidt H: Indications for high-dose chemotherapy with autologous stem cell support in patients with systemic amyloid light chain amyloidosis. Transplantation 2005;80:S160-–S163.

42. Chow LQ, Bahlis N, Russell J, Chaudhry A, Morris D, Brown C, Stewart DA: Autologous transplantation for primary systemic AL amyloidosis is feasible outside a major amyloidosis referral centre: the Calgary BMT Program experience. Bone Marrow Transplant 2005;36:591-–596.

43. Moreau P, Leblond V, Bourquelot P, Facon T, Huynh A, Caillot D, Hermine O, Attal M, Hamidou M, Nedellec G, Ferrant A, Audhuy B, Bataille R, Milpied N, Harousseau JL: Prognostic factors for survival and response after high-dose therapy and autologous stem cell transplantation in systemic AL amyloidosis: a report on 21 patients. Br J Haematol 1998;101:766-–769.

44. Gertz MA, Blood E, Vesole DH, Abonour R, Lazarus HM, Greipp PR: A multicenter phase 2 trial of stem cell transplantation for immunoglobulin light-chain amyloidosis (E4A97): an Eastern Cooperative Oncology Group Study. Bone Marrow Transplant 2004;34:149-–154.

45. Goodman HJ, Gillmore JD, Lachmann HJ, Wechalekar AD, Bradwell AR, Hawkins PN: Outcome of autologous stem cell transplantation for AL amyloidosis in the UK. Br J Haematol 2006;134:417-–425.

46. Vesole DH, Perez WS, Akasheh M, Boudreau C, Reece DE, Bredeson CN: High-dose therapy and autologous hematopoietic stem cell transplantation for patients with primary systemic amyloidosis: a Center for International Blood and Marrow Transplant Research Study. Mayo Clin Proc 2006;81:880-–888.

47. Dispenzieri A, Kyle RA, Lacy MQ, Therneau TM, Larson DR, Plevak MF, Rajkumar SV, Fonseca R, Greipp PR, Witzig TE, Lust JA, Zeldenrust SR, Snow DS, Hayman SR, Litzow MR, Gastineau DA, Tefferi A, Inwards DJ, Micallef IN, Ansell SM, Porrata LF, Elliott MA, Gertz MA: Superior survival in primary systemic amyloidosis patients undergoing peripheral blood stem cell transplantation: a case-control study. Blood 2004;103:3960-–3963.

48. Comenzo RL, Gertz MA: Autologous stem cell transplantation for primary systemic amyloidosis. Blood 2002;99:4276-–4282.

49. Perfetti V, Siena S, Palladini G, Bregni M, Di Nicola M, Obici L, Magni M, Brunetti L, Gianni AM, Merlini G: Long-term results of a risk-adapted approach to melphalan conditioning in autologous peripheral blood stem cell transplantation for primary (AL) amyloidosis. Haematologica 2006;91:1635--1643.

50. Comenzo RL, Michelle D, LeBlanc M, Wally J, Zhang Y, Kica G, Karandish S, Arkin CF, Wright DG, Skinner M, McMannis J: Mobilized CD34 + cells selected as autografts in patients with primary light-chain amyloidosis: rationale and application. Transfusion 1998;38:60--69.

51. Sanchorawala V, Wright DG, Seldin DC, Falk RH, Finn KT, Dember LM, Berk JL, Quillen K, Anderson JJ, Comenzo RL, Skinner M: High-dose intravenous melphalan and autologous stem cell transplantation as initial therapy or following two cycles of oral chemotherapy for the treatment of AL amyloidosis: results of a prospective randomized trial. Bone Marrow Transplant 2004;33:381--388.

52. Gillmore JD, Goodman HJ, Lachmann HJ, Offer M, Wechalekar AD, Joshi J, Pepys MB, Hawkins PN: Sequential heart and autologous stem cell transplantation for systemic AL amyloidosis. In Blood. 2006:1227--1229.

53. Schonland SO, Lokhorst H, Buzyn A, Leblond V, Hegenbart U, Bandini G, Campbell A, Carreras E, Ferrant A, Grommisch L, Jacobs P, Kroger N, La Nasa G, Russell N, Zachee P, Goldschmidt H, Iacobelli S, Niederwieser D, Gahrton G: Allogeneic and syngeneic hematopoietic cell transplantation in patients with amyloid light-chain amyloidosis: a report from the European Group for Blood and Marrow Transplantation. Blood 2006;107:2578--2584.

54. Skinner M, Anderson J, Simms R, Falk R, Wang M, Libbey C, Jones LA, Cohen AS: Treatment of 100 patients with primary amyloidosis: a randomized trial of melphalan, prednisone, and colchicine versus colchicine only. Am J Med 1996;100:290--298.

55. Kyle RA, Gertz MA, Greipp PR, Witzig TE, Lust JA, Lacy MQ, Therneau TM: A trial of three regimens for primary amyloidosis: colchicine alone, melphalan and prednisone, and melphalan, prednisone, and colchicine. N Engl J Med 1997;336:1202--1207.

56. Sanchorawala V, Wright DG, Seldin DC, Falk RH, Berk JL, Dember LM, Finn KT, Skinner M: Low-dose continuous oral melphalan for the treatment of primary systemic (AL) amyloidosis. Br J Haematol 2002;117:886--889.

57. Perz JB, Schonland SO, Hundemer M, Kristen AV, Dengler TJ, Zeier M, Linke RP, Ho AD, Goldschmidt H: High-dose melphalan with autologous stem cell transplantation after VAD induction chemotherapy for treatment of amyloid light chain amyloidosis: a single centre prospective phase II study. Br J Haematol 2004;127:543--551.

58. Dhodapkar MV, Hussein MA, Rasmussen E, Solomon A, Larson RA, Crowley JJ, Barlogie B: Clinical efficacy of high-dose dexamethasone with maintenance dexamethasone/alpha interferon in patients with primary systemic amyloidosis: results of United States Intergroup Trial Southwest Oncology Group (SWOG) S9628. Blood 2004;104:3520--3526.

59. Palladini G, Anesi E, Perfetti V, Obici L, Invernizzi R, Balduini C, Ascari E, Merlini G: A modified high-dose dexamethasone regimen for primary systemic (AL) amyloidosis. Br J Haematol 2001;113:1044--1046.

60. Palladini G, Perfetti V, Obici L, Caccialanza R, Semino A, Adami F, Cavallero G, Rustichelli R, Virga G, Merlini G: Association of melphalan and high-dose dexamethasone is effective and well tolerated in patients with AL (primary) amyloidosis who are ineligible for stem cell transplantation. Blood 2004;103:2936--2938.

61. Seldin DC, Choufani EB, Dember LM, Wiesman JF, Berk JL, Falk RH, O'Hara O'Hara C, Fennessey S, Finn KT, Wright DG, Skinner M, Sanchorawala V: Tolerability and efficacy of thalidomide for the treatment of patients with light chain-associated (AL) amyloidosis. Clin Lymphoma 2003;3:241--246.

62. Dispenzieri A, Lacy MQ, Rajkumar SV, Geyer SM, Witzig TE, Fonseca R, Lust JA, Greipp PR, Kyle RA, Gertz MA: Poor tolerance to high doses of thalidomide in patients with primary systemic amyloidosis. Amyloid 2003;10:257--261.

63. Palladini G, Perfetti V, Perlini S, Obici L, Lavatelli F, Caccialanza R, Invernizzi R, Comotti B, Merlini G: The combination of thalidomide and intermediate-dose dexamethasone is an effective but toxic treatment for patients with primary amyloidosis (AL). Blood 2005;105:2949--2951.

64. Wechalekar AD, Goodman HJ, Lachmann HJ, Offer M, Hawkins PN, Gillmore JD: Safety and efficacy of risk-adapted cyclophosphamide, thalidomide, and dexamethasone in systemic AL amyloidosis. Blood 2007;109:457--464.

65. Sanchorawala V, Wright DG, Rosenzweig M, Finn KT, Fennessey S, Zeldis JB, Skinner M, Seldin DC: Lenalidomide and dexamethasone in the treatment of AL amyloidosis: results of a phase 2 trial. Blood 2007;109:492--496.

66. Dispenzieri A, Lacy MQ, Zeldenrust SR, Hayman SR, Kumar SK, Geyer SM, Lust JA, Allred JB, Witzig TE, Rajkumar SV, Greipp PR, Russell SJ, Kabat B, Gertz MA: The activity of lenalidomide with or without dexamethasone in patients with primary systemic amyloidosis. Blood 2007;109:465--470.

67. Gertz MA, Lacy MQ, Dispenzieri A, Cheson BD, Barlogie B, Kyle RA, Palladini G, Geyer SM, Merlini G: A multicenter phase II trial of 4¢'-iodo-4'¢deoxydoxorubicindeoxydoxorubicin (IDOX) in primary amyloidosis (AL). Amyloid 2002;9:24--30.

68. Gianni L, Bellotti V, Gianni AM, Merlini G: New drug therapy of amyloidoses: resorption of AL-type deposits with 4¢'-iodo-4¢'-deoxydoxorubicin. Blood 1995;86:855--861.

69. Pepys MB, Herbert J, Hutchinson WL, Tennent GA, Lachmann HJ, Gallimore JR, Lovat LB, Bartfai T, Alanine A, Hertel C, Hoffmann T, Jakob-Roetne R, Norcross RD, Kemp JA, Yamamura K, Suzuki M, Taylor GW, Murray S, Thompson D, Purvis A, Kolstoe S, Wood SP, Hawkins PN: Targeted pharmacological depletion of serum amyloid P component for treatment of human amyloidosis. Nature 2002;417:254--259.

70. Hussein MA, Juturi JV, Rybicki L, Lutton S, Murphy BR, Karam MA: Etanercept therapy in patients with advanced primary amyloidosis. Med Oncol 2003;20:283--290.

71. Hrncic R, Wall J, Wolfenbarger DA, Murphy CL, Schell M, Weiss DT, Solomon A: Antibody-mediated resolution of light chain-associated amyloid deposits. Am J Pathol 2000;157:1239--1246.

Chapter 34

POEMS Syndrome and Other Atypical Plasma Cell Disorders

Angela Dispenzieri

Atypical PCD Associated with Peripheral Neuropathy as Dominant Phenotype

Other important peripheral neuropathies (PNs)-associated plasma cell disorders (PCDs) include those induced by chemotherapy and those related to Waldenström macroglobulinemia, multiple myeloma, and light-chain amyloid, but these are beyond the scope of this chapter. Disorders like cryoglobulinemia, scleromyxedema can also be associated with PN, but those entities will be reviewed in later sections since PN is not their dominant phenotype. In this section, the focus will be on POEMS (*p*olyneuropathy, *o*rganomegaly, *e*ndocrinopathy, *M* protein, and *s*kin changes) syndrome and MGUS (*m*onoclonal *g*ammopathy of *u*ndetermined *s*ignificance)-associated PN.

POEMS Syndrome

The complexity of the interaction with plasma cell dyscrasia and PN became increasingly evident in 1956 with Crow's description of two patients with osteosclerotic plasmacytomas with neuropathy, and other "striking features," which included clubbing, skin pigmentation, dusky discoloration of skin, white finger nails, mild lymphadenopathy, and ankle edema.[1] As many as 50% of patients with osteosclerotic myeloma were noted to have PN[2–4] in contrast to 1–8% of patients with multiple myeloma.[5,6] A syndrome distinct from multiple myeloma-associated neuropathy came to be recognized.

In 1980, Bardswick described two patients and coined the acronym POEMS.[7] In 1981, Kelly et al. reported on 16 cases seen at Mayo,[8] and in 1983[9] and 1984,[10] two large series of cases collected from Japan were reported solidifying the existence of a distinct pathologic entity. Another series from France further bolstered these concepts in the early 1990s with a report of 25 patients.[11]

The acronym POEMS captures several dominant features of the syndrome. The major clinical feature of the syndrome is a chronic progressive polyneuropathy with a predominant motor disability.[7,12] Important characteristics not included in the acronym include elevated levels of vascular endothelial growth factor (VEGF), sclerotic bone lesions, Castleman's disease, papilledema,

From: *Contemporary Hematology Myeloma Therapy*
Edited by: S. Lonial © Humana Press, Totowa, NJ

peripheral edema, ascites, effusions, thrombocytosis, polycythemia, fatigue, and clubbing. Other names for the syndrome include osteosclerotic myeloma, Crow-Fukase syndrome, and Takatsuki syndrome.[9,10] Although the majority of patients have osteosclerotic myeloma, these same patients usually have only 5% bone marrow plasma cells or less (almost always monoclonal lambda), and rarely have anemia, hypercalcemia, or renal insufficiency. Castleman's disease may also be a part of the disease. These characteristics and the superior median survival differentiate POEMS syndrome from multiple myeloma.

Pathogenesis

The pathogenesis of this multisystem disease is complex. Elevation of proangiogenic[13–22] and proinflammatory[13,15,16,21] cytokines is a hallmark of the disorder. Little is known about the plasma cells except that more than 95% of the time they are lambda light chain restricted. Prior hypotheses have included implication of hyperestrogenemia[11] and human herpesvirus 8 (HHV-8).[23–25] Although the cytokine network is highly complex and interrelated, VEGF appears to be the dominant driving cytokine in this disorder.[13,22,26] VEGF normally targets endothelial cells and induces a rapid and reversible increase in vascular permeability. It is important in angiogenesis, and osteogenesis is strongly dependent on angiogenesis. VEGF is expressed by osteoblasts, in bone tissue, macrophages, tumor cells (including plasma cells), and megakaryocytes/platelets. Both interleukin (IL)-1β and IL-6 have been shown to stimulate VEGF production.

Although patients with POEMS have higher levels of IL-1β, tumor necrosis factor-α (TNF-α), and IL-6 than do patients with classic multiple myeloma [13,27] and controls,[15,16,21,27] this relationship appears to be less consistent.[15–20] For some patients, levels of IL-6 correlate with disease activity,[15] and increased levels have been found in the cerebrospinal fluid (CSF),[17] pericardium,[28] and ascites.[18] Transforming growth factor-β1 (TGF-β1) is lower in POEMS than in multiple myeloma.[13] IL-1β is expressed in the lymph nodes of these patients,[27] typically by the macrophages.[16] Moreover, levels of IL-1 receptor antagonist and sTNF-receptor are also increased in POEMS.[13,21,29]

Plasma and serum levels of VEGF are markedly elevated in patients with POEMS[13,22,26] and correlate with the activity of the disease.[13,30,31] Serum VEGF levels are 10–50 times higher than plasma levels of VEGF,[32] making it ambiguous to decide which test is better. The principal isoform of VEGF expressed is VEGF165.[30] VEGF levels are independent of M protein size.[30] Increased VEGF could account for the organomegaly, edema, skin hemangiomata, and the occasional mesangioproliferative changes found on renal biopsy. It could be an important regulator of osteoblastic differentiation.[13]

Little is known about the plasma cell clone in this disease, but aneuploidy[16] and deletion of chromosome 13[33] have been described. The light-chain variable gene usage of two patients' clones has been described; both belonged to the Vλ1 family and had 92–93% identity with the 1e gene.[34] Although at least 95% of all patients with POEMS have monoclonal lambda plasma cells, there are no convincing data to support that POEMS is a deposition disease like primary systemic amyloidosis.[10]

Clinical Features

The peak incidence of the POEMS syndrome is in the fifth and sixth decades of life, one to two decades earlier than patients with multiple myeloma. Symptoms of PN usually dominate the clinical picture.[8] Symptoms begin in the feet and consist of tingling, paresthesias, and coldness. Motor involvement follows the sensory symptoms. Some patients have a painful neuropathy. Neuropathic symptoms are distal, symmetric, and progressive with a gradual proximal spread. Severe weakness occurs in more than one-half of patients and results in inability to climb stairs, arise from a chair, or grip objects firmly with their hands. The course is usually progressive and patients may be confined to a wheelchair. Impotence occurs but autonomic symptoms are not a feature. Bone pain and fractures rarely occur. Weight loss and fatigue are common features as the disease progresses. Because patients become so restricted in their movement due to their neuropathy, it is rare for them to report dyspnea despite markedly abnormal pulmonary testing.

As time progresses, muscle weakness is more marked than sensory loss. Touch, pressure, vibratory, and joint position senses are usually involved. Loss of temperature discrimination and nociception is less frequent. The cranial nerves are not involved except for papilledema. Nerve conduction studies and electromyelography demonstrate a polyneuropathy with prominent demyelination as well as features of axonal degeneration, which are similar to the findings of patients with chronic inflammatory demyelinating polyradiculoneuropathy (CIDP).[8,35,36] Biopsy of the sural nerve usually shows both axonal degeneration and demyelination. VEGF is highly expressed in blood vessels and some nonmyelin-forming Schwann cells, but the expression of VEGF receptor 2 is downregulated as compared to normals.[31] In most cases of POEMS syndrome, the nerve biopsy shows typical features of uncompacted myelin lamellae. At ultrastructural examination, there are no features of macrophage-associated demyelination, which are seen in some cases of chronic inflammatory demyelinating polyneuropathy.[17,37–39]

Hyperpigmentation is common. Coarse black hair may appear on the extremities. Other skin changes include skin thickening, rapid accumulation of glomeruloid angiomata, flushing, dependent rubor or acrocyanosis, white nails, and clubbing. Testicular atrophy and gynecomastia may be present. Pitting edema of the lower extremities is common. Ascites and pleural effusion occur in approximately one-third of patients. The liver is palpable in almost one-half of patients, but splenomegaly and lymphadenopathy is found in fewer patients. On lymph node biopsy, the histology is frequently angiofollicular lymph node hyperplasia (Castleman's disease) or Castleman's -like disease.[10,12] Between 11% and 30% of patients with POEMS have documented Castleman's disease or Castleman's-like disease.[10,11] This estimate may be conservative since most patients do not undergo lymph node biopsies. In some cases of POEMS with lymphadenopathy, the lymph nodes do not meet the criteria to be called frank Castleman's disease, but are said to have Castleman's-like histology.[10,40]

Patients may develop arterial and/or venous thromboses during their course. Lesprit et al. observed 4 of 20 patients to have arterial occlusion.[41] In the Mayo series, there were 18 patients suffering serious events such as stroke, myocardial infarction, and Budd-Chiari syndrome.[12] Affected vessels include carotid, iliac, celiac, subclavian, mesenteric, and femoral.[42–45] The POEMS-associated strokes tend to be end artery border-zone infarctions.[45] Gangrene of lower extremities can occur.[44] It seems likely that VEGF and platelets play a role in arterial occlusion. VEGF protein is present in platelets and megakaryocytes. When vascular injury occurs at endothelial cells, platelets aggregate to repair damaged vascular intima and to release VEGF.[46]

Thrombocytosis is common, and polycythemia may be seen.[8,12] Anemia and thrombocytopenia are not characteristic unless there is coexisting Castleman's disease. Hypercalcemia and renal insufficiency are rarely present. The size of the M protein on electrophoresis is small (median 1.1 g/dL) and is rarely more than 3.0 g/dL. The M protein is usually IgG or IgA and almost always of the lambda type.[9,12] Levels of serum erythropoietin are low and are inversely correlated with VEGF levels.[31] Protein levels in the CSF are elevated in virtually all patients. Bone marrow usually contains less than 5% of plasma cells, and when clonal cells are found they are almost always monoclonal lambda. Osteosclerotic lesions occur in ~95% of patients, and can be confused with benign bone islands, aneurysmal bone cysts, nonossifying fibromas, and fibrous dysplasia. Lesions may be densely sclerotic, be lytic with a sclerotic rim, have a mixed soap-bubble appearance, or any such combination (Fig. 1). Bone windows of computed cotomography (CT) body images are often very informative. Fluorodeoxyglucose (FDG)-avidity is variable.

Endocrinopathy is a central but poorly understood feature of POEMS. In a recent large series from the Mayo Clinic,[47] ~84% of patients have a recognized endocrinopathy, with hypogonadism as the most common endocrine abnormality, followed by thyroid abnormalities, glucose metabolism abnormalities, and lastly by adrenal insufficiency. The majority of patients had evidence of multiple endocrinopathies in the four major endocrine axes (gonadal, thyroid, glucose, and adrenal).

Renal dysfunction is usually not a dominant feature of this syndrome. A slight excess in urinary protein is not unusual. In our experience, ~9% of patients have proteinuria exceeding 0.5 g/24 h and only 6% have a serum creatinine greater than or equal to 1.5 mg/dL. A total of four patients in our series developed

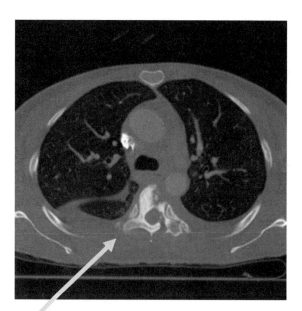

Sclerotic and lytic lesion T5

Fig. 1 POEMS (polyneuropathy, organomegaly, endocrinopathy, M protein, skin changes) Syndrome. Densely sclerotic lesion with adjacent lytic lesion. Also seen are pleural effusions and compressive atelectasis.

renal failure as preterminal events.[12] Renal disease is more likely to occur in patients who have coexisting Castleman's disease. The renal histology is diverse with membranoproliferative features and evidence of endothelial injury being most common.[48] On both light and electron microscopy, mesangial expansion, narrowing of capillary lumina, basement membrane thickening, subendothelial deposits, widening of the subendothelial space, swelling and vacuolization of endothelial cells, and mesangiolysis predominate.[49–55] Standard immunofluorescence is negative,[50,56] and this differentiates it from primary membranoproliferative glomerulitis.[48] Rarely, infiltration by plasma cell nests or Castleman's-like lymphoma can be seen.[55]

The pulmonary manifestations are protean, including pulmonary hypertension, restrictive lung disease, impaired neuromuscular respiratory function, and impaired diffuse capacity of carbon monoxide but improve with effective therapy (Fig. 2).[57–61] In a series of 20 patients with POEMS, followed over a 10-year period, 25% manifested pulmonary hypertension.[59] Findings on autopsy[59] or biopsy[62] are those of classic pulmonary hypertension, including eccentric intimal fibrosis, medial hypertrophy, and marked dilatation of arteries and arterioles. Whether the digital clubbing seen in POEMS is a reflection of underlying pulmonary hypertension and/or parenchymal disease is yet to be determined.

Diagnosis and Differential Diagnosis

Establishing diagnostic criteria for any syndrome is fraught with difficulty, POEMS notwithstanding. They must be broad enough to diagnose patients early to avoid cumulative morbidity, but narrow enough that patients without the syndrome are not mislabeled as having the syndrome. Soubrier et al.

Transplant date 8/26/02

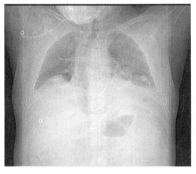 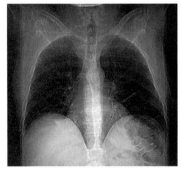

July 9, 2002

TLC 60%

FEV1 45%

PI max 42%

DLCO 55%

January 12, 2005

TLC 93%

FEV1 80%

PI max 111%

DLCO 92%

Fig. 2 POEMS (polyneuropathy, organomegaly, endocrinopathy, M protein, skin changes) Syndrome. Restrictive lung disease secondary to neuromuscular weakness, chest radiographs, and pulmonary function tests. **a**. Pretreatment. **b**. Posttreatment.

demonstrated that prognosis was not dependent on the number of features present in these patients.[11] We confirmed that in our series of 99 patients and proposed criteria, which were later criticized for being too broad.[63] With increasing information about the role of cytokines in this disorder, Arimura et al. have suggested including elevated levels of VEGF as one of the diagnostic criteria.[64] Table 1 includes revised criteria for a diagnosis of POEMS syndrome, based on our experience and that of the literature.[9,11,12,14,30,64]

The dominant feature of this syndrome is typically the PN, and not infrequently patients are initially diagnosed with chronic inflammatory demyelinating polyneuropathy (CIDP) or, less frequently, Guillain-Barré syndrome. If a monoclonal protein is detected, monoclonal gammopathy-associated PN and AL amyloidosis enter the differential diagnosis. The two best ways to distinguish POEMS from these entities are to measure a plasma or serum VEGF level and to determine whether there are other POEMS syndrome symptoms or signs. Watanabe et al. studied serum levels of VEGF in 10 patients with POEMS and compared them to measurements from normal controls ($n = 25$), CIDP ($n = 7$), Guillan-Barré syndrome ($n = 12$), and other neurologic disorders ($n = 20$).[30] Seventy percent of patients with POEMS had elevated levels while all other patients had normal levels. VEGF levels are higher in patients with POEMS than in patients with MGUS[13] and multiple myeloma.[13,14]

Table 1 Proposed criteria for the diagnosis of POEMS syndrome[a].

Major criteria	1. Polyneuropathy
	2. Monoclonal plasma cell-proliferative disorder (almost always λ)
	3. Sclerotic bone lesions
	4. Castleman's disease
	5. VEGF elevation
Minor criteria	6. Organomegaly (splenomegaly, hepatomegaly, or lymphadenopathy)
	7. Extravascular volume overload (edema, pleural effusion, or ascites)
	8. Endocrinopathy (adrenal, thyroid,[b] pituitary, gonadal, parathyroid, pancreatic[b])
	9. Skin changes (hyperpigmentation, hypertrichosis, glomeruloid hemangiomata, plethora, acrocyanosis, flushing, and white nails)
	10. Papilledema
	11. Thrombocytosis/polycythemia[c]
Other symptoms and signs	Clubbing, weight loss, hyperhidrosis, pulmonary hypertension/restrictive lung disease, thrombotic diatheses, diarrhea, and low vitamin B12 values
Possible associations	Arthralgias, cardiomyopathy (systolic dysfunction), and fever

POEMS polyneuropathy, organomegaly, endocrinopathy, M protein, skin changes, *VEGF* vascular endothelial growth factor

[a]Polyneuropathy and monoclonal plasma cell disorder present in all patients; to make diagnosis *at least* one other major criterion and one minor criterion is required to make diagnosis after exclusion of other causes

[b]Because of the high prevalence of diabetes mellitus and thyroid abnormalities, this diagnosis alone is not sufficient to meet this minor criterion

[c]Anemia and/or thrombocytopenia are distinctively unusual in this syndrome unless Castleman's disease is present

Treatment and Prognosis

The course of POEMS syndrome is chronic and patients typically survive for more than a decade in contrast to multiple myeloma. In our experience, the median survival was 13.8 years.[12] Individual reports of patients with the disease for more than 5 years are not unusual and in one French study, at least 7 of 15 patients were alive for more than 5 years.[11] In Nakanishi's series of 102 patients, the median survival was 33 months[10] though in Takatsuki's study of 109 patient, the authors stated that the "clinical course is very chronic ... some patients survived greater than 10 years."[9] In our experience, only fingernail clubbing and extravascular volume overload, that is, effusions, edema, and ascites, were significantly associated with a shorter overall survival. Other variables like number of POEMS features, age, alkylator use, number of bone lesions, endocrine involvement, weight loss, lymphadenopathy, Castleman's disease, organomegaly, papilledema, skin, gender, serum M protein, urine M protein, thrombocytosis, or hemoglobin had no predictive value for overall survival in the Mayo series.[12] More recently, we have identified respiratory symptoms to be predictive of adverse outcome.[61] In the French series, patients without plasmocytoma or bone lesions had a worse prognosis than those with other types of plasma cell dyscrasia in the absence of bone lesions.[11]

Additional features typically arise over time if treatment is unsuccessful or if the diagnosis is delayed.[12] The most common causes of death are cardiorespiratory failure, progressive inanition, infection, capillary-leak-like syndrome, and renal failure. Even those patients with multiple bone lesions or more than 10% plasma cells do not progress to classic multiple myeloma. The renal pathology in the occasional patient who develops renal failure is different from that of patients with classic myeloma. Stroke and myocardial infarction are also observed causes of death.

There are no randomized controlled trials in patients with POEMS. Information about benefits of therapy is most typically derived retrospectively (Table 2). Given these limitations, however, there are therapies which benefit patients with POEMS syndrome, including radiation therapy,[3,12,65,66,96,97] alkylator-based therapies,[6,10,12,54,67,98] and corticosteroids.[12] Intensive supportive care measures must also be instituted. Single or multiple osteosclerotic lesions in a limited area should be treated with radiation. If a patient has widespread osteosclerotic lesions or diffuse bone marrow plasmacytosis, systemic therapy is warranted. In contrast to CIDP, plasmapheresis and intravenous immunoglobulin do not produce clinical benefit. High-dose chemotherapy with peripheral blood transplant is yielding very promising results.[95] When the selected therapy is effective, response of systemic symptoms and skin changes typically precede those of the neuropathy, with the former beginning to respond within a month, and the latter within 3–6 months with maximum benefit frequently not seen before 2–3 years. Clinical response to therapy correlates better with VEGF level than with M protein level,[64,99] and complete hematologic response is not required to derive substantial clinical benefit.

Melphalan is among the most effective agents against plasmaproliferative disorders. Based on retrospective data, ~40% of patients with POEMS syndrome will respond to melphalan and prednisone.[12] The optimal duration of therapy has not been established, but borrowing from the experience of

Table 2 POEMS syndrome response to therapy.

Response to standard therapies

Reference	Treatment	Improvement rates (%)
3,6,12,65,66	Radiation	50
6,12,67–69	Standard dose alkylator-based therapy	40
10,12,17,51,70	Corticosteroids	15
48,71–84	High-dose chemotherapy with PBSCT	90

Response to experimental therapies

Reference	Treatment	No. of patients	Outcomes
85	Tamoxifen	1	Disappearance of edema, effusions and regression of PN
86	Ticlopidine	1	Improved edema, ascites, effusions, and VEGF for "several months"; no improvement in PN, other labs, or thyroid function.
32	Argatroban	2	1 improvement; 1 no response
87	IFN + argatroban	2	Improvement in paraprotein, neuropathy, and coagulation parameters – doing well at 2 years
88	IFN-α	1	POEMS + CD: Begun after radiation. Remarkable improvement in PN and organomegaly and lymphadenopathy after 3 months
89	Trans-retinoic acid	1	Improved cytokines, platelet count, but worsening PN
90	Strontium-89	1	Improvement in LA, hepatomegaly, PN, platelets
91	Thalidomide + dexamethasone	1	POEMS + CD: Improved PN, ascites, pleural effusion, dyspnea, creatinine, CBC, IL-6 within 2 months
92	Thalidomide	1a	Improved ascites, anemia, leukopenia, thrombocytopenia, ESR, and sense of well being
93	Bevacizumab	1	Patient also receiving melphalan + dexamethasone; improved edema, pain, weakness, VEGF
94	Bevacizumab	1	Worsening PN, anasarca, MOF; died of pneumonia 5 weeks after treatment
94	Bevacizumab	1	Initial worsening, dose repeated with cyclophosphamide resulted in improvement of pulmonary HTN, anasarca, skin changes
95	Lenalidomide + low-dose dexamethasone	1	Improvement in ascites, performance status, PN, VEGF levels, testosterone levels, pulmonary function tests

POEMS polyneuropathy, organomegaly, endocrinopathy, M protein, skin changes, *PN* peripheral neuropathy, *VEGF* vascular endothelial growth factor, *IFN* interferon, *CD* Castleman's disease, *HTN* hypertension, *IL-6* interleukin-6, *LA* lymphadenopathy, *MOF* multiorgan failure, *PBSCT* peripheral blood stem cell transplant, *ESR* erythrocyte sedimentation rateaPOEMS (w/ nl IL-6 and no bone lesions), but CD-like since anemia, leukopenia, thrombocytopenia, increased ESR multiple myeloma, 12–24 months of treatment is reasonable.100 Limiting the melphalan exposure is important because secondary myelodysplastic syndrome or acute leukemia can occur.101Cyclophosphamide is another alkylator that can control the disease in a limited number of patients. If the patient is considered to be a candidate for peripheral blood stem cell transplantation, melphalan-containing regimens should be avoided until after stem cell harvest.

High-dose chemotherapy with peripheral blood stem cell transplant is an emerging therapy for patients with POEMS. The first report was that of a 25-year-old woman who was treated with high-dose chemotherapy followed by bone marrow transplantation; she died of multiorgan failure 63 days after her stem cell transplant.71 Subsequently, there have been an additional 38 transplanted patients published.[48,72–84] All patients had improvement in their neuropathy over time; as in the case with radiation therapy and other chemotherapy, improvement in the PN takes months to years. Other clinical features improve after stem cell transplant, including levels of VEGF in several of the patients studied.[74,76]

Among the first 16 patients we transplanted, the treatment-related morbidity was higher than expected.[78] Thirty-seven percent of our patients spent time in the intensive care unit and thirty-seven percent required mechanical ventilation. Although only one of our patients died (6.2% mortality rate), if the published experience of transplanted patients with POEMS is pooled, the mortality figure is 2 of 27 or 7.4%. These numbers appear higher than the 2% transplant-related mortality observed in patients with multiple myeloma but lower than the 14% transplant-related mortality observed in patients with primary systemic amyloidosis.[102]

Other treatments which have been reported are shown in Table 2, and include plasmapheresis,[67,103,104] intravenous immunoglobulin,[105] interferon-α (IFN-α),[88,87] tamoxifen,[85,106] trans-retinoic acid,[89] thalidomide,[92] ticlopidine,[86] argatroban,[32,87] strontium-89,[90] bevacizumab,[93,94] and lenalidomide.[95] Plasmapheresis is not an effective treatment in this disorder.[103] Those reports purporting efficacy of plasma exchange combine the treatment with corticosteroids and/or other therapies confounding interpretation.[67,104] Intravenous immunoglobulin also cannot be recommended based on our experience or on a review of the literature.[105] Once again the few reports claiming effectiveness simultaneously use other immunosuppressants or treatments.[107–110] Although there is a theoretical rationale (anti-VEGF and antiTNF effects) for using the thalidomide in patients with POEMS , enthusiasm for its use should be tempered by the high rate of PN induced by the drug.[111] In contrast, the next-generation immune-modulatory drug, lenalidomide, has a much lower risk of PN. We have observed dramatic improvements in one patient treated with this drug.[95] Bevacizumab has been tried with mixed results. Two patients who had also received alkylator during and/or predating the bevacizumab had benefit. One who received it after radiation died.[93,94]

All-trans-retinoic acid (ATRA) has been tried based on the theory that it represses the AP-1 (a protein complex of c-jun and c-fos proto-onocgene products)-mediated induction of gene expression. AP-1-responsive elements are present on the IL-6, IL-1, and TNF-α genes, suggesting a possible inhibition of these cytokines by ATRA.[89] A patient was treated with ATRA, and 26 days into treatment, radiation therapy was also begun. Before the radiation therapy began, there was an insignificant drop in the serum IgA lambda level, a significant drop in the platelet and lymphocyte count, and the levels of IL-1β, IL-6 and TNF-α. However, there was only worsening of the neuropathy during therapy.

The physical limitations of the patient should not be overlooked while evaluating and/or treating the underlying PCD. As always a multidisciplinary, thoughtful treatment program will improve a complex patient's treatment outcome. A physical therapy and occupational therapy program is essential to maintain flexibility and assist in lifestyle management despite the neuropathy. In those patients with respiratory muscle weakness and/or pulmonary hypertension, overnight oxygen or continuous positive airway pressure (CPAP) may be useful.

MGUS-Associated Peripheral Neuropathy

MGUS is found in ~2–3% of patients older than 50 years of age and in 3–5% of persons older than 70 years.[112] It is defined by the presence of a serum M protein less than 3 g/dL and fewer than 10% plasma cells in the bone marrow in the absence of multiple myeloma, Waldenström macroglobulinemia, primary amyloidosis, cryoglobulinemia, or POEMS syndrome.[113]

The most convincing data for the connection of MGUS and PN was published in the 1980s.[114,115] Kahn and colleagues detected 58 cases of monoclonal gammopathy without evidence of myeloma or Waldenström macroglobulinemia in 14,000 serum samples (0.4%) obtained from patients admitted to a neurologic tertiary care center[114]; 16 of those 58 patients (28%) had PN. The second published study of import establishing a relationship between MGUS and PN was by Kelly et al. This study was conducted over a 1-year period in 692 patients with a clinically apparent PN who were identified in the electromyography (EMG) laboratory at the Mayo Clinic.[115] Three hundred and fifty-eight patients had an identifiable systemic disease known to cause PN such as diabetes mellitus, or alcoholism (secondary neuropathy group); 334 were apparently idiopathic. Approximately 80% of patients in each group had serum protein electrophoretic studies. In the secondary group, 2.5% of the patients had an M protein, while in the idiopathic group, 10% had an M protein: MGUS (16 patients); primary systemic amyloidosis (7 patients); Waldenström macroglobulinemia (1 patient); and gamma heavy chain disease (1 patient). The age-matched rate of monoclonal gammopathy was statistically significant higher in patients with PN as compared to normal populations in Minnesota and Sweden. Not all studies support the association,[116] but others do.[117–120]

Pathogenesis

The pathogenesis of MGUS neuropathy (especially IgM) is sometimes related to the reactivity of the monoclonal immunoglobulins to specific antigens expressed on peripheral nerves such as myelin-associated glycoprotein (MAG), gangliosides, chondroitin sulfate, and sulfatide. The most convincing pathogenic relationship is between IgM MGUS neuropathy and MAG antibodies, although there is still some controversy. In 1980, Latov et al. described a patient with sensorimotor PN and a monoclonal IgM protein that was directed against peripheral nerve myelin.[121] Dellagi et al. also reported that the IgM monoclonal protein with anti-MAG activity bound to the myelin sheaths of patients with PN.[122] Direct electron microscopic immunohistochemical studies with colloidal gold revealed deposition of IgM within the myelin and extending throughout the compact myelin in both large and small myelinated fibers. Complement-mediated damage to the sheath can be demonstrated resulting in separation of the outer lamellae of myelin.[123,124] Quarles and Weiss provide a comprehensive review of autoantibodies associated with PN.[125]

In approximately one-half of patients with an IgM MGUS and PN, the M protein binds to MAG.[122,124] There is no correlation between the size of the M protein and the anti-MAG titers. Low antibody titers (1:200 or less) to MAG can be found in 17% of control patients without MGUS.[126] In a series of 52 asymptomatic patients with IgM MGUS, symptomatic neuropathy eventually occurred in 3 of 4 patients with a high anti-MAG titer and in 3 of 21 patients with low anti-MAG titer.[127]

Clinical Course

Typically, MGUS-associated neuropathy has the following features: (1) there is an M protein in the serum, most commonly IgM, followed in frequency by IgG and then IgA; (2) there is a symmetric sensorimotor polyradiculopathy or neuropathy which begins insidiously and is usually slowly progressive; (3) cranial nerves are not involved; (4) it occurs more often in the sixth to seventh decade of life; (5) it affects men more frequently than women; (6) POEMS syndrome is not present.[128] Paresthesias, ataxia, and pain may be predominant features, but predisposition for these symptoms depends on the type of monoclonal protein present and whether there are anti-MAG antibodies present. Symptoms usually begin with paresthesias and numbness distally in the feet or hands, and early motor symptoms are rare or minor. The neuropathy then progresses proximally in stocking/glove distribution and may involve motor as well as sensory functions. Ataxia and tremor may be present and sometimes predominate. There is no correlation between the size of the monoclonal protein and the severity of the neuropathy. Roughly 50% of MGUS neuropathies are associated with IgM gammopathy; about one-half to two-thirds of these monoclonal proteins will have anti-MAG activity.[129,130]

IgM with Anti-MAG: Anti-MAG neuropathy has a fairly homogeneous clinical presentation.[130–133] Patients present in their sixth to ninth decades with a slowly progressive and relatively painless sensory neuropathy, which gradually ascends proximally. Patients report a symmetric numbness and paresthesias of the feet and distal legs along with gradually increasing unsteadiness due to sensory ataxia. A minority of patients will have an intention tremor of the hands.[133] On physical exam, they have discriminative sensory loss, including loss of vibration and position sense and a positive Romberg's sign. Pain and temperature sense is less severely affected. Clinically evident autonomic dysfunction rarely occurs. Loss of motor strength is typically minor and overshadowed by the sensory loss. Reflexes are typically absent in the lower extremities.

EMG shows the classic findings of a demyelinating polyneuropathy with marked slowing of motor conduction velocities, very prolonged distal latencies, and areas of conduction block and dispersal on proximal stimulation, with secondary axonal degenerative changes.[133] Sensory potentials are absent or severely attenuated. CSF has a high protein concentration, with normal glucose and cell count. Nerve biopsy typically shows IgM deposition on the myelin sheath using imunofluorescent techniques, and splitting and separation of the outer layers of compacted myelin on electron microscopy. The serum protein electrophoresis (SPEP) usually shows a small monoclonal protein, but immunofixation should always be ordered since these small proteins can be buried in a normal background that can be missed on SPEP alone. Specialized testing using enzyme-linked immunosorbent assay (ELISA) or immunoblotting shows that the IgM antibody reacts with MAG and other sphinogoglycolipid epitopes.

IgM Without Anti-MAG: IgM MGUS-associated PN without anti-MAG reactivity tends to be more heterogeneous than the anti-MAG-associated PN.[129] Some of these patients will have a demyelinating presentation, while others will have an axonal degeneration presentation. Patients with the demyelinating type resemble the anti-MAG neuropathy based on clinical and electrophysiologic attributes. Serologic studies may show antibodies against sulfatides.[134] However, the nerve biopsy does not show the typical myelin deposition of antibodies or the characteristic myelin splitting of the anti-MAG neuropathy. Patients may also present with an axonal form of PN reporting dysesthesia. Antisulfatide antibodies may be present. Amyloidosis and cryoglobulinemia need to be excluded.

IgG or IgA: The neuropathy associated with IgG or IgA is different and should be distinguished from those with IgM.[129] The IgG- and IgA-associated PNs account for ~40–50% of the MGUS-associated neuropathies, with IgG more common than IgA. Most patients in this group will have axonal neuropathies, which are mild, affecting mainly the feet and the legs, potentially causing dysethesias with little functional deficit.

Diagnosis and Differential Diagnosis

MGUS neuropathy must be distinguished from the entities in Table 3 as well as chronic inflammatory demyelinating polyneuropathy (CIDP), paraneoplastic neuropathies, and metabolic and toxic neuropathies. The relationship between chronic inflammatory demyelinating polyradiculopathy and CIDP with MGUS is unclear. In contrast to patients with CIDP, patients with a CIDP-like presentation and MGUS have a more indolent course,[135,136] less severe weakness,[135–137] more of a sensory deficit including vibration loss in the hands,[137] more ataxia,[137] no cranial nerve involvement,[136] and symmetrical involvement.[136] The clinical course tends to be progressive in most patients with MGUS whereas those with CIDP were more likely to have a relapsing course.[135] On electrophysiologic examination, the MGUS group is more likely to have absent median and ulnar sensory potentials[136,137] and abnormal sural nerve action potentials.[136] POEMS syndrome should be excluded in this patient population, especially if the immunoglobulin light chain is lambda.

In those cases with axonal features, amyloidosis should be excluded, although the neuropathy associated with amyloidosis tends to be more severe and is often associated with autonomic and other organ dysfunction.

Treatment and Prognosis

Initiation of treatment is largely based on comparing the potential risk of therapy to its potential benefit. Nobile-Orazio et al. analyzed the long-term

Table 3 System involvement by various atypical plasma cell disorders.

	Peripheral nerves	Kidney	Skin	Heart	Liver	LN	Intestines	Eyes	Lungs
Amyloidosis	+	++	++	++	+	+	+	+a	+
POEMS	+++	− to +	++	− to +	++	++	− to +	++	++
MGUS-associated PN	+++	−	−	−	−	−	−	−	−
Cryoglobulinemia	+ to ++	+	+++	−	++	+	−	+	−
Scleromyxedema	+	−	+++	+	−	−	++	−	+
Xanthogranuloma necrobiotica	−	− to +	+++	− to +	−	−	− to +	+, +++a	− to +
Schnitzler's syndrome	−	−	+++	−	+	++	−	−	−
Light-chain deposition disease	−	+++	−	+	+	−	−	−	+
Fanconi's syndrome	−	+++	−	−	−	−	−	−	−
Fibrillary glomerulonephritis	−	+++	−	−	−	−	−	−	−
α-heavy-chain disease	−	−	−	−	−	+	+++	−	−
μ-heavy-chain disease	−	−	−	−	++	+	−	−	−
γ-heavy-chain disease	−	−	−	−	+ to ++	+	−	−	−

POEMS polyneuropathy, organomegaly, endocrinopathy, M protein, skin changes, *MGUS* monoclonal gammopathy of undetermined significance, *PN* peripheral neuropathy−, ~0%; +, 1–39%; ++, 40–99%; +++, ~100%
aPeriorbital tissues only

outcome of 25 of the 26 patients (mean age at entry 65 years, range 45–85 years) with neuropathy and high anti-MAG IgM.[138] After a mean follow-up of 8.5 years (range 2-13 years) and a mean duration of neuropathy symptoms of 11.8 years (range 3–18, > 10 years in 16), 17 patients (68%) were alive. The eight (32%) who died did so 3–15 years (mean 10.6) after neuropathy onset; in none of them was death caused by the neuropathy, although in three it was possibly related to the therapy for the neuropathy. The authors also found that at last follow-up or before death, 11 patients (44%) were disabled by severe hand tremor, gait ataxia or both, with disability rates at 5, 10, and 15 years from neuropathy onset of 16%, 24%, and 50%, respectively. Of the 19 patients treated during the follow-up for 0.5–11 years (mean 4 years) with various immune therapies, only five (26%) reported a consistent and four (21%) a slight improvement in the neuropathy after one treatment or more; only one patient had persistent improvement throughout the follow-up period. Severe adverse events, possibly related to therapy, occurred during treatment in ten patients (53%).[138]

To date, treatment strategies have been directed toward reducing the IgM paraprotein level either by removing the antibody or targeting the presumed monoclonal B-cell clone, or toward interfering with the presumed effector mechanisms such as complement activation or macrophage recruitment. There are limited published data regarding efficacy of the various immunosuppressive regimes in IgM paraproteinaemic neuropathies and only six randomized controlled trials (Table 4).[139,140,142–144] Most case series are small, include diverse groups of patients and measurements of efficacy differ between trials.

Table 4 Randomized trials to treat MGUS-associated peripheral neuropathy.

Reference	No. of Patients	Treatment	Outcome
139	39	Double-blind plasma exchange vs sham	Improvement in NDS with protein electrophoresis ; especially in IgA and IgG patients
140	24	Chlorambucil vs chlorambucil and plasma exchange	Sensory component of NDS improved slightly in both arms. No difference between treatments
141	20	Open randomized IFN-α vs IV IG	8/10 vs 1/10 improved NDS at 6 months, persistent at 12 months. Sensory improvement only. Decreased IgM in 2 IFN-α patients. MAG Ab persist
142	22	IV Ig vs placebo	Improved handgrip, 10 m walking time, and sensory symptom score in IV Ig group as compared to baseline. Only difference at 4 weeks was hand grip
143	24	Double-blind randomized IFN-α vs placebo	3/12 patients in each arm improved clinically. No benefit to IFN-α

MGUS monoclonal gammopathy of undetermined significance, *IFN* interferon, *NDS* neuropathy disability score, *MAG* myelin-associated glycoprotein, *IV* intravenously

The first of these randomized trials in patients with MGUS-associated PN was a comparison of plasma exchange with sham exchange in 39 patients, 21 of whom had an IgM paraprotein.[139] Patients received either plasma exchange twice weekly or sham-plasma exchange in a double-blind trial. Sham-plasma exchange patients subsequently underwent plasma exchange in an open trial. The average neuropathy disability score improved significantly in the plasma exchange group. In both the double blind and open trials IgG or IgA gammopathy had a better response to plasma exchange than those with IgM gammopathy.[139] In multiple small studies of plasma exchange used as monotherapy, improvement has been reported in more than 50% of cases of MGUS-associated neuropathy.[137,138,145] Improvement with plasma exchange in combination with other drugs has been described. However, in a prospective study of 44 patients with an IgM MGUS and PN, patients were randomized to receive either chlorambucil orally or chlorambucil plus 15 courses of plasma exchange during the first 4 months of therapy. There was no difference in the two treatment groups.[140]

Alylators may be used, with the knowledge that secondary myelodysplastic syndrome or acute leukemia are possible complications. Small studies indicate response rates of ~33%.[121,124,132,138,140] Corticosteroids are not usually effective in patients with neuropathy and IgM MGUS.[146]

Based on the results of a small open label randomized study in which patients were randomized to either IFN-α or IV Ig, it was thought that IFN-α was an effective therapy in patients with IgM MAG-associated PN. A successor study, which was a blinded comparison of IFN-α and placebo, however, was negative.[143]

Intravenous gammaglobulin produces benefit in some patients with CIDP and may be used for patients with sensorimotor PN and MGUS. Intravenous immunoglobulin is beneficial in 25–50% of patients.[144,143] Dalakas et al. randomized 11 patients with IgM MAG-associated PN to either intravenous gammaglobulin or placebo; at 3 months patients crossed over to the other therapy. There was improvement in 27% of the patients, improved strength in two patients and improved sensory symptoms in another, without any change in MAG or SGPG titers.[144] Comi et al. treated 22 patients with IgM MAG-associated PN with either intravenous gammaglobulin or placebo, and found short-term intrapatient improvement.[142]

Novel therapies such as purine nucleoside analogs[147] and rituximab[148–150] may be useful. Fludarabine, a purine analog, produced benefit in 3 of 4 patients with an IgM MGUS and PN obtained clinical and neurophysiologic benefit from fludarabine.[147] Thirty-five patients have been treated with anti-CD20 antibodies in three open studies with response rates of 66–100%.[148–150] Lowering of both IgM levels and anti-MAG antibody titers is observed.[149] Pestronk et al. treated 21 patients with IgM MAG (7 patients)- or IgM ganglioside (14 patients)-associated neuropathy with rituximab, with an option to retreat, followed by a maintenance course of a dose every 10 weeks for 2 years. Eighty-one percent had improvement in the functional scores over baseline at the conclusion of the study.[150]

Atypical PCD with Dermopathy as Dominant Phenotype

Cryoglobulinemia

In 1933, Wintrobe and Buell[151] reported observing cryoglobulins in a serum sample from a patient with multiple myeloma. The term "cryoglobulin" was coined by Lerner and Watson[152] in 1947. Precipitation of cryoglobulins is dependent on temperature, pH, cryoglobulin concentration, and weak non-covalent factors.[153] Meltzer and others delineated a distinct syndrome of purpura, arthralgias, asthenia, renal disease, and neuropathy – often occurring with immune complex deposition or vasculitis, or both.[154,155] Brouet et al.[156] popularized a system of classifying cryoglobulinemia on the basis of the components of the cryoprecipitate: type I, isolated monoclonal immunoglobulins; type II, a monoclonal component, usually IgM, possessing activity toward polyclonal immunoglobulins, usually IgG; and type III, polyclonal immunoglobulins of more than one isotype.[156] This classification provided a framework by which clinical correlations could be made. Associated conditions, such as lymphoproliferative disorders, connective tissue disorders, infection, and liver disease, were observed in some patients.[157,158] In several large series, 34–71% of cryoglobulinemia cases were not associated with other specific disease states and were termed "essential" or primary cryoglobulinemia.[156,157,159] In 1990, hepatitis C virus (HCV) was recognized as an etiologic factor for the majority of these cases.[160,161]

Pathogenesis

Cryoglobulinemia is driven primarily by four classes of disease: liver disease (predominantly HCV), infection (again, predominantly HCV), connective tissue disease, and lymphoproliferative disease. These diseases induce a seemingly nonspecific stimulation of B cells, frequently resulting in polyclonal hypergammaglobulinemia. When these various antibodies are produced, antibodies to autoantigens may also result. In animal models, a strong B-cell stimulus disrupts the sequential order of idiotype–anti-idiotype interactions, resulting in both immunosuppression and idiotype–anti-idiotype immune complexes.[162] Furthermore, poorly regulated production and clearance of IgM rheumatoid factor contribute to immune complex formation[153,157] and pathologic conditions, which include vasculitis, nephritis, and vascular occlusion.

Complement components, fibronectin, and lipoproteins have been found along with antigen–antibody complexes within cryoprecipitates. Although hepatitis B virus, Epstein-Barr virus, and bacterial products may also be present, by far the most common pathogen within cryoprecipitates is HCV.[163] HCV RNA, HCV-specific proteins, and anti-HCV antibodies are found in the supernatant of the cryoprecipitate and in the cryoprecipitate itself in 42–98% of patients with essential mixed cryoglobulinemia[164–170] Cryoprecipitates contain 20–1,000 times more HCV RNA than is present in the supernatant.[171] The IgG component to which the IgM-rhematoid factor fraction binds is directed against the HCV proteins.[172]

Clinical Course

The prevalence of cryoglobulinemia is difficult to estimate both because of its clinical polymorphism and because of the necessity of separating the laboratory finding of cryoglobulins from the symptomatic disease state. Although only a minority of patients with serum cryoglobulins have symptoms referable to them, cryoglobulins may be found in patients with cirrhosis (up to 45%), alcoholic hepatitis (32%), autoimmune hepatitis (40%), subacute bacterial endocarditis (90%), rheumatoid arthritis (47%), IgG myeloma (10%), and Waldenström macroglobulinemia (19%).[156–158,173,174]

Results of most studies show that the median age at diagnosis is the early to mid-1950s. In some studies, the woman predominance for cryoglobulinemia is greater than 2:1. No racial preference has been noted, but the incidence is higher in regions where HCV occurs at higher frequencies (e.g., southern Europe).

Involvement of the skin, peripheral nerves, kidneys, and liver is common (Table 5). Lymphadenopathy is present in ~17% of patients.[155,157] On autopsy, widespread vasculitis involving small and medium vessels in the heart, gastrointestinal tract, central nervous system, muscles, lungs, and adrenal glands may also be seen.[157,182] The interval between the onset of symptoms and the time of diagnosis varies considerably (range, 0–10 years).[157] Type I cryoglobulinemia is usually asymptomatic. When symptomatic, it most commonly causes occlusive symptoms rather than the vasculitis of types II and III.[155–156,157] Symptoms of hyperviscosity may occur. Type II cryoglobulinemia is more frequently symptomatic (61% of patients) than type III (21% of patients).[183]

Skin: Purpura is the most frequent symptom of mixed cryoglobulinemia, being present in 55–100% of patients with mixed cryoglobulinemia.[156,157,159,176] The incidence varies from 15% to 33% in type I, from 60% to 93% in type II,

Table 5 Clinical features of cryoglobulinemia at diagnosis.

Reference[a]	N	Essential[b]	Cryo type			LPD	Liver[c]	Sicca	Skin	Raynaud	Renal	Arthralgia	Neuro
			I	II	III								
Meltzer et al.[155]	29	41	59	41d	41d	31	72e	17e	92e	–	25e	92e	17e
Brouet et al.[156]	86	34	25	25	50	44	–	9	55	50	21	35	17
	40	100	0	32	68	–	70	15	100	25	55	72	12
Tarantino et al.[156]	44	82	–	–	–	0f	14	2	59	7	100	57	7
Singer et al.[176]	16	–	12	63	25	6	–	–	94	–	63	63	56
Monti et al.[177]	891	72	6	62	32	6	39	5	76	19	20	–	21
Ferri et al.[156]	231	<8	–	62	38	10	77	53	98	48	30	98	80
Trejo et al.[179]	206g	–	–	–	–	10	–	–	51	11	39	40	14
Rieu et al.[180]	49	12	6h	49	33	0	43	35	82	35	24	51	55
Bryce[181]	66	15	–	100	–	9	50	2	55	12	26	21	18

Abd abdominal, *cryo* cryoglobulinemia, *LPD* lymphoproliferative disorder, *neuro* neurologic disease

[a] Publications are listed chronologically, from oldest to most recent

[b] Cryoglobulinemia without any identified predisposing condition. These values do not represent actual incidence but rather the makeup of the population analyzed for symptoms

[c] Patients with abnormal liver function tests or hepatomegaly, or both

[d] Value is for types II and III combined

[e] Symptoms of the essential mixed cryoglobulinemia (types II and III) population only

[f] Patients with multiple myeloma, Waldenström macroglobulinemia, and infection were excluded from this study by design

[g] Only patients with a cryocrit value of 1% or greater were included. The percentages were calculated on the basis of the 206 symptomatic patients described by the authors

[h] In this study, 12% of the patients were not typed

[i] Series restricted to patients with renal involvement

and from 70% to 83% in type III.[184] Petechiae and palpable purpura are the most common lesions (Fig. 3a), although ecchymoses, erythematous spots, and dermal nodules occur in as many as 20% of patients. Bullous or vesicular lesions are distinctly uncommon.[156] Successive purpuric rashes, which may be preceded by a burning or itching sensation, occur most commonly on the lower extremities, gradually extending to the thighs and lower abdomen. Occasionally the arms are involved, but the face and trunk are generally spared.[156] Head and mucosal involvement, livedoid vasculitis, and cold-induced acrocyanosis of the helices of the ears are more frequently observed in type I; infarction, hemorrhagic crusts, or ulcers occur in 10–25% of all patients with mixed cryoglobulinemia (Fig. 3b).[185] Showers of purpura last for 1–2 weeks and occur once or twice a month. Cold precipitates these types of lesions in only 10%–30% of the patients.[156,185] Raynaud phenomenon occurs in about 19–50% of patients[156,157,159,176]; in a quarter of these, the symptoms may be severe, including necrosis of fingertips.[156] Skin necrosis, urticaria, and livedo, which are all rare, are more commonly associated with exposure to cold.

Arthralgias:

Arthralgias are common, affecting 35–92% of patients with cryoglobulinemia, with the highest incidence in type III cryoglobulinemia (Table 1). The small distal joints are affected more frequently than the larger proximal joints. Symmetrical polyarthralgia is often exacerbated by the cold. Frank arthritis is rare.[156,157,159,176,179]

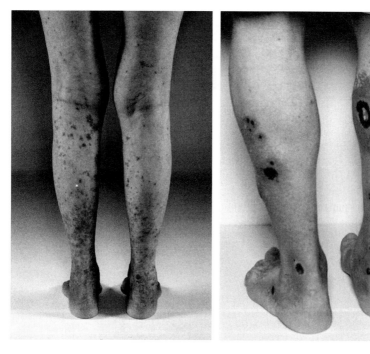

A   B

Fig. 3 Cryoglobulinemic skin changes. **a**. Purpura. **b**. Vaculitic ulcers (*see* Plate 22).

Nervous System:

PN is the most common presentation, although central nervous system involvement may occur. In the largest clinical series, peripheral nerve involvement is described in 12–56% of patients (Table 1).[156,157,159,176,179] Signs and symptoms of sensory neuropathy usually precede those of motor neuropathy.[156,186] The presentation may be an acute or subacute distal symmetric polyneuropathy or a mononeuritis multiplex[186–188] with a chronic or chronic-relapsing evolution.[189] The neuropathy in essential mixed cryoglobulinemia is most often characterized by axonal degeneration. Epineurial vasculitis is a common finding on sural nerve biopsy.[187,188,190–192] Even when other manifestations of mixed cryoglobulinemia are stable over time, there is typically worsening of the PN.[193]

More recently, there have been documented central nervous system abnormalities in patients with mixed cryoglobulinemia. Casato et al. reported on 40 patients with mixed cryoglobulinemia vasculitis and chronic active HCV infection, whom they compared to normal controls and patients with HCV without mixed cryoglobulinemia. Twenty-four of the 27 (89%) evaluated patients with HCV-mixed cryoglobulinemia had a deficiency in one or more of the ten cognitive domains examined.[194]

Kidney: Approximately 21–39% of patients with mixed cryoglobulinemia have renal involvement.[156,179,195] The incidence of renal injury is highest in patients with type II cryoglobulins.[159,196] Although renal and extrarenal manifestations may occur concurrently, renal involvement usually follows the onset of purpura by ~4 years.[157,197] Proteinuria greater than 0.5 g/day and hematuria are the most common features of renal disease at diagnosis (present in 50% of patients)[198]; nephrotic syndrome affects ~20% of patients and acute nephritic syndrome affects ~25% of patients.[197,198] Although cryopathic membranoproliferative glomerulonephritis portends a poor prognosis[157,173,196,198,199] progression to end-stage renal failure due to sclerosing nephritis is uncommon.[199] Among patients with mixed cryoglobulinemia-associated membranoproliferative glomerulonephritis followed up for a median of 11 years, 15% had disease progression to end-stage renal failure, and 43% died of cardiovascular, hepatic, or infectious causes.[198]

Liver: Approximately 39% of patients with symptomatic cryoglobulinemia[159] and as many as 77% with mixed cryoglobulinemia[157,200] have documented liver abnormalities at the time of diagnosis (Table 5). Furthermore, hepatomegaly is present in up to 70% of patients, and splenomegaly is present in up to 52% of patients.[154,157,175] Among patients with symptomatic cryoglobulinemia, liver failure is the cause of death in 2.5–7.6% of patients[157,198,177] and in 5.6–29% of all reported deaths.[157,198,177]

Histologic findings include portal fibrosis, chronic persistent hepatitis, chronic active hepatitis, chronic active hepatitis with cirrhosis, and postnecrotic cirrhosis.[200] Most specimens are characterized by a diffuse lymphocytic infiltrate ranging from minimal periportal to extensive infiltration with nodule formation. These changes correlate with the severity of other pathologic findings. Plasma cell infiltration has also been noted in several specimens.[183,200] The lymphoid population in the liver may show the histologic and immunophenotypic findings of lymphoplasmacytoid lymphoma/immunocytoma, and frequently the lymphoid elements arrange in pseudo-follicular structures in the liver with morphologic features similar to those previously reported in chronic HCV without cryoglobulinemia.[201] These liver lymphoid nodules contain B cells predominantly with a CD5[+]/Bcl-2[+]/Ki67[-] phenotype – that is, low apoptotic and proliferative rates.[202]

Serologic Testing: The type or quantity of the cryoglobulin does not reliably predict the presence or nature of symptoms. On SPEP, polyclonal hypergammaglobulinemia is the most common finding, although normal patterns or hypogammaglobulinemia may also be seen.[155,157,181] Even among patients with type II cryoglobulinemia, only 15% have a visible monoclonal spike on SPEP. Frequently, serum[157] IgM levels are elevated; cryoprecipitable IgM may comprise up to one-third of the total serum IgM concentration.[157] Hyperviscosity occurs only occasionally.[154] Marked depression of complement CH50, C1q, and C4 in the presence of relatively normal C3 levels is usual.[157,179,203] Neither C4 concentrations nor cryoglobulin levels correlate with overall clinical severity, although for individual patients the cryoglobulin level can sometimes serve as a marker for disease activity.[157,203–205] Rheumatoid factor activity – that is, anti-Fc activity – is detectable in the sera in 87–100% of patients with mixed cryoglobulinemia,[155,156,177] and levels may decrease with response to therapy.[206] An elevated erythrocyte sedimentation rate (ESR) and a mild normochromic, normocytic anemia are fairly common.[157,205]

Diagnosis and Differential Diagnosis

By definition, all patients with cryoglobulinemia have serum cryoglobulins, but they should also have symptoms of the syndrome. Within the differential diagnosis for cryoglobulinemia are vasculitides, connective tissue diseases, and HCV with extrahepatic manifestations, but without cryoglobulinemia.

Treatment and Prognosis

It is well recognized that cryoglobulinemia has a fluctuating course with spontaneous exacerbation and remission. This feature makes controlled clinical trials essential in evaluating the response to therapy. Unfortunately, such studies are rare in the field of cryoglobulinemia. With the exception of the IFN-α trials of the 1990s[207–211] and the small low-antigen diet trial performed in the 1980s,[212] the remainder of the information about the treatment of symptomatic cryoglobulinemia is anecdotal (Table 6).

Fortunately, the prognosis for most is good. In a large series by Ferri et al. of 231 patients seen from 1972 to 2001, the mixed cryoglobulinemia syndrome followed a relatively benign clinical course in over 50% of cases, whereas a moderate–severe clinical course was observed in one-third of patients whose prognosis was severely affected by renal and/or liver failure. For 15% of individuals, the disease was complicated by malignancy: B-cell more common than hepatocellular and thyroid malignancies. Ten year overall survival was 56%. Lower survival rates were seen in men and in individuals with renal involvement.[178] The most common causes of death include renal failure, infection, lymphoproliferative disorders, liver failure, cardiovascular complications, and hemorrhage.[156,157,159,176,180]

For years, the standard treatment of mild symptomatic cryoglobulinemia (purpura, asthenia, arthralgia, and mild sensory neuropathy) has included bed rest, analgesics, low-dose corticosteroid therapy, low-antigen content diet, and

Table 6 Treatment strategies for symptomatic cryoglobulinemia.

Reference	Treatment	Effective?
See text	IFN	Yes
213	Ribavirin	Probably
212	Low-antigen diet	Probably (mild disease)
205,214–216,217–219	Plasmapheresis, plasma exchange	Probably
154,157,173,175,220,221	Low-dose corticosteroids	Probably
222,223	High-dose corticosteroids	Probably
214	Chlorambucil	Probably
224,219,225,226	Cyclophosphamide	Probably
220	Melphalan	Probably
227–233	Anti-CD20	Probably
234,235	Thalidomide	Probably
157	Azathioprine	Possibly
201,236	Cyclosporin	Possibly
237	Anti-TNF-α antibody	Probably not
238	Colchicine	Probably not
239,240	Immunoglobulin IV	Variablea
241,242	Cladribine and fludarabine	Variable
154,224	Splenectomy	Variable
154	Chloroquine	Probably not
156	H1 and H2 blockers	Probably not
157	Penicillamine	Probably not

IFN interfeon, *TNF*-α tumor necrosis factor-α, *IV* intravenouslyaOne case report of precipitating acute renal failure[239] and another of systemic vasculitis[243]

protective measures against cold; the treatment of severe disease (glomerulonephritis, motor neuropathy, and systemic vasculitis) has included plasmapheresis, high-dose corticosteroid therapy, and cytotoxic therapy. Since the association was made between HCV and mixed cryoglobulinemia, immunosuppressive therapy has been viewed less favorably, and IFN is generally considered to be first-line therapy for HCV-positive patients who are in nonemergent situations.[207–211,244] For patients with symptomatic type I cryoglobulinemia, anti-CD20 therapy and/or cytotoxic therapy appropriate for the lymphoproliferative disorder remains the therapy of choice. Similarly, treatment of underlying connective tissue disease or infection would be first-line therapy in appropriate situations. The importance of not over treating patients must be emphasized. Clinical trials are needed to clarify these issues.

For emergent situations (acute nephritis or severe vasculitis), authors have suggested initially using measures aimed at reducing the inflammatory activity of renal lesions (corticosteroids), removing circulating cryoglobulins (plasmapheresis), and reducing the formation of new antibodies (e.g., cyclophosphamide)[197,245,246] is the dogma, although no randomized clinical trials support this strategy. Plasma exchange or plasmapheresis alone can reverse serious complications, but most authors have reported use of these procedures in combination with cytotoxic agents or corticosteroids for more durable responses.[204,214–216] According to case reports, responses may be seen in 60–100% of patients.[204,214–216] Skin manifestations and arthralgias usually respond the quickest, whereas the degree of neural and renal responses depends on the acuity of their occurrence, with poorer responses occurring in chronic cases.[215] With combination immunosuppressive therapy and plasma exchange, reversal of catastrophic complications such as encephalopathy and acute glomerulone-phritis has been documented.[204,215,247] High-dose pulse therapy with methyl-prednisolone is also a favored therapeutic intervention for acute events, with 90% response rates in rapidly progressive glomerulo-nephritis.[197,222] Once the acute exacerbation has been mitigated, those patients who are HCV positive antiviral strategies are implemented in HCV-positive patients to consolidate and maintain response. There is mounting evidence that the ribavirin and IFN-α combination are effective in the setting of renal disease.[245,248] One should be cognoscente of reports of PN (personal observation) and,[249] nephritis,[250] vasculitis,[251] and ischemic manifestations being exacerbated by IFN-α.[252]

Antiviral Therapy: Five randomized trials evaluating the efficacy of IFN therapy in HCV-positive patients with symptomatic type II mixed cryoglob-ulinemia conducted in the 1990s documented clinical responses in 60–89% of the patients.[207–211] However, when compared with HCV-related chronic hepatitis, treatment of mixed cryoglobulinemia with IFN monotherapy was associated with a relatively poorer response and a high relapse rate, especially in severe cases.[246] A majority of patients relapsed within 6 months of discon-tinuation.[208–211,244] Lack of response after 3–4 months predicted for mono-therapy failure.[244] Factors associated with a poorer response to therapy or rapid relapse include liver cirrhosis, advanced age,[211] male sex gender,[244] and high levels of HCV RNA at the onset of therapy.[209,253] Purpuric lesions and liver function abnormalities are the features that tend to respond rapidly (within weeks), but neuropathy and nephropathy respond more slowly.[244,249]

The frequent relapse of both HCV replication and mixed cryoglobulinemia syndrome at the end of IFN treatment suggested the combination with ribavirin: this therapeutic option appeared valid in several studies.[254–257] Even ribavirin monotherapy has been shown to decrease transaminase levels and mixed cryoglobulinemia-related symptoms. IFN-α and ribavirin is now the preferred strategy for patients with symptomatic HCV-associated cryoglobulinemia.[254,256,258] More than 60% of patients with symptomatic mixed cryoglobulinemia who do not respond to IFN therapy alone respond to combined therapy, and 80% of patients who relapse with IFN-α therapy alone respond to combined therapy.[254]

For those who cannot tolerate the combination therapy and relapse or do not respond to standard schedules of IFN-α more frequent dosing[249,259] and longer duration of therapy (at least 1 year) may result in more rapid[249,259] and durable responses.[207,208,244] The use of prednisone in the induction strategy may result in quicker and more durable responses, but care must be taken because serum HCV RNA levels may increase with the use of prednisone.[209] If relapse occurs during therapy, resistance may result from antibodies to IFN; reinduction may be possible.[249]

Ribavirin plus weekly pegylated IFN-α is at least as effective than the com-bination using standard thrice weekly IFN-α.[260,261] Saadoun et al. compared the outcomes of 72 consecutive patients who received treatment with IFN-α (*n* = 32 patients) or pegylated IFN-α (*n* = 40 patients), both in combination with oral ribavirin, for at least 6 months. Compared with patients treated with

IFN-α plus ribavirin, those receiving pegylated IFN-α plus ribavirin had a higher sustained clinical (67.5% vs 56.3%), virologic (62.5% vs 53.1%), and immunologic (57.5% vs 31.3%) response, regardless of HCV genotype and viral load. In multivariate analyses, an early virologic response was independently associated with a complete clinical response of mixed cryoglobulinemia. A glomerular filtration rate less than or equal to 70 ml/min was negatively associated with a complete clinical response of mixed cryoglobulinemia.[261]

Rituximab Therapy: Anti-CD20 therapy with rituximab has been shown to produce responses in patients with all types of cryoglobulinemia[227–229]; however, those patients with HCV are at risk for increased HCV replication.[227,228]

Zaja et al. reported on 15 patients with type II mixed cryoglobulinemia (HCV-related in 12 of 15) who were treated with rituximab. Skin vasculitis manifestations (ulcers, purpura, or urticaria), subjective symptoms of PN, low-grade B-cell lymphoma, arthralgias, and fever improved and nephritis of recent onset went into remission in one case. Laboratory features, that is, significantly decreased serum rheumatoid factor and cryoglobulins and increased C4, were consistent with the clinical efficacy.[227]

In another report, Sansanno and coworkers treated 20 patients with mixed cryoglobulinemia and HCV-positive chronic active liver disease, resistant to IFN-α therapy. Sixteen patients (80%) showed a complete response, characterized by rapid improvement in clinical signs (disappearance of purpura and weakness arthralgia and improvement in PN), and decline of cryocrit. Complete response was associated with a significant reduction in rheumatoid factor activity and anti-HCV antibody titers. However, HCV RNA increased approximately twice the baseline levels in the responders, whereas it remained much the same in the nonresponders.[228]

Others have seen similar clinical results.[229,230] Basse and coworkers studied seven patients with type III cryoglobulin-related renal graft dysfunction, five of whom were HCV positive. Rituximab resulted in a dramatic improvement in all renal parameters, but two patients experienced serious infectious complications as well.[231] The initial increase in the cryoglobulin level after rituximab therapy for type II cryoglobulinemia secondary to Waldenström macroglobulinemia does not indicate failure of response.[262]

Other Therapies: Although not formally studied, high-dose therapy with autologous stem cell transplantation may be considered for patients with symptomatic, refractory cryoglobulinemia that results from a plasmaproliferative disorder. There is an increased risk of lethal veno-occlusive disease in patients with chronic hepatitis C who are undergoing stem cell transplantation;[263] for these patients, there are no data to support implementation of this therapy.

Dramatic reductions in the cryocrit and the cryoglobulinemic symptoms, including membranoproliferative glomerulonephritis, have been reported in several patients who underwent splenectomy for hypersplenism.[224,264] In contrast, in the series reported by Meltzer and Franklin the one patient who underwent splenectomy died of acute renal failure.[154] Because this intervention has not been studied thoroughly, and because of the high risk involved, it should not be considered as a standard therapy but rather as a potential option for patients without cirrhosis who have disease that is difficult to manage because of cytopenias resulting from hypersplenism.

Scleromyxedema

Scleromyxedema is a cutaneous mucinosis characterized by a generalized papular and sclerodermoid eruption, mucin deposition, increased fibroblast proliferation, fibrosis, and monoclonal gammopathy in the absence of thyroid disease. Extracutaneous manifestations may involve the cardiovascular, gastrointestinal, pulmonary, rheumatologic, and central nervous systems. See recent review by Cokonis Georgakis et al.[265]

The disorder was previously described by Dubruilh in 1906 under the alternate name of lichen myxedematosis and distinguished from sclerederma and generalized myxedema by Montgomery and Underwood in 1953. More recently, scleromyxedema has been used as the generalized form of lichen myxedematosus while papular mucinosis is thought to be the localized form of the disease.[265]

Pathogenesis and Histology

The pathogenesis of the disorder is not understood. In vitro serum from patients with scleromyxedema stimulates dermal fibroblast proliferation with resultant hyaluronic acid and protaglandin E production.[266] Isolated serum IgG does not stimulate this effect despite the fact that 83% of patients with the disorder have an IgG monoclonal protein.[265]

There is a fibroblastic proliferation that usually shows immunoreactiveity with CD34 and procollagen-I. There is an increased small vessel proliferation, increased dermal mucin, and increased numbers of CD68 cells. A mild perivascular mononuclear cell inflammatory infiltrate may be present.

Clinical Presentation

This rare disorder appears to affect men at a slightly higher rate than women, with a mean age of the sixth decade.[267] The hallmark of the disorder is the rash, which consists of small (2–3 mm), waxy, firm papules (Fig. 4a.) that are closely spaced and often arranged linearly. They may be dome shaped or flat topped, and they most commonly affect the face, neck, distal forearms, and hands. The skin may exhibit diffuse erythema, edema, and a brownish discoloration and there is often loss of skin appendages. In those patients with diffuse mucin deposition within the glabella, there is a leonine facies appearance. Pruritis may or may not be present.

The mucin infiltration in the skin results in stiffening of the skin and decreased range of motion in the hands, lips, and extremities (Fig. 4b). The infiltration is not limited to skin, however, and mucin deposition in adventitia around vessels in many organ systems can cause life-threatening extracutaneous complications.

The majority of patients have extracutaneous manifestations, the most common of which is gastrointestinal.[267] Dysphagia is commonly seen. Patients not infrequently have esophageal dysmotility, aspiration, and vocal hoarseness. Approximately 25% of patients develop proximal weakness and myopathy. Histologically, the most common muscle feature is vacular myopathy. Mucin deposits in the muscle are rare, and occasionally there are interstitial inflammatory infiltrates. Very rarely, patients may have an inflammatory arthritis. Carpal tunnel has been reported in association with the disease as well.

Neurologic and psychiatric disorders have been described with scleromyxedema.[268] Central nervous system findings including seizures, stroke, encephalopathy, stroke, and psychosis have been reported. Reported peripheral nervous system associations include PN and mononeuritis multiplex.

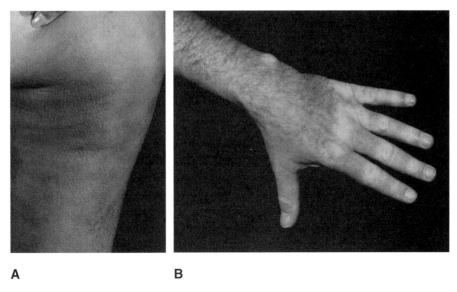

Fig. 4 Scleromyxedema skin changes. **a**. Small waxy papules. **b**. Stiffening of the skin and decreased range of motion in the hands (*see* Plate 23).

Myopathy, myositis, and rhabdomyolysis have also been reported. Dyspnea is not unusual, and upon testing obstructive and/or restrictive pulmonary disease can be seen in about one-fourth of patients.[267] In one study, 10% of patients had cardiac manifestations.[269]

Diagnosis and Differential Diagnosis

Diagnosis of scleromyxedema should fulfill the following criteria: (1) generalized papular and sclerodermoid eruption; (2) mucin deposition, fibroblast proliferation, and fibrosis; (3) monoclonal gammopathy; and (4) the absence of thyroid disease.[270]

The connective tissue diseases that are in the differential diagnosis are systemic sclerosis, dermatomyositis, and rheumatoid arthritis. Nephrogenic fibrosing dermopathy, also known as nephrogenic systemic fibrosus, shares dermatologic features with scleromyexedema. The main differences between these two disorders include the following. First, patients with the former disorder all have serious renal dysfunction. Second, more than 80% of patients with scleromyxedema have an IgG lambda monoclonal protein in their serum. Third, facial involvement is not common in nephrogenic firbrosing dermopathy. Histologically and immunophenotypically, there are some differences as well. In scleromyxedema, there may be a sparse lymphoplasmacytic infiltrate, whereas in nephrogenic firbrosing dermopathy there is a paucity of inflammation.[266] Procollagen-I is more highly expressed in scleromyxedema as well.

Treatment and Prognosis

The most commonly used upfront therapies have included systemic corticosteroids, melphalan, and plasmapheresis. More recently, novel treatments like high-dose chemotherapy with peripheral blood stem cell transplantation and thalidomide have shown to be effective, at least in the short term.[271,272] Other agents with variable utility include isotretinonin, etretinate, intralesional corticosteroids, intravenous gammaglobulin, purine nucleoside analogs, IFN-α, PUVA (psoralen and ultraviolet irradiation), radiation, surgery, and methotexate.[265] Although it may improve the skin manifestations, low-dose alkylator therapy should be used with caution since secondary acute leukemia has been reported.[267] In one series, more than half of the patients treated with oral melphalan died of treatment-related causes.

As the case with any individual with a monoclonal gammopathy, these patients have a small risk of evolving into multiple myeloma. Cases of non-Hodgkin's lymphoma have also been reported.[267]

Necrobiotic Xanthogranuloma

Necrobiotic xanthogranuloma (NXG) is a rare chronic granlomatous disease of the skin and extracutaneous tissues. It was originally described in 1980 by Kossard and Winkelmann as a distinctive disorder consisting of cutaneous and subcutaneous xanthomatous plaques, which frequently were associated with monoclonal protein and/or lymphoproliferative diseases. See recent review by Fernandez-Herrera and Pedraz.[273]

Pathogenesis

The pathogenesis of the disorder is poorly understood. Approximately 80–90% of cases have a monoclonal gammopathy, IgG kappa in ~60% and IgG lambda in nearly 30%.[274] One theory is that the monoclonal protein has functional features of a lipoprotein, binding to lipoprotein receptors of monocytes, thereby inducing xanthoma formation.[275] The activation of monocytes may contribute to an intracellular accumulation of lipoprotein-derived lipids in the skin.[273] Matsura et al. observed one patient who had increased serum levels of macrophage colony-stimulating factor.[276]

On light microscopy, changes are seen in the deep dermis and subcutaneous tissue. The superficial dermis and epidermis are typically spared. There are large areas of hyaline necrobiosis with degenerated collagen bundles, neuclear debris, and granulamatous inflammation. The granulomas are composed of sheets of xanthomatized histiocytes, multinucleate giant cells, and a few lymphocytes. Cholesterol clefts may also be seen. Vasculitis is not usually present.

Besides MGUS, other hematologic disorders seen with NXG include multiple myeloma, amyloidosis, Waldenström macroglobulinemia, cryoglobulinemia, chronic lymphocytic leukemia, Hodgkin's disease, non-Hodgkin's lymphoma, and myelodysplastic syndrome.[273]

Clinical Course

It is a progressive multiple-organ disease with an indolent course for most patients. NXG is a progressive, histiocytic disease characterized by destructive cutaneous lesions, a monoclonal protein, and extracutaneous manifestations. It tends to occur in the sixth decade and is without sex predilection.[273]

The skin manifestations consist of multiple indurated yellow-red plaques or nodules, most commonly collecting around the periorbital region (Fig. 5a). The symmetric involvement around the eyes may produce a variety of symptoms including pain and blurred vision. There can be conjunctival involvement, keratitis, scleritis, episcleritis, corneal perforation, and uveitis.[273]

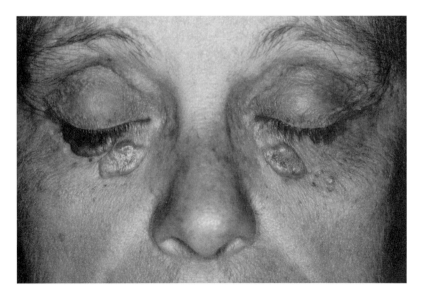

A

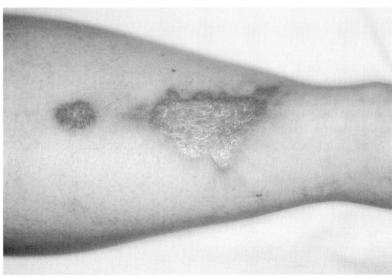

B

Fig. 5 Xanthogranuloma necrobiotica skin changes. **a**. Periorbital lesions. **b**. Cutaneous involvement (*see* Plate 24).

The lesions start as papules, but become confluent, as indurated plaques (Fig. 5b). The plaques often have a yellowish hue and may have telangectasia; they can become atrophied and ulcerate. Nearly half of the cases ulcerate. Extracutaneous sites of involvement include the spleen, heart, lung, kidney, intestine, larynx, pharanx, skeletal muscle, and central nervous system.[274] Most of the visceral lesions are asymptomatic and only discovered postmortem.

Diagnosis and Differential Diagnosis

Within the histopathologic differential diagnosis of NXG is necrobiosis lipoidica, granuloma annulare, juvenile xanthogranuloma, erythema induratum of Baxin, foreign body granuloma, atypical sarcoid, and other xanthomas. NXG can be differentiated from necrobiosis lipoidica by the fact that the latter condition does not contain xanthogranulomatous changes, lymphoid follicles, or cholesterol clefts. In addition, the NXG infiltration is deeper, often extending to subcutaneous tissues.[273]

Treatment and Prognosis

There are no standardized treatments of NXG. Alkylator-based therapies like low-dose melphalan, cyclophosphamide, or chlorambucil with or without prednisone have been used [274] as has IFN with some response.[277] Other agents like azathioprine and methotrexate have not been useful.[274] We recently reported a case of a patient treated with high-dose chemotherapy with peripheral blood stem cell transplant who had an excellent response.[278] He had a transient response to splenectomy predating his transplant. Intralesional steroid injections, radiation therapy, plasmapheresis, and surgical removal have all been tried with limited efficacy.[273]

The course tends to be indolent, but progressive. The prognosis is dependent on extracutaneous involvement and whether the disease is associated with a hematologic malignancy or not.

Schnitzler's Syndrome

Schnitzler's syndrome is a poorly defined syndrome characterized by chronic urticaria, IgM monoclonal gammopathy, bone pain, elevated ESR, lymphadenopathy, and recurrent fever. See two excellent reviews by Lipsker et al. and by de Koning et al..[279,280] A variant with a similar phenotype, but an IgG monoclonal protein has also been described, and is now recognized as a variant of the syndrome.[280]

Pathogenesis and Histology

The pathophysiology of this disorder is not well understood. It has been postulated that the monoclonal protein serves as an autoantibody that deposits triggering a local inflammatory response that could induce the skin lesions.

The typical histologic appearance of a skin lesion is that of neutrophilic urticaria.[281] There is edema and a perivascular infiltrate of neutrophils and eosinophils in the papillary dermis. Fibrinoid deposits may be seen around dilated superficial blood vessels. However, fibrinoid necrosis, the hallmark of fully developed leukocytoclastic vasculitis, is not seen and immunofluorescence studies are usually negative, although IgM has been seen along the dermal–epidermal junction.[282]

Cytokine aberrations have been implicated including elevations in IL-6 and antibodies again IL-1. The demonstrated clinical efficacy of the IL-1b inhibitor anakinra against this disorder would suggest that IL-1b plays an important role in the pathophysiology.[280,283–285]

Clinical Course

Because it is a rare disorder, it is underrecognized and the time from symptoms to diagnosis is usually more than 5 years.[279] de Koning et al. have recently published a review of 94 cases of scleromyxedema. The mean age of onset was 51 years.[280]

The rash is pale rose, slightly elevated papules, and plaques. Individual lesions measure 0.5–3 cm in diameter. New lesions appear daily and disappear in 12–24 h. It can be chronic and unrelenting, but patients can go 1–2 weeks without eruptions. Head and neck are usually spared, and the trunk and extremities are most commonly affected. Approximately 45% of patients experience pruritis, but this tends to be a later finding. Angioedema is rare.

Extradermatologic manifestations include fever (88%), arthralgia/arthritis (82%), bone pain (72%), weight loss (64%), lymphadenopathy (44%), hepatomegaly (29%), and splenomegaly (12%).[280]

Typical laboratory findings include a moderately increased ESR, leukocytosis, mild anemia, and an elevated C-reactive protein. On immunofixation, an IgM monoclonal protein will be found. Since the monoclonal protein is typically small, it can be missed by merely measuring quantitative immunoglobulins by nephelometry or by screening with a SPEP. Occasionally, there will be a monoclonal IgG monoclonal protein instead. Completment levels are normal. The bone marrow biopsy may be "negative" and lymph nodes tend to show only reactive hyperplasia.

Bone radiographs are most commonly normal, but increased bone density, lytic lesions, and periosteal appostion have been discribed.[279,280]

Diagnosis and Differential Diagnosis

It was first described in 1972.[279,286] Shown in Table 7 are diagnostic criteria by Lipsker et al. for a diagnosis of Schnitzler's syndrome.

The differential diagnosis includes idiopathic chronic urticaria, cryoglobulinemia, mastocytosis, hypocomplemetic urticarial vasculitis, acquired C1 inhibitor deficiency, hyper-IgD syndrome, adult-onset Still's disease, systemic lupus erythematosus, Behcet's disease, and hereditary autoinflammatory syndromes (e.g., cryopyrin-associated syndrome, familial cold urticaria, Muckle-Wells syndrome, and chronic infantile neurologic cutaneous and articular syndrome).[279,280]

Treatment and Prognosis

Treatments that have provided varying degrees of relief include anakinra (an IL- receptor antagonist), oral glucocorticoids, thalidomide, PUVA, antihistamines, nonsteroidal antiinflammatory drugs, IFN, rituximab, intravenous

Table 7 Diagnostic criteria[a] of the Schnitzler's syndrome.[280,287]

Major criteria:
Chronic urticarial rash
Monoclonal IgM (or IgG: variant type)
Minor criteria:
Intermittent fever
Arthragia or arthritis
Bone pain
Lymphadenopathy
Hepato- and/or splenomegaly
Elevated ESR and/or leukocytosis
Bone abnormalities (radiologic or histologic)

ESR erythrocyte sedimentation rate.
[a]To meet criteria, patient must have both major criteria, and at least two minor criteria after exclusion of other causes

gammaglobulin, colchicine, dapsone, cyclosporin, alkylating agents purine nucleoside analogs, methotrexate, and plasma exchange.[279,280]

This constellation of symptoms can severely interfere with normal function. Patients are at risk for both progression to Waldenström macroglobulinemia and AA amyloidosis. AL amyloidosis has not been reported. In a recent study of 94 patients, the 15 year survival rate was 91%.[280] In this same series, 11 pateints developed Waldenström macroglobulinemia.

Atypical PCD with Nephropathy as Dominant Phenotype

The most common atypical PCD with nephropathy as the dominant phenotype is light-chain (AL) amyloidosis. This topic, however, is beyond the scope of this chapter and is discussed in Chapter XX. The other disorders are listed in Table 3 and described in greated detail below.

Nonamyloidogenic Light-Chain Deposition Disease

Light-chain deposition disease (LCDD) is a systemic disorder first described by Randall and coworkers in 1976.[288] The light chains are produced by clonal plasma cells, which are most typically few in number; however, this disorder can also occur in the context of active multiple myeloma.

Pathogenesis and Histology

LCDD is due to pathologic protein deposition in various tissues and organs. Even less commonly, the immunoglobulin heavy chain can deposit either alone or in combination with light chains. These conditions are referred to as heavy-chain deposition disease and light- and heavy-chain deposition disease, respectively.[289,290] Unlike the light-chain deposits observed in patients with primary systemic amyloidosis, these infiltrates are not congophilic by light microscopy, nor are they fibrillar on electron microscopy. Instead, amorphous nodular deposits are seen.

The organ most commonly involved is the kidney. Nodular glomerulosclerosis is commonly seen. The light chains most frequently found within these deposits are κ I and κ IV. It has been suggested that somatic mutations of specific amino acid sequences in the light chains affecting the three-dimensional confirmation of the protein.[291,292] Ultrastructurally, light-chain deposits may be seen as punctuate, granular, electron-dense materials in the glomeruli, the interstituium, along the tubular basement membranes, and in blood vessel walls.[293] Herrera's group has shown that the mesangial cells in LCDD acquire a prominent rough endoplasmic reticulum, overexpress α-smooth muscle actin produce a variety of extracellular matrix proteins including fibrillary collagens and underexpress matrix metalloproteinases.[293]

Clinical Course

The most common area of involvement is the kidney, but other organs like the heart, liver,[294] and lung,[295] have been described. Patients may be asymptomatic and have an incidental finding of renal insufficiency or proteinuria. In one series of 63 cases of LCDD, the median age was 52 years with approximately two-thirds of patients being man.[296] Ninety-six percent presented with renal insufficiency and 84% with proteinuria greater than 1 g/day. Approximately two-thirds of patients will have monoclonal kappa deposition, with the other-third being lambda. The size of the serum and/or urine monoclonal protein is often small with approximately one-third of patients meeting criteria for MGUS rather than multiple myeloma. Not uncommonly, the clinical phenotype of these patients is more akin to AL amyloidosis than multiple myeloma.

Diagnosis and Differential Diagnosis

Any dieasease causing glomerular damage is in the differential diagnosis including AL amyloidosis. The diagnosis is made by light and electron microscopy.

Treatment and Prognosis

The prognosis of patients who have this disorder depends on whether there is underlying multiple myeloma. In two retrospective studies of patients with LCDD, 5-year actuarial patient survival and survival free of end-stage renal disease were 40–70% and 37%, respectively.[296,297] Renal prognosis was linked to age and presenting creatinine, while overall survival was tied to age and extrarenal sites of involvement.

There is no standard therapy. For those who meet criteria for active multiple myeloma, chemotherapy is appropriate. During the era in which low-dose alkylators were the only therapies available, a common strategy was to avoid therapy with the understanding that renal failure would ensue; this risk was felt to be preferable over the risk alkylator-induced myelodysplasia. Salvage renal allografting is feasible, but allograft survival is short if measures to significantly reduce light-chain production have not been employed.[298] High-dose chemotherapy and peripheral blood stem cell transplant, however, offers a treatment option for these patients with a lower risk of secondary myelodysplasia, but with a risk of precipitating renal failure.[299,300] It is not known what role novel agents like thalidomide and bortezomib may play in the care of these patients. The use of lenalidomide may be curtailed by the extent of renal failure in these patients.

Acquired Fanconi's Syndrome

Fanconi's syndrome is a rare complication of plasma cell dyscrasias characterized by diffuse failure in reabsorption at the level of the proximal renal tubule and resulting in glycosuria, generalized aminoaciduria, and hypophosphatemia.[301] Fanconi first described the syndrome in children. Subsequently, acquired forms were described in adults.

Clinical Course

Acquired Fanconi's syndrome is usually associated with MGUS. Overt hematologic malignancies like multiple myeloma, Waldenström macroglobulinemia, or other lymphoproliferative disorders may be present at diagnosis or with further follow-up. In the Mayo series of 32 patients with Fanconi's syndrome, nearly 50% of patients presented with bone pain as their main complaint.[301] Approximately one third had asymptomatic renal insufficiency, proteinuria, or glycosuria while the remainder presented with fatigue. Hypokalemia, hypophosphatemia, and hypouricemia were present in 44%, 50%, and 66% respectively. All patients tested had aminoaciduria and glucosuria. Bence-Jones proteinuria is usually present and is almost always of the κ type.

Pathogenesis

The crystals that deposit in the proximal renal tubules are composed of a portion of the variable region of the monoclonal light chain. The κ-variable domains from patients with this syndrome have been shown to be hightly resistant to protease degradation and to have unusual self-reactivity to form crystals. It is thought that these light chains do not undergo complete proteolysis, and therefore accumulate in the lysosomal compartment of the cells in the renal tubules.[302–304]

Diagnosis

The diagnosis of Fanconi's syndrome can be made when a patient with a monoclonal PCD presents with aminoaciduria, phosphaturia, and glycosuria. On renal biopsy, crystals are seen in the epithelial cells of the proximal tubes, but interstitial fibrosis and nonspecific changes may also be seen.

Treatment and Prognosis

Treatment consists of supplementation with phosphorus, calcium, and vitamin D. The prognosis is good in the absence of overt malignant disease. The median time from diagnosis to end-stage renal failure was 196 months in one series.[301] Chemotherapy may benefit patients with rapidly progressive renal failure or symptomatic malignancy, but patients treated with alkylators are at risk for secondary myelodysplastic syndrome or acute leukemia.

Fibrillary Glomerulonephritis

Fibrillary glomerulonephritis may occur in association with monoclonal gammopathy.[305–308] The causal relationship is not always iron-clad. The clinical presentation includes hematuria, proteinuira, and renal insufficiency. Extrarenal manifestations have been reported. On electron microcroscopy, randomly arranged extracellular Congo red fibrils with diameter ranging from 13 to 29 mm are found. Common histologies include membranoproliferative glomerulonephritis, diffuse proliferative glomerulonephritis, and cresents. The deposits more commonly contain IgG1 and IgG4. Immunotactoid glomerulonephritis is probably a subgroup of fibrillary GN. The size range of fibrils for this disorder tend to be larger (20–55 nm) and have a hollow center. These deposits often stain positive for monoclonal immunoglobulins.

Other Atypical Plasma Cell Disorders

The heavy-chain diseases are a rare group of disorders with diverse clinical presentations. The three conditions (α-, γ-, and μ-HCD) are discussed together because they are lymphoproliferative or plasmaproliferative disorders that share the generation and secretion of an isolated heavy-chain fragment. α-HCD (Mediterranean lymphoma or immunoproliferative small intestinal disease, IPSID) is the most common and has the most uniform presentation; γ- and μ-HCD have variable clinical presentations and histopathologic features. In the majority of cases, the heavy-chain fragment is not secreted in large quantities and immunofixation or immunoelectrophoresis is required to detect the abnormality. Screening the serum and urine of patients with lymphoplasmacytoid NHL would most likely identify more patients with γ- or μ-HCD. Cases of γ- and μ-heavy-chain monoclonal gammopathy of unknown significance have been reported.[309–311]

α-Heavy-Chain Disease

Mediterranean lymphoma, originally described in the 1960s as a condition in young adults, is a primary small intestinal lymphoma coupled with intestinal malabsorption.[312] An isolated IgA immunoglobulin heavy-chain fragment was recognized in association with this condition. Because some patients had benign-appearing lymphocytes in their small bowel, the term "α-HCD" was preferred over "Mediterranean lymphoma" by some authors.[313] A consensus panel in 1976 concluded that α-HCD and Mediterranean lymphoma represented a spectrum of disease with benign, intermediate, and overtly malignant stages, and the term "immunoproliferative small intestinal disease" came into use.[314] This entity has been recently reviewed.[315]

Pathogenesis and Histology

Histologic features of IPSID range from early lymphoplasmacytic intestinal infiltration to overt malignant diffuse large B-cell lymphoma. This entity shares morphologic features of mucosa-associated lymphoid tissue (MALT) in that there are lympho-epithelial lesions, centroyte-like cells, and plasma cell differentiation.[316] The histologic findings are classified into stages A, B, and C. Stage A includes a diffuse, dense, compact, and apparently benign lymphoplasmacytic infiltration of mucosal lamina propria. Stage B has features of stage A but also has circumscribed "immunoblastic" lymphoma in either the intestinal or mesenteric lymph nodes. Stage C comprises a diffuse "immunoblastic" lymphoma with or without demonstrable lymphoplasmacytic infiltration.[314] Villous broadening or effacement and shortened sparse crypts are also observed. These histopathologic findings can be distinguished from those of celiac sprue because celiac sprue includes total villous atrophy, hyperplastic and elongated crypts, intraepithelial lymphocytosis, and surface epithelial flattening. The lymphoma that arises from celiac sprue is T-cell lymphoma[317] rather than B-cell lymphoma, as in the case of α-HCD. A recent study of 11 cases of IPSID demonstrated higher expression of syndecan-1 in stage A samples relative to stage B; conversely, stage B samples showed higher expression of BCL-6 and p53.[318] IPSID lacks the (11;18) translocation which is not uncommon in other MALT lymphomas. Other cytogenetic abnormalities have been seen including t(9;14), t(2;14), and t(5;9).[315]

The hypothesis that chronic antigenic stimulation by intestinal organisms is the cause of this disorder is credible and can be modeled after the MALT lymphoma paradigm. This hypothesis is further supported by the fact that the incidence of α-HCD (or IPSID) is most common in patients who live in areas with poor sanitation and who also have a high prevalence of intestinal microbial infestation. *Helicobacter pylori* had been a candidate organism,[319] but its association was subsequently challenged.[316] *Campylobacter jejuni* is now considered to be a possible offending organism,[320] but this will need to be confirmed.

Clinical Presentation

The majority of reported patients with α-HCD are from northern Africa, Israel, and surrounding Middle Eastern or Mediterranean countries, with fewer patients from central and southern Africa, eastern Asia, and South and Central America.[321]

Patients present with malabsorption syndrome, weight loss, and abdominal pain. On physical examination, peripheral edema, clubbing, and an abdominal mass are not uncommon findings.[314,315,321,322] On endoscopy of the small intestine, one may find thickened mucosal folds, nodules, ulcers, a mosaic pattern, or submucosal infiltration. Intestinal parasites and bacterial overgrowth in the small intestine are common. Anemia, vitamin deficiencies, and hypogammaglobulinemia are also common. The IgA level is generally not increased, but on immunofixation or immunoelectrophoresis, a monoclonal component is present, especially in the earlier phases of the disease. An immunoglobulin light chain is not found. The monoclonal IgA fragment may be found in jejunal secretions as well as in blood and urine.[322] The monoclonal protein in patients with α-HCD is of the α1 subclass and consists of multiple polymers. The length of the basic polypeptide subunit is typically between one half and three fourths that of a normal α-heavy chain; the shortening results from an internal deletion involving most of the V_H and the C_H^1 domain.[323] In about one-half of the cases, the electrophoretic pattern of α-HCD protein contains a broad band extending from the α2 region to the β-globulin region because of the tendency of these chains to polymerize. The remainder of the patients may have a normal SPEP pattern.

Treatment and Prognosis

Although no data exist from randomized prospective studies, the standard accepted treatment of the early stage is broad-spectrum antibiotics, with or without corticosteroids. This protocol has resulted in clinical or histologic remission (in 33–71% of cases), which is generally short-lived but occasionally durable.[315,321] In the absence of a documented parasite or an intestinal bacterial overgrowth, therapy with tetracycline or metronidazole and ampicillin is appropriate.[324,325] Any documented parasite should be eradicated. Treatment of *H. pylori* has led to complete remission in two patients with α-HCD,[326] one of whom was unresponsive to prior combination chemotherapy. Lecuit et al. demonstrated response of IPSID after clearance of *C. jejuni*.[320] Response to antibiotics usually occurs promptly; however, a minimum 6-month trial of tetracycline (1–2 g/day) is recommended for establishing responsiveness of the lesion.[327] In patients with more advanced stages, or unresponsive early stages, total abdominal radiation or combination chemotherapy, or both, have been used (remission rate, 64%).[315,328-333] Overall 5-year survival rates are 60–70%. Immunotherapy with rituximab, an anti-CD20 monoclonal antibody, has been a major advance in the treatment of indolent NHL,[334] but to date there have been no reports of rituximab use in patients with α-HCD.

γ-Heavy-Chain Disease

First described in 1964 by Franklin et al.[335], γ-HCD has a diverse clinical phenotype.

Clinical Presentation

The median age of patients with γ-HCD is 61 years, with 54% of the patients being man.[336,337] Originally, γ-HCD was considered to be merely a lymphoma-like illness; Kyle et al.[336] challenged this concept. Since the original description, there have been ~100 cases reported in the literature.[310] Although most patients present with weakness, fatigue, fever, lymphadenopathy (62%), hepatomegaly (58%), splenomegaly (59%), and lymphoma, other features, such as autoimmune hemolytic anemia and idiopathic thrombocytopenic purpura, may also be seen.[310,336] Cutaneous and subcutaneous involvement is not uncommon.[338] Several cases have arisen in patients with long-standing connective tissue disorders such as rheumatoid arthritis,[310,339–341] lupus,[310,342] keratoconjunctivitis sicca,[343,344] vasculitis,[344] and myasthenia gravis.[310] A normochromic anemia is a presenting feature in about 79% of patients. About 10% have either a Coombs-positive or Coombs-negative autoimmune hemolytic anemia.[309,310,344] Lymphopenia and lymphocytosis each occur in less than 10% of patients. Thrombocytopenia may be present in as many as 22% of patients.[310]

The γ chain in this disorder is truncated with deletions at the $C_H{}^1$ domain.[345,346] The mobility pattern of the immunoglobulin fragment on protein electrophoresis is quite variable, with the band present anywhere from the α1-globulin region to the slow γ-globulin region; most commonly, however, it runs in the β region.[310] The subclass is IgG1 in 76%, IgG2 in 19%, and IgG4 in 5% of cases. With the normal distribution of subclasses, one would expect a higher occurrence of IgG2 and a lower occurrence of IgG3 and IgG1. Proteinuria can range from none to 20 g/day.

Bone marrow most commonly demonstrates an increase in plasma cells, lymphocytes, or plasmacytoid lymphocytes; occasionally eosinophilia is seen. The lymphoproliferative disorders range from benign lymphoplasma cell proliferative disorder to plasmacytoma, to chronic lymphocytic leukemia, to angioimmunoblastic lymphoma to diffuse large cell lymphoma.[310,347] Lytic bone disease occurs rarely. Amyloid deposits may be present.[336]

Treatment and Prognosis

The median survival is 7.4 years, with a range of 1 month to more than 25 years.[310] Treatment is not standardized. Single-agent therapy with prednisone and combination chemotherapy with cyclophosphamide, vincristine, and prednisone have been used with benefit. Wahner-Roedler et al. reported a rituximab response in one patient.[310] Patients with aggressive lymphomas should receive a regimen containing anthracycline.

µ-Heavy-Chain Disease

First described in 1970, µ-HCD is a rare poorly understood condition.[348,349]

Clinical Presentation

The median age of patients with µ-HCD is about 57 years and equal numbers of men and women are affected.[209,336,350] Common clinical presentations include splenomegaly and hepatomegaly. Lymphadenopathy is less common. About one-third of patients have chronic lymphocytic leukemia. Some patients with µ-HCD have features resembling those of lymphoma or multiple myeloma with amyloid arthropathy.[351]

Hypogammaglobulinemia is present in about one-half of the patients and a free monoclonal IgM fragment is found in the serum of all patients. The µ-heavy chain is missing most, if not all, of its VH region.[352] A free monoclonal light chain has been described in the urine in about one-half of the cases.[309,353] Lytic bone lesions or osteoporosis occur in a minority of patients. Bone marrow plasma cells tend to be vacuolated. Survival ranges from less than 1 month to 11 years (median, 24 months).[309]

Treatment and Prognosis

There is no standard treatment for this disorder, but it is generally treated as a low-grade lymphoproliferative disease with observation alone for asymptomatic patients and low-intensity chemotherapy for symptomatic patients.

Acknowledgments: *Financial support:* AD was supported in part by grants CA125614, CA062242, CA107476, CA15083, and CA11345 from the National Cancer Institute.

Financial disclosures: Clinical trial support from Celgene, Cytogen, Neurochem.

References

1. Crow R. Peripheral neuritis in myelomatosis. Brit Med J 1956;2:802–4.
2. Driedger H, Pruzanski W. Plasma cell neoplasia with osteosclerotic lesions. A study of five cases and a review of the literature. Arch Intern Med 1979;139(8):892–6.
3. Iwashita H, Ohnishi A, Asada M, Kanazawa Y, Kuroiwa Y. Polyneuropathy, skin hyperpigmentation, edema, and hypertrichosis in localized osteosclerotic myeloma. Neurology 1977;27(7):675–81.
4. Mangalik A, Veliath AJ. Osteosclerotic myeloma and peripheral neuropathy. A case report. Cancer 1971;28(4):1040–5.
5. Evison G, Evans KT. Sclerotic bone deposits in multiple myeloma [letter]. Br J Radiol 1983;56(662):145.
6. Reitan JB, Pape E, Fossa SD, Julsrud OJ, Slettnes ON, Solheim OP. Osteosclerotic myeloma with polyneuropathy. Acta Medica Scandinavica 1980;208(1–2):137–44.
7. Bardwick PA, Zvaifler NJ, Gill GN, Newman D, Greenway GD, Resnick DL. Plasma cell dyscrasia with polyneuropathy, organomegaly, endocrinopathy, M protein, and skin changes: the POEMS syndrome. Report on two cases and a review of the literature. Medicine 1980;59(4):311–22.
8. Kelly JJ, Jr., Kyle RA, Miles JM, Dyck PJ. Osteosclerotic myeloma and peripheral neuropathy. Neurology 1983;33(2):202–10.
9. Takatsuki K, Sanada I. Plasma cell dyscrasia with polyneuropathy and endocrine disorder: clinical and laboratory features of 109 reported cases. Jpn J Clin Oncol 1983;13(3):543–55.
10. Nakanishi T, Sobue I, Toyokura Y, et al. The Crow-Fukase syndrome: a study of 102 cases in Japan. Neurology 1984;34(6):712–20.
11. Soubrier MJ, Dubost JJ, Sauvezie BJ. POEMS syndrome: a study of 25 cases and a review of the literature. French Study Group on POEMS Syndrome. Am J Med 1994;97(6):543–53.
12. Dispenzieri A, Kyle RA, Lacy MQ, et al. POEMS syndrome: definitions and long-term outcome. Blood 2003;101(7):2496–506.
13. Soubrier M, Dubost JJ, Serre AF, et al. Growth factors in POEMS syndrome: evidence for a marked increase in circulating vascular endothelial growth factor. Arthritis Rheum 1997;40(4):786–7.
14. Gherardi RK, Belec L, Soubrier M, et al. Overproduction of proinflammatory cytokines imbalanced by their antagonists in POEMS syndrome. Blood 1996;87(4):1458–65.
15. Hitoshi S, Suzuki K, Sakuta M. Elevated serum interleukin-6 in POEMS syndrome reflects the activity of the disease. Intern Med 1994;33(10):583–7.
16. Rose C, Zandecki M, Copin MC, et al. POEMS syndrome: report on six patients with unusual clinical signs, elevated levels of cytokines, macrophage involvement and chromosomal aberrations of bone marrow plasma cells. Leukemia 1997;11(8):1318–23.
17. Orefice G, Morra VB, De Michele G, et al. POEMS syndrome: clinical, pathological and immunological study of a case. Neurol Res 1994;16(6):477–80.

18. Nakazawa K, Itoh N, Shigematsu H, Koh CS. An autopsy case of Crow-Fukase (POEMS) syndrome with a high level of IL-6 in the ascites. Special reference to glomerular lesions. Acta Pathologica Japonica 1992;42(9):651–6.

19. Emile C, Danon F, Fermand JP, Clauvel JP. Castleman disease in POEMS syndrome with elevated interleukin-6 [letter; comment]. Cancer 1993;71(3):874.

20. Saida K, Ohta M, Kawakami H, Saida T. Cytokines and myelin antibodies in Crow-Fukase syndrome. Muscle Nerve 1996;19(12):1620–2.

21. Feinberg L, Temple D, de Marchena E, Patarca R, Mitrani A. Soluble immune mediators in POEMS syndrome with pulmonary hypertension: case report and review of the literature. Crit Rev Oncog 1999;10(4):293–302.

22. Hashiguchi T, Arimura K, Matsumuro K, et al. Highly concentrated vascular endothelial growth factor in platelets in Crow-Fukase syndrome. Muscle Nerve 2000;23(7):1051–6.

23. Belec L, Mohamed AS, Authier FJ, et al. Human herpesvirus 8 infection in patients with POEMS syndrome-associated multicentric Castleman's disease. Blood 1999;93(11):3643–53.

24. Belec L, Authier FJ, Mohamed AS, Soubrier M, Gherardi RK. Antibodies to human herpesvirus 8 in POEMS (polyneuropathy, organomegaly, endocrinopathy, M protein, skin changes) syndrome with multicentric Castleman's disease. Clin Infect Dis 1999;28(3):678–9.

25. Bosch EP, Smith BE. Peripheral neuropathies associated with monoclonal proteins. [Review] [63 refs]. Med Clin North Am 1993;77(1):125–39.

26. Watanabe O, Arimura K, Kitajima I, Osame M, Maruyama I. Greatly raised vascular endothelial growth factor (VEGF) in POEMS syndrome [letter]. Lancet 1996;347(9002):702.

27. Gherardi RK, Belec L, Fromont G, et al. Elevated levels of interleukin-1 beta (IL-1 beta) and IL-6 in serum and increased production of IL-1 beta mRNA in lymph nodes of patients with polyneuropathy, organomegaly, endocrinopathy, M protein, and skin changes (POEMS) syndrome. Blood 1994;83(9):2587–93.

28. Shikama N, Isono A, Otsuka Y, Terano T, Hirai A. A case of POEMS syndrome with high concentrations of interleukin-6 in pericardial fluid. J Intern Med 2001;250(2):170–3.

29. Gherardi RK, Chouaib S, Malapert D, Belec L, Intrator L, Degos JD. Early weight loss and high serum tumor necrosis factor-alpha levels in polyneuropathy, organomegaly, endocrinopathy, M protein, skin changes syndrome. Ann Neurol 1994;35(4):501–5.

30. Watanabe O, Maruyama I, Arimura K, et al. Overproduction of vascular endothelial growth factor/vascular permeability factor is causative in Crow-Fukase (POEMS) syndrome. Muscle Nerve 1998;21(11):1390–7.

31. Scarlato M, Previtali SC, Carpo M, et al. Polyneuropathy in POEMS syndrome: role of angiogenic factors in the pathogenesis. Brain 2005;128(Pt 8):1911–20.

32. Tokashiki T, Hashiguchi T, Arimura K, Eiraku N, Maruyama I, Osame M. Predictive value of serial platelet count and VEGF determination for the management of DIC in the Crow-Fukase (POEMS) syndrome. Intern Med 2003;42(12):1240–3.

33. Bryce AH, Ketterling RP, Gertz MA, et al Cytogenetic analysis using multiple myeloma targets in POEMS syndrome. In: Proceedings of American Society of Oncology Meeting; 2007; Chicago, IL.

34. Soubrier M, Labauge P, Jouanel P, Viallard JL, Piette JC, Sauvezie B. Restricted use of Vlambda genes in POEMS syndrome. Haematologica 2004;89(4):ECR02.

35. Sung JY, Kuwabara S, Ogawara K, Kanai K, Hattori T. Patterns of nerve conduction abnormalities in POEMS syndrome. Muscle Nerve 2002;26(2):189–93.

36. Suarez GA, Dispenzieri A, Gertz MA, Kyle RA. The electrophysiologic findings of the peripheral neuropathy associated with POEMS. Clin Neurophysiol 2002;113(Suppl 1):S9.

37. Vital C, Vital A, Ferrer X, et al. Crow-Fukase (POEMS) syndrome: a study of peripheral nerve biopsy in five new cases. J Peripher Nerv Syst 2003;8(3):136–44.

38. Crisci C, Barbieri F, Parente D, Pappone N, Caruso G. POEMS syndrome: follow-up study of a case. Clin Neurol Neurosurg 1992;94(1):65–8.

39. Bergouignan FX, Massonnat R, Vital C, . Uncompacted lamellae in three patients with POEMS syndrome. Eur Neurol 1987;27(3):173–81.

40. Bardwick PA, Zvaifler NJ, Gill GN, Newman D, Greenway GD, Resnick DL. Plasma cell dyscrasia with polyneuropathy, organomegaly, endocrinopathy, M protein, and skin changes: the POEMS syndrome. Report on two cases and a review of the literature. Medicine (Baltimore) 1980;59(4):311–22.

41. Lesprit P, Authier FJ, Gherardi R, et al. Acute arterial obliteration: a new feature of the POEMS syndrome? Medicine 1996;75(4):226–32.

42. Zenone T, Bastion Y, Salles G, et al. POEMS syndrome, arterial thrombosis and thrombocythaemia. J Intern Med 1996;240(2):107–9.

43. Soubrier M, Guillon R, Dubost JJ, et al. Arterial obliteration in POEMS syndrome: possible role of vascular endothelial growth factor. J Rheumatol 1998;25(4):813–5.

44. Bova G, Pasqui AL, Saletti M, Bruni F, Auteri A. POEMS syndrome with vascular lesions: a role for interleukin-1beta and interleukin-6 increase—a case report. Angiology 1998;49(11):937–40.

45. Kang K, Chu K, Kim DE, Jeong SW, Lee JW, Roh JK. POEMS syndrome associated with ischemic stroke. Arch Neurol 2003;60(5):745–9.

46. Koga H, Tokunaga Y, Hisamoto T, et al. Ratio of serum vascular endothelial growth factor to platelet count correlates with disease activity in a patient with POEMS syndrome. Eur J Intern Med 2002;13(1):70–4.

47. Ghandi GY, Basu R, Dispenzieri A, Basu A, Montori V, Brennan MD. Endocrinopathy in POEMS syndrome: the Mayo Clinic Experience. Mayo Clin Proc;(In press).

48. Sanada S, Ookawara S, Karube H, et al. Marked recovery of severe renal lesions in POEMS syndrome with high-dose melphalan therapy supported by autologous blood stem cell transplantation. Am J Kidney Dis 2006;47(4):672–9.

49. Navis GJ, Dullaart RP, Vellenga E, Elema JD, de Jong PE. Renal disease in POEMS syndrome: report on a case and review of the literature. [Review] [25 refs]. Nephrol Dial Transplant 1994;9(10):1477–81.

50. Viard JP, Lesavre P, Boitard C, et al. POEMS syndrome presenting as systemic sclerosis. Clinical and pathologic study of a case with microangiopathic glomerular lesions. Am J Med 1988;84(3 Pt 1):524–8.

51. Sano M, Terasaki T, Koyama A, Narita M, Tojo S. Glomerular lesions associated with the Crow-Fukase syndrome. Virchows Arch A Pathol Anat Histopathol 1986;409(1):3–9.

52. Takazoe K, Shimada T, Kawamura T, et al. Possible mechanism of progressive renal failure in Crow-Fukase syndrome [letter]. Clin Nephrol 1997;47(1):66–7.

53. Mizuiri S, Mitsuo K, Sakai K, . Renal involvement in POEMS syndrome. Nephron 1991;59(1):153–6.

54. Stewart PM, McIntyre MA, Edwards CR. The endocrinopathy of POEMS syndrome. Scott Med J 1989;34(5):520–2.

55. Nakamoto Y, Imai H, Yasuda T, Wakui H, Miura AB. A spectrum of clinicopathological features of nephropathy associated with POEMS syndrome. Nephrol Dial Transplant 1999;14(10):2370–8.

56. Fukatsu A, Ito Y, Yuzawa Y, et al. A case of POEMS syndrome showing elevated serum interleukin 6 and abnormal expression of interleukin 6 in the kidney. Nephron 1992;62(1):47–51.

57. Mufti GJ, Hamblin TJ, Gordon J. Melphalan-induced pulmonary fibrosis in osteosclerotic myeloma [letter]. Acta Haematol 1983;69(2):140–1.

58. Iwasaki H, Ogawa K, Yoshida H, et al. Crow-Fukase syndrome associated with pulmonary hypertension. Intern Med 1993;32(7):556–60.

59. Lesprit P, Godeau B, Authier FJ, et al. Pulmonary hypertension in POEMS syndrome: a new feature mediated by cytokines. Am J Respir Crit Care Med 1998;157(3 Pt 1):907–11.

60. Dispenzieri A, Moreno-Aspitia A, Suarez GA, . Peripheral blood stem cell transplantation in 16 patients with POEMS syndrome, and a review of the literature. Blood 2004;104(10):3400–7.

61. Allam JS, Kennedy CC, Aksamit TR, Dispenzieri A. Pulmonary manifestations are common and associated with shortened survival in POEMS syndrome: a retrospective review of 141 patients. Submitted.

62. Lewerenz J, Gocht A, Hoeger PH, et al. Multiple vascular abnormalities and a paradoxical combination of vitamin B(12) deficiency and thrombocytosis in a case with POEMS syndrome. J Neurol 2003;250(12):1488–91.

63. Yishay O, Eran E. POEMS syndrome: failure of newly suggested diagnostic criteria to anticipate the development of the syndrome. Am J Hematol 2005;79(4):316–8.

64. Mineta M, Hatori M, Sano H, et al. Recurrent Crow-Fukase syndrome associated with increased serum levels of vascular endothelial growth factor: a case report and review of the literature. Tohoku J Exp Med 2006;210(3):269–77.

65. Morley JB, Schwieger AC. The relation between chronic polyneuropathy and osteosclerotic myeloma. J Neurol Neurosurg Psychiatry 1967;30(5):432–42.

66. Davis L, Drachman D. Myeloma neuropathy. Arch Neurol 1972;27:507–11.

67. Ku A, Lachmann E, Tunkel R, Nagler W. Severe polyneuropathy: initial manifestation of Castleman's disease associated with POEMS syndrome. Arch Phys Med Rehabil 1995;76(7):692–4.

68. Judge MR, McGibbon DH, Thompson RP. Angioendotheliomatosis associated with Castleman's lymphoma and POEMS syndrome. Clin Exp Dermatol 1993;18(4):360–2.

69. Kuwabara S, Hattori T, Shimoe Y, Kamitsukasa I. Long term melphalan-prednisolone chemotherapy for POEMS syndrome. J Neurol Neurosurg Psychiatry 1997;63(3):385–7.

70. Arima F, Dohmen K, Yamano Y, et al. [Five cases of Crow-Fukase syndrome]. [Japanese]. Fukuoka Igaku Zasshi Fukuoka Acta Medica 1992;83(2):112–20.

71. Wong VA, Wade NK. POEMS syndrome: an unusual cause of bilateral optic disk swelling. Am J Ophthalmol 1998;126(3):452–4.

72. Hogan WJ, Lacy MQ, Wiseman GA, Fealey RD, Dispenzieri A, Gertz MA. Successful treatment of POEMS syndrome with autologous hematopoietic progenitor cell transplantation. Bone Marrow Transplant 2001;28(3):305–9.

73. Rovira M, Carreras E, Blade J, et al. Dramatic improvement of POEMS syndrome following autologous haematopoietic cell transplantation. Br J Haematol 2001;115(2):373–5.

74. Jaccard A, Royer B, Bordessoule D, Brouet JC, Fermand JP. High-dose therapy and autologous blood stem cell transplantation in POEMS syndrome. Blood 2002;99(8):3057–9.

75. Peggs KS, Paneesha S, Kottaridis PD, et al. Peripheral blood stem cell transplantation for POEMS syndrome. Bone Marrow Transplant 2002;30(6):401–4.

76. Soubrier M, Ruivard M, Dubost JJ, Sauvezie B, Philippe P. Successful use of autologous bone marrow transplantation in treating a patient with POEMS syndrome. Bone Marrow Transplant 2002;30(1):61–2.

77. Wiesmann A, Weissert R, Kanz L, Einsele H. Long-term follow-up on a patient with incomplete POEMS syndrome undergoing high-dose therapy and autologous blood stem cell transplantation. Blood 2002;100(7):2679–80.

78. Dispenzieri A, Kyle RA, Lacy MQ, et al. Superior survival in primary systemic amyloidosis patients undergoing peripheral blood stem cell transplantation: a case-control study. Blood 2004;103(10):3960–3.

79. Takai K, Niikuni K, Kurasaki T. [Successful treatment of POEMS syndrome with high-dose chemotherapy and autologous peripheral blood stem cell transplantation]. Rinsho Ketsueki 2004;45(10):1111–4.

80. Ganti AK, Pipinos I, Culcea E, Armitage JO, Tarantolo S. Successful hematopoietic stem-cell transplantation in multicentric Castleman disease complicated by POEMS syndrome. Am J Hematol 2005;79(3):206–10.

81. Kastritis E, Terpos E, Anagnostopoulos A, Xilouri I, Dimopoulos MA. Angiogenetic factors and biochemical markers of bone metabolism in POEMS syndrome treated with high-dose therapy and autologous stem cell support. Clin Lymphoma Myeloma 2006;7(1):73–6.

82. Kuwabara S, Misawa S, Kanai K, et al. Autologous peripheral blood stem cell transplantation for POEMS syndrome. Neurology 2006;66(1):105–7.

83. Kojima H, Katsuoka Y, Katsura Y, et al. Successful treatment of a patient with POEMS syndrome by tandem high-dose chemotherapy with autologous CD34+ purged stem cell rescue. Int J Hematol 2006;84(2):182–5.

84. Imai N, Kitamura E, Tachibana T, et al. Efficacy of autologous peripheral blood stem cell transplantation in POEMS syndrome with polyneuropathy. Intern Med 2007;46(3):135–8.

85. Barrier JH, Le Noan H, Mussini JM, Brisseau JM. Stabilisation of a severe case of P.O.E.M.S. syndrome after tamoxifen administration [letter]. J Neurol Neurosurg Psychiatry 1989;52(2):286.

86. Matsui H, Udaka F, Kubori T, Oda M, Nishinaka K, Kameyama M. POEMS syndrome demonstrating VEGF decrease by ticlopidine. Intern Med 2004;43(11):1082–3.

87. Saida K, Kawakami H, Ohta M, Iwamura K. Coagulation and vascular abnormalities in Crow-Fukase syndrome. Muscle Nerve 1997;20(4):486–92.

88. Coto V, Auletta M, Oliviero U, et al. POEMS syndrome: an Italian case with diagnostic and therapeutic implications. Annali Italiani di Medicina Interna 1991;6(4):416–9.

89. Authier FJ, Belec L, Levy Y, et al. All-trans-retinoic acid in POEMS syndrome. Therapeutic effect associated with decreased circulating levels of proinflammatory cytokines. Arthritis Rheum 1996;39(8):1423–6.

90. Sternberg AJ, Davies P, Macmillan C, Abdul-Cader A, Swart S. Strontium-89: a novel treatment for a case of osteosclerotic myeloma associated with life-threatening neuropathy. Br J Haematol 2002;118(3):821–4.

91. Kim SY, Lee SA, Ryoo HM, Lee KH, Hyun MS, Bae SH. Thalidomide for POEMS syndrome. Ann Hematol 2006;85(8):545–6.

92. Sinisalo M, Hietaharju A, Sauranen J, Wirta O. Thalidomide in POEMS syndrome: case report. Am J Hematol 2004;76(1):66–8.

93. Badros A, Porter N, Zimrin A. Bevacizumab therapy for POEMS syndrome. Blood 2005;106(3):1135.

94. Straume O, Bergheim J, Ernst P. Bevacizumab therapy for POEMS syndrome. Blood 2006;107(12):4972–3; author reply 3–4.

95. Dispenzieri A, Klein CJ, Mauermann ML. Letter to the editor: lenalidomide therapy in a patient with POEMS syndrome. Blood In press.

96. Philips ED, el-Mahdi AM, Humphrey RL, Furlong MB, Jr. The effect of the radiation treatment on the polyneuropathy of multiple myeloma. J Can Assoc Radiol 1972;23(2):103–6.

97. Broussolle E, Vighetto A, Bancel B, Confavreux C, Pialat J, Aimard G. P.O.E.M.S. syndrome with complete recovery after treatment of a solitary plasmocytoma. Clin Neurol Neurosurg 1991;93(2):165–70.

98. Cabezas-Agricola JM, Lado-Abeal JJ, Otero-Anton E, Sanchez-Leira J, Cabezas-Cerrato J. Hypoparathyroidism in POEMS syndrome [letter]. Lancet 1996;347(9002):701–2.

99. Nakano A, Mitsui T, Endo I, Takeda Y, Ozaki S, Matsumoto T. Solitary plasmacytoma with VEGF overproduction: report of a patient with polyneuropathy. Neurology 2001;56(6):818–9.

100. Anonymous. Combination chemotherapy versus melphalan plus prednisone as treatment for multiple myeloma: an overview of 6,633 patients from 27 randomized trials. Myeloma Trialists' Collaborative Group. J Clin Oncol 1998;16(12):3832–42.

101. Satoh K, Miura I, Chubachi A, Utsumi S, Imai H, Miura AB. Development of secondary leukemia associated with (1;7)(q10;p10) in a patient with Crow-Fukase syndrome. Intern Med 1996;35(8):660–2.

102. Gertz MA, Lacy MQ, Dispenzieri A, et al. Stem cell transplantation for the management of primary systemic amyloidosis. Am J Med 2002;113(7):549–55.

103. Silberstein LE, Duggan D, Berkman EM. Therapeutic trial of plasma exchange in osteosclerotic myeloma associated with the POEMS syndrome. J Clin Apher 1985;2(3):253–7.

104. Atsumi T, Kato K, Kurosawa S, Abe M, Fujisaku A. A case of Crow-Fukase syndrome with elevated soluble interleukin-6 receptor in cerebrospinal fluid. Response to double-filtration plasmapheresis and corticosteroids. Acta Haematol 1995;94(2):90–4.

105. Chang YJ, Huang CC, Chu CC. Intravenous immunoglobulin therapy in POEMS syndrome: a case report. Chung Hua i Hsueh Tsa Chih Chinese Medical Journal 1996;58(5):366–9.

106. Enevoldson TP, Harding AE. Improvement in the POEMS syndrome after administration of tamoxifen [letter]. J Neurol Neurosurg Psychiatry 1992;55(1):71–2.

107. Benito-Leon J, Lopez-Rios F, Rodriguez-Martin FJ, Madero S, Ruiz J. Rapidly deteriorating polyneuropathy associated with osteosclerotic myeloma responsive to intravenous immunoglobulin and radiotherapy. J Neurol Sci 1998;158(1):113–7.

108. Henze T, Krieger G. Combined high-dose 7S-IgG and dexamethasone is effective in severe polyneuropathy of the POEMS syndrome [letter] [see comments]. J Neurol 1995;242(7):482–3.

109. Rotta FT, Bradley WG. Marked improvement of severe polyneuropathy associated with multifocal osteosclerotic myeloma following surgery, radiation, and chemotherapy. Muscle Nerve 1997;20(8):1035–7.

110. Huang CC, Chu CC. Poor response to intravenous immunoglobulin therapy in patients with Castleman's disease and the POEMS syndrome [letter; comment]. J Neurol 1996;243(10):726–7.

111. Singhal S, Mehta J, Desikan R, et al. Antitumor activity of thalidomide in refractory multiple myeloma. N Engl J Med 1999;341(21):1565–71.

112. Kyle RA, Therneau TM, Rajkumar SV, et al. A long-term study of prognosis in monoclonal gammopathy of undetermined significance. N Engl J Med 2002;346(8):564–9.

113. Criteria for the classification of monoclonal gammopathies, multiple myeloma and related disorders: a report of the International Myeloma Working Group. Br J Haematol 2003;121(5):749–57.

114. Kahn SN, Riches PG, Kohn J. Paraproteinaemia in neurological disease: incidence, associations, and classification of monoclonal immunoglobulins. J Clin Pathol 1980;33(7):617–21.

115. Kelly JJ, Jr., Kyle RA, O'Brien PC, Dyck PJ. Prevalence of monoclonal protein in peripheral neuropathy. Neurology 1981;31(11):1480–3.

116. Johansen P, Leegaard OF. Peripheral neuropathy and paraproteinemia: an immunohistochemical and serologic study. Clin Neuropathol 1985;4(3):99–104.

117. Isobe T, Osserman EF. Pathologic conditions associated with plasma cell dyscrasias: a study of 806 cases. Ann N Y Acad Sci 1971;190:507–18.

118. Nobile-Orazio E, Barbieri S, Baldini L, et al. Peripheral neuropathy in monoclonal gammopathy of undetermined significance: prevalence and immunopathogenetic studies. Acta Neurol Scand 1992;85(6):383–90.

119. Vrethem M, Cruz M, Wen-Xin H, Malm C, Holmgren H, Ernerudh J. Clinical, neurophysiological and immunological evidence of polyneuropathy in patients with monoclonal gammopathies. J Neurol Sci 1993;114(2):193–9.

120. Baldini L, Nobile-Orazio E, Guffanti A, et al. Peripheral neuropathy in IgM monoclonal gammopathy and Waldenstrom's macroglobulinemia: a frequent complication

in elderly males with low MAG-reactive serum monoclonal component. Am J Hematol 1994;45(1):25–31.

121. Latov N, Sherman WH, Nemni R, et al. Plasma-cell dyscrasia and peripheral neuropathy with a monoclonal antibody to peripheral-nerve myelin. N Engl J Med 1980;303(11):618–21.

122. Dellagi K, Dupouey P, Brouet JC, et al. Waldenstrom's macroglobulinemia and peripheral neuropathy: a clinical and immunologic study of 25 patients. Blood 1983;62(2):280–5.

123. Nemni R, Galassi G, Latov N, Sherman WH, Olarte MR, Hays AP. Polyneuropathy in nonmalignant IgM plasma cell dyscrasia: a morphological study. Ann Neurol 1983;14(1):43–54.

124. Latov N, Hays AP, Sherman WH. Peripheral neuropathy and anti-MAG antibodies. Crit Rev Neurobiol 1988;3(4):301–32.

125. Quarles RH, Weiss MD. Autoantibodies associated with peripheral neuropathy. Muscle Nerve 1999;22(7):800–22.

126. Nobile-Orazio E, Francomano E, Daverio R, et al. Anti-myelin-associated glycoprotein IgM antibody titers in neuropathy associated with macroglobulinemia. Ann Neurol 1989;26(4):543–50.

127. Meucci N, Baldini L, Cappellari A, et al. Anti-myelin-associated glycoprotein antibodies predict the development of neuropathy in asymptomatic patients with IgM monoclonal gammopathy. Ann Neurol 1999;46(1):119–22.

128. Dispenzieri A, Kyle RA. Neurological aspects of multiple myeloma and related disorders. Best Pract Res Clin Haematol 2005;18(4):673–88.

129. Suarez GA, Kelly JJ, Jr. Polyneuropathy associated with monoclonal gammopathy of undetermined significance: further evidence that IgM-MGUS neuropathies are different than IgG-MGUS. Neurology 1993;43(7):1304–8.

130. Chassande B, Leger JM, Younes-Chennoufi AB, et al. Peripheral neuropathy associated with IgM monoclonal gammopathy: correlations between M-protein antibody activity and clinical/electrophysiological features in 40 cases. Muscle Nerve 1998;21(1):55–62.

131. Melmed C, Frail D, Duncan I, et al. Peripheral neuropathy with IgM kappa monoclonal immunoglobulin directed against myelin-associated glycoprotein. Neurology 1983;33(11):1397–405.

132. Kelly JJ, Adelman LS, Berkman E, Bhan I. Polyneuropathies associated with IgM monoclonal gammopathies. Arch Neurol 1988;45(12):1355–9.

133. Kelly JJ, Jr. The electrodiagnostic findings in polyneuropathies associated with IgM monoclonal gammopathies. Muscle Nerve 1990;13(12):1113–7.

134. Ilyas AA, Cook SD, Dalakas MC, Mithen FA. Anti-MAG IgM paraproteins from some patients with polyneuropathy associated with IgM paraproteinemia also react with sulfatide. J Neuroimmunol 1992;37(1–2):85–92.

135. Simmons Z, Albers JW, Bromberg MB, Feldman EL. Long-term follow-up of patients with chronic inflammatory demyelinating polyradiculoneuropathy, without and with monoclonal gammopathy. Brain 1995;118(Pt 2):359–68.

136. Notermans NC, Franssen H, Eurelings M, Van der Graaf Y, Wokke JH. Diagnostic criteria for demyelinating polyneuropathy associated with monoclonal gammopathy. Muscle Nerve 2000;23(1):73–9.

137. Gorson KC, Allam G, Ropper AH. Chronic inflammatory demyelinating polyneuropathy: clinical features and response to treatment in 67 consecutive patients with and without a monoclonal gammopathy. Neurology 1997;48(2):321–8.

138. Nobile-Orazio E, Meucci N, Baldini L, Di Troia A, Scarlato G. Long-term prognosis of neuropathy associated with anti-MAG IgM M- proteins and its relationship to immune therapies. Brain 2000;123(Pt 4):710–7.

139. Dyck PJ, Low PA, Windebank AJ, et al. Plasma exchange in polyneuropathy associated with monoclonal gammopathy of undetermined significance. N Engl J Med 1991;325(21):1482–6.

140. Oksenhendler E, Chevret S, Leger JM, Louboutin JP, Bussel A, Brouet JC. Plasma exchange and chlorambucil in polyneuropathy associated with monoclonal IgM gammopathy. IgM-associated Polyneuropathy Study Group. J Neurol Neurosurg Psychiatry 1995;59(3):243–7.

141. Mariette X, Chastang C, Clavelou P, Louboutin JP, Leger JM, Brouet JC. A randomised clinical trial comparing interferon-alpha and intravenous immunoglobulin in polyneuropathy associated with monoclonal IgM. The IgM-associated Polyneuropathy Study Group. J Neurol Neurosurg Psychiatry 1997;63(1):28–34.

142. Comi G, Roveri L, Swan A, . A randomised controlled trial of intravenous immunoglobulin in IgM paraprotein associated demyelinating neuropathy. J Neurol 2002;249(10):1370–7.

143. Mariette X, Brouet JC, Chevret S, et al. A randomised double blind trial versus placebo does not confirm the benefit of alpha-interferon in polyneuropathy associated with monoclonal IgM [letter]. J Neurol Neurosurg Psychiatry 2000;69(2):279–80.

144. Dalakas MC, Quarles RH, Farrer RG, et al. A controlled study of intravenous immunoglobulin in demyelinating neuropathy with IgM gammopathy. Ann Neurol 1996;40(5):792–5.

145. Sherman WH, Olarte MR, McKiernan G, Sweeney K, Latov N, Hays AP. Plasma exchange treatment of peripheral neuropathy associated with plasma cell dyscrasia. J Neurol Neurosurg Psychiatry 1984;47(8):813–9.

146. Yeung KB, Thomas PK, King RH, et al. The clinical spectrum of peripheral neuropathies associated with benign monoclonal IgM, IgG and IgA paraproteinaemia. Comparative clinical, immunological and nerve biopsy findings. J Neurol 1991;238(7):383–91.

147. Wilson HC, Lunn MP, Schey S, Hughes RA. Successful treatment of IgM paraproteinaemic neuropathy with fludarabine. J Neurol Neurosurg Psychiatry 1999;66(5):575–80.

148. Levine TD, Pestronk A. IgM antibody-related polyneuropathies: B-cell depletion chemotherapy using rituximab. Neurology 1999;52(8):1701–4.

149. Renaud S, Gregor M, Fuhr P. Rituximab in the treatment of polyneuropathy associated with anti-MAG antibodies. Muscle Nerve 2003; 27(5):611–5.

150. Pestronk A, Florence J, Miller T, Choksi R, Al-Lozi MT, Levine TD. Treatment of IgM antibody associated polyneuropathies using rituximab. J Neurol Neurosurg Psychiatry 2003;74(4):485–9.

151. Wintrobe M, Buell M. Hyperproteinemia associated with multiple myeloma. Bull Johns Hopkins Hosp 1933;52:156–165.

152. Lerner A, Watson C. Studies of cryoglobulins. Unusual purpura associated with the presence of a high concentration of cryoglobulin (cold precipitable serum globulin). Am J Med Sci 1947;214:410.

153. Grey HM, Kohler PF. Cryoimmunoglobulins. Semin Hematol 1973;10(2):87–112.

154. Meltzer M, Franklin EC. Cryoglobulinemia—a study of twenty-nine patients. I. IgG and IgM cryoglobulins and factors affecting cryoprecipitability. Am J Med 1966;40:828–56.

155. Meltzer M, Franklin EC, Elias K, McCluskey RT, Cooper N. Cryoglobulinemia— a clinical and laboratory study. II. Cryoglobulins with rheumatoid factor activity. Am J Med 1966;40(6):837–56.

156. Brouet J, Clauvel J, Danon F, Klein M, Seligmann M. Biological and clinical significance of cryoglobulins. A report of 86 cases. Am J Med 1974;57:775–88.

157. Gorevic PD, Kassab HJ, Levo Y, et al. Mixed cryoglobulinemia: clinical aspects and long-term follow-up of 40 patients. Am J Med 1980;69(2):287–308.

158. Dispenzieri A, Gorevic PD. Cryoglobulinemia. Hematol Oncol Clin North Am 1999;13(6):1315–49.

159. Monti G, Galli M, Invernizzi F, et al. Cryoglobulinaemias: a multi-centre study of the early clinical and laboratory manifestations of primary and secondary disease. GISC. Italian Group for the Study of Cryoglobulinaemias. Qjm 1995;88(2):115–26.

160. Pascual M, Perrin L, Giostra E, Schifferli JA. Hepatitis C virus in patients with cryoglobulinemia type II. J Infect Dis 1990;162(2):569–70.

161. Ferri C, Greco F, Longombardo G, et al. Antibodies to hepatitis C virus in patients with mixed cryoglobulinemia. Arthritis Rheum 1991;34(12):1606–10.

162. Goldman M, Renversez JC, Lambert PH. Pathological expression of idiotypic interactions: immune complexes and cryoglobulins. [33 refs]. Springer Semin Immunopathol 1983;6(1):33–49.

163. Wilson MR, Arroyave CM, Miles L, Tan EM. Immune reactants in cryoproteins. Relationship to complement activation. Ann Rheum Dis 1977;36(6):540–8.

164. Agnello V, Chung R, Kaplan L. A role for hepatitis C virus infection in type II cryoglobulinemia. N Engl J Med 1992;327(21):1490–5.

165. Misiani R, Bellavita P, Fenili D, et al. Hepatitis C virus infection in patients with essential mixed cryoglobulinemia. Ann Intern Med 1992;117(7):573–7.

166. Pechere-Bertschi A, Perrin L, de Saussure P, Widmann JJ, Giostra E, Schifferli JA. Hepatitis C: a possible etiology for cryoglobulinaemia type II. Clin Exp Immunol 1992;89(3):419–22.

167. Bichard P, Ounanian A, Girard M, et al. High prevalence of hepatitis C virus RNA in the supernatant and the cryoprecipitate of patients with essential and secondary type II mixed cryoglobulinemia. J Hepatol 1994;21(1):58–63.

168. Cacoub P, Fabiani FL, Musset L, et al. Mixed cryoglobulinemia and hepatitis C virus. Am J Med 1994;96(2):124–32.

169. Munoz-Fernandez S, Barbado FJ, Martin Mola E, et al. Evidence of hepatitis C virus antibodies in the cryoprecipitate of patients with mixed cryoglobulinemia. J Rheumatol 1994;21(2):229–33.

170. Tanaka K, Aiyama T, Imai J, Morishita Y, Fukatsu T, Kakumu S. Serum cryoglobulin and chronic hepatitis C virus disease among Japanese patients. Am J Gastroenterol 1995;90(10):1847–52.

171. Lunel F, Musset L, Cacoub P, et al. Cryoglobulinemia in chronic liver diseases: role of hepatitis C virus and liver damage. Gastroenterology 1994;106(5):1291–300.

172. Sansonno D, Iacobelli AR, Cornacchiulo V, et al. Immunochemical and biomolecular studies of circulating immune complexes isolated from patients with acute and chronic hepatitis C virus infection. Eur J Clin Invest 1996;26(6):465–75.

173. Invernizzi F, Galli M, Serino G, et al. Secondary and essential cryoglobulinemias. Frequency, nosological classification, and long-term follow-up. Acta Haematol 1983;70(2):73–82.

174. Osserman E. Plasma cell myeloma. N Eng J Med 1959;261:952–60.

175. Tarantino A, De Vecchi A, Montagnino G, et al. Renal disease in essential mixed cryoglobulinaemia. Long-term follow-up of 44 patients. Q J Med 1981;50:1.

176. Singer DR, Venning MC, Lockwood CM, Pusey CD. Cryoglobulinaemia: clinical features and response to treatment. Ann Med Interne 1986;137(3):251–3.

177. Monti G, Saccardo F, Pioltelli P, Rinaldi G. The natural history of cryoglobulinemia: symptoms at onset and during follow-up. A report by the Italian Group for the Study of Cryoglobulinemias (GISC). Clin Exp Rheumatol 1995;13(13):S129–33.

178. Ferri C, Sebastiani M, Giuggioli D, et al. Mixed cryoglobulinemia: demographic, clinical, and serologic features and survival in 231 patients. Semin Arthritis Rheum 2004;33(6):355–74.

179. Trejo O, Ramos-Casals M, Garcia-Carrasco M, et al. Cryoglobulinemia: study of etiologic factors and clinical and immunologic features in 443 patients from a single center. Medicine (Baltimore) 2001;80(4):252–62.

180. Rieu V, Cohen P, Andre MH, et al. Characteristics and outcome of 49 patients with symptomatic cryoglobulinaemia. Rheumatology (Oxford) 2002;41(3):290–300.

181. Bryce AH, Kyle RA, Dispenzieri A, Gertz MA. Natural history and therapy of 66 patients with mixed cryoglobulinemia. Am J Hematol 2006;81(7):511–8.

182. Mendez P, Saeian K, Reddy KR, et al. Hepatitis C, cryoglobulinemia, and cutaneous vasculitis associated with unusual and serious manifestations. Am J Gastroenterol 2001;96(8):2489–93.

183. Donada C, Crucitti A, Donadon V, et al. Systemic manifestations and liver disease in patients with chronic hepatitis C and type II or III mixed cryoglobulinaemia. J Viral Hepat 1998;5(3):179–85.

184. Montagnino G. Reappraisal of the clinical expression of mixed cryoglobulinemia. Springer Semin Immunopathol 1988;10(1):1–19.

185. Cohen SJ, Pittelkow MR, Su WP. Cutaneous manifestations of cryoglobulinemia: clinical and histopathologic study of seventy-two patients. J Am Acad Dermatol 1991;25(1 Pt 1):21–7.

186. Gemignani F, Brindani F, Alfieri S, et al. Clinical spectrum of cryoglobulinaemic neuropathy. J Neurol Neurosurg Psychiatry 2005;76(10):1410–4.

187. Chad D, Pariser K, Bradley WG, Adelman LS, Pinn VW. The pathogenesis of cryoglobulinemic neuropathy. Neurology 1982;32(7):725–9.

188. Nemni R, Corbo M, Fazio R, Quattrini A, Comi G, Canal N. Cryoglobulinaemic neuropathy. A clinical, morphological and immunocytochemical study of 8 cases. Brain 1988;111(Pt 3):541–52.

189. Cavaletti G, Petruccioli MG, Crespi V, Pioltelli P, Marmiroli P, Tredici G. A clinico-pathological and follow up study of 10 cases of essential type II cryoglobulinaemic neuropathy. J Neurol Neurosurg Psychiatry 1990;53(10):886–9.

190. Khella SL, Frost S, Hermann GA, et al. Hepatitis C infection, cryoglobulinemia, and vasculitic neuropathy. Treatment with interferon alfa: case report and literature review. Neurology 1995;45(3 Pt 1):407–11.

191. Garcia-Bragado F, Fernandez JM, Navarro C, Villar M, Bonaventura I. Peripheral neuropathy in essential mixed cryoglobulinemia. Arch Neurol 1988;45(11):1210–4.

192. Valli G, De Vecchi A, Gaddi L, Nobile-Orazio E, Tarantino A, Barbieri S. Peripheral nervous system involvement in essential cryoglobulinemia and nephropathy. Clin Exp Rheumatol 1989;7(5):479–83.

193. Ammendola A, Sampaolo S, Ambrosone L, et al. Peripheral neuropathy in hepatitis-related mixed cryoglobulinemia: electrophysiologic follow-up study. Muscle Nerve 2005;31(3):382–5.

194. Casato M, Saadoun D, Marchetti A, et al. Central nervous system involvement in hepatitis C virus cryoglobulinemia vasculitis: a multicenter case-control study using magnetic resonance imaging and neuropsychological tests. J Rheumatol 2005;32(3):484–8.

195. Ferri C, La Civita L, Longombardo G, Zignego AL, Pasero G. Mixed cryoglobulinaemia: a cross-road between autoimmune and lymphoproliferative disorders. Lupus 1998;7(4):275–9.

196. Cordonnier D, Vialtel P, Renversez JC, et al. Renal diseases in 18 patients with mixed type II IgM-IgG cryoglobulinemia: monoclonal lymphoid infiltration (2 cases) and membranoproliferative glomerulonephritis (14 cases). Adv Nephrol Necker Hosp 1983;12:177–204.

197. D' Amico G. Renal involvement in hepatitis C infection: cryoglobulinemic glomerulonephritis. Kidney Int 1998;54(2):650–71.

198. Tarantino A, Campise M, Banfi G, et al. Long-term predictors of survival in essential mixed cryoglobulinemic glomerulonephritis. Kidney Int 1995;47(2):618–23.

199. Gorevic PD, Frangione B. Mixed cryoglobulinemia cross-reactive idiotypes: implications for the relationship of MC to rheumatic and lymphoproliferative diseases. Semin Hematol 1991;28(2):79–94.

200. Levo Y, Gorevic PD, Kassab HJ, Tobias H, Franklin EC. Liver involvement in the syndrome of mixed cryoglobulinemia. Ann Intern Med 1977;87(3):287–92.

201. Monteverde A, Ballare M, Bertoncelli MC, et al. Lymphoproliferation in type II mixed cryoglobulinemia. Clin Exp Rheumatol 1995;13(13):S141–7.

202. Monteverde A, Ballare M, Pileri S. Hepatic lymphoid aggregates in chronic hepatitis C and mixed cryoglobulinemia. Springer Semin Immunopathol 1997;19(1):99–110.

203. Tarantino A, Anelli A, Costantino A, De Vecchi A, Monti G, Massaro L. Serum complement pattern in essential mixed cryoglobulinaemia. Clin Exp Immunol 1978;32(1):77–85.

204. Ferri C, Moriconi L, Gremignai G, et al. Treatment of the renal involvement in mixed cryoglobulinemia with prolonged plasma exchange. Nephron 1986;43(4):246–53.

205. Frankel AH, Singer DR, Winearls CG, Evans DJ, Rees AJ, Pusey CD. Type II essential mixed cryoglobulinaemia: presentation, treatment and outcome in 13 patients. Q J Med 1992;82(298):101–24.

206. Ferri C, Marzo E, Longombardo G, et al. Interferon-alpha in mixed cryoglobulinemia patients: a randomized, crossover-controlled trial. Blood 1993;81(5):1132–6.

207. Ferri C, Marzo E, Longombardo G, et al. Interferon alfa-2b in mixed cryoglobulinaemia: a controlled crossover trial. Gut 1993;34(2 Suppl):S144–5.

208. Misiani R, Bellavita P, Fenili D, et al. Interferon alfa-2a therapy in cryoglobulinemia associated with hepatitis C virus. N Engl J Med 1994;330(11):751–6.

209. Dammacco F, Sansonno D, Han JH, et al. Natural interferon-alpha versus its combination with 6-methyl-prednisolone in the therapy of type II mixed cryoglobulinemia: a long-term, randomized, controlled study. Blood 1994;84(10):3336–43.

210. Lauta VM, De Sangro MA. Long-term results regarding the use of recombinant interferon alpha-2b in the treatment of II type mixed essential cryoglobulinemia. Med Oncol 1995;12(4):223–30.

211. Mazzaro C, Lacchin T, Moretti M, et al. Effects of two different alpha-interferon regimens on clinical and virological findings in mixed cryoglobulinemia. Clin Exp Rheumatol 1995;13(13):S181–5.

212. Ferri C, Pietrogrande M, Cecchetti R, et al. Low-antigen-content diet in the treatment of patients with mixed cryoglobulinemia. Am J Med 1989;87(5):519–24.

213. Durand JM, Cacoub P, Lunel-Fabiani F, et al. Ribavirin in hepatitis C related cryoglobulinemia. J Rheumatol 1998;25(6):1115–7.

214. Geltner D, Kohn RW, Gorevic P, Franklin EC. The effect of combination therapy (steroids, immunosuppressives, and plasmapheresis) on 5 mixed cryoglobulinemia patients with renal, neurologic, and vascular involvement. Arthritis Rheum 1981;24(9):1121–7.

215. Valbonesi M, Montani F, Mosconi L, Florio G, Vecchi C. Plasmapheresis and cytotoxic drugs for mixed cryoglobulinemia. Haematologia 1984;17(3):341–51.

216. Sinico RA, Fornasieri A, Fiorini G, et al. Plasma exchange in the treatment of essential mixed cryoglobulinemia nephropathy. Long-term follow up. Int J Artif Organs 1985;2:15–8.

217. Berkman EM, Orlin JB. Use of plasmapheresis and partial plasma exchange in the management of patients with cryoglobulinemia. Transfusion 1980;20(2):171–8.

218. McLeod BC, Sassetti RJ. Plasmapheresis with return of cryoglobulin-depleted autologous plasma (cryoglobulinpheresis) in cryoglobulinemia. Blood 1980;55(5):866–70.

219. Reik L, Jr., Korn JH. Cryoglobulinemia with encephalopathy: successful treatment by plasma exchange. Ann Neurol 1981;10(5):488–90.

220. Ristow SC, Griner PF, Abraham GN, Shoulson I. Reversal of systemic manifestations of cryoglobulinemia. Ach Intern Med 1976;136:467–70.

221. Volpe R, Bruce-Robertson A, Fletcher A, et al. Essential cryoglobulinemia: review of the literature and report of a case treated with ACTH and cortisone. Am J Med 1956;20:533–53.

222. De Vecchi A, Montagnino G, Pozzi C, Tarantino A, Locatelli F, Ponticelli C. Intravenous methylprednisolone pulse therapy in essential mixed cryoglobulinemia nephropathy. Clin Nephrol 1983;19(5):221–7.

223. Ponticelli C, Imbasciati E, Tarantino A, Pietrogrande M. Acute anuric glomerulone-phritis in monoclonal cryoglobulinaemia. Br Med J 1977;1(6066):948.

224. Mathison DA, Condemi JJ, Leddy JP, Callerame ML, Panner BJ, Vaughan JH. Purpura, arthralgia, and IgM-IgM cryoglobulinemia with rheumatoid factor acrivity. Response to cyclophosphamide and splenectomy. Ann Intern Med 1971;74(3):383–90.

225. Germain MJ, Anderson RW, Keane WF. Renal disease in cryoglobulinemia type II: response to therapy. A case report and review of the literature. Am J Nephrol 1982;2(4):221–6.

226. Quigg RJ, Brathwaite M, Gardner DF, Gretch DR, Ruddy S. Successful cyclophosphamide treatment of cryoglobulinemic membranoproliferative glomerulonephritis associated with hepatitis C virus infection. Am J Kidney Dis 1995;25(5):798–800.

227. Zaja F, De Vita S, Mazzaro C, et al. Efficacy and safety of rituximab in type II mixed cryoglobulinemia. Blood 2003;101(10):3827–34.

228. Sansonno D, De Re V, Lauletta G, Tucci FA, Boiocchi M, Dammacco F. Monoclonal antibody treatment of mixed cryoglobulinemia resistant to interferon alpha with an anti-CD20. Blood 2003;101(10):3818–26.

229. Bryce AH, Dispenzieri A, Kyle RA, et al. Response to rituximab in patients with type II cryoglobulinemia. Clin Lymphoma Myeloma 2006;7(2):140–4.

230. Roccatello D, Baldovino S, Rossi D, . Long-term effects of anti-CD20 monoclonal antibody treatment of cryoglobulinaemic glomerulonephritis. Nephrol Dial Transplant 2004;19(12):3054–61.

231. Basse G, Ribes D, Kamar N, et al. Rituximab therapy for mixed cryoglobulinemia in seven renal transplant patients. Transplant Proc 2006;38(7):2308–10.

232. Lamprecht P, Lerin-Lozano C, Merz H, et al. Rituximab induces remission in refractory HCV associated cryoglobulinaemic vasculitis. Ann Rheum Dis 2003;62(12):1230–3.

233. Ghijsels E, Lerut E, Vanrenterghem Y, Kuypers D. Anti-CD20 monoclonal antibody (rituximab) treatment for hepatitis C-negative therapy-resistant essential mixed cryoglobulinemia with renal and cardiac failure. Am J Kidney Dis 2004;43(5):e34–8.

234. Sampson A, Callen JP. The cutting edge: thalidomide for type 1 cryoglobulinemic vasculopathy. Arch Dermatol 2006;142(8):972–4.

235. Cem Ar M, Soysal T, Hatemi G, Salihoglu A, Yazici H, Ulku B. Successful management of cryoglobulinemia-induced leukocytoclastic vasculitis with thalidomide in a patient with multiple myeloma. Ann Hematol 2005;84(9):609–13.

236. Ballare M, Bobbio F, Poggi G, . A pilot study on the effectiveness of cyclosporine in type II mixed cryoglobulinemia. Clin Exp Rheumatol 1995;13(13):S201–3.

237. Chandesris MO, Gayet S, Schleinitz N, Doudier B, Harle JR, Kaplanski G. Infliximab in the treatment of refractory vasculitis secondary to hepatitis C-associated mixed cryoglobulinaemia. Rheumatology (Oxford) 2004;43(4):532–3.

238. Monti G, Saccardo F, Rinaldi G, Petrozzino MR, Gomitoni A, Invernizzi F. Colchicine in the treatment of mixed cryoglobulinemia. Clin Exp Rheumatol 1995;13(13):S197–9.

239. Barton JC, Herrera GA, Galla JH, Bertoli LF, Work J, Koopman WJ. Acute cryoglobulinemic renal failure after intravenous infusion of gamma globulin. Am J Med 1987;82(3 Spec No):624–9.

240. Boom BW, Brand A, Bavinck JN, Eernisse JG, Daha MR, Vermeer BJ. Severe leukocytoclastic vasculitis of the skin in a patient with essential mixed cryoglobulinemia treated with high-dose gamma-globulin intravenously. Arch Dermatol 1988;124(10):1550–3.

241. Enzenauer RJ, Judson PH. Type II mixed cryoglobulinemia treated with fludarabine. J Rheumatol 1996;23(4):794–5.

242. Zaja F. Fludarabine in the treatment of essential mixed cryoglobulinaemia. Eur J Haematol 1996;57(3):259–60.

243. Odum J, D'Costa D, Freeth M, Taylor D, Smith N, MacWhannell A. Cryoglobulinaemic vasculitis caused by intravenous immunoglobulin treatment. Nephrol Dial Transplant 2001;16(2):403–6.

244. Migliaresi S, Tirri G. Interferon in the treatment of mixed cryoglobulinemia. Clin Exp Rheumatol 1995;13(13):S175–80.

245. Alric L, Plaisier E, Thebault S, et al. Influence of antiviral therapy in hepatitis C virus-associated cryoglobulinemic MPGN. Am J Kidney Dis 2004;43(4):617–23.

246. Zignego AL, Ferri C, Pileri SA, Caini P, Bianchi FB. Extrahepatic manifestations of hepatitis C virus infection: a general overview and guidelines for a clinical approach. Dig Liver Dis 2006.

247. Dispenzieri A. Symptomatic cryoglobulinemia. Curr Treat Options Oncol 1999;1(2):105–18.

248. Bruchfeld A, Lindahl K, Stahle L, Soderberg M, Schvarcz R. Interferon and ribavirin treatment in patients with hepatitis C-associated renal disease and renal insufficiency. Nephrol Dial Transplant 2003;18(8):1573–80.

249. Casato M, Lagana B, Antonelli G, Dianzani F, Bonomo L. Long-term results of therapy with interferon-alpha for type II essential mixed cryoglobulinemia. Blood 1991;78(12):3142–7.

250. Ohta S, Yokoyama H, Wada T, et al. Exacerbation of glomerulonephritis in subjects with chronic hepatitis C virus infection after interferon therapy. Am J Kidney Dis 1999;33(6):1040–8.

251. Beuthien W, Mellinghoff HU, Kempis J. Vasculitic complications of interferon-alpha treatment for chronic hepatitis C virus infection: case report and review of the literature. Clin Rheumatol 2005;24(5):507–15.

252. Cid MC, Hernandez-Rodriguez J, Robert J, et al. Interferon-alpha may exacerbate cryoblobulinemia-related ischemic manifestations: an adverse effect potentially related to its anti-angiogenic activity. Arthritis Rheum 1999;42(5):1051–5.

253. Cresta P, Musset L, Cacoub P, et al. Response to interferon alpha treatment and disappearance of cryoglobulinaemia in patients infected by hepatitis C virus [see comments]. Gut 1999;45(1):122–8.

254. Calleja JL, Albillos A, Moreno-Otero R, et al. Sustained response to interferon-alpha or to interferon-alpha plus ribavirin in hepatitis C virus-associated symptomatic mixed cryoglobulinaemia. Aliment Pharmacol Ther 1999;13(9):1179–86.

255. Zuckerman E, Keren D, Slobodin G, et al. Treatment of refractory, symptomatic, hepatitis C virus related mixed cryoglobulinemia with ribavirin and interferon-alpha. J Rheumatol 2000;27(9):2172–8.

256. Mazzaro C, Zorat F, Comar C, et al. Interferon plus ribavirin in patients with hepatitis C virus positive mixed cryoglobulinemia resistant to interferon. J Rheumatol 2003;30(8):1775–81.

257. Cacoub P, Lidove O, Maisonobe T, et al. Interferon-alpha and ribavirin treatment in patients with hepatitis C virus-related systemic vasculitis. Arthritis Rheum 2002;46(12):3317–26.

258. Donada C, Crucitti A, Donadon V, Chemello L, Alberti A. Interferon and ribavirin combination therapy in patients with chronic hepatitis C and mixed cryoglobulinemia. Blood 1998;92(8):2983–4.

259. Bonomo L, Casato M, Afeltra A, Caccavo D. Treatment of idiopathic mixed cryoglobulinemia with alpha interferon. Am J Med 1987;83(4):726–30.

260. Mazzaro C, Zorat F, Caizzi M, et al. Treatment with peg-interferon alfa-2b and ribavirin of hepatitis C virus-associated mixed cryoglobulinemia: a pilot study. J Hepatol 2005;42(5):632–8.

261. Saadoun D, Resche-Rigon M, Thibault V, Piette JC, Cacoub P. Antiviral therapy for hepatitis C virus-associated mixed cryoglobulinemia vasculitis: a long-term follow-up study. Arthritis Rheum 2006;54(11):3696–706.

262. Ghobrial IM, Uslan DZ, Call TG, Witzig TE, Gertz MA. Initial increase in the cryoglobulin level after rituximab therapy for type II cryoglobulinemia secondary to Waldenström macroglobulinemia does not indicate failure of response. Am J Hematol 2004;77(4):329–30.

263. Frickhofen N, Wiesneth M, Jainta C, et al. Hepatitis C virus infection is a risk factor for liver failure from veno-occlusive disease after bone marrow transplantation. Blood 1994;83(7):1998–2004.

264. Ubara Y, Hara S, Katori H, et al. Splenectomy may improve the glomerulopathy of type II mixed cryoglobulinemia. Am J Kidney Dis 2000;35(6):1186–92.

265. Cokonis Georgakis CD, Falasca G, Georgakis A, Heymann WR. Scleromyxedema. Clin Dermatol 2006;24(6):493–7.

266. Kucher C, Xu X, Pasha T, Elenitsas R. Histopathologic comparison of nephrogenic fibrosing dermopathy and scleromyxedema. J Cutan Pathol 2005;32(7):484–90.

267. Dinneen AM, Dicken CH. Scleromyxedema. J Am Acad Dermatol 1995;33(1):37–43.

268. Berger JR, Dobbs MR, Terhune MH, Maragos WF. The neurologic complications of scleromyxedema. Medicine (Baltimore) 2001;80(5):313–9.

269. Pomann JJ, Rudner EJ. Scleromyxedema revisited. Int J Dermatol 2003;42(1):31–5.

270. Rongioletti F, Rebora A. Updated classification of papular mucinosis, lichen myxedematosus, and scleromyxedema. J Am Acad Dermatol 2001;44(2):273–81.

271. Lacy MQ, Hogan WJ, Gertz MA, . Successful treatment of scleromyxedema with autologous peripheral blood stem cell transplantation. Arch Dermatol 2005;141(10):1277–82.

272. Sansbury JC, Cocuroccia B, Jorizzo JL, Gubinelli E, Gisondi P, Girolomoni G. Treatment of recalcitrant scleromyxedema with thalidomide in 3 patients. J Am Acad Dermatol 2004;51(1):126–31.

273. Fernandez-Herrera J, Pedraz J. Necrobiotic xanthogranuloma. Semin Cutan Med Surg 2007;26(2):108–13.

274. Finan MC, Winkelmann RK. Necrobiotic xanthogranuloma with paraproteinemia. A review of 22 cases. Medicine (Baltimore) 1986;65(6):376–88.

275. Bullock JD, Bartley GB, Campbell RJ, Yanes B, Connelly PJ, Funkhouser JW. Necrobiotic xanthogranuloma with paraproteinemia: case report and a pathogenetic theory. Trans Am Ophthalmol Soc 1986;84:342–54.

276. Matsuura F, Yamashita S, Hirano K, et al. Activation of monocytes in vivo causes intracellular accumulation of lipoprotein-derived lipids and marked hypocholesterolemia—a possible pathogenesis of necrobiotic xanthogranuloma. Atherosclerosis 1999;142(2):355–65.

277. Venencie PY, Le Bras P, Toan ND, Tchernia G, Delfraissy JF. Recombinant interferon alfa-2b treatment of necrobiotic xanthogranuloma with paraproteinemia. J Am Acad Dermatol 1995;32(4):666–7.

278. Goede JS, Misselwitz B, Taverna C, et al. Necrobiotic xanthogranuloma successfully treated with autologous stem cell transplantation. Ann Hematol 2007;86(4):303–6.

279. Lipsker D, Veran Y, Grunenberger F, Cribier B, Heid E, Grosshans E. The Schnitzler syndrome. Four new cases and review of the literature. Medicine (Baltimore) 2001;80(1):37–44.

280. de Koning HD, Bodar EJ, van der Meer JW, Simon A. Schnitzler syndrome: beyond the case reports: review and follow-up of 94 patients with an emphasis on prognosis and treatment. Semin Arthritis Rheum 2007.

281. de Castro FR, Masouye I, Winkelmann RK, Saurat JH. Urticarial pathology in Schnitzler's (hyper-IgM) syndrome. Dermatology 1996;193(2):94–9.

282. Lipsker D, Spehner D, Drillien R, et al. Schnitzler syndrome: heterogeneous immunopathological findings involving IgM-skin interactions. Br J Dermatol 2000;142(5):954–9.

283. Schneider SW, Gaubitz M, Luger TA, Bonsmann G. Prompt response of refractory Schnitzler syndrome to treatment with anakinra. J Am Acad Dermatol 2007;56(5 Suppl):S120–2.

284. Eiling E, Moller M, Kreiselmaier I, Brasch J, Schwarz T. Schnitzler syndrome: treatment failure to rituximab but response to anakinra. J Am Acad Dermatol 2007.

285. Martinez-Taboada VM, Fontalba A, Blanco R, Fernandez-Luna JL. Successful treatment of refractory Schnitzler syndrome with anakinra: comment on the article by Hawkins et al. Arthritis Rheum 2005;52(7):2226–7.

286. Schnitzler L, Schubert B, Boasson M, Gardais J, Tourmen A. Urticaire chronique, lesions osseuses, macroglobulinemie IgM: maladie de Waldenstrom-IIe presentation. Bull Soc Fr Dermatol Syphiligr 1974;81:363.

287. Lipsker D, Imrie K, Simon A, Sullivan KE. Hot and hobbling with hives: Schnitzler syndrome. Clin Immunol 2006;119(2):131–4.

288. Randall RE, Williamson WC, Jr., Mullinax F, Tung MY, Still WJ. Manifestations of systemic light chain deposition. Am J Med 1976;60(2):293–9.

289. Gallo G, Picken M, Frangione B, Buxbaum J. Nonamyloidotic monoclonal immunoglobulin deposits lack amyloid P component. Mod Pathol 1988;1(6):453–6.

290. Kambham N, Markowitz GS, Appel GB, Kleiner MJ, Aucouturier P, D'Agati VD. Heavy chain deposition disease: the disease spectrum. Am J Kidney Dis 1999;33(5):954–62.

291. Vidal R, Goni F, Stevens F, et al. Somatic mutations of the L12a gene in V-kappa(1) light chain deposition disease: potential effects on aberrant protein conformation and deposition. Am J Pathol 1999;155(6):2009–17.

292. Gallo GR, Lazowski P, Kumar A, Vidal R, Baldwin DS, Buxbaum JN. Renal and cardiac manifestations of B-cell dyscrasias with nonamyloidotic monoclonal light chain and light and heavy chain deposition diseases. Adv Nephrol Necker Hosp 1998;28:355–82.

293. Keeling J, Teng J, Herrera GA. AL-amyloidosis and light-chain deposition disease light chains induce divergent phenotypic transformations of human mesangial cells. Lab Invest 2004;84(10):1322–38.

294. Pozzi C, Locatelli F. Kidney and liver involvement in monoclonal light chain disorders. Semin Nephrol 2002;22(4):319–30.

295. Bhargava P, Rushin JM, Rusnock EJ, et al. Pulmonary light chain deposition disease: report of five cases and review of the literature. Am J Surg Pathol 2007;31(2):267–76.

296. Pozzi C, D'Amico M, Fogazzi GB, et al. Light chain deposition disease with renal involvement: clinical characteristics and prognostic factors. Am J Kidney Dis 2003;42(6):1154–63.

297. Heilman RL, Velosa JA, Holley KE, Offord KP, Kyle RA. Long-term follow-up and response to chemotherapy in patients with light-chain deposition disease. Am J Kidney Dis 1992;20(1):34–41.

298. Leung N, Lager DJ, Gertz MA, Wilson K, Kanakiriya S, Fervenza FC. Long-term outcome of renal transplantation in light-chain deposition disease. Am J Kidney Dis 2004;43(1):147–53.

299. Royer B, Arnulf B, Martinez F, et al. High dose chemotherapy in light chain or light and heavy chain deposition disease. Kidney Int 2004;65(2):642–8.

300. Weichman K, Dember LM, Prokaeva T, et al. Clinical and molecular characteristics of patients with non-amyloid light chain deposition disorders, and outcome following treatment with high-dose melphalan and autologous stem cell transplantation. Bone Marrow Transplant 2006;38(5):339–43.

301. Ma CX, Lacy MQ, Rompala JF, et al. Acquired Fanconi syndrome is an indolent disorder in the absence of overt multiple myeloma. Blood 2004;104(1):40–2.

302. Messiaen T, Deret S, Mougenot B, et al. Adult Fanconi syndrome secondary to light chain gammopathy. Clinicopathologic heterogeneity and unusual features in 11 patients. Medicine (Baltimore) 2000;79(3):135–54.

303. Aucouturier P, Bauwens M, Khamlichi AA, et al. Monoclonal Ig L chain and L chain V domain fragment crystallization in myeloma-associated Fanconi's syndrome. J Immunol 1993;150(8 Pt 1):3561–8.

304. Rocca A, Khamlichi AA, Touchard G, et al. Sequences of V kappa L subgroup light chains in Fanconi's syndrome. Light chain V region gene usage restriction and peculiarities in myeloma-associated Fanconi's syndrome. J Immunol 1995;155(6):3245–52.

305. Pronovost PH, Brady HR, Gunning ME, Espinoza O, Rennke HG. Clinical features, predictors of disease progression and results of renal transplantation in fibrillary/immunotactoid glomerulopathy. Nephrol Dial Transplant 1996;11(5):837–42.

306. Strom EH, Hurwitz N, Mayr AC, Krause PH, Mihatsch MJ. Immunotactoid-like glomerulopathy with massive fibrillary deposits in liver and bone marrow in monoclonal gammopathy. Am J Nephrol 1996;16(6):523–8.

307. Rosenstock JL, Markowitz GS, Valeri AM, Sacchi G, Appel GB, D'Agati VD. Fibrillary and immunotactoid glomerulonephritis: distinct entities with different clinical and pathologic features. Kidney Int 2003;63(4):1450–61.

308. Takemura T, Yoshioka K, Akano N, et al. Immunotactoid glomerulopathy in a child with Down syndrome. Pediatr Nephrol 1993;7(1):86–8.

309. Wahner-Roedler DL, Kyle RA. Mu-heavy chain disease: presentation as a benign monoclonal gammopathy. Am J Hematol 1992;40(1):56–60.

310. Wahner-Roedler DL, Witzig TE, Loehrer LL, Kyle RA. Gamma-heavy chain disease: review of 23 cases. Medicine (Baltimore) 2003;82(4):236–50.

311. Galanti LM, Doyen C, Vander Maelen C, et al. Biological diagnosis of a gamma-1-heavy chain disease in an asymptomatic patient. Eur J Haematol 1995;54(3):202–4.

312. Seijffers MJ, Levy M, Hermann G. Intractable watery diarrhea, hypokalemia, and malabsorption in a patient with Mediterranean type of abdominal lymphoma. Gastroenterology 1968;55(1):118–24.

313. Rambaud JC, Galian A, Matuchansky C, et al. Natural history of alpha-chain disease and the so-called Mediterranean lymphoma. Recent Results Cancer Res 1978;64:271–6.

314. Alpha-chain disease and related small-intestinal lymphoma: a memorandum. Bull World Health Organ 1976;54(6):615–24.

315. Al-Saleem T, Al-Mondhiry H. Immunoproliferative small intestinal disease (IPSID): a model for mature B-cell neoplasms. Blood 2005;105(6):2274–80.

316. Suarez F, Lortholary O, Hermine O, Lecuit M. Infection-associated lymphomas derived from marginal zone B cells: a model of antigen-driven lymphoproliferation. Blood 2006;107(8):3034–44.

317. Loughran TP, Jr., Kadin ME, Deeg HJ. T-cell intestinal lymphoma associated with celiac sprue. Ann Intern Med 1986;104(1):44–7.

318. Vaiphei K, Kumari N, Sinha SK, et al. Roles of syndecan-1, bcl6 and p53 in diagnosis and prognostication of immunoproliferative small intestinal disease. World J Gastroenterol 2006;12(22):3602–8.

319. Fischbach W, Tacke W, Greiner A, Konrad H, Muller H. Regression of immunoproliferative small intestinal disease after eradication of Helicobacter pylori. Lancet 1997;349(9044):31–2.

320. Lecuit M, Abachin E, Martin A, et al. Immunoproliferative small intestinal disease associated with Campylobacter jejuni. N Engl J Med 2004;350(3):239–48.

321. Fine KD, Stone MJ. Alpha-heavy chain disease, Mediterranean lymphoma, and immunoproliferative small intestinal disease: a review of clinicopathological features, pathogenesis, and differential diagnosis. Am J Gastroenterol 1999;94(5):1139–52.

322. Rambaud JC, Halphen M, Galian A, Tsapis A. Immunoproliferative small intestinal disease (IPSID): relationships with alpha-chain disease and "Mediterranean" lymphomas. Springer Semin Immunopathol 1990;12(2–3):239–50.

323. Goossens T, Klein U, Kuppers R. Frequent occurrence of deletions and duplications during somatic hypermutation: implications for oncogene translocations and heavy chain disease. Proc Natl Acad Sci U S A 1998;95(5):2463–8.

324. Galian A, Lecestre MJ, Scotto J, Bognel C, Matuchansky C, Rambaud JC. Pathological study of alpha-chain disease, with special emphasis on evolution. Cancer 1977;39(5):2081–101.

325. Mir-Madjlessi SH, Mir-Ahmadian M. Alpha-chain disease—a report of eleven patients from Iran. J Trop Med Hyg 1979;82(11–12):229–36.

326. Zamir A, Parasher G, Moukarzel AA, Guarini L, Zeien L, Feldman F. Immunoproliferative small intestinal disease in a 16-year-old boy presenting as severe malabsorption with excellent response to tetracycline treatment. J Clin Gastroenterol 1998;27(1):85–9.

327. Martin IG, Aldoori MI. Immunoproliferative small intestinal disease: Mediterranean lymphoma and alpha heavy chain disease. Br J Surg 1994;81(1):20–4.

328. Salimi M, Spinelli JJ. Chemotherapy of Mediterranean abdominal lymphoma. Retrospective comparison of chemotherapy protocols in Iranian patients. Am J Clin Oncol 1996;19(1):18–22.

329. Ben-Ayed F, Halphen M, Najjar T, et al. Treatment of alpha chain disease. Results of a prospective study in 21 Tunisian patients by the Tunisian-French intestinal Lymphoma Study Group. Cancer 1989;63(7):1251–6.

330. Akbulut H, Soykan I, Yakaryilmaz F, et al. Five-year results of the treatment of 23 patients with immunoproliferative small intestinal disease: a Turkish experience. Cancer 1997;80(1):8–14.

331. Price SK. Immunoproliferative small intestinal disease: a study of 13 cases with alpha heavy-chain disease. Histopathology 1990;17(1):7–17.

332. Shih LY, Liaw SJ, Hsueh S, Kuo TT. Alpha-chain disease. Report of a case from Taiwan. Cancer 1987;59(3):545–8.

333. Malik IA, Shamsi Z, Shafquat A, et al. Clinicopathological features and management of immunoproliferative small intestinal disease and primary small intestinal lymphoma in Pakistan. Med Pediatr Oncol 1995;25(5):400–6.

334. McLaughlin P, Grillo-Lopez AJ, Link BK, et al. Rituximab chimeric anti-CD20 monoclonal antibody therapy for relapsed indolent lymphoma: half of patients respond to a four-dose treatment program. J Clin Oncol 1998;16(8):2825–33.

335. Franklin EC, Lowenstein J, Bigelow B, Meltzer M. Heavy chain disease—a new disorder of serum γ-globulins: report of the first case. Am J Med 1964;37:332.

336. Kyle RA, Greipp PR, Banks PM. The diverse picture of gamma heavy-chain disease. Report of seven cases and review of literature. Mayo Clin Proc 1981;56(7):439–51.

337. Fermand JP, Brouet JC. Heavy-chain diseases. Hematol Oncol Clin North Am 1999;13(6):1281–94.

338. Lassoued K, Picard C, Danon F, et al. Cutaneous manifestations associated with gamma heavy chain disease. Report of an unusual case and review of literature. J Am Acad Dermatol 1990;23(5 Pt 2):988–91.

339. Zawadzki ZA, Benedek TG, Ein D, Easton JM. Rheumatoid arthritis terminating in heavy-chain disease. Ann Intern Med 1969;70(2):335–47.

340. Jacqueline F, Renversez JC, Groslambert P, Fine JM. Gamma heavy chain disease during rheumatoid polyarthritis. A clinical and immunochemical study [French]. Rev Rhum Mal Osteoartic 1978;45(11):661–5.

341. Gaucher A, Bertrand F, Brouet JC, et al. Gamma heavy chain disease associated with rheumatoid arthritis. Spontaneous disappearance of the pathologic protein [French]. Sem Hop 1977;53(38):2117–20.

342. Westin J, Eyrich R, Falsen E, et al. Gamma heavy chain disease. Reports of three patients. Acta Med Scand 1972;192(4):281–92.

343. Lyons RM, Chaplin H, Tillack TW, Majerus PW. Gamma heavy chain disease: rapid, sustained response to cyclophosphamide and prednisone. Blood 1975;46(1):1–9.

344. Wager O, Rasanen JA, Lindeberg L, Makela V. Two cases of IgG heavy-chain disease. Acta Pathol Microbiol Scand 1969;75(2):350–2.

345. Frangione B, Franklin EC. Heavy chain diseases: clinical features and molecular significance of the disordered immunoglobulin structure. Semin Hematol 1973;10(1):53–64.

346. Fermand JP, Brouet JC, Danon F, Seligmann M. Gamma heavy chain "disease": heterogeneity of the clinicopathologic features. Report of 16 cases and review of the literature. Medicine (Baltimore) 1989;68(6):321–35.

347. Wester SM, Banks PM, Li CY. The histopathology of gamma heavy-chain disease. Am J Clin Pathol 1982;78(4):427–36.

348. Forte FA, Prelli F, Yount WJ, et al. Heavy chain disease of the gamma (gamma M) type: report of the first case. Blood 1970;36(2):137–44.

349. Ballard HS, Hamilton LM, Marcus AJ, Illes CH. A new variant of heavy-chain disease (mu-chain disease). N Engl J Med 1970;282(19):1060–2.

350. Wahner-Roedler DL, Kyle RA. Heavy chain diseases. Best Pract Res Clin Haematol 2005;18(4):729–46.

351. Pruzanski W, Hasselback R, Katz A, Parr DM. Multiple myeloma (light chain disease) with rheumatoid-like amyloid arthropathy and mu-heavy chain fragment in the serum. Am J Med 1978;65(2):334–41.

352. Mihaesco E, Barnikol-Watanabe S, Barnikol HU, Mihaesco C, Hilschmann N. The primary structure of the constant part of mu-chain-disease protein BOT. Eur J Biochem 1980;111(1):275–86.

353. Brouet JC, Seligmann M, Danon F, Belpomme D, Fine JM. mu-chain disease. Report of two new cases. Arch Intern Med 1979;139(6):672–4.

Chapter 35

Monoclonal Gammopathy of Undetermined Significance

Robert A. Kyle and S. Vincent Rajkumar

Introduction

Waldenström introduced the term "essential hyperglobulinemia" 55 years ago to describe patients who had a small serum protein electrophoretic spike but no evidence of multiple myeloma (MM), Waldenstrom's macroglobulinemia (WM), primary amyloidosis (AL), or related disorders.[1] Since then, other terms including benign, asymptomatic, idiopathic, nonmyelomatous, and idiopathic paraproteinemia have been used. He stressed the stability of the size of the protein peak and contrasted it with the increasing quantity of the spike in MM. The term "benign monoclonal gammopathy" was also commonly used but it is misleading because some patients will progress to symptomatic MM, WM, AL, or a related monoclonal plasma cell proliferative disorder. The term "monoclonal gammopathy of undetermined significance" (MGUS) was introduced almost 3 decades ago. It was defined as a serum monoclonal (M) protein < 3.0 g/dL; <10% plasma cells in the bone marrow, if performed; little or no M protein in the urine; and no lytic bone lesions, renal insufficiency, hypercalcemia, or anemia.

The monoclonal gammopathies are characterized by the proliferation of a single clone of plasma cells that produces a homogeneous M protein. Each M protein consists of two heavy polypeptide chains of the same class: Gamma (γ) in immunoglobulin G (IgG), alpha (α) in IgA, mu (μ) in IgM, delta (δ) in IgD, epsilon (ϵ) in IgE, and two light chains of the same type (kappa [κ] or lambda [λ]). Monoclonal gammopathies are characterized by the proliferation of one clone of plasma cells that produces an M protein while polyclonal gammopathies contain all types of the heavy chain classes and both light-chain types. A monoclonal increase in immunoglobulins results from a clonal process that is malignant or potentially malignant while a polyclonal increase in immunoglobulins is caused by a reactive or inflammatory process.[2]

Diagnosis of Monoclonal Proteins

The recommended method of detection is electrophoresis on agarose gel. After recognition of a localized band on electrophoresis, immunofixation must be

From: *Contemporary Hematology Myeloma Therapy*
Edited by: S. Lonial © Humana Press, Totowa, NJ

done to confirm the presence of an M protein and to determine its immunoglobulin heavy- and light-chain type.[3] In addition, immunofixation should be performed when MM, WM, AL, or a related disorder is suspected because a small M protein may not be detected on serum protein electrophoresis.[4]

Serum protein electrophoresis should be done in any patient who has unexplained weakness/fatigue, anemia, unexplained back pain, osteoporosis, osteolytic lesions or fractures, renal insufficiency, Bence-Jones proteinuria, or hypercalcemia. In addition, serum protein electrophoresis should be done in adults with unexplained sensorimotor peripheral neuropathy, carpal tunnel syndrome, refractory congestive heart failure, nephrotic syndrome, orthostatic hypotension, or malabsorption because a localized band or spike suggests AL. Changes in the tongue or voice, increased bruising or bleeding, and steatorrhea are additional indications for serum protein electrophoresis. Electrophoresis and immunofixation of a 24-h urine specimen should be performed in all patients with MM, WM, AL, and the heavy chain diseases or when these entities are expected. The amount of M protein in the urine provides an indirect measurement of the patient's tumor mass.

An M protein is usually seen as a localized band on the agarose gel electrophoretic strip or as a tall, narrow spike in the β or λ region or, rarely, in the α-2 globulin area of the densitometer tracing. A polyclonal increase in immunoglobulins is seen as a broad band or broad-based peak that migrates in the λ region.

Quantitation of immunoglobulins should be performed with a rate nephelometer because it is not affected by molecular size and accurately measures 7S IgM, polymers of IgA, and aggregates of IgG. However, levels of IgM, IgG, or IgA obtained by nephelometry may be 1000–2000 mg/dL higher than that expected on the basis of the serum protein electrophoretic tracing. On the contrary, a very large M protein may not be completely bound by the dye and underestimate the amount of M protein. Ideally, both serum protein electrophoresis and nephelometry should be performed.

The serum free light chain (FLC) assay is an automated nephelometric test which measures the level of free κ and free λ light chains in the serum. The normal / ratio for FLC is 0.26–1.65. This test is useful for monitoring patients with plasma cell disorders who do not have a measurable M spike in the serum or urine. It is particularly useful in following patients with nonsecretory MM. The FLC assay is of prognostic value in MGUS and solitary plasmacytoma of bone.

Between January 1960 and December 2006, 36,392 patients with monoclonal plasma cell disorders were identified at Mayo Clinic. MGUS accounted for 21,256 (58.5%); MM for 6,408 (18%), AL for 3,389 (9%), lymphoproliferative disorders for 1157 (3%), smolderingMM (SMM) for 1,359; solitary or extramedullary plasmacytoma for 740 (2%), WM for 824 (2%), while other conditions including POEMS syndrome, idiopathic Bence-Jones proteinuria, cryoglobulinemia, and light chain deposition disease accounted for 1,259 patients (3.5%) (Fig. 1; Table 1).

Prevalence of MGUS

M proteins have been reported without evidence of MM or WM in ~1.5% of persons in Sweden,[5] in the United States,[6] in western France,[7] and in ~1.5% of patients older than 50 years of age. The frequency of M proteins is higher

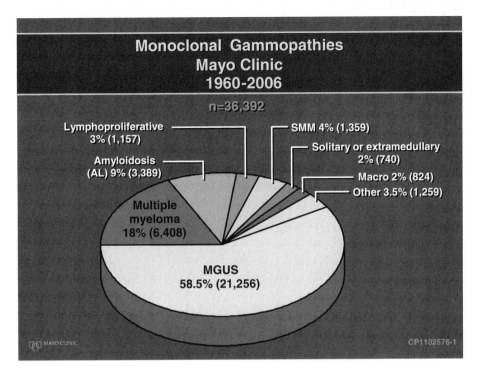

Fig. 1 Monoclonal (*M*) gammopathies diagnosed at the Mayo Clinic during 2006. Macroglobulinemia; *MGUS* monoclonal gammopathy of undetermined significance, *SMM* smoldering multiple myeloma (*see* Plate 25).

among older patients. The incidence is higher in African American patients than in white patients.[8] In a study of 4 million males admitted to Veterans Affairs Hospitals in the United States, 0.9% of African Americans and 0.4% of Caucasians had MGUS. The age-adjusted prevalence of MGUS in the African Americans was threefold greater than that in the Caucasian population.[9]

The first population-based study using agarose gel electrophoresis and immunofixation to detect M proteins has been reported.[10] Serum samples were obtained from 21,463 (77%) of the 28,038 enumerated residents of Olmsted County, Minnesota, who were 50 years of age or older. MGUS was found in 694 (3.2%) of these patients (3.7% of men and 2.9% of women, $p < 0.001$) (Table 2). The rate among men was similar to that among women a decade older; 97.3% were Caucasian. The prevalence increased with advancing age and was almost 4 times higher among patients 80 years of age or older compared to those 50–59 years of age. The prevalence of MGUS was 8.9% in men older than 85 years of age. There was no significant difference in the concentration of the M protein among the age groups.

IgG was found in 69% of the 694 patients with MGUS, IgM in 17%, IgA in 11%, and biclonal in 3%. The light chain class was κ in 62% and λ in 38%. The M protein concentration was modest in size, with 63% having an M spike < 1.0 g/dL. The M spike was 2.0 g/dL or greater in 4.5% and was too low to measure in 13%. The median size of the M spike was 0.7 g/dL if the unmeasurable proteins were excluded. The level of uninvolved (normal, polyclonal, or background) immunoglobulins was reduced in 124 (28%) of the 447 patients

Table 1 Classification of monoclonal gammopathies.

Monoclonal gammopathy of undetermined significance
  -Benign (IgG, IgA, IgD, IgM, and rarely, free light chains)

  -Associated with neoplasms of cell types not known to produce M proteins
  -Biclonal and triclonal gammopathies
  -Idiopathic Bence Jones proteinuria

Malignant monoclonal gammopathies
  -Multiple myeloma (IgG, IgA, IgD, IgE, and free κ or λ light chains)
    -Overt multiple myeloma
    -Smoldering multiple myeloma
    -Plasma cell leukemia
    -Nonsecretory myeloma
    -IgD myeloma
    -POEMS (polyneuropathy, organomegaly, endocrinopathy, monoclonal protein, skin changes; osteosclerotic myeloma)
  Plasmacytoma
    -Solitary plasmacytoma of bone
    -Extramedullary plasmacytoma
  -Malignant lymphoproliferative disorders
  -Waldenström's macroglobulinemia (primary macroglobulinemia)
  -Malignant lymphoma
  -Chronic lymphocytic leukemia or lymphoproliferative disorders
  -Heavy-chain diseases
    -γ Heavy-chain disease
    -α Heavy-chain disease
    -μ Heavy-chain disease
  -Amyloidosis
    -Primary amyloidosis (AL)
    -With multiple myeloma (secondary, localized, and familial amyloidosis have no M protein)

From Kyle RA, Rajkumar SV. Monoclonal gammopathies of undetermined significance. Permissions requested from *Rev Clin Exp Hematol* 2002;6:225–52

Table 2 Prevalence of MGUS according to age group and sex among residents of Olmsted County, Minnesota.

Age (year)	Men	Women number/total number (%)[a]	Total
50–59	82/4038 (2.0)	59/4335 (1.4)	141/8373 (1.7)
60–69	105/2864 (3.7)	73/3155 (2.3)	178/6019 (3.0)
70–79	104/1858 (5.6)	101/2650 (3.8)	205/4508 (4.6)
80	59/709 (8.3)	110/1854 (6.0)	170/2563 (6.6)
Total	350/9469 (3.7)[b]	343/11,994 (2.9)[b]	694/21,463 (3.2)[c]

MGUS monoclonal gammopathy of undetermined significance
[a]The percentage was calculated as the number of patients with MGUS divided by the number who were tested
[b]Prevalence was age-adjusted to the 2000 US total population as follows: men, 4.0% (95% confidence interval, 3.5–4.4); women, 2.7% (95% confidence interval, 2.4–3.0); and total, 3.2% (95% confidence interval, 3.0–3.5)
[c]Prevalence was age adjusted and sex adjusted to the 2000 US total population

Permission requested from N Engl J Med 354:13, 2006

whose immunoglobulin concentration was measured. One of the two immunoglobulins was reduced in 22%, and both were decreased in 6% of patients. An M urinary protein was found in 21.5% of the 79 patients who were tested. Kappa was found in 16.5% and λ in 5.0%.

Long-Term Follow-up of MGUS

MGUS is a common finding in the medical practice of all physicians. It produces no symptoms and is found during laboratory testing of an apparently normal patient or during evaluation of an unrelated disorder. All practicing physicians see patients with MGUS and, consequently, it is important for both the physician and the patient to know whether the M protein will remain stable and benign or progress to MM or a related disorder.

Mayo Clinic Referral Patients

We reviewed the medical records of all patients with monoclonal gammopathy who were seen at Mayo Clinic from 1956 through 1970.[11] Patients with MM, WM, AL, lymphoma, or related disorders were excluded. Two hundred and forty-one patients were eligible for long-term study. After 3,579 patient-years of follow-up (median 13.7 years, range 0–39 years), patients were divided into one of four groups: Group 1: Patients who were still living and whose M-protein level had remained stable and could be classified as having benign monoclonal gammopathy, 14 (6%); Group 2: Patients in whom the M protein had increased to 3.0 g/dL or greater but symptomatic MM, WM, and AL did not develop, n = 25 (10%); Group 3: Patients who died of unrelated causes without development of MM or related disorders, n = 138 (57%); and Group 4: Patients in whom MM, AL, WM, or a related disorder had developed, n = 64 (27%) [12](Table 3). The actuarial rate at 10 years was 17%; at 20 years 34%; and at 25 years 39%, which is ~1.5% per year (Fig. 2).

There were 141 men (58%) and 101 women (42%). The median age was 64 years when MGUS was recognized. Four percent were younger than 40 years of age, while one-third were 70 years or older. IgG accounted for 73.5%, IgA 10.5%, IgM 14%, and biclonal 2%. The uninvolved immunoglobulins were reduced in 38%.

Table 3 Course of 241 patients with MGUS.[a]

Patient group	Description	No. (%) of patients at follow-up[b]
1	Living patients with no substantial increase in monoclonal protein	14 (6)
2	Monoclonal protein value ≥ 3.0 g/dL but no myeloma or related disorder	25 (10)
3	Died of unrelated causes	138 (57)
4	Developed multiple myeloma, macroglobulinemia, amyloidosis, or related disorder	64 (27)
Total		241 (100)

[a]The patient groups are described in the "Patients and Methods" section. *MGUS* monoclonal gammopathy of undetermined significance

[b]Person-years follow-up = 3579 (median 13.7 year per patient; range, 0–39 years). Permission requested from Kyle[12]

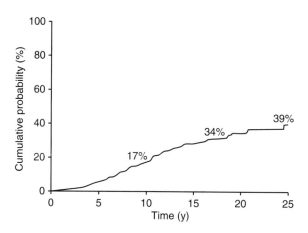

Fig. 2 Rate of development of multiple myeloma (*MM*) or related disorder in 241 patients with monoclonal gammopathy of undetermined significance (*MGUS*).

Of the 64 patients with progression, 44 (69%) had MM with intervals from recognition of the M protein to the diagnosis of MM in the 44 patients ranging from 1 to 32 years (median 10.6 years) (Table 4). In ten patients, the diagnosis was made 20 years after recognition of the serum M protein. Median duration of survival after diagnosis of MM was 33 months, which is similar to that expected. Systemic AL was found in eight patients 6–19 years (median 9 years) after recognition of an M protein in the serum. WM developed in seven patients, all of whom had a serum IgM κ protein level ranging from 3.1 to 8.1 g/dL at diagnosis. A malignant lymphoproliferative process (malignant lymphoma, 3; chronic lymphocytic leukemia, 1; an atypical malignant lymphoproliferative disorder, 1) developed in five patients 4–19 years (median 10.5 years) after detection of the M protein.

Long-Term Follow-up in 1,384 Patients with MGUS from Southeastern Minnesota

A population-based study was done to confirm the findings of the original Mayo Clinic study which consisted mainly of patients referred to a tertiary care center. A total of 1,384 patients who resided in the 11 counties of southeastern Minnesota were identified as having MGUS, defined as a serum M protein value of 3.0 g/dL or less; <10% plasma cells in the bone marrow (if the test was done); little or no M protein in the urine; and the absence of lytic bone lesions, anemia, hypercalcemia, or renal insufficiency related to the M protein. The patients were evaluated at Mayo Clinic from January 1, 1960, through December 31, 1994.[13] The median age at diagnosis of MGUS was 72 years, which was 8 years older than that in the 241 cohort. This indicates that older patients are less likely to visit tertiary referral centers. There were 753 men (54%) and 631 women (46%). Only 2% were younger than 40 years at diagnosis, while 59% were aged 70 years or older. The serum M-protein level at diagnosis ranged from unmeasurable to 3.0 g/dL. Seventy percent of the M proteins were IgG, 12% IgA, 15% IgM, and 3% were biclonal. The light-chain type was κ in 61% and λ in 39%. A reduction of uninvolved

Table 4 Development of multiple myeloma (MM) or related disorder in 64 patients with MGUS.[a]

| | No. (%) of patients | Interval to disease (year) | |
		Median	Range
Multiple myeloma	44 (69)	10.6	1–32
Macroglobulinemia	7 (11)	10.3	4–16
Amyloidosis	8 (12)	9.0	6–19
Lymphoproliferative disease	5 (8)	8.0	4–19
Total	64 (100)	10.4	1–32

[a]*MGUS* monoclonal gammopathy of undetermined significancePermission requested from Kyle[12]

(normal or background) immunoglobulins was found in 38% of 840 patients in whom quantitation of immunoglobulins was determined. Electrophoresis, immunoelectrophoresis, and immunofixation of urine were performed in 418 patients. Twenty-one percent had a monoclonal κ light chain and 10% had λ at the time of recognition of MGUS, and 69% were negative. Only 71 of 418 patients (17%) had an M-protein level > 150 mg/24 h. The median percentage of bone marrow plasma cells was 3% (range 0–10% in the 160 patients with a bone marrow examination). The initial hemoglobin values ranged from 5.7 to 18.9 g/dL, but were <10 g/dL in only 7%. The anemia was due to causes other than the plasma cell proliferative process in all instances. The serum creatinine level was >2 mg/dL in 6%, but was not related to the plasma cell proliferative process.

During a follow-up of 11,009 person-years (median 15.4 years, range 0–35 years), 963 patients (70%) died. During follow-up, MM, AL, lymphoma with an IgM serum protein, WM, plasmacytoma, or chronic lymphocytic leukemia developed in 115 patients (8%) (Table 5). The cumulative probability of progression to one of these disorders was 10% at 10 years, 21% at 20 years, and 26% at 25 years, which is ~1% per year (Fig. 3). However, these patients were at risk for progression even after 25 years or more of stable MGUS. In addition, 32 patients had an increase to >3 g/dL in the M protein or the percentage of bone marrow plasma cells increased to more than 10%, but in whom symptomatic MM or WM did not develop. These findings confirmed the results of the initial Mayo Clinic study.

The number of patients with progression to a plasma cell disorder (115 patients) was 7.3 times the number expected on the basis of the incidence rates for those conditions in the general population.[14] The risk of MM developing was increased 25-fold; WM, 46-fold; and AL, 8.4-fold.[15] The risk of development of lymphoma was only modestly increased at 2.4-fold, but this risk was underestimated because only lymphomas associated with a M IgM protein were counted in the observed number, whereas the incidence rates for lymphomas associated with IgG, IgA, and IgM proteins were used to calculate the expected number. The risk of development of chronic lymphocytic leukemia was only slightly increased.

The 75 patients in whom MM developed accounted for 65% of the 115 patients who had progressed. A diagnosis of MM was made more than 10 years after detection of the M protein in 24 patients (32%), while 5 (7%)

Table 5 Risk of progression among 1384 residents of southeastern Minnesota in whom monoclonal gammopathy of undetermined significance was diagnosed in 1960 through 1994.[a]

Type of progression	Observed no. of patients	Expected no. of patients[b]	Relative risk (95% CI)
Multiple myeloma	75	3.0	25.0 (20–32)
Lymphoma	19[c]	7.8	2.4 (2–4)
Primary amyloidosis	10	1.2	8.4 (4–16)
Macroglobulinemia	7	0.2	46.0 (19–95)
Chronic lymphocytic leukemia	3[d]	3.5	0.9 (0.2–3)
Plasmacytoma	1	0.1	8.5 (0.2–47)
Total	115	15.8	7.3 (6–9)

[a]CI denotes confidence interval

[b]Expected numbers of cases were derived from the age- and sex-matched white population of the surveillance, epidemiology, and end results program in Iowa, except for primary amyloidosis for which data are from Kyle et al"

[c]All 19 patients had serum IgM monoclonal protein. If the 30 patients with IgM, IgA, or IgG monoclonal protein and lymphoma were included, the relative risk would be 3.9 (95% confidence interval, 2.6–5.5)

[d]All three patients had serum IgM monoclonal protein. If all six patients with IgM, IgA, or IgG monoclonal protein and chronic lymphocytic leukemia were included, the relative risk would be 1.7 (95% confidence interval, 0.6–3.7)This table is reprinted with permissions from Kyle[13]

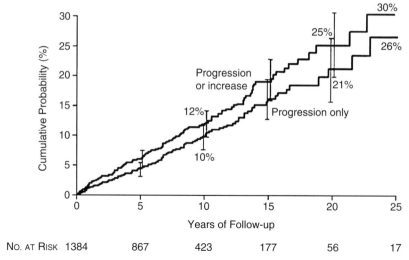

Fig. 3 Probability of progression among 1384 residents of Southeastern Minnesota in whom monoclonal gammopathy of undetermined significance (*MGUS*) was diagnosed from 1960 through 1994. The top curve shows the probability of progression to a plasma cell cancer (115 patients) or of an increase in the monoclonal (*M*) protein concentration to more than 3 g/dL or the proportion of plasma cells in bone marrow to more than 10% (32 patients). The bottom curve shows only the probability of progression of MGUS to multiple myeloma (*MM*), IgM lymphoma, primary amyloidosis (*AL*), macroglobulinemia, chronic lymphocytic leukemia, or plasmacytoma (115 patients). The bars show 95% confidence intervals.

were recognized after 20 years of follow-up. The characteristics of these 75 patients with MM were comparable to those of the 1,027 patients with newly diagnosed MM referred to Mayo Clinic from 1985 to 1998, except that the southeastern Minnesota patients were older (median 72 vs 66 years) and less likely to be male (46% vs 60%).[16]

The mode of development of MM among patients with MGUS was quite variable (Table 6). The M protein disappeared without an apparent cause in 27 patients (2%). Only 6 of these 27 patients (0.4% of all patients) had a discrete spike on the densitometer tracing. The spontaneous disappearance of M protein after the diagnosis of MGUS is rare.

Patients with MGUS had shorter median survival than expected for Minnesota residents of matched age and sex (8.1 vs 11.8 years, $P<0.001$). The rates of death due to other diseases such as cardiovascular or cerebrovascular diseases and non-plasma cell malignancies were 53% at 10 years, 72% at 20 years, and 76% at 25 years as compared with 6% at 10 years, 10% at 20 years, and 11% at 25 years for death due to plasma cell disorders (Fig. 4).

Table 6 Patterns of increase in the level of M protein among residents of southeastern Minnesota with MGUS and progression to multiple myeloma or macroglobulinemia.

	No. of patients	
Pattern	Multiple myeloma	Macroglobulinemia
Stable, with sudden increase	19	2
Stable, with gradual increase	9	0
Gradual increase	9	3
Sudden increase	11	0
Stable	10	0
Indeterminate	17	2
Total	75	7

MGUS monoclonal gammopathy of undetermined significance

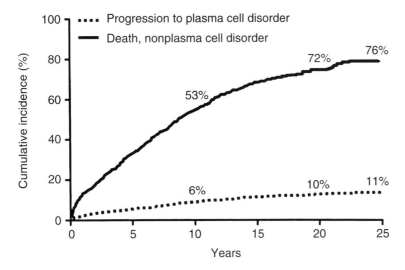

Fig. 4 Rate of death from nonplasma cell disorders compared with progression to plasma cell disorders in 1384 patients with monoclonal gammopathy of undetermined significance (*MGUS*) from southeastern Minnesota. Permission requested from Immunological Reviews 194:125, 2003, Kyle & Rajkumar, monoclonal gammopathies of undetermined significance.

Follow-up in Other Series

During a 20-year follow-up, Axelsson[17] reported that 2 of 64 patients with MGUS had died of MM and 1 died of lymphoma. Eleven percent of the patients had some evidence of progression. Van de Poel[18] reported that 6.6% of 332 patients with MGUS had a malignant transformation after a median follow-up of 8.4 years. Baldini et al.[19] noted that 6.8% of 335 patients with MGUS had progressed during a median follow-up of 70 months. In a cohort of 1,324 patients with MGUS in North Jutland, Denmark, malignant transformation was the cause of death in 97 patients compared with 4.9 deaths expected.[20] Sixty-four new cases of malignancy (5 expected, relative risk 12.9) were found among 1,229 patients with MGUS in the Danish Cancer Registry. The risk for development of MM was 34.3-fold; WM, 63.8-fold; and non-Hodgkin lymphoma, 5.9-fold. In a cohort of 504 patients with MGUS from Iceland, a plasma cell malignancy developed in 51 of 504 patients (10%).[21] In summary, multiple studies confirm that the risk of progression from MGUS to MM or related disorders is ~1% per year.

Pathophysiology of Progression of MGUS

The events responsible for malignant transformation of MGUS to MM or a related plasma cell proliferative disorder are poorly understood. Genetic changes, bone marrow angiogenesis, cytokines related to myeloma bone disease, and infectious agents may all play a role in the progression of MGUS to MM or a related disorder. However, the specific role of these possibilities is not clear.[22]

Genetic Changes

Cytogenetic changes are common in MM as well as MGUS. On the basis of fluorescence in situ hybridization (FISH) studies, 60% of patients with myeloma have IgH (14q32 translocations),[23] while 46% of patients with MGUS have IgH translocations.[24] In a series of 59 patients with MGUS studied with FISH, 27 (46%) had IgH translocations consisting of t(11;14)(q13;q32) in 25%, t(4;14)(p16.3;q32) in 9%, and t(14;16)(q32;q23) in 5%.[25] These translocations may lead to the dysregulation of oncogenes such as cyclin D1 (11q13), C-*maf* (16q23), FGFR3/MMSET (fibroblastic growth factor receptor 3/MMSET domain) (4p16.3), and cyclin D3 (6p21) but may be involved with initiation of the MGUS clone rather than progression of MGUS to MM. Recently, Chng et al.[26] reported that 11 of 28 patients (40%) with SMM or MGUS had hyperdiploidy. This percentage is similar to that of hyperdiploid MM reported in the literature. It is apparent that MGUS is associated with genomic instability that is manifested as IgH translocations in approximately one-half and hyperdiploidy in most of the remaining patients.

Deletions of chromosome 13 have been found to have an adverse prognostic effect in MM, but are also present in MGUS.[27] Although deletions of chromosome 13 produce an adverse effect on myeloma, it is not known whether the rate of progression from MGUS to MM is accelerated because the frequency of deletion of chromosome 13 is similar in both MGUS and MM.

K-*ras* and N-*ras* mutations were noted in 5% of 20 patients with MGUS, in contrast to 31% of 58 patients with MM.[28] Aberrant methylation of the 5' gene-promoter regions of tumor suppression genes has been found in

MGUS, although aberrant methylation is lower in frequency compared with myeloma.[29] The role of methylation in the progression of MGUS is not clear.

Angiogenesis

Bone marrow angiogenesis was studied in 400 patients with plasma cell disorders. The median microvessel density (vessels per high-power field) was 1.3 in 42 normal controls, 1.7 in AL, 3 in MGUS, 4 in SMM, 11 in MM, and 20 in relapsed myeloma. The bone marrow angiogenesis increased progressively from the more benign MGUS to advanced MM.[30] The increase in angiogenesis that occurs with progression does not seem to be related to overexpression of any single proangiogenetic cytokine by neoplastic plasma cells but rather to an alteration in the balance between pro- and antiangiogenetic effects. In addition, there appears to be a loss of angiogenesis inhibitory activity with disease progression from MGUS to MM. In one study, 63% of MGUS sera inhibited angiogenesis, whereas 43% of SMM and 4% of MM serum samples ($P < .001$) did so.[31] Therefore, loss of an angiogenesis inhibitor may be involved in the increased angiogenesis that occurs with disease progression.

Cytokines Associated with Myeloma Bone Disease

Clinically, lytic bone lesions, osteopenia, hypercalcemia, and pathologic fractures differentiate MM from MGUS. However, in a study of 488 Olmsted County residents with MGUS, we found a 2.7-fold increase in axial fractures but no increase in limb fractures.[32]

The development of bone lesions with progression of MGUS to MM is caused by osteoclastic activation and inhibition of osteoblastic differentiation. Osteoclast activation is caused by overexpression of various cytokines such as receptor activator of nuclear factor $\kappa\beta$ ligand (RANKL) and macrophage inflammatory protein-1α (MIP-1α).[33] RANKL is modulated by a decoy receptor, osteoprotegerin. Myeloma bone disease may occur from excess RANKL or reduced levels of osteoprotegerin.[34] Interleukin-1-β induces osteoclast formation and may play a role in the transformation of MGUS to MM.[35] Tumor necrosis factor-α and interleukin-6 may also play a role in myeloma bone disease.

Infectious Agents

In one report, 39 of 59 patients (68% with MGUS) had *Helicobacter pylori* infection.[36] Erradication of *H. pylori* led to the resolution of monoclonal gammopathy in 11 of these 39 patients. In another report, serologic testing for *H. pylori* showed that 30% of 93 patients with MGUS who were residents of Olmsted County, Minnesota, had positive results, as did 32% of 98 control subjects from the same population. In addition, 51 of 154 patients (33%) from Mayo Clinic with MGUS were positive for *H. pylori* as were 365 of 1103 (33%) without MGUS. Thus, controversy exists about the role, if any, of *H. pylori* infection in MGUS.[37]

Predictors of Malignant Transformation in MGUS

No findings at diagnosis of MGUS can distinguish patients whose condition will remain stable from those in whom a malignant condition may develop.[38]

Size of Monoclonal Protein

In a series of 1,384 patients with MGUS, the size of the M protein at recognition of MGUS was the most important predictor of progression (Fig. 5).[13] The risk of progression to MM or a related disorder 20 years after recognition of MGUS was 14% for patients with an initial M-protein level of 0.5 g/dL or less, 16% for 1 g/dL, 25% for 1.5 g/dL, 41% for 2 g/dL, 49% for 2.5 g/dL, and 64% for 3.0 g/dL. The risk of progression with an M-protein level of 1.5 g/dL was almost twice that in a patient with an M-protein level of 0.5 g/dL, while the risk of progression with an M-protein level of 2.5 g/dL was 4.6 times that of a patient with a 0.5 g/dL spike.

Type of Immunoglobulin

In the southeastern Minnesota series, patients with IgM or IgA M protein had an increased risk of progression compared to those with an IgG M protein ($P = 0.001$) (Fig. 5). Blade et al. also noted that MM developed more commonly in patients with an IgA M protein than in the remainder.[39]

Number of Bone Marrow Plasma Cells

The number of plasma cells in the bone marrow is helpful in predicting progression. Cesana et al.[40] reported that having more than 5% bone marrow plasma cells was an independent risk factor for progression. Baldini et al.[19] noted that the malignant transformation rate was 6.8% when the bone marrow plasma cell level was <10% and 37% in those with MGUS with a bone marrow plasma cell level of 10–30%.

Abnormal Free Light Chain Ratio

An abnormal FLC ratio was detected in 33% of 1148 patients with MGUS from southeastern Minnesota. At a median follow-up of 15 years, malignant

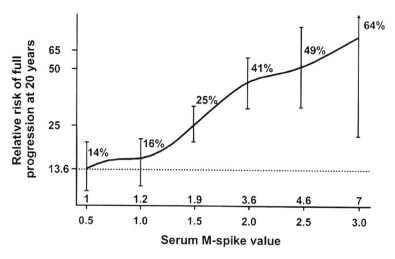

Fig. 5 Actuarial risk of full progression by serum monoclonal protein (*M*-protein) value at diagnosis of monoclonal gammopathy of undetermined significance (*MGUS*) in persons from southeastern Minnesota.

progression occurred in 7.6%. The risk of progression in patients with an abnormal FLC ratio was significantly higher than in patients with a normal ratio (hazard ratio 3.5; $P < 0.001$) and was independent of the size and type of M protein.[41]

Risk-Stratification Model for MGUS

A new risk-stratification model for determining the risk of progression of MGUS was developed (Table 7). Patients with risk factors consisting of an abnormal serum FLC ratio, IgA or IgM MGUS, and a serum M protein value of ≥1.5 g/dL had a risk of progression of 58%, at 20 years whereas the risk was only 5% when none of the risk factors were present. When competing causes of death were taken into account, the risk of progression was only 2% at 20 years in those without a risk factor.

Differential Diagnosis

The differentiation of a patient with MGUS from one with MM may be difficult at the time of presentation and is based on the clinical and laboratory findings. A radiographic bone survey and a bone marrow aspirate and biopsy are indicated in all patients with an M protein value of 1.5 g/dL or more, those with an IgA or an IgM MGUS, patients with an abnormal free FLC ratio, and all who have an abnormality in the blood counts, creatinine, or calcium values. The serum M protein value is of help because higher levels are associated with a greater likelihood of malignancy. Reduction in levels of uninvolved (background, normal) immunoglobulins or the presence of an M protein in the urine (Bence-Jones proteinuria) may occur in MGUS and are of little help in differentiation. Patients with more than 10% bone marrow plasma cells or an M spike > 3 g/dL are classified as having SMM. These patients have a higher risk of progression to malignancy than patients with MGUS, but should be observed and not treated until progression occurs. The presence of osteolytic lesions suggests MM, but metastatic carcinoma may also produce lytic lesions. If there is doubt, a biopsy is required to make the distinction. An elevated plasma cell labeling index usually indicates symptomatic MM, but one-third of patients with symptomatic MM have a normal labeling index and, furthermore, the test is not widely available. Circulating plasma cells in the peripheral blood suggest symptomatic MM.[42]

Conventional cytogenetic studies are not useful for the differentiation of MGUS and MM because abnormal karyotypes are rare in MGUS because of the small number of plasma cells and the lower proliferative rate. FISH studies show that abnormalities including deletion of chromosome 13q occur in MGUS as well as MM.

Ocqueteau et al.[43] identified a population of polyclonal plasma cells with CD38 expression and low forward light scatter. The plasma cells expressed CD19, but were negative for CD56. The monoclonal plasma cell population showed a lower CD38 expression and a higher forward light scatter population and expressed CD56, but not CD19. Ninety-eight percent of patients with MGUS had more than 3% normal polyclonal plasma cells but only 1.5% of patients with MM had the same findings. Serum levels of interleukin-6 and interleukin-1β are increased commonly in MM, but not MGUS. Beta-2 microglobulin levels are not helpful for differentiating MGUS from low-grade MM.[44]

Ultimately, the differentiation of active MM requiring therapy from MGUS or SMM depends on the presence or absence of end organ damage (CRAB: hypercalcemia, renal insufficiency, anemia, bone lesions) that is felt to be attributable to the underlying plasma cell proliferative disorder. MGUS and SMM are differentiated from each other on the basis of the size of the serum M protein and the bone marrow plasma cell percentage.

Management

Regardless of the results of sophisticated laboratory tests, the differentiation between MGUS and MM is based on clinical factors such as symptoms, anemia, hypercalcemia, renal insufficiency, and lytic bone lesions. However, the presence of a high plasma cell labeling index in a patient with MGUS or SMM needs to be followed up more frequently for other evidence of progression. No single factor can differentiate a patient with a stable monoclonal gammopathy from one in whom a malignant plasma cell disorder will develop. A 24-h urine specimen should be collected for electrophoresis, and immunofixation, a metastatic bone radiographic survey, and a bone marrow examination should be done if there is suspicion of MM or a related malignant disorder.

Serum protein electrophoresis should be repeated in 3 months to exclude MM; if the results are stable and the patient has no clinical features of MM, WM, or AL and a serum M protein value of <1.5 g/dL, IgG type, and normal FLC ratio, serum protein electrophoresis should be repeated at intervals of every 2–3 years. In this setting, bone marrow examination is rarely necessary.

If the asymptomatic MGUS patient has an M protein value > 1.5 g/dL, IgA or IgM protein, or an abnormal FLC ratio, a bone marrow examination should be done. It should also be performed in patients who have unexplained anemia, renal insufficiency, hypercalcemia, or bone lesions. Cytogenetic studies (conventional and FISH), determination of the plasma cell labeling index, and a search for circulating plasma cells in the peripheral blood should be done if possible. If an IgM M protein is present, a bone marrow examination and a computed tomographic scan of the abdomen may be useful for recognizing retroperitoneal lymph nodes. If there is evidence of MM or WM, levels of β-2 microglobulin, lactate dehydrogenase, and C-reactive protein should be determined. If the results of these tests are satisfactory, serum protein electrophoresis should be repeated at 6-month intervals for a year and then at annual intervals. If there is any change in the clinical condition, the patient must contact the physician immediately.

Variants of MGUS

Smoldering (Asymptomatic) Multiple Myeloma

Patients with SMM have a serum M protein of 3 g/dL or higher and/or 10% or more plasma cells in the bone marrow, but no evidence of end organ damage (hypercalcemia, renal insufficiency, anemia, or bone lesions).

The International Myeloma Working Group criteria for the classification of monoclonal gammopathies has been published.[45] Patients may have a small amount of monoclonal light chains in the urine and a reduction of uninvolved immunoglobulins in the serum. These findings are consistent with a diagnosis of MM. However, these patients have MGUS from the biological standpoint. The diagnosis of SMM is difficult when the patient is seen initially because most patients with this level of bone marrow plasma cell infiltration and size of M protein in the serum have symptomatic MM.[46]

SMM accounts for ~15% of all cases of newly diagnosed MM.[47] The prevalence of SMM is unknown because many reports include asymptomatic patients with lytic bone lesions on skeletal survey while others exclude those with bone lesions on skeletal surveys but include patients who have lytic lesions on magnetic resonance imaging.

Two subsets of SMM have been described: (1) Evolving SMM, characterized by a progressive increase in the serum M-protein level in a patient with MGUS, and (2) Nonevolving SMM, characterized by a stable M protein value that abruptly increases when symptomatic MM develops.[48]

Almost all patients with SMM have evidence of genomic instability manifested as IgH translocations or hyperdiploidy on molecular genetic testing. SMM is differentiated from MM in the same manner as MGUS and is based on the presence or absence of end-organ damage.

SMM is an asymptomatic condition, but the risk of progression to MM or a related malignancy is much higher compared to MGUS. In a recent study of 276 patients with SMM, we found that the risk of progression was 10% per year for the first 5 years, 3% per year for the next 5 years, and then 1% per year for the following 10 years.[49] The median duration from recognition of SMM to the development of SMM was 4.8 years. One should recognize that the decrease in risk of progression with time in SMM is different from the fixed 1% per year risk of progression in MGUS. The type of serum M protein, the amount of Bence-Jones proteinuria, and the presence of circulating plasma cells in the peripheral blood are all risk factors for progression.

Management of SMM
The current standard of care for SMM is close follow-up every 3–6 months without chemotherapy. This recommendation is based on results of trials demonstrating no significant improvement in overall survival in patients who received immediate treatment with melphalan plus prednisone compared to those who received treatment at progression of stage I or asymptomatic MM.[50,51]

Preliminary data suggests that thalidomide may delay time to progression,[52] but data are needed from randomized trials before such therapy can be recommended because of the adverse effects associated with thalidomide. Clinical trials are ongoing to determine whether the use of other agents such as bisphosphonates, interleukin-1β inhibitors, clarithromycin, or dehydroepiandrosterone can delay progression to symptomatic MM. However, phase 3 randomized trials to determine the durability of response and effect on overall survival without harm to the patient must be proven before new agents can be recommended for standard clinical practice. The recommendation to observe closely without treatment until progression is also based on the toxic effects of therapy and the fact that the disease may not progress for years.

Biclonal Gammopathy

Biclonal gammopathies are characterized by the presence of two different M proteins and occur in 3–6% of patients with monoclonal gammopathies. The two M proteins may be caused by the proliferation of two different clones of plasma cells, each producing an unrelated M protein, or by the production of two M proteins by a single clone of plasma cells. In a report of 57 patients with biclonal gammopathy, 37 had biclonal gammopathy of undetermined significance.[53] The age range was 39–93 years (median 67 years). Two localized bands were found in only 18 patients with electrophoresis on cellulose acetate; in the others, a second M protein was not recognized until immunoelectrophoresis or immunofixation was performed. The clinical findings of biclonal gammopathies were similar to those of monoclonal gammopathies. Thirty-five percent of the 57 patients had MM, WM, or another malignant lymphoproliferative disorder.

Triclonal Gammopathy

In a review of 24 patients with triclonal gammopathy, 16 were associated with a malignant immunolymphoproliferative disorder, 5 occurred in nonhematologic diseases, and 3 were of undetermined significance.[54] In a case report of a patient with non-Hodgkin lymphoma, IgG κ, IgG λ, and IgM λ monoclonal components were described. Three separate populations of M protein-producing cells were identified.[55]

Idiopathic Bence-Jones Proteinuria

Benign monoclonal gammopathy of the light-chain type must be considered even though Bence-Jones proteinuria is a recognized feature of MM, AL, WM, and other lymphoproliferative disorders. In one study, two patients with stable serum M-protein levels excreted 0.8 g/dL or more of Bence-Jones proteinuria for over 17 years without disease progression.[56] Seven additional patients have been described who presented with Bence-Jones proteinuria (>1 g/24 h), but in whom no M protein was found in the serum and had no evidence of MM or a related disorder.[57] During follow-up, MM developed in two of the seven patients, SMM in one, AL in one, and two died of unrelated causes. One of these patients had excreted up to 1.8 g/24 h of κ light chain for 37 years without development of symptomatic MM or renal insufficiency. This patient died of a sudden cardiac arrhythmia, and no evidence of systemic AL or MM was found at autopsy. Although idiopathic Bence-Jones proteinuria may remain stable for many years, MM or AL often results. Consequently, patients must be followed up indefinitely.

IgM MGUS

Patients with a serum IgM M-protein value < 3 g/dL, bone marrow lymphoplasmacytic infiltration < 10%, and no evidence of anemia, constitutional symptoms, hyperviscosity, lymphadenopathy, or hepatosplenomegaly are considered to have IgM MGUS, not WM. Of 430 patients in whom an IgM serum M protein was detected on laboratory testing at Mayo Clinic between 1956 and 1978, 56% had MGUS.[58] In a more recent study, Gobbi et al.[59] recognized IgM MGUS in ~20% of patients with MGUS and in 30% of patients who had an IgM M protein.

IgM MGUS was diagnosed in 213 Mayo Clinic patients who resided in the 11 counties of southeastern Minnesota.[60] Twenty-nine (14%) of these 213 patients subsequently developed non-Hodgkin lymphoma (17), WM (6), chronic lymphocytic leukemia (3), or AL (3), with relative risks of 15-, 262-, 6-, and 16-fold, respectively. The risk of progression was 1.5% per year, which persisted even after 20 years of follow-up. A higher initial level of the serum M protein and a lower serum albumin level at diagnosis were independent predictors of progression.

In another series of 138 patients with IgM MGUS who had remained stable for 12 months, 14 (10%) progressed after a median follow-up of 75 months.[61] In another series of 83 patients with an IgM-related disorder, type-I cryoglobulinemia was present in 19, type-II cryoglobulinemia in 56, peripheral neuropathy in 5, and idiopathic thrombocytopenia in 3. Overt WM or a related disorder developed in 8 (9.6%) during a median follow-up of 62 months.[62] In a retrospective evaluation of 217 patients with IgM MGUS and 201 with indolent WM, 15 of those with IgM MGUS and 45 of those with indolent WM progressed to non-Hodgkin lymphoma. The median time to progression was not reached for MGUS and was 141.5 months for indolent WM. The variables adversely related to progression were initial IgM values, hemoglobin value, and gender in both groups.[63]

IgD MGUS

The presence of an IgD M protein almost always indicates MM, AL, or plasma cell leukemia. However, IgD MGUS has been reported. O'Connor et al.[64] described a patient with an IgD protein level of 0.5 g/dL who was followed up for more than 6 years without evidence of progressive disease. We have seen a patient with an IgD λ MGUS at Mayo Clinic who was followed up for more than 8 years without development of MM or AL.[65]

Association of Monoclonal Gammopathy with Other Diseases

Many diseases are associated with MGUS, as would be expected in an older population. The association of two diseases depends on the frequency with which each occurs independently. In addition, an apparent association may occur because of differences in the referral practice or in other selected patient groups. Valid epidemiologic and statistical methods are necessary in evaluating these associations. Appropriate controls are essential. For a more detailed review of the association of M proteins, the reader is encouraged to consult more extensive reviews.[66,67]

Lymphoproliferative Disorders

Azar et al.[68] reported that malignant lymphoma and lymphatic leukemia were associated with a myeloma-type serum protein. Kyle et al.[69] described six patients with lymphoma who had serum electrophoretic patterns consistent with those of MM. Among 1,150 patients with lymphoma or chronic lymphocytic leukemia, Alexanian[70] found an M protein in 49 patients. Among 292 patients with nodular lymphoma, 4 had an M protein, whereas only 1 of

218 patients with Hodgkin disease had an M protein. In contrast, 7%[44] of 640 patients with diffuse non-Hodgkin lymphoma or chronic lymphocytic leukemia had an M protein.

We reviewed the medical records of 430 patients in whom a serum IgM monoclonal gammopathy had been identified between 1956 and 1978 at Mayo Clinic. The patients were classified as follows: MGUS (56%), WM (17%), lymphoproliferative disorder (14%), non-Hodgkin lymphoma (7%), chronic lymphocytic leukemia (5%), and AL (1%).[58] Lin et al.[71] described 382 patients with a lymphoid neoplasm and an associated IgM M protein. Fifty-nine percent had lymphoplasmacytic lymphoma/WM, chronic lymphocytic leukemia/small lymphocytic lymphoma (20%), malignant zone lymphoma (7%), follicular lymphoma (5%), mantle cell lymphoma (3%), diffuse large B-cell lymphoma (2%), and miscellaneous (4%). In another study, 7 (27%) of 26 patients with an extranodal marginal zone lymphoma had an M protein. There was a strong correlation of the presence of an M protein with involvement of the bone marrow.[72]

Leukemia

We described 100 patients with chronic lymphocytic leukemia and an M protein in the serum or urine.[73] IgM accounted for 38%, IgG 51%, IgA 1%, and light chain only 10%. No major differences were apparent in patients with chronic lymphocytic leukemia, whether or not they had an M protein. Hairy cell leukemia, adult T-cell leukemia, chronic myelocytic leukemia, Sezary syndrome, mycosis fungoides, Kaposi sarcoma, and erythema elevatum diutinum have all been reported with a monoclonal gammopathy.

Other Hematologic Disorders

Monoclonal gammopathy has been reported with refractory anemia, myelodysplastic syndrome, chronic neutrophilic leukemia, idiopathic myelofibrosis, and Gaucher's disease.[74,75] Von Willebrand's disease,[76] pernicious anemia, pure red blood cell aplasia, and polycythemia vera have all been associated with monoclonal gammopathies. Thromboembolic disease has been reported with MGUS. In 310 patients with MGUS, 19 (6%) developed venous thromboembolic disease.[77]

Connective Tissue Disorders

Rheumatoid arthritis, lupus erythematosus, scleroderma, polymyalgia rheumatica, polymyositis, and discoid lupus erythematosus have all been reported with M proteins.

Neurologic Disorders

We found 16 cases (6%) of MGUS in 279 patients with a sensorimotor peripheral neuropathy of unknown cause. An association exists between MGUS and sensorimotor peripheral neuropathy, but the incidence is variable and depends on the vigor with which an M protein is sought and whether the diagnosis of peripheral neuropathy is made on clinical or electrophysiologic grounds. IgM is the most common M protein associated with peripheral neuropathy. In approximately one-half of patients, the M protein binds to myelin-associated glycoprotein (MAG). However, the role of antibodies in peripheral neuropathy is not clear. We reviewed our experience with 65 patients with MGUS and sensorimotor peripheral neuropathy at Mayo Clinic.[78] Thirty-one had IgM, 24 had IgG, and 10 had an IgA M protein. Neither the size of the M protein nor anti-MAG activity influenced the type and severity of neuropathy. The neuropathy was progressive in the majority of patients.

Treatment of patients with peripheral neuropathy and monoclonal gammopathy is challenging, but often disappointing. Plasmapheresis was of some value in a randomized plasmapheresis or sham plasmapheresis in a double-blind trial.[79] The role of plasma exchange in neurologic disorders has recently been reviewed.[80] Patients who do not respond to plasmapheresis may be given chlorambucil when the M protein is of the IgM type or melphalan and prednisone for IgG and IgA gammopathies. However, there is risk of myelodysplasia, particularly in younger patients with chronic disease. Rituximab, fludarabine, and intravenous immunoglobulin have all been used. Therapy of neuropathies associated with monoclonal gammopathies has recently been reviewed.[81] Guidelines on the management of M protein-associated neuropathies have been published.[82,83] Monoclonal gammopathies have been reported with motor neuron disease, myasthenia gravis, nemaline myopathy, and ataxia-telangiectasia.

POEMS Syndrome (Osteosclerotic Myeloma)

POEMS syndrome (osteosclerotic myeloma) is characterized by a chronic sensorimotor peripheral neuropathy with predominating motor disability. It is characterized by polyneuropathy, organomegaly, endocrinopathy, M protein, and skin changes. The syndrome is defined by the presence of a monoclonal plasma cell proliferative disorder, peripheral neuropathy, and at least one of the following seven features: osteosclerotic lesions, Castleman's disease, organomegaly, endocrinopathy (except diabetes mellitus or hypothyroidism), edema, typical skin changes, and papilledema. Respiratory problems include neuromuscular weakness, reduced diffusion capacity, or pulmonary hypertension. Hyperpigmentation, hypertrichosis, gynecomastia, and testicular atrophy may be seen. Polycythemia or thrombocytosis may be a prominent feature. Almost all patients have an M protein of the λ light-chain type. This syndrome is rarely associated with Bence-Jones proteinuria, renal insufficiency, hypercalcemia, large serum M spike, or skeletal fractures. Patients do not develop the features of classic symptomatic MM. In our report of 99 patients, the median duration of survival was 13.8 years.[84] Radiation therapy in tumorcidal doses is indicated if single or multiple sclerotic lesions are found in a limited area. If the lesions are widespread, systemic therapy similar to myeloma, such as autologous stem cell transplantation or alkylating therapy, is indicated.[85]

Endocrine Disorders

The association of MGUS and hyperparathyroidism is controversial. In one report, 9 (1%) of 911 patients at Mayo Clinic had MGUS which is similar to that in a normal population.[86] On the contrary, 20 of 101 patients with hyperparathyroidism had an M protein compared with only 2 of 127 controls.[87]

Dermatologic Diseases

Lichen myxedematosus (papular mucinosis, scleromyxedema) is a rare dermatologic condition frequently associated with a cathodal IgG λ protein. Pyoderma gangrenosum, necrobiotic xanthogranuloma, Schnitzler syndrome, subcorneal pustular dermatoses, and diffuse plane xanthomatosis may be associated with a monoclonal gammopathy. The association of monoclonal gammopathies and skin disorders has been reviewed.[88]

Immunosuppression

M proteins are frequently seen following renal, liver, heart, or autologous bone marrow transplantation.[89] In a report of five patients with MGUS undergoing transplantation, smoldering MM developed in two and one other had an increase in the serum M protein.[90]

Miscellaneous Conditions

Acquired C1 inhibitor deficiency[91] and capillary leak syndrome[92] have been reported with monoclonal gammopathy. Idiopathic segmental glomerulosclerosis also appears to be associated with MGUS.[93] MGUS has been reported following silicone breast implants, but the frequency does not appear to be increased.[94] M proteins may be bound to calcium, copper, transferrin, or serum phosphorus. M proteins may be associated with antibody activity.[95]

Acknowledgment: Supported in part by grants (CA 62242 and CA 107476) from the National Cancer Institute.

References

1. Waldenstrom J. Abnormal proteins in myeloma. Adv Intern Med 1952;5:398–440.
2. Kyle RA, Rajkumar SV. Monoclonal gammopathies of undetermined significance: a review. [Review] [237 refs]. Immunol Rev 2003;194:112–39.
3. Kyle RA. Sequence of testing for monoclonal gammopathies. Arch Pathol Lab Med 1999;123(2):114–8.
4. Keren DF, Alexanian R, Goeken JA, Gorevic PD, Kyle RA, Tomar RH. Guidelines for clinical and laboratory evaluation patients with monoclonal gammopathies. Arch Pathol Lab Med 1999;123(2):106–7.
5. Axelsson U, Bachmann R, Hallen J. Frequency of pathological proteins (M-components) om 6,995 sera from an adult population. Acta Med Scand 1966;179(2):235–47.
6. Kyle RA, Finkelstein S, Elveback LR, Kurland LT. Incidence of monoclonal proteins in a Minnesota community with a cluster of multiple myeloma. Blood 1972;40(5):719–24.
7. Saleun JP, Vicariot M, Deroff P, Morin JF. Monoclonal gammopathies in the adult population of Finistere, France. J Clin Pathol 1982;35(1):63–8.
8. Cohen HJ, Crawford J, Rao MK, Pieper CF, Currie MS. Racial differences in the prevalence of monoclonal gammopathy in a community-based sample of the elderly.[erratum appears in Am J Med 1998 Oct;105(4):362]. Am J Med 1998;104(5):439–44.
9. Landgren O, Gridley G, Turesson I,et al. Risk of monoclonal gammopathy of undetermined significance (MGUS) and subsequent multiple myeloma among African American and white veterans in the United States. Blood 2006;107(3):904–6.

10. Kyle RA, Therneau TM, Rajkumar SV, et al . Prevalence of monoclonal gammopathy of undetermined significance. N Engl J Med 2006;354(13):1362–9.

11. Kyle RA. Monoclonal gammopathy of undetermined significance. Natural history in 241 cases. Am J Med 1978;64(5):814–26.

12. Kyle RA, Therneau TM, Rajkumar SV, Larson DR, Plevak MF, Melton LJ, 3rd. Long-term follow-up of 241 patients with monoclonal gammopathy of undetermined significance: the original Mayo Clinic series 25 years later.[see comment]. Mayo Clin Proc 2004;79(7):859–66.

13. Kyle RA, Therneau TM, Rajkumar SV,et al. A long-term study of prognosis in monoclonal gammopathy of undetermined significance.[see comment]. N Engl J Med 2002;346(8):564–9.

14. Surveillance, Epidemiology, and End Results (SEER) Program Public-Use Data CD Rom (1973–1998). In. Bethesda, MD: National Cancer Institute, Cancer Statistitics Branch; 2001.

15. Kyle RA, Linos A, Beard CM,et al. Incidence and natural history of primary systemic amyloidosis in Olmsted County, Minnesota, 1950 through 1989.[see comment]. Blood 1992;79(7):1817–22.

16. Kyle RA, Gertz MA, Witzig TE, . Review of 1027 patients with newly diagnosed multiple myeloma.[see comment]. Mayo Clin Proc 2003;78(1):21–33.

17. Axelsson U. A 20-year follow-up study of 64 subjects with M-components. Acta Med Scand 1986;219(5):519–22.

18. van de Poel MH, Coebergh JW, Hillen HF. Malignant transformation of monoclonal gammopathy of undetermined significance among out-patients of a community hospital in southeastern Netherlands. Br J Haematol 1995;91(1):121–5.

19. Baldini L, Guffanti A, Cesana BM,et al . Role of different hematologic variables in defining the risk of malignant transformation in monoclonal gammopathy. Blood 1996;87(3):912–8.

20. Gregersen H, Ibsen J, Mellemkjoer L, Dahlerup J, Olsen J, Sorensen H. Mortality and causes of death in patients with monoclonal gammopathy of undetermined significance. Br J Haematol 2001;112(2):353–7.

21. Ogmundsdottir HM, Haraldsdottir V, Gu mundur MJ, . Monoclonal gammopathy in Iceland: a population-based registry and follow-up. Br J Haematol 2002;118(1):166–73.

22. Kyle RA, Rajkumar SV. Monoclonal gammopathy of undetermined significance. Clin Lymphoma Myeloma 2005;6(2):102–14.

23. Avet-Loiseau H, Li JY, Facon T, . High incidence of translocations t(11;14)(q13;q32) and t(4;14)(p16;q32) in patients with plasma cell malignancies. Cancer Res 1998;58(24):5640–5.

24. Avet-Loiseau H, Facon T, Daviet A,   14q32 translocations and monosomy 13 observed in monoclonal gammopathy of undetermined significance delineate a multistep process for the oncogenesis of multiple myeloma. Intergroupe Francophone du Myelome. Cancer Res 1999;59(18):4546–50.

25. Fonseca R, Bailey RJ, Ahmann GJ,et al. Genomic abnormalities in monoclonal gammopathy of undetermined significance. Blood 2002;100(4):1417–24.

26. Chng WJ, Van Wier SA, Ahmann GJ,et al. A validated FISH trisomy index demonstrates the hyperdiploid and nonhyperdiploid dichotomy in MGUS. Blood 2005;106(6):2156–61.

27. Avet-Loiseau H, Li JY, Morineau N, Monosomy 13 is associated with the transition of monoclonal gammopathy of undetermined significance to multiple myeloma. Intergroupe Francophone du Myelome. Blood 1999;94(8):2583–9.

28. Rasmussen T, Kuehl M, Lodahl M, Johnsen HE, Dahl IMS. Possible roles for activating RAS mutations in the MGUS to MM transition and in the intramedullary to extramedullary transition in some plasma cell tumors. Blood 2005;105(1):317–23.

29. Takahashi T, Shivapurkar N, Reddy J,et al . DNA methylation profiles of lymphoid and hematopoietic malignancies. Clin Cancer Res 2004;10(9):2928–35.

30. Rajkumar SV, Mesa RA, Fonseca R,et al. Bone marrow angiogenesis in 400 patients with monoclonal gammopathy of undetermined significance, multiple myeloma, and primary amyloidosis. Clin Cancer Res 2002;8(7):2210–6.

31. Kumar S, Witzig TE, Timm M, et al. Bone marrow angiogenic ability and expression of angiogenic cytokines in myeloma: evidence favoring loss of marrow angiogenesis inhibitory activity with disease progression. Blood 2004;104(4):1159–65.

32. Melton LJ, 3rd, Rajkumar SV, Khosla S,et al. Fracture risk in monoclonal gammopathy of undetermined significance. J Bone Miner Res 2004;19(1):25–30.

33. Roodman GD, III. Biology of myeloma bone disease. In: Broudy VC, Abkowitz JL, Vose JM, eds. Hematology 2002: American Society of Hematology Education Program Book. Washington, DC; 2002:227–32.

34. Croucher PI, Shipman CM, Lippitt J,et al. Osteoprotegerin inhibits the development of osteolytic bone disease in multiple myeloma. Blood 2001;98(13):3534–40.

35. Lust JA, Donovan KA. Biology of the transition of monoclonal gammopathy of undetermined significance (MGUS) to multiple myeloma. Cancer Control 1998;5(3):209–17.

36. Malik AA, Ganti AK, Potti A, Levitt R, Hanley JF. Role of Helicobacter pylori infection in the incidence and clinical course of monoclonal gammopathy of undetermined significance. Am J Gastroenterol 2002;97(6):1371–4.

37. Rajkumar SV, Kyle RA, Plevak MF, Murray JA, Therneau TM. Helicobacter pylori infection and monoclonal gammopathy of undetermined significance. Br J Haematol 2002;119(3):706–8.

38. Kyle RA. "Benign" monoclonal gammopathy – after 20 to 35 years of follow-up. Mayo Clin Proc 1993;68(1):26–36.

39. Blade J, Lopez-Guillermo A, Rozman C,et al. Malignant transformation and life expectancy in monoclonal gammopathy of undetermined significance. Br J Haematol 1992;81(3):391–4.

40. Cesana C, Klersy C, Barbarano L,et al. Prognostic factors for malignant transformation in monoclonal gammopathy of undetermined significance and smoldering multiple myeloma. J Clin Oncol 2002;20(6):1625–34.

41. Rajkumar SV, Kyle RA, Therneau TM, . Serum free light chain ratio is an independent risk factor for progression in monoclonal gammopathy of undetermined significance. Blood 2005;106(3):812–7.

42. Kumar S, Rajkumar SV, Kyle RA,et al. Prognostic value of circulating plasma cells in monoclonal gammopathy of undetermined significance. J Clin Oncol 2005;23(24):5668–74.

43. Ocqueteau M, Orfao A, Almeida J, Immunophenotypic characterization of plasma cells from monoclonal gammopathy of undetermined significance patients. Implications for the differential diagnosis between MGUS and multiple myeloma. Am J Pathol 1998;152(6):1655–65.

44. Garewal H, Durie BG, Kyle RA, Finley P, Bower B, Serokman R. Serum beta 2-microglobulin in the initial staging and subsequent monitoring of monoclonal plasma cell disorders. J Clin Oncol 1984;2(1):51–7.

45. Criteria for the classification of monoclonal gammopathies, multiple myeloma and related disorders: a report of the International Myeloma Working Group. Br J Haematol 2003;121(5):749–57.

46. Kyle RA, Greipp PR. Smoldering multiple myeloma. N Engl J Med 1980;302(24):1347–9.

47. Dimopoulos MA, Moulopoulos LA, Maniatis A, Alexanian R. Solitary plasmacytoma of bone and asymptomatic multiple myeloma. Blood 2000;96(6):2037–44.

48. Rosinol L, Blade J, Esteve J,et al. Smoldering multiple myeloma: natural history and recognition of an evolving type. Br J Haematol 2003;123(4):631–6.

49. Kyle RA, Remstein ED, Therneau TM,et al. Clinical course and prognosis of smoldering (asymptomatic) multiple myeloma. N Engl J Med 2007;356(25):2582–90.

50. Hjorth M, Hellquist L, Holmberg E, Magnusson B, Rodjer S, Westin J. Initial versus deferred melphalan-prednisone therapy for asymptomatic multiple myeloma stage I – a randomized study. Myeloma Group of Western Sweden. Eur J Haematol 1993;50(2):95–102.

51. Grignani G, Gobbi PG, Formisano R, et al. A prognostic index for multiple myeloma. Br J Cancer 1996;73(9):1101–7.

52. Rajkumar SV, Gertz MA, Lacy MQ, . Thalidomide as initial therapy for early-stage myeloma.[see comment]. Leukemia 2003;17(4):775–9.

53. Kyle RA, Robinson RA, Katzmann JA. The clinical aspects of biclonal gammopathies. Review of 57 cases. Am J Med 1981;71(6):999–1008.

54. Grosbois B, Jego P, de Rosa H, Triclonal gammopathy and malignant immunoproliferative syndrome. [Review] [25 refs] [French]. Rev Med Interne 1997;18(6):470–3.

55. Tirelli A, Guastafierro S, Cava B, Lucivero G. Triclonal gammopathy in an extranodal non-Hodgkin lymphoma patient. Am J Hematol 2003;73(4):273–5.

56. Kyle RA, Maldonado JE, Bayrd ED. Idiopathic Bence Jones proteinuria – a distinct entity? Am J Med 1973;55(2):222–6.

57. Kyle RA, Greipp PR. "Idiopathic" Bence Jones proteinuria: long-term follow-up in seven patients. N Engl J Med 1982;306(10):564–7.

58. Kyle RA, Garton JP. The spectrum of IgM monoclonal gammopathy in 430 cases. Mayo Clin Proc 1987;62(8):719–31.

59. Gobbi PG, Baldini L, Broglia C, et al. Prognostic validation of the international classification of immunoglobulin M gammopathies: a survival advantage for patients with immunoglobulin M monoclonal gammopathy of undetermined significance? Clin Cancer Res 2005;11(5):1786–90.

60. Kyle RA, Therneau TM, Rajkumar SV, . Long-term follow-up of IgM monoclonal gammopathy of undetermined significance. Blood 2003;102(10):3759–64.

61. Morra E, Cesana C, Klersy C, et al. Prognostic factors for transformation in asymptomatic immunoglobulin m monoclonal gammopathies. Clin Lymphoma 2005;5(4):265–9.

62. Cesana C, Barbarano L, Miqueleiz S, et al. Clinical characteristics and outcome of immunoglobulin M-related disorders. Clin Lymphoma 2005;5(4):261–4.

63. Baldini L, Goldaniga M, Guffanti A, et al. Immunoglobulin M monoclonal gammopathies of undetermined significance and indolent Waldenstrom's macroglobulinemia recognize the same determinants of evolution into symptomatic lymphoid disorders: proposal for a common prognostic scoring system. J Clin Oncol 2005;23(21):4662–8.

64. O'Connor ML, Rice DT, Buss DH, Muss HB. Immunoglobulin D benign monoclonal gammopathy. A case report. [Review] [16 refs]. Cancer 1991;68(3):611–6.

65. Blade J, Kyle RA. IgD monoclonal gammopathy with long-term follow-up. Br J Haematol 1994;88(2):395–6.

66. Kyle RA, Rajkumar SV. Monoclonal gammopathies of undetermined significance. In: Malpas J, ,eds. Myeloma: Biology and Management, 3rd Ed. Philadelphia, PS: Saunders; 2004:315–52.

67. Kyle RA, Rajkumar SV. Monoclonal gammopathy of undetermined significance. Br J Haematol 2006;134(6):573–89.

68. Azar HA, Hill WT, Osserman EF. Malignant lymphoma and lymphatic leukemia. Am J Med 1957;23:239–49.

69. Kyle RA, Bayrd ED, McKenzie BF, Heck FJ. Diagnostic Criteria for electrophoretic patterns of serum and urinary proteins in multiple myeloma: study of one hundred and sixty-five multiple myeloma patients with similar electrophoretic patterns. JAMA 1960;174:245–51.

70. Alexanian R. Monoclonal gammopathy in lymphoma. Arch Intern Med 1975;135(1):62–6.

71. Lin P, Hao S, Handy BC, Bueso-Ramos CE, Medeiros LJ. Lymphoid neoplasms associated with IgM paraprotein: a study of 382 patients. Am J Clin Pathol 2005;123(2):200–5.

72. Asatiani E, Cohen P, Ozdemirli M, Kessler CM, Mavromatis B, Cheson BD. Monoclonal gammopathy in extranodal marginal zone lymphoma (ENMZL) correlates with advanced disease and bone marrow involvement. Am J Hematol 2004;77(2):144–6.

73. Noel P, Kyle RA. Monoclonal proteins in chronic lymphocytic leukemia. Am J Clin Pathol 1987;87(3):385–8.

74. Rosenbloom BE, Weinreb NJ, Zimran A, Kacena KA, Charrow J, Ward E. Gaucher disease and cancer incidence: a study from the Gaucher Registry. Blood 2005;105(12):4569–72.

75. Zimran A, Liphshitz I, Barchana M, Abrahamov A, Elstein D. Incidence of malignancies among patients with type I Gaucher disease from a single referral clinic. Blood Cells Mol Dis 2005;34(3):197–200.

76. Lamboley V, Zabraniecki L, Sie P, Pourrat J, Fournie B. Myeloma and monoclonal gammopathy of uncertain significance associated with acquired von Willebrand's syndrome. Seven new cases with a literature review. Joint, Bone, Spine: Revue du Rhumatisme 2002;69(1):62–7.

77. Sallah S, Husain A, Wan J, Vos P, Nguyen NP. The risk of venous thromboembolic disease in patients with monoclonal gammopathy of undetermined significance. Ann Oncol 2004;15(10):1490–4.

78. Gosselin S, Kyle RA, Dyck PJ. Neuropathy associated with monoclonal gammopathies of undetermined significance.[see comment]. Ann Neurol 1991;30(1):54–61.

79. Dyck PJ, Low PA, Windebank AJ, et al. Plasma exchange in polyneuropathy associated with monoclonal gammopathy of undetermined significance. N Engl J Med 1991;325(21):1482–6.

80. Lehmann HC, Hartung HP, Hetzel GR, Stuve O, Kieseier BC. Plasma exchange in neuroimmunological disorders: part 2. Treatment of neuromuscular disorders. Arch Neurol 2006;63(8):1066–71.

81. Nobile-Orazio E. Treatment of dys-immune neuropathies. J Neurol 2005;252(4):385–95.

82. Hadden RD, Nobile-Orazio E, Sommer C, et al. European Federation of Neurological Societies/Peripheral Nerve Society guideline on management of paraproteinaemic demyelinating neuropathies: report of a joint task force of the European Federation of Neurological Societies and the Peripheral Nerve Society. Eur J Neurol 2006;13(8):809–18.

83. European Federation of Neurological Societies/Peripheral Nerve Society Guideline on management of paraproteinemic demyelinating neuropathies. Report of a joint task force of the European Federation of Neurological Societies and the Peripheral Nerve Society. J Peripher Nerv Syst 2006;11(1):9–19.

84. Dispenzieri A, Kyle RA, Lacy MQ, et al. POEMS syndrome: definitions and long-term outcome. Blood 2003;101(7):2496–506.

85. Dispenzieri A, Moreno-Aspitia A, Suarez GA, et al. Peripheral blood stem cell transplantation in 16 patients with POEMS syndrome, and a review of the literature. Blood 2004;104(10):3400–7.

86. Mundis RJ, Kyle RA. Primary hyperparathyroidism and monoclonal gammopathy of undetermined significance. Am J Clin Pathol 1982;77(5):619–21.

87. Arnulf B, Bengoufa D, Sarfati E, . Prevalence of monoclonal gammopathy in patients with primary hyperparathyroidism: a prospective study. Arch Intern Med 2002;162(4):464–7.

88. Daoud MS, Lust JA, Kyle RA, Pittelkow MR. Monoclonal gammopathies and associated skin disorders. [Review] [214 refs]. J Am Acad Dermatol 1999;40(4):507–35; quiz 36–8.

89. Zent CS, Wilson CS, Tricot G, et al. Oligoclonal protein bands and Ig isotype switching in multiple myeloma treated with high-dose therapy and hematopoietic cell transplantation. Blood 1998;91(9):3518–23.

90. Rostaing L, Modesto A, Abbal M, Durand D. Long-term follow-up of monoclonal gammopathy of undetermined significance in transplant patients. Am J Nephrol 1994;14(3):187–91.

91. Pascual M, Mach-Pascual S, Schifferli JA. Paraproteins and complement depletion: pathogenesis and clinical syndromes. Semin Hematol 1997;34(1 Suppl 1):40–8.
92. Droder RM, Kyle RA, Greipp PR. Control of systemic capillary leak syndrome with aminophylline and terbutaline. Am J Med 1992;92(5):523–6.
93. Dingli D, Larson DR, Plevak MF, Grande JP, Kyle RA. Focal and segmental glomerulosclerosis and plasma cell proliferative disorders. Am J Kidney Dis 2005;46(2):278–82.
94. Karlson EW, Tanasijevic M, Hankinson SE, . Monoclonal gammopathy of undetermined significance and exposure to breast implants. Arch Intern Med 2001;161(6):864–7.
95. Merlini G, Farhangi M, Osserman EF. Monoclonal immunoglobulins with antibody activity in myeloma, macroglobulinemia and related plasma cell dyscrasias. [Review] [202 refs]. Semin Oncol 1986;13(3):350–65.

Index

Printed in the United States of America